Heart Diseases and Covid-19: An Issue of Cardiology Clinics

Heart Diseases and Covid-19: An Issue of Cardiology Clinics

Editor: Reece Hogan

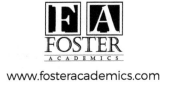

www.fosteracademics.com

www.fosteracademics.com

Cataloging-in-Publication Data

Heart diseases and covid-19 : an issue of cardiology clinics / edited by Reece Hogan.
   p. cm.
Includes bibliographical references and index.
ISBN 978-1-64646-585-9
1. Heart--Diseases. 2. COVID-19 (Disease). 3. COVID-19 (Disease)--Complications.
4. Cardiology. I. Hogan, Reece.
RC681 .H43 2023
616.12--dc23

Foster Academics,
118-35 Queens Blvd., Suite 400,
Forest Hills, NY 11375, USA

ISBN 978-1-64646-585-9 (Hardback)

Contents

Preface

This book aims to highlight the current researches and provides a platform to further the scope of innovations in this area. This book is a product of the combined efforts of many researchers and scientists, after going through thorough studies and analysis from different parts of the world. The objective of this book is to provide the readers with the latest information of the field.

Heart disease refers to a type of disease that primarily impacts the heart or blood vessels. There are several risk factors of these diseases, including high cholesterol, smoking, insufficient exercise, high blood pressure, obesity and a poor diet. Coronavirus disease (Covid-19) is a type of infectious disease caused by the SARS-CoV-2 virus. Covid-19 patients are more likely to develop a wide variety of cardiovascular disorders, such as ischemic and non-ischemic heart disease, myocarditis, thromboembolic disease, heart failure, dysrhythmias, pericarditis and cerebrovascular disorders. Inflammation linked to Covid-19 increases the risk of heart attack through the disruption of the blood vessel lining and activation of the body's clotting system. The patients of Covid-19 may also experience symptoms similar to a heart attack, such as changes on their echocardiogram, chest pain and shortness of breath. This book explores all the important aspects of heart diseases and Covid-19. It will help new researchers by foregrounding their knowledge in these medical conditions.

I would like to express my sincere thanks to the authors for their dedicated efforts in the completion of this book. I acknowledge the efforts of the publisher for providing constant support. Lastly, I would like to thank my family for their support in all academic endeavors.

Editor

B-Type Natriuretic Peptide Concentrations, COVID-19 Severity and Mortality

Angelo Zinellu[1], Salvatore Sotgia[1], Ciriaco Carru[1,2] and Arduino A. Mangoni[3,4]*

[1] Department of Biomedical Sciences, University of Sassari, Sassari, Italy, [2] Quality Control Unit, University Hospital of Sassari, Sassari, Italy, [3] Discipline of Clinical Pharmacology, College of Medicine and Public Health, Flinders University, Adelaide, SA, Australia, [4] Department of Clinical Pharmacology, Flinders Medical Centre, Southern Adelaide Local Health Network, Adelaide, SA, Australia

*Correspondence:
Arduino A. Mangoni
arduino.mangoni@flinders.edu.au

Alterations in cardiac biomarkers have been reported in patients with coronavirus disease 2019 (COVID-19) in relation to disease severity and mortality. We conducted a systematic review and meta-analysis with meta-regression of studies reporting B-type natriuretic peptide (BNP) or N-terminal proBNP (NT-proBNP) plasma concentrations in COVID-19. We searched PubMed, Web of Science, and Scopus, between January 2020 and 2021, for studies reporting BNP/NT-proBNP concentrations, measures of COVID-19 severity, and survival status (PROSPERO registration number: CRD42021239190). Forty-four studies in 18,856 COVID-19 patients were included in the meta-analysis and meta-regression. In pooled results, BNP/NT-proBNP concentrations were significantly higher in patients with high severity or non-survivor status when compared to patients with low severity or survivor status during follow up (SMD = 1.07, 95% CI: 0.89–1.24, and $p < 0.001$). We observed extreme between-study heterogeneity ($I^2 = 93.9\%$, $p < 0.001$). In sensitivity analysis, the magnitude and the direction of the effect size were not substantially modified after sequentially removing individual studies and re-assessing the pooled estimates, (effect size range, 0.99 – 1.10). No publication bias was observed with the Begg's ($p = 0.26$) and Egger's ($p = 0.40$) t-tests. In meta-regression analysis, the SMD was significantly and positively associated with D-dimer ($t = 2.22$, $p = 0.03$), myoglobin ($t = 2.40$, $p = 0.04$), LDH ($t = 2.38$, $p = 0.02$), and procalcitonin ($t = 2.56$, $p = 0.01$) concentrations. Therefore, higher BNP/NT-proBNP plasma concentrations were significantly associated with severe disease and mortality in COVID-19 patients.

Keywords: B-type natriuretic peptide, COVID-19, disease severity, mortality, biomarkers

INTRODUCTION

A significant number of clinical and demographic factors have been studied in patients with coronavirus disease 19 (COVID-19) in regard to their association with specific clinical presentations and measures of clinical severity (1, 2). The evidence of an excessive activation of inflammatory and immunomodulating pathways in patients with the more severe forms of the disease, typically characterized by the development of respiratory failure with or without multi-organ dysfunction, have prompted the search for specific biomarkers of inflammation and immuno-activation in order to develop better predictive models to assist with management (3). The increasing evidence of significant alterations of different organs and/or systems in patients with COVID-19 has also led to the investigation of the predictive capacity of additional, organ-specific, biomarkers. For example, the presence of myocardial injury, associated with several cardiac manifestations, including myocarditis, acute coronary syndrome, and arrhythmias, has been well-documented in COVID-19 patients with or without pre-existing cardiovascular history (4). Notably, cardiac abnormalities in this group are independently associated with an increased risk of mortality (5). While the exact mechanisms involved in the onset and progression of COVID-19 related myocardial injury remain to be elucidated, several circulating markers of myocardial damage, particularly creatine kinase (CK), and troponin, are being increasingly studied in terms of their predictive capacity (6). Another cardiac complication, heart failure, has been observed in about a quarter of patients with COVID-19 and has been associated with an increased risk of adverse outcomes (7, 8). The active peptide B-type natriuretic peptide (BNP) and the inactive peptide N-terminal proBNP (NT-proBNP) are both derived from the human BNP precursor proBNP in the ventricular myocytes. The increased secretion of BNP and NT-proBNP from the heart, in response to high ventricular filling pressures, is routinely used as a diagnostic and prognostic marker in heart failure and, by some, as a marker of the size or severity of ischaemic insults (9–11). However, its biological and clinical role in patients with COVID-19 is not well-established. We addressed this issue by conducting a systematic review and meta-analysis with meta-regression of studies reporting plasma BNP or NT-proBNP concentrations in COVID-19 patients with different disease severity, based on clinical guidelines or need for hospitalization, mechanical ventilation, or transfer to the intensive care unit (ICU), and clinical outcomes, particularly survival status during follow up.

MATERIALS AND METHODS

Search Strategy, Eligibility Criteria, and Study Selection

We conducted a systematic literature search, using the terms "brain natriuretic peptide" or "BNP" or "NT-proBNP" or "N-terminal pro-brain natriuretic peptide" and "coronavirus disease 19" or "COVID-19," in PubMed, Web of Science and Scopus, from January 2020 to January 2021, to identify peer-reviewed studies reporting BNP/NT-proBNP concentrations in COVID-19 patients according to disease severity and/or mortality. We accessed the references of the retrieved articles to identify additional studies. Eligibility criteria were (a) reporting continuous data on plasma BNP/NT-proBNP concentrations in COVID-19 patients, (b) investigating COVID-19 patients with different disease severity or survival status during follow up, (c) adult patients, (d) English language, (e) >10 patients, and (f) full-text available. Two investigators independently screened individual abstracts. If relevant, they independently reviewed the full articles (PROSPERO registration number: CRD42021239190). We used the Newcastle-Ottawa scale to assess study quality, with a score ≥6 indicating high quality (12).

Statistical Analysis

We calculated standardized mean differences (SMD) and 95% confidence intervals (CIs) in BNP/NT-proBNP concentrations between COVID-19 patients with low vs. high severity or survivor vs. non-survivor status. A $p < 0.05$ was considered statistically significant. When studies reported medians and interquartile ranges (IQR) the corresponding means and standard deviations were estimated (13). We assessed between-study heterogeneity in SMD values using the Q-statistic (significance level at $p < 0.10$). Inconsistency across studies

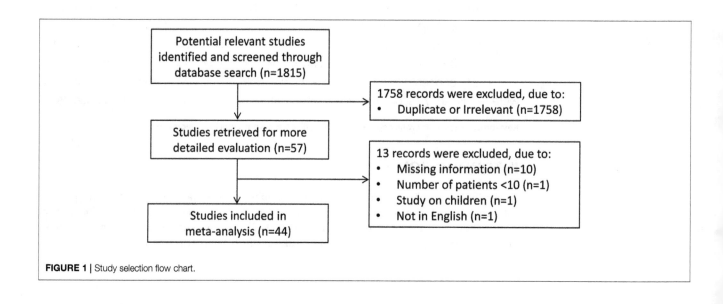

FIGURE 1 | Study selection flow chart.

TABLE 1 | Characteristics of the selected studies.

References	Country	Study design	Endpoint	NOS (stars)	Low severity or survivor				High severity or non-survivor			
					n	Age (Years)	Gender (M/F)	BNP pg/mL (Mean ± SD)	n	Age (Years)	Gender (M/F)	BNP pg/mL (Mean ± SD)
Abdeladim et al. (21)	Morocco	R	Disease severity	6	39	50	11/28	81 ± 50*	34	61	12/22	2,982 ± 3,172*
Aladag et al. (22)	Turkey	R	Survival status	7	35	68	22/13	3,318 ± 5,054*	15	68	6/9	15,511 ± 13,638*
Almeida Junior et al. (23)	Brazil	R	Survival status or MV	7	139	64	86/53	73 ± 90	44	76	34/10	287 ± 485
Bao et al. (24)	China	P	Disease severity	5	129	NR	NR	11 ± 25	49	NR	NR	53 ± 85
Belarte-Tornero et al. (25)	Spain	NR	Survival status	7	82	77	45/37	518 ± 528*	47	86	18/29	5,192 ± 6,673*
Chen et al. (26)	China	NR	Survival status	8	1,651	57	781/870	67 ± 93	208	70	153/55	685 ± 987
Chen et al. (7)	China	R	Survival status	6	161	51	88/73	92 ± 122*	113	68	83/30	1,002 ± 1,058*
Chen et al. (27)	China	R	Survival status	8	53	64	27/26	336 ± 298*	20	69	15/5	840 ± 898*
Ciceri et al. (28)	Italy	NR	Survival status	8	291	62	207/84	206 ± 259*	95	76	70/25	1,583 ± 2,176*
Cui et al. (29)	China	R	Survival status	8	699	61	353/346	153 ± 158*	137	70	86/51	1,244 ± 1,649*
D'Alto et al. (30)	Italy	P	Survival status	8	69	62	53/16	686 ± 1,224*	25	68	17/8	3,375 ± 3,891*
Deng et al. (31)	China	R	Survival status	8	212	63	97/115	227 ± 293*	52	75	33/19	1,248 ± 1,478*
Du et al. (32)	China	R	Transfer to ICU	6	58	73	31/27	852 ± 620*	51	68	40/11	564 ± 654*
Feng et al. (33)	China	R	Disease severity	6	352	51	190/162	41 ± 64	124	60	81/43	65 ± 67
Ferrari et al. (34)	Italy	R	Survival status	6	40	60	27/13	690 ± 1,075*	42	74	30/12	6,296 ± 17,528*
Gan et al. (35)	China	R	Survival status	8	56	62	30/26	1,653 ± 289	39	70	28/11	1,848 ± 784
Gavin et al. (36)	USA	R	Survival status	6	118	57	58/60	160 ± 51	18	73	11/7	587 ± 184
Gottlieb et al. (37)	USA	R	Hospitalization	8	7,190	38	3,935/3,255	33 ± 35	1,483	58	792/691	73 ± 74
Guo et al. (38)	China	R	Survival status	8	28	59	NR	1,741 ± 2,363*	46	72	NR	3,544 ± 7,998*
Han et al. (39)	China	R	Disease severity	6	198	59	127/71	145 ± 169*	75	59	26/49	624 ± 1,027*
He et al. (40)	China	NR	Disease severity	6	32	42	15/17	42 ± 66*	21	57	13/8	822 ± 1,100*
He et al. (41)	China	R	Disease severity	8	530	60	241/289	83 ± 95*	501	66	297/204	381 ± 498*
Hui et al. (42)	China	R	Survival status	8	65	55	42/23	176 ± 178*	47	66	29/18	1,631 ± 2,453*
Koc et al. (43)	Turkey	R	Disease severity	6	60	65	37/23	53 ± 35*	30	61	20/10	267 ± 339*
Li et al. (44)	China	R	Transfer to ICU	8	312	49	131/181	100 ± 129*	211	62	119/92	103 ± 132*
Li et al. (45)	China	R	Survival status	6	60	62	33/27	327 ± 455	14	71	11/3	854 ± 849
Liu et al. (46)	China	P	Survival status	8	21	64	15/6	1,859 ± 2,599*	22	65	7/15	7,530 ± 8,820*
Lorente et al. (47)	Spain	P	Survival status	7	118	64	53/65	538 ± 789*	25	71	7/18	3,370 ± 4,218*
Ma et al. (48)	China	R	Disease severity	6	429	42	230/199	180 ± 273	94	50	59/35	663 ± 641
Myhre et al. (49)	Norway	P	Survival status or transfer to ICU	8	88	58	46/42	126 ± 170*	35	64	25/10	186 ± 181*
Pan et al. (50)	China	R	Survival status	8	35	65	18/17	63 ± 73	89	69	67/22	107 ± 113
Qin et al. (51)	China	R	Survival status	8	239	63	113/126	93 ± 102	23	69	10/13	499 ± 468
Rath et al. (52)	Germany	P	Survival status	7	107	67	65/42	808 ± 1,320*	16	73	12/4	3,376 ± 5,410*

(Continued)

TABLE 1 | Continued

References	Country	Study design	Endpoint	NOS (stars)	Low severity or survivor				High severity or non-survivor			
					n	Age (Years)	Gender (M/F)	BNP pg/mL (Mean ± SD)	n	Age (Years)	Gender (M/F)	BNP pg/mL (Mean ± SD)
Sun et al. (53)	China	R	Survival status	8	123	67	51/72	2 ± 2*	121	72	82/39	13 ± 16*
Sun et al. (54)	China	P	Disease severity	7	49	52	26/23	9 ± 6	50	71	34/16	163 ± 232
Tao et al. (55)	China	R	Disease severity	7	202	54	72/130	198 ± 352*	20	65	8/12	811 ± 1,367*
Vrillon et al. (56)	France	P	Survival status	8	54	90	19/35	184 ± 242	22	90	15/7	367 ± 371
Wang et al. (57)	China	R	Disease severity	6	72	NR	24/48	48 ± 46	38	NR	24/14	206 ± 228
Xie et al. (58)	China	R	Disease severity	7	38	61	26/12	29 ± 29	24	72	12/12	97 ± 106
Yang et al. (59)	China	R	Disease severity	6	99	44	49/50	1,705 ± 2,326*	15	60	7/8	243 ± 165*
Yu et al. (60)	China	R	Survival status	8	123	80	46/77	299 ± 287*	18	84	11/7	2 ± 349,941*
Zhang et al. (61)	China	R	Survival status	6	62	60	35/27	310 ± 441*	36	71	23/13	3,200 ± 5,144*
Zhao et al. (62)	China	R	Disease severity	8	19	49	7/12	97 ± 115	31	60	23/8	703 ± 641
Zheng et al. (63)	China	R	Disease severity	6	32	44	NR	67 ± 91*	67	64	NR	1,086 ± 3,217*

ICU, intensive care unit; MV, mechanical ventilation; NOS, Newcastle-Ottawa quality assessment scale for case-control studies; NR, not reported; P, prospective; R, retrospective; *, NT-proBNP.

was evaluated using the I^2 statistic, where $I^2 < 25\%$ indicated no heterogeneity, between 25 and 50% moderate heterogeneity, between 50 and 75% large heterogeneity, and >75% extreme heterogeneity (14, 15). Random-effect models were used to calculate the pooled SMD and 95% CIs if significant heterogeneity was present. In sensitivity analyses, the influence of individual studies on the overall effect size was assessed using the leave-one-out method (16). The presence of publication bias was assessed using the Begg's and the Egger's test, at the $p < 0.05$ level of significance (17, 18), and the Duval and Tweedie "trim and fill" procedure (19). To identify factors contributing to the between-study variance, we investigated the effects of several biologically and/or clinically plausible factors on the SMD by univariate meta-regression analysis. These factors included age, gender, clinical endpoint, study design (retrospective or prospective), geographical area where the study was conducted, aspartate aminotransferase (AST), alanine aminotransferase (ALT), D-dimer, serum creatinine, myoglobin, troponin, CK, albumin, ferritin, lactate dehydrogenase (LDH), procalcitonin, C-reactive protein (CRP), white blood cell count (WBC), diabetes, hypertension and cardiovascular disease. Statistical analyses were performed using Stata 14 (STATA Corp., College Station, TX, USA). The study was fully compliant with the PRISMA statement (20).

RESULTS

Literature Search and Study Selection

We initially identified 1,815 studies. A total of 1,758 studies were excluded after the first screening because they were duplicates or irrelevant. Following full-text revision of the remaining 57 articles, 13 were further excluded because they did not meet the inclusion criteria. Thus, 44 studies in 18,856 COVID-19 patients, 14,569 (53% males, mean age 48 years) with low severity or survivor status and 4,287 (59% males, mean age 61 years) with high severity or non-survivor status, were included in the final analysis (**Figure 1** and **Table 1**) (7, 21–63). Thirty-two studies were conducted in Asia (7, 22, 24, 26, 27, 29, 31–33, 35, 38–46, 48, 50, 51, 53–55, 57–63), eight in Europe (25, 28, 30, 34, 47, 49, 52, 56), three in America (23, 36, 37), and one in Africa (21). Thirty-two studies were retrospective (7, 21–23, 27, 29, 31–39, 41–45, 48, 50, 51, 53, 55, 57–63), eight prospective (24, 30, 46, 47, 49, 52, 54, 56), whereas the remaining four did not report the study design (25, 26, 28, 40). Clinical endpoints included disease severity based on current clinical guidelines in 15 studies (21, 24, 33, 39–41, 43, 48, 54, 55, 57–59, 62, 63), hospitalization in one (37), ICU transfer in three (32, 44, 49), or need for mechanical ventilation in one (23), and survival status in 24 studies (7, 22, 25–31, 34–36, 38, 42, 45–47, 50–53, 56, 60, 61). Sixteen studies reported plasma BNP concentrations (23, 24, 26, 33, 35–37, 45, 48, 50, 51, 54, 56–58, 62), whereas the remaining 28 reported plasma NT-proBNP concentrations (7, 21, 22, 25, 27–32, 34, 38–44, 46, 47, 49, 52, 53, 55, 59–61, 63). Only one study reported cumulative 7-day mean plasma NT-proBNP concentrations (34), whereas another reported BNP concentrations on initial presentation to the emergency department (37). The remaining 42 studies

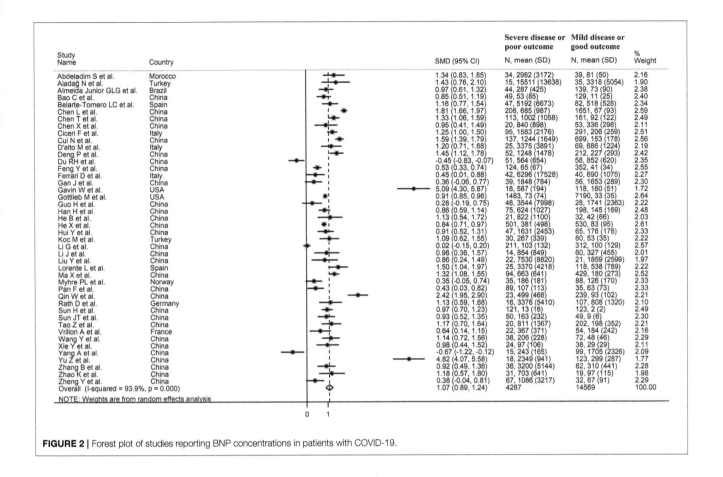

FIGURE 2 | Forest plot of studies reporting BNP concentrations in patients with COVID-19.

reported BNP or NT-proBNP concentrations within the first 24–48 h from admission.

Meta-Analysis

The overall SMD in BNP/NT-proBNP concentrations between COVID-19 patients with low vs. high severity or survivor vs. non-survivor status is shown in **Figure 2**. In two studies, patients with high severity or non-survivor status had significantly lower BNP/NT-proBNP concentrations when compared to those with low severity or survivor status (mean difference range, −0.45 to −0.67) (31, 59). By contrast, in the remaining studies BNP/NT-proBNP concentrations were lower in patients with low severity or survivor status (mean difference range, 0.02 – 5.09), with a non-significant difference in five studies (35, 38, 44, 50, 63). Pooled results confirmed that BNP/NT-proBNP concentrations were significantly higher in patients with severe disease or non-survivor status (SMD = 1.07, 95% CI: 0.89 – 1.24, and $p < 0.001$; **Figure 2**). There was extreme between-study heterogeneity (I^2 = 93.9%, $p < 0.001$). BNP/NT-proBNP concentrations remained significantly higher (SMD = 1.06, 95% CI: 0.86 – 1.26, and $p < 0.001$; I^2 = 93.0%, $p < 0.001$) in patients with high severity or non-survivor status after excluding two relatively large studies, accounting for nearly 56% of the overall sample size (26, 37).

In sensitivity analysis, the magnitude and the direction of the effect size were not substantially modified after sequentially removing each study and re-assessing the pooled estimates (effect size range, 0.99 – 1.10; **Figure 3**). No publication bias was observed with the Begg's ($p = 0.26$) and Egger's ($p = 0.40$) t-tests. However, using the trim-and-fill method, we identified three potential missing studies to be added to the left side of the funnel plot to ensure symmetry (**Figure 4**). The adjusted SMD, albeit attenuated, remained significant (SMD = 0.90, 95% CI: 0.70 – 1.09, and $p < 0.001$).

Sub-group analysis of the 42 studies reporting BNP/NT-proBNP concentrations on admission showed that the SMD remained significantly higher in patients with high severity or non-survivor status (SMD = 1.10, 95% CI: 0.88 – 1.31, and $p < 0.001$) with an extreme between-study variance (I^2 = 94.1%, $p < 0.001$). Additionally, the pooled SMD value in studies assessing disease severity (SMD = 0.87, 95% CI: 0.68 – 1.07, and $p < 0.001$; $I^2 = 79.5, p < 0.001$) was non-significantly lower than those investigating survivor status (SMD = 1.37, 95% CI: 1.08 – 1.66, $p < 0.001$; $I^2 = 92.3, p < 0.001$; $t = 1.63, p = 0.11$; **Figure 5**). Similarly, non-significantly higher SMD values were observed in retrospective (SMD = 1.06, 95% CI: 0.86 – 1.27, $p < 0.001$; I^2 = 94.5, $p < 0.001$) vs. prospective studies (SMD = 0.92, 95% CI: 0.67 – 1.18, $p < 0.001$; $I^2 = 59.4, p = 0.016$; $t = −0.41, p = 0.69$; **Figure 6**). The pooled SMD value in European studies (SMD = 0.96, 95% CI: 0.67 – 1.26, $p < 0.002$; $I^2 = 75.5\%, p < 0.001$) was non-significantly lower than that observed in Asian (SMD = 1.01, 95% CI: 0.77 – 1.24, $p < 0.001$; $I^2 = 94.5\%, p < 0.001$) and American studies (SMD = 2.24, 95% CI: 0.83 – 3.64, $p < 0.001$;

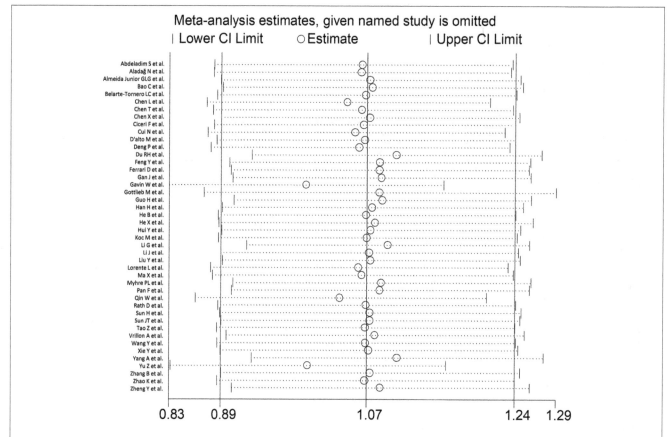

FIGURE 3 | Sensitivity analysis of the association between BNP and COVID-19 disease, assessed by investigating the influence of individual studies on the overall standardized mean difference (SMD). The SMD and the 95% confidence intervals (CIs) are indicated by the middle and the lateral vertical axes, respectively. The pooled SMD and the 95% CIs are indicated by the hollow circles and the two ends of each broken line, respectively.

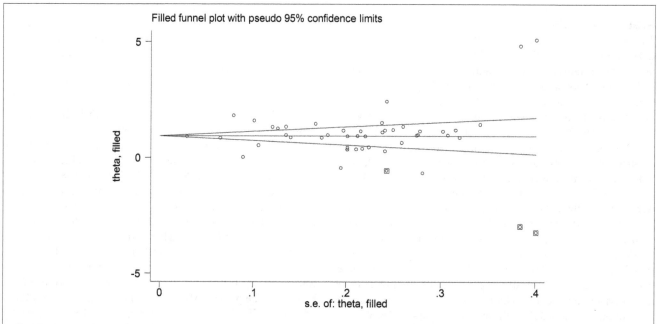

FIGURE 4 | Funnel plot of studies investigating disease severity or survival status after trimming and filling. Enclosed and free circles indicate dummy and genuine studies, respectively.

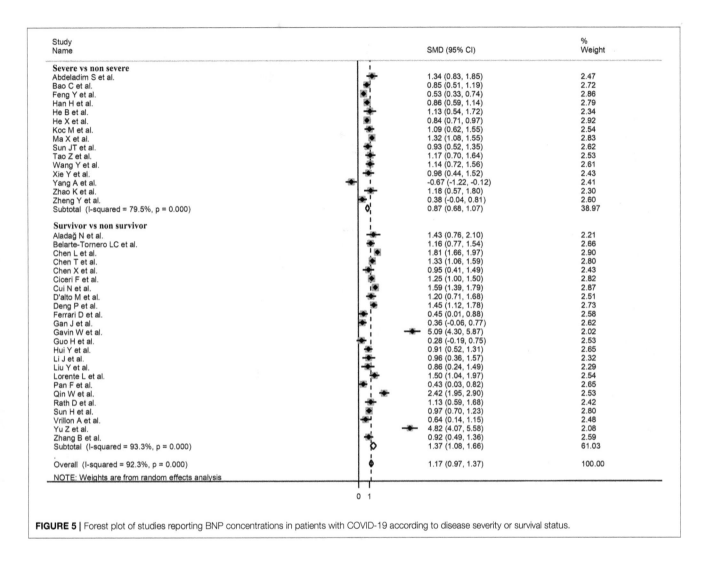

FIGURE 5 | Forest plot of studies reporting BNP concentrations in patients with COVID-19 according to disease severity or survival status.

$I^2 = 98.2\%$, $p < 0.001$; $t = 1.36$, $p = 0.18$; **Figure 7**). Finally, the pooled SMD value in studies reporting plasma NT-proBNP concentrations (SMD = 0.98, 95% CI: 0.74 – 1.23, $p < 0.001$; $I^2 = 93.2\%$, $p < 0.001$) was non-significantly lower than that observed in studies reporting plasma BNP concentrations (SMD = 1.22, 95% CI: 0.93 – 1.52, $p < 0.001$; $I^2 = 95.0\%$, $p < 0.001$; $t = -0.85$, $p = 0.40$; **Figure 8**). A relatively lower heterogeneity was observed in prospective ($I^2 = 59.4\%$) and European studies ($I^2 = 75.5\%$), and in those investigating disease severity ($I^2 = 79.5\%$).

Meta-Regression

The D-dimer ($t = 2.22$, $p = 0.03$), myoglobin ($t = 2.40$, $p = 0.04$), LDH ($t = 2.38$, $p = 0.02$), and procalcitonin ($t = 2.56$, $p = 0.01$) concentrations were significantly and positively associated with the pooled SMD. By contrast, no significant correlations were observed between the SMD and age ($t = -0.30$, $p = 0.76$), gender ($t = 0.26$, $p = 0.80$), AST ($t = 0.25$, $p = 0.81$), ALT ($t = -0.89$, $p = 0.38$), creatinine ($t = 0.93$, $p = 0.36$), troponin ($t = 0.18$, $p = 0.86$), CK ($t = 0.85$, $p = 0.41$), albumin ($t = 0.70$, $p = 0.49$), ferritin ($t = -1.29$, $p = 0.22$), CRP ($t = 0.96$, $p = 0.34$), WBC ($t = 0.08$, $p = 0.94$), diabetes ($t = -0.59$, $p = 0.56$), hypertension ($t = -0.01$, $p = 0.99$), and cardiovascular disease ($t = -0.53$, $p = 0.60$).

DISCUSSION

In our study, plasma concentrations of BNP and NT-proBNP, generally measured within the first 24–48 h from admission, were significantly higher in COVID-19 patients with severe disease, based on clinical assessment or the need for hospitalization, mechanical ventilation, or ICU transfer, and in those who did not survive when compared to patients with mild disease or who survived during follow up. The observed SMD values for combined natriuretic peptide concentrations or BNP and NT-proBNP separately, 1.07, 1.22, and 0.98, respectively, suggest a biologically and clinically significant effect size (64). Although between-study heterogeneity was extreme, in sensitivity analysis the effect size was not influenced when individual studies were sequentially removed. The Begg's and Egger's t-tests did not show any evidence of publication bias. In meta-regression analysis, significant associations were observed between the SMD value and D-dimer, myoglobin, LDH, and procalcitonin,

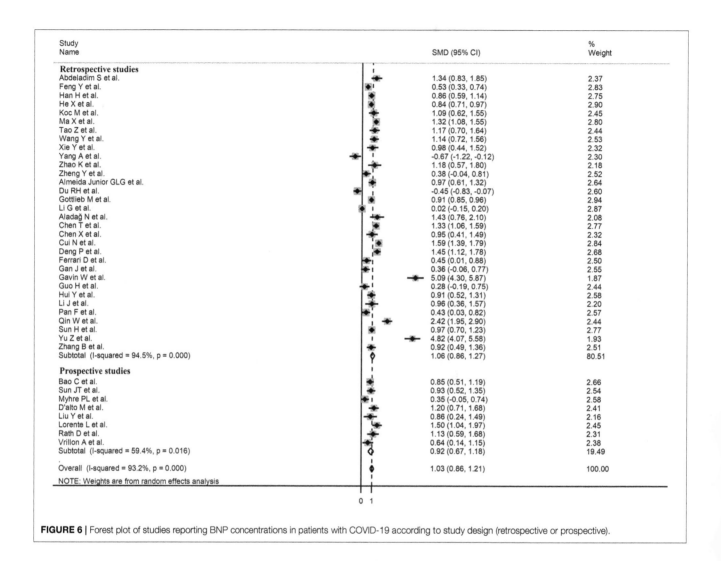

Study Name	SMD (95% CI)	% Weight
Retrospective studies		
Abdeladim S et al.	1.34 (0.83, 1.85)	2.37
Feng Y et al.	0.53 (0.33, 0.74)	2.83
Han H et al.	0.86 (0.59, 1.14)	2.75
He X et al.	0.84 (0.71, 0.97)	2.90
Koc M et al.	1.09 (0.62, 1.55)	2.45
Ma X et al.	1.32 (1.08, 1.55)	2.80
Tao Z et al.	1.17 (0.70, 1.64)	2.44
Wang Y et al.	1.14 (0.72, 1.56)	2.53
Xie Y et al.	0.98 (0.44, 1.52)	2.32
Yang A et al.	-0.67 (-1.22, -0.12)	2.30
Zhao K et al.	1.18 (0.57, 1.80)	2.18
Zheng Y et al.	0.38 (-0.04, 0.81)	2.52
Almeida Junior GLG et al.	0.97 (0.61, 1.32)	2.64
Du RH et al.	-0.45 (-0.83, -0.07)	2.60
Gottlieb M et al.	0.91 (0.85, 0.96)	2.94
Li G et al.	0.02 (-0.15, 0.20)	2.87
Aladağ N et al.	1.43 (0.76, 2.10)	2.08
Chen T et al.	1.33 (1.06, 1.59)	2.77
Chen X et al.	0.95 (0.41, 1.49)	2.32
Cui N et al.	1.59 (1.39, 1.79)	2.84
Deng P et al.	1.45 (1.12, 1.78)	2.68
Ferrari D et al.	0.45 (0.01, 0.88)	2.50
Gan J et al.	0.36 (-0.06, 0.77)	2.55
Gavin W et al.	5.09 (4.30, 5.87)	1.87
Guo H et al.	0.28 (-0.19, 0.75)	2.44
Hui Y et al.	0.91 (0.52, 1.31)	2.58
Li J et al.	0.96 (0.36, 1.57)	2.20
Pan F et al.	0.43 (0.03, 0.82)	2.57
Qin W et al.	2.42 (1.95, 2.90)	2.44
Sun H et al.	0.97 (0.70, 1.23)	2.77
Yu Z et al.	4.82 (4.07, 5.58)	1.93
Zhang B et al.	0.92 (0.49, 1.36)	2.51
Subtotal (I-squared = 94.5%, p = 0.000)	1.06 (0.86, 1.27)	80.51
Prospective studies		
Bao C et al.	0.85 (0.51, 1.19)	2.66
Sun JT et al.	0.93 (0.52, 1.35)	2.54
Myhre PL et al.	0.35 (-0.05, 0.74)	2.58
D'alto M et al.	1.20 (0.71, 1.68)	2.41
Liu Y et al.	0.86 (0.24, 1.49)	2.16
Lorente L et al.	1.50 (1.04, 1.97)	2.45
Rath D et al.	1.13 (0.59, 1.68)	2.31
Vrillon A et al.	0.64 (0.14, 1.15)	2.38
Subtotal (I-squared = 59.4%, p = 0.016)	0.92 (0.67, 1.18)	19.49
Overall (I-squared = 93.2%, p = 0.000)	1.03 (0.86, 1.21)	100.00

NOTE: Weights are from random effects analysis

0   1

FIGURE 6 | Forest plot of studies reporting BNP concentrations in patients with COVID-19 according to study design (retrospective or prospective).

but not with age, gender, AST, ALT, creatinine, troponin, CK, albumin, ferritin, CRP, WBC, diabetes, hypertension, or cardiovascular disease.

Differently from the inactive NT-proBNP, the BNP exerts significant biological effects through its binding to the guanylyl cyclase-coupled natriuretic receptors A and B. The consequent increase in cyclic guanosine monophosphate causes vasodilatation, diuresis, natriuresis, inhibition of the renin-angiotensin-aldosterone system, inhibition of fibrosis, hypertrophy, cell apoptosis and inflammation, including suppression of superoxide generation by neutrophils, and improvement in myocardial relaxation (10). Notably, there is no evidence of significant associations between BNP and cyclic guanosine monophosphate concentrations in human studies. Furthermore, specific BNP-mediated protective effects, particularly the suppression of neutrophil-mediated generation of superoxide via nicotinamide adenine dinucleotide phosphate oxidase, are impaired in the context of acute heart failure, even in the presence of increased BNP concentrations (65). Whilst such effects are partially restored with pharmacological treatment, the failure of BNP-related suppression of superoxide release might

lead to sustained tissue inflammation in heart failure, with or without concomitant COVID-19. There are other differences between the BNP and the NT-proBNP, with the latter being characterized by a higher molecular mass, a longer half-life (>60 vs. 15–20 min), a higher degree of *in vivo* glycosylation, and a lower degree of intra-individual biological variation (66). The better analytical characteristics of the available immunoassay methods for the measurement of NT-proBNP concentrations, when compared to those for the assessment of the BNP, have prompted some experts to advocate the measurement and monitoring of NT-proBNP concentrations as the best strategy for the management of patients with heart failure (66). These issues notwithstanding, in our meta-analysis the studies reporting BNP vs. NT-proBNP plasma concentrations had similar SMD values and degrees of heterogeneity.

The significant association observed between plasma BNP/NT-proBNP concentrations, disease severity and mortality in patients with COVID-19 is likely to reflect the presence of heart failure and its adverse sequelae in this group. In this context, these routine and relatively inexpensive biomarkers might assist the clinician with the early diagnosis of cardiac dysfunction

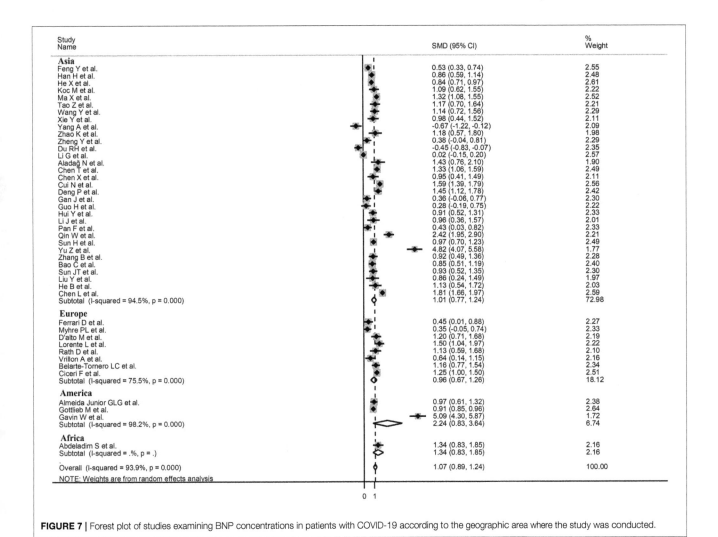

FIGURE 7 | Forest plot of studies examining BNP concentrations in patients with COVID-19 according to the geographic area where the study was conducted.

and the prompt initiation of appropriate pharmacological and non-pharmacological therapies (67). Further research is warranted to determine whether the assessment of BNP/NT-proBNP might also be incorporated into predictive tools that are specifically developed and validated in COVID-19 patients. The reported associations, in meta-regression analysis, between the SMD of BNP/NT-proBNP and D-dimer, myoglobin, LDH, and pro-calcitonin suggests that the effect size is particularly correlated with markers of pro-coagulant activity, skeletal muscle and other tissue damage, and severe sepsis, respectively. Notably, these markers have, in turn, been shown to have significant associations with COVID-19 severity and outcomes (68–70). By contrast, the lack of associations observed with other cardiac biomarkers, e.g., troponin and CK, suggests that the measurement of BNP/NT-proBNP may provide complementary, rather than redundant, information regarding the presence of cardiac abnormalities in patients with COVID-19.

The extreme between-study heterogeneity represents a limitation of our study. However, we did not observe significant publication bias and the overall effect size was not substantially

affected in sensitivity analyses. The lack of significant associations between the SMD and several patient and study characteristics, except for D-dimer, myoglobin, LDH, and procalcitonin concentrations, suggests that other unreported factors might have contributed to the observed heterogeneity. Such factors may include the relationship between the SMD values and the presence of new onset vs. acute on chronic heart failure and the information regarding the specific analytical methods used for the determination of BNP and NT-proBNP plasma concentrations (66). In this context, the lack of available information on indexes of left ventricular function prevented the conduct of further meta-regression analyses of the association between such indexes and the SMD values. Furthermore, virtually all selected studies reported isolated, rather than serial, measurements of natriuretic peptide shortly after hospital admission. This issue is particularly important as the routine monitoring of BNP/NT-proBNP concentrations has been shown to be beneficial in heart failure (71). Further studies should investigate the prognostic value of single vs. serial BNP/NT-proBNP measurements also in patients with COVID-19.

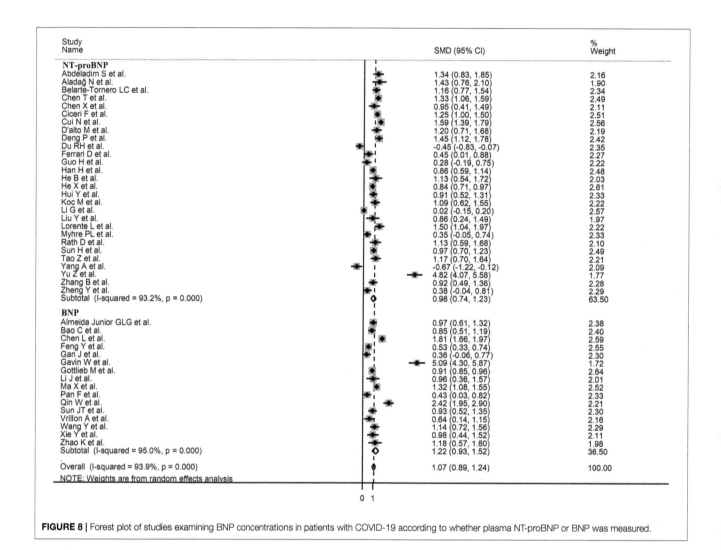

FIGURE 8 | Forest plot of studies examining BNP concentrations in patients with COVID-19 according to whether plasma NT-proBNP or BNP was measured.

In conclusion, higher plasma concentrations of BNP or NT-proBNP are significantly associated with higher disease severity and increased mortality in COVID-19. Additional studies are required to determine whether these cardiac biomarkers can be incorporated into robust predictive tools that further assist with early management and monitoring in this patient group.

AUTHOR CONTRIBUTIONS

AZ: initial idea. AZ and SS: data collection and analysis. AZ, SS, CC, and AM: data interpretation and writing—review and editing. AM: writing—first draft. All authors contributed to the article and approved the submitted version.

REFERENCES

1. Huang C, Soleimani J, Herasevich S, Pinevich Y, Pennington KM, Dong Y, et al. Clinical characteristics, treatment, and outcomes of critically ill patients with COVID-19: a scoping review. *Mayo Clin Proc.* (2021) 96:183–202. doi: 10.1016/j.mayocp.2020.10.022

2. Pijls BG, Jolani S, Atherley A, Derckx RT, Dijkstra JIR, Franssen GHL, et al. Demographic risk factors for COVID-19 infection, severity, ICU admission and death: a meta-analysis of 59 studies. *BMJ Open.* (2021) 11:e044640. doi: 10.1136/bmjopen-2020-044640

3. Fajgenbaum DC, June CH. Cytokine Storm. *N Engl J Med.* (2020) 383:2255–73. doi: 10.1056/NEJMra2026131

4. Nishiga M, Wang DW, Han Y, Lewis DB, Wu JC. COVID-19 and cardiovascular disease: from basic mechanisms to clinical perspectives. *Nat Rev Cardiol.* (2020) 17:543–58. doi: 10.1038/s41569-020-0413-9

5. Shi S, Qin M, Shen B, Cai Y, Liu T, Yang F, et al. Association of cardiac injury with mortality in hospitalized patients with COVID-19 in Wuhan, China. *JAMA Cardiol.* (2020) 5:802–10. doi: 10.1001/jamacardio.2020.0950

6. Yang J, Liao X, Yin W, Wang B, Yue J, Bai L, et al. Elevated cardiac biomarkers may be effective prognostic predictors for patients with COVID-19: a multicenter, observational study. *Am J Emerg Med.* (2021) 39:34–41. doi: 10.1016/j.ajem.2020.10.013

7. Chen T, Wu D, Chen H, Yan W, Yang D, Chen G, et al. Clinical characteristics of 113 deceased patients with coronavirus disease 2019: retrospective study. *BMJ.* (2020) 368:m1091. doi: 10.1136/bmj.m1091

8. Zhou F, Yu T, Du R, Fan G, Liu Y, Liu Z, et al. Clinical course and risk factors for mortality of adult inpatients with COVID-19 in Wuhan, China: a retrospective cohort study. *Lancet.* (2020) 395:1054–62. doi: 10.1016/S0140-6736(20)30566-3

9. Maisel AS, Duran JM, Wettersten N. Natriuretic peptides in heart failure: atrial and B-type natriuretic peptides. *Heart Fail Clin.* (2018) 14:13–25. doi: 10.1016/j.hfc.2017.08.002

10. Potter LR, Yoder AR, Flora DR, Antos LK, Dickey DM. Natriuretic peptides: their structures, receptors, physiologic functions and therapeutic applications. *Handb Exp Pharmacol.* (2009) 191:341–66. doi: 10.1007/978-3-540-68964-5_15

11. Omland T, Persson A, Ng L, O'Brien R, Karlsson T, Herlitz J, et al. N-terminal pro-B-type natriuretic peptide and long-term mortality in acute coronary syndromes. *Circulation.* (2002) 106:2913–8. doi: 10.1161/01.CIR.0000041661.63285.AE

12. Wells GA, Shea B, O'Connell D, Peterson J, Welch V, Losos M, et al. *The Newcastle-Ottawa Scale (NOS) for Assessing the Quality of Nonrandomised Studies in Meta-Analyses.* The Ottawa Hospital Research Institute (2013). Available online at: http://www.ohri.ca/programs/clinical_epidemiology/oxford.asp (accessed June 11, 2021).

13. Wan X, Wang W, Liu J, Tong T. Estimating the sample mean and standard deviation from the sample size, median, range and/or interquartile range. *BMC Med Res Methodol.* (2014) 14:135. doi: 10.1186/1471-2288-14-135

14. Bowden J, Tierney JF, Copas AJ, Burdett S. Quantifying, displaying and accounting for heterogeneity in the meta-analysis of RCTs using standard and generalised Q statistics. *BMC Med Res Methodol.* (2011) 11:41. doi: 10.1186/1471-2288-11-41

15. Higgins JP, Thompson SG. Quantifying heterogeneity in a meta-analysis. *Stat Med.* (2002) 21:1539–58. doi: 10.1002/sim.1186

16. Tobias A. Assessing the influence of a single study in the meta-analysis estimate. *Stata Tech Bull.* (1999) 47:15–7.

17. Begg CB, Mazumdar M. Operating characteristics of a rank correlation test for publication bias. *Biometrics.* (1994) 50:1088–101. doi: 10.2307/2533446

18. Sterne JA, Egger M. Funnel plots for detecting bias in meta-analysis: guidelines on choice of axis. *J Clin Epidemiol.* (2001) 54:1046–55. doi: 10.1016/S0895-4356(01)00377-8

19. Duval S, Tweedie R. Trim and fill: a simple funnel-plot-based method of testing and adjusting for publication bias in meta-analysis. *Biometrics.* (2000) 56:455–63. doi: 10.1111/j.0006-341X.2000.00455.x

20. Liberati A, Altman DG, Tetzlaff J, Mulrow C, Gotzsche PC, Ioannidis JP, et al. The PRISMA statement for reporting systematic reviews and meta-analyses of studies that evaluate healthcare interventions: explanation and elaboration. *BMJ.* (2009) 339:b2700. doi: 10.1136/bmj.b2700

21. Abdeladim S, Oualim S, Elouarradi A, Bensahi I, Aniq Filali R, El Harras M, et al. Analysis of cardiac injury biomarkers in COVID-19 patients. *Arch Clin Infect Dis.* (2020) 15:e105515. doi: 10.5812/archcid.105515

22. Aladag N, Atabey RD. The role of concomitant cardiovascular diseases and cardiac biomarkers for predicting mortality in critical COVID-19 patients. *Acta Cardiol.* (2021) 76:132–9. doi: 10.1080/00015385.2020.1810914

23. Almeida Junior GLG, Braga F, Jorge JK, Nobre GF, Kalichsztein M, Faria PMP, et al. Prognostic value of troponin-T and B-type natriuretic peptide in patients hospitalized for COVID-19. *Arq Bras Cardiol.* (2020) 115:660–6. doi: 10.36660/abc.20200385

24. Bao C, Tao X, Cui W, Yi B, Pan T, Young KH, et al. SARS-CoV-2 induced thrombocytopenia as an important biomarker significantly correlated with abnormal coagulation function, increased intravascular blood clot risk and mortality in COVID-19 patients. *Exp Hematol Oncol.* (2020) 9:16. doi: 10.1186/s40164-020-00172-4

25. Belarte-Tornero LC, Valdivielso-More S, Vicente Elcano M, Sole-Gonzalez E, Ruiz-Bustillo S, Calvo-Fernandez A, et al. Prognostic implications of chronic heart failure and utility of NT-proBNP levels in heart failure patients with SARS-CoV-2 infection. *J Clin Med.* (2021) 10:323. doi: 10.3390/jcm10020323

26. Chen L, Yu J, He W, Chen L, Yuan G, Dong F, et al. Risk factors for death in 1859 subjects with COVID-19. *Leukemia.* (2020) 34:2173–83. doi: 10.1038/s41375-020-0911-0

27. Chen X, Yan L, Fei Y, Zhang C. Laboratory abnormalities and risk factors associated with in-hospital death in patients with severe COVID-19. *J Clin Lab Anal.* (2020) 34:e23467. doi: 10.1002/jcla.23467

28. Ciceri F, Castagna A, Rovere-Querini P, De Cobelli F, Ruggeri A, Galli L, et al. Early predictors of clinical outcomes of COVID-19 outbreak in Milan, Italy. *Clin Immunol.* (2020) 217:108509. doi: 10.1016/j.clim.2020.108509

29. Cui N, Yan R, Qin C, Zhao J. Clinical characteristics and immune responses of 137 deceased patients with COVID-19: a retrospective study. *Front Cell Infect Microbiol.* (2020) 10:595333. doi: 10.3389/fcimb.2020.595333

30. D'Alto M, Marra AM, Severino S, Salzano A, Romeo E, De Rosa R, et al. Right ventricular-arterial uncoupling independently predicts survival in COVID-19 ARDS. *Crit Care.* (2020) 24:670. doi: 10.1186/s13054-020-03385-5

31. Deng P, Ke Z, Ying B, Qiao B, Yuan L. The diagnostic and prognostic role of myocardial injury biomarkers in hospitalized patients with COVID-19. *Clin Chim Acta.* (2020) 510:186–90. doi: 10.1016/j.cca.2020.07.018

32. Du RH, Liu LM, Yin W, Wang W, Guan LL, Yuan ML, et al. Hospitalization and critical care of 109 decedents with COVID-19 pneumonia in Wuhan, China. *Ann Am Thorac Soc.* (2020) 17:839–46. doi: 10.1513/AnnalsATS.202003-225OC

33. Feng Y, Ling Y, Bai T, Xie Y, Huang J, Li J, et al. COVID-19 with different severities: a multicenter study of clinical features. *Am J Respir Crit Care Med.* (2020) 201:1380–8. doi: 10.1164/rccm.202002-0445OC

34. Ferrari D, Seveso A, Sabetta E, Ceriotti D, Carobene A, Banfi G, et al. Role of time-normalized laboratory findings in predicting COVID-19 outcome. *Diagnosis (Berl).* (2020) 7:387–94. doi: 10.1515/dx-2020-0095

35. Gan J, Li J, Li S, Yang C. Leucocyte subsets effectively predict the clinical outcome of patients with COVID-19 pneumonia: a retrospective case-control study. *Front Public Health.* (2020) 8:299. doi: 10.3389/fpubh.2020.00299

36. Gavin W, Campbell E, Zaidi SA, Gavin N, Dbeibo L, Beeler C, et al. Clinical characteristics, outcomes and prognosticators in adult patients hospitalized with COVID-19. *Am J Infect Control.* (2021) 49:158–65. doi: 10.1016/j.ajic.2020.07.005

37. Gottlieb M, Sansom S, Frankenberger C, Ward E, Hota B. Clinical course and factors associated with hospitalization and critical illness among COVID-19 patients in Chicago, Illinois. *Acad Emerg Med.* (2020) 27:963–73. doi: 10.1111/acem.14104

38. Guo H, Shen Y, Wu N, Sun X. Myocardial injury in severe and critical coronavirus disease 2019 patients. *J Card Surg.* (2021) 36:82–8. doi: 10.1111/jocs.15164

39. Han H, Xie L, Liu R, Yang J, Liu F, Wu K, et al. Analysis of heart injury laboratory parameters in 273 COVID-19 patients in one hospital in Wuhan, China. *J Med Virol.* (2020) 92:819–23. doi: 10.1002/jmv.25809

40. He B, Wang J, Wang Y, Zhao J, Huang J, Tian Y, et al. The metabolic changes and immune profiles in patients with COVID-19. *Front Immunol.* (2020) 11:2075. doi: 10.3389/fimmu.2020.02075

41. He X, Wang L, Wang H, Xie Y, Yu Y, Sun J, et al. Factors associated with acute cardiac injury and their effects on mortality in patients with COVID-19. *Sci Rep.* (2020) 10:20452. doi: 10.1038/s41598-020-77172-1

42. Hui Y, Li Y, Tong X, Wang Z, Mao X, Huang L, et al. The risk factors for mortality of diabetic patients with severe COVID-19: a retrospective study of 167 severe COVID-19 cases in Wuhan. *PLoS One.* (2020) 15:e0243602. doi: 10.1371/journal.pone.0243602

43. Koc M, Sumbul HE, Gulumsek E, Koca H, Bulut Y, Karakoc E, et al. Disease severity affects ventricular repolarization parameters in patients with COVID-19. *Arq Bras Cardiol.* (2020) 115:907–13. doi: 10.36660/abc.20200482

44. Li G, Zhou CL, Ba YM, Wang YM, Song B, Cheng XB, et al. Nutritional risk and therapy for severe and critical COVID-19 patients: a multicenter retrospective observational study. *Clin Nutr.* (2021) 40:2154–61. doi: 10.1016/j.clnu.2020.09.040

45. Li J, Xu G, Yu H, Peng X, Luo Y, Cao C. Clinical characteristics and outcomes of 74 patients with severe or critical COVID-19. *Am J Med Sci.* (2020) 360:229–35. doi: 10.1016/j.amjms.2020.05.040

46. Liu Y, Xie J, Gao P, Tian R, Qian H, Guo F, et al. Swollen heart in COVID-19 patients who progress to critical illness: a perspective from echo-cardiologists. *ESC Heart Fail.* (2020) 7:3621–32. doi: 10.1002/ehf2.12873

47. Lorente L, Martin MM, Argueso M, Sole-Violan J, Perez A, Marcos YRJA, et al. Association between red blood cell distribution width and mortality of COVID-19 patients. *Anaesth Crit Care Pain Med.* (2020) 40:100777. doi: 10.1016/j.accpm.2020.10.013

48. Ma X, Li A, Jiao M, Shi Q, An X, Feng Y, et al. Characteristic of 523 COVID-19 in henan province and a death prediction model. *Front Public Health.* (2020) 8:475. doi: 10.3389/fpubh.2020.00475

49. Myhre PL, Prebensen C, Strand H, Roysland R, Jonassen CM, Rangberg A, et al. Growth differentiation factor 15 provides prognostic information superior to established cardiovascular and inflammatory biomarkers in unselected patients hospitalized with COVID-19. *Circulation.* (2020) 142:2128–37. doi: 10.1161/CIRCULATIONAHA.120.050360

50. Pan F, Yang L, Li Y, Liang B, Li L, Ye T, et al. Factors associated with death outcome in patients with severe coronavirus disease-19 (COVID-19): a case-control study. *Int J Med Sci.* (2020) 17:1281–92. doi: 10.7150/ijms.46614

51. Qin WD, Bai W, Liu K, Liu Y, Meng X, Zhang K, et al. Clinical course and risk factors of disease deterioration in critically ill patients with COVID-19. *Hum Gene Ther.* (2021) 32:310–5. doi: 10.1089/hum.2020.255

52. Rath D, Petersen-Uribe A, Avdiu A, Witzel K, Jaeger P, Zdanyte M, et al. Impaired cardiac function is associated with mortality in patients with acute COVID-19 infection. *Clin Res Cardiol.* (2020) 109:1491–9. doi: 10.1007/s00392-020-01683-0

53. Sun H, Ning R, Tao Y, Yu C, Deng X, Zhao C, et al. Risk factors for mortality in 244 older adults with COVID-19 in Wuhan, China: a retrospective study. *J Am Geriatr Soc.* (2020) 68:E19–E23. doi: 10.1111/jgs.16533

54. Sun JT, Chen Z, Nie P, Ge H, Shen L, Yang F, et al. Lipid profile features and their associations with disease severity and mortality in patients with COVID-19. *Front Cardiovasc Med.* (2020) 7:584987. doi: 10.3389/fcvm.2020.584987

55. Tao Z, Xu J, Chen W, Yang Z, Xu X, Liu L, et al. Anemia is associated with severe illness in COVID-19: a retrospective cohort study. *J Med Virol.* (2021) 93:1478–88. doi: 10.21203/rs.3.rs-39184/v1

56. Vrillon A, Hourregue C, Azuar J, Grosset L, Boutelier A, Tan S, et al. COVID-19 in older adults: a series of 76 patients aged 85 years and older with COVID-19. *J Am Geriatr Soc.* (2020) 68:2735–43. doi: 10.1111/jgs.16894

57. Wang Y, Zhou Y, Yang Z, Xia D, Hu Y, Geng S. Clinical characteristics of patients with severe pneumonia caused by the SARS-CoV-2 in Wuhan, China. *Respiration.* (2020) 99:649–57. doi: 10.1159/000507940

58. Xie Y, You Q, Wu C, Cao S, Qu G, Yan X, et al. Impact of cardiovascular disease on clinical characteristics and outcomes of coronavirus disease 2019 (COVID-19). *Circ J.* (2020) 84:1277–83. doi: 10.1253/circj.CJ-20-0348

59. Yang A, Qiu Q, Kong X, Sun Y, Chen T, Zuo Y, et al. Clinical and Epidemiological Characteristics of COVID-19 Patients in Chongqing China. *Front Public Health.* (2020) 8:244. doi: 10.3389/fpubh.2020.00244

60. Yu Z, Ke Y, Xie J, Yu H, Zhu W, He L, et al. Clinical characteristics on admission predict in-hospital fatal outcome in patients aged >/=75 years with novel coronavirus disease (COVID-19): a retrospective cohort study. *BMC Geriatr.* (2020) 20:514. doi: 10.1186/s12877-020-01921-0

61. Zhang B, Dong C, Li S, Song X, Wei W, Liu L. Triglyceride to high-density lipoprotein cholesterol ratio is an important determinant of cardiovascular risk and poor prognosis in coronavirus disease-19: a retrospective case series study. *Diabetes Metab Syndr Obes.* (2020) 13:3925–36. doi: 10.2147/DMSO.S268992

62. Zhao K, Huang J, Dai D, Feng Y, Liu L, Nie S. Serum iron level as a potential predictor of coronavirus disease 2019 severity and mortality: a retrospective study. *Open Forum Infect Dis.* (2020) 7:ofaa250. doi: 10.1093/ofid/ofaa250

63. Zheng Y, Xu H, Yang M, Zeng Y, Chen H, Liu R, et al. Epidemiological characteristics and clinical features of 32 critical and 67 noncritical cases of COVID-19 in Chengdu. *J Clin Virol.* (2020) 127:104366. doi: 10.1016/j.jcv.2020.104366

64. Cohen J. *Statistical Power Analysis for the Behavioral Sciences, 2nd Edn.* Hillsdale, NJ: Erlbaum (1988).

65. Liu S, Ngo DT, Chong CR, Amarasekera AT, Procter NE, Licari G, et al. Suppression of neutrophil superoxide generation by BNP is attenuated in acute heart failure: a case for 'BNP resistance'. *Eur J Heart Fail.* (2015) 17:475–83. doi: 10.1002/ejhf.242

66. Clerico A, Zaninotto M, Passino C, Plebani M. New issues on measurement of B-type natriuretic peptides. *Clin Chem Lab Med.* (2017) 56:32–9. doi: 10.1515/cclm-2017-0433

67. Zhang Y, Coats AJS, Zheng Z, Adamo M, Ambrosio G, Anker SD, et al. Management of heart failure patients with COVID-19: a joint position paper of the Chinese Heart Failure Association & National Heart Failure Committee and the Heart Failure Association of the European Society of Cardiology. *Eur J Heart Fail.* (2020) 22:941–56. doi: 10.1002/ejhf.1915

68. Paliogiannis P, Mangoni AA, Dettori P, Nasrallah GK, Pintus G, Zinellu A. D-Dimer Concentrations and COVID-19 severity: a systematic review and meta-analysis. *Front Public Health.* (2020) 8:432. doi: 10.3389/fpubh.2020.00432

69. Ghahramani S, Tabrizi R, Lankarani KB, Kashani SMA, Rezaei S, Zeidi N, et al. Laboratory features of severe vs. non-severe COVID-19 patients in Asian populations: a systematic review and meta-analysis. *Eur J Med Res.* (2020) 25:30. doi: 10.1186/s40001-020-00432-3

70. Qin JJ, Cheng X, Zhou F, Lei F, Akolkar G, Cai J, et al. Redefining cardiac biomarkers in predicting mortality of inpatients with COVID-19. *Hypertension.* (2020) 76:1104–12. doi: 10.1161/HYPERTENSIONAHA.120.15528

71. Januzzi JL, Troughton R. Are serial BNP measurements useful in heart failure management? Serial natriuretic peptide measurements are useful in heart failure management. *Circulation.* (2013) 127:500–7; discussion 8. doi: 10.1161/CIRCULATIONAHA.112.120485

2

Late Cardiac Pathology in Severe Covid-19: A Postmortem Series of 30 Patients

Ana Ferrer-Gómez [1,2†], Héctor Pian-Arias [1†], Irene Carretero-Barrio [1,2],
Antonia Navarro-Cantero [1,2], David Pestaña [2,3], Raúl de Pablo [2,4,5],
José Luis Zamorano [2,4,6,7], Juan Carlos Galán [4,8,9], Belén Pérez-Mies [1,2,4,10],
Ignacio Ruz-Caracuel [1,4] and José Palacios [1,2,10*]

[1] Pathology Department, University Hospital Ramón y Cajal, Madrid, Spain, [2] Faculty of Medicine, Alcalá University, Alcalá de Henares, Spain, [3] Anaesthesiology and Surgical Critical Care Department, Hospital Universitario Ramón y Cajal, Madrid, Spain, [4] Instituto Ramón y Cajal for Health Research (IRYCIS), Madrid, Spain, [5] Medical Intensive Care Unit, Hospital Universitario Ramón y Cajal, Madrid, Spain, [6] Cardiology Department, Hospital Universitario Ramón y Cajal, Madrid, Spain, [7] Centro de Investigación Biomédica en Red de Enfermedades Cardiovasculares (CIBERCV), Instituto de Salud Carlos III, Madrid, Spain, [8] Microbiology Department, Hospital Universitario Ramón y Cajal, Madrid, Spain, [9] Centro de Investigación Biomédica en Red en Epidemiología y Salud Pública (CIBERESP), Madrid, Spain, [10] Centro de Investigación Biomédica en Red de Cáncer (CIBERONC), Instituto de Salud Carlos III, Madrid, Spain

*Correspondence:
José Palacios
jose.palacios@salud.madrid.org

† These authors have contributed
equally to this work

The role of SARS-CoV-2 as a direct cause in the cardiac lesions in patients with severe COVID-19 remains to be established. Our objective is to report the pathological findings in cardiac samples of 30 patients who died after a prolonged hospital stay due to Sars-Cov-2 infection. We performed macroscopic, histological and immunohistochemical analysis of the hearts of 30 patients; and detected Sars-Cov-2 RNA by RT-PCR in the cardiac tissue samples. The median age of our cohort was 69.5 years and 76.6% were male. The median time between symptoms onset and death was 36.5 days. The main comorbidities were arterial hypertension (13 patients, 43.3%), dyslipidemia (11 patients, 36.7%), cardiovascular conditions (8 patients, 26.7%), and obesity (8 patients, 26.7%). Cardiovascular conditions included ischemic cardiopathy in 4 patients (13.3%), hypertrophic cardiomyopathy in 2 patients (6.7%) and valve replacement and chronic heart failure in one patient each (3.3%). At autopsy, the most frequent histopathological findings were coronary artery atherosclerosis (8 patients, 26.7%), left ventricular hypertrophy (4 patients, 13.3%), chronic epicardial inflammation (3 patients, 10%) and adipose metaplasia (2 patients, 6.7%). Two patients showed focal myocarditis, one due to invasive aspergillosis. One additional patient showed senile amyloidosis. Sars-Cov-2 RNA was detected in the heart of only one out of 30 patients, who had the shortest disease evolution of the series (9 days). However, no relevant cardiac histological alterations were identified. In present series, cardiac pathology was only modest in most patients with severe COVID-19. At present, the contribution of a direct effect of SARS-CoV-2 on cardiac lesions remains to be established.

Keywords: COVID-19, SARS-CoV-2, heart, cardiac pathology, autopsy

INTRODUCTION

Coronavirus-19 disease (COVID-19), caused by the new coronavirus SARS-CoV-2 has become a global health challenge in our time (1). It is known that SARS-CoV-2 affects mainly the respiratory system, with a spectrum of clinical manifestations ranging from asymptomatic to mild illness with fever and fatigue (80% of symptomatic patients) (2). However, in the most severe cases, which represent around 5%, it can lead to respiratory distress syndrome that requires ventilatory support (3, 4). As cardiovascular complications including myocarditis, acute myocardial infarction, and exacerbation of heart failure are present in patients suffering from other respiratory viral infections, such as influenza virus each annual epidemic period, special attention has been paid to a possible heart involvement by SARS-CoV-2 since the beginning of the pandemic (5). In fact, reported clinical cardiac manifestation in COVID-19 patients included right heart dilatation and dysfunction, myocarditis, cardiac fibrosis, arrhythmias, endothelial dysfunction, dysautonomia, and thrombotic events (6). Moreover, it has been suggested that patients with a history of cardiovascular disease or cardiovascular risk factors such as hypertension, dyslipidemia or obesity are strongly associated to severe symptoms and higher mortality rate in patients infected by SARS-CoV-2 (2, 7). The possible pathophysiological mechanisms by which SARS-CoV-2 would cause damage to the myocardium and vascular endothelium include a direct myocardial injury due to viral invasion, a damage secondary to hypoxemia as consequence of respiratory failure, infarct secondary to thrombosis, as well as a dysregulated immunological response (known as cytokine storm) (8).

Since autopsies are the gold standard procedure to settle the underlying pathophysiology of the diseases (9), several autopsy series of patients who died from COVID-19 have been reported in the last months. In addition, some studies have reviewed the cardiac lesions reported in those series (10–12). However, our information regarding cardiac pathology is limited to about 700 hearts and, despite these studies, there is still limited and controversial data about the histopathological cardiac findings in patients with SARS-CoV-2 infection. Previous series are mostly formed by patients who died during the acute illness. Thus, the longest duration of illness in the cohorts reviewed by Roshdy et al. (10) was 52 days with a median duration from symptoms onset to death of 12 days (range, 0–52 days, $n = 98$), which means that the long-term evolution or complications of the disease were not covered by this review.

The objective of our study is to present the histopathological cardiac lesions in a series of 30 autopsies performed in patients who died by severe COVID-19 with relative long-term evolution from symptoms onset (median 36.5 days, range 9–108 days).

MATERIALS AND METHODS
Autopsy Procedure and Clinical Data

This is a retrospective analysis of the macroscopic and histological findings in the hearts of all autopsies performed on patients with COVID-19 in University Hospital Ramón y Cajal (Madrid, Spain), from April 2020 to April 2021 ($n = 30$), representing ∼3% of patients who died from COVID-19 during this period. The Research Ethics Committee approved the study (reference: Necropsias_Covid19; 355_20). All the deceased patients were diagnosed of SARS-CoV-2 infection confirmed by RT-PCR nasopharyngeal swab test. Demographic and clinical data were collected from the electronic medical records.

These consecutive autopsies were requested by the medical staff according to clinical interest. Most autopsies ($n = 25$, 83%) corresponded to patients with severe respiratory diseases and were requested by ICU staffs. Consequently, the series does not represent the complete spectrum of causes of death attributable to COVID-19 (**Table 1**). All autopsies were consented by patients' relatives and carried out according to safety protocols, in a negative pressure autopsy room, using personal protection equipment, as previously reported (13).

In the first 14 consecutive decedents, we took *in-corpore* representative sections from the heart, lungs, liver, kidney, pancreas, and bone marrow. In the rest of the patients, due to improved technical training, we extracted the complete heart and lung block, left kidney, spleen, and sections from the liver, pancreas and bone marrow. We extracted the brain in 10 patients.

After each procedure, the hearts were fixed in formalin for 24–48 h.

Histopathology and Immunohistochemistry

For histological study, in the 14 first autopsies, we only took 5 representative sections corresponding to the anterior, lateral and posterior left ventricle walls, the septum, and right ventricle wall. In the rest of the patients, the complete heart and great proximal vessels were studied following the protocol depicted in **Figure 1**.

Hematoxylin and eosin stain was performed in all sections. In addition, when inflammatory infiltrates were present, special histochemical stains such as PAS, Grocott or Gram were done to rule out microorganisms such as bacteria or fungi. Congo red stain was performed in suspected cases of amyloid deposit.

To analyze the immune infiltrates, we performed immunohistochemistry for CD20, CD3, CD8, CD4, and CD68 (Agilent, Santa Clara, CA, USA) in sections with inflammation. Transthyretin immunohistochemistry (Agilent, Santa Clara, CA, USA) was also done to confirm senile amyloidosis.

Sars-Cov-2 RNA Analysis

To investigate the presence of Sars-Cov-2 RNA, we took swabs samples from the left ventricle in 28 patients. In addition, we tested Sars-Cov-2 RNA in paraffin blocks from the left ventricle in all 30 patients, selecting those blocks with inflammatory infiltrates.

All swab samples were sent on the same day to the Microbiology Department for the detection of genomic SARS-CoV-2 RNA (gRNA). RNA extraction and reverse-transcription-polymerase-chain-reaction (RT-PCR) amplification were performed within 3 h after reception in the laboratory. RNA extraction was performed using MagmaxTM Core Nucleic Acid Purification Kit (Thermo Fisher, Waltham, United States) and gRNA SARS-CoV-2 was detected using TaqmanTM 2019 nCoV assay (Thermo Fisher, Waltham, United States).

TABLE 1 | Demographic, clinical, and laboratory findings.

Demographics	Total	30 (100%)
Male, n (%)		23 (76.67%)
Age	Median (IQR)	69.5 (12.25)
	Min, Max	52, 91
Weight	Median (IQR)	76.5 (14)
	Min, Max	53, 109
Days from initial symptoms	Median (IQR)	36.5 (17.5)
	Min, Max	9, 108
Hospitalization days	Median (IQR)	29.5 (18)
	Min, Max	3, 102
Patients admitted to ICU, n (%)		26 (86.67%)
ICU days	Median (IQR)	21 (15)
	Min, Max	12, 95
Mechanical ventilation, n (%)		26 (86.67%)
Comorbidities		
Hypertension, n (%)		13 (43.33%)
Dyslipidemia, n (%)		11 (36.67%)
Cardiovascular condition, n (%)		8 (26.67%)
• Ischemic cardiopathy		4 (50.00%, n = 8)
• Hypertrophic cardiomyopathy		2 (18.18%, n = 8)
• Valve replacement		1 (12.50%, n = 8)
• Heart failure		1 (12.50%, n = 8)
Obesity, n (%)		8 (26.67%)
Malignancy, n (%)		6 (20.00%)
Chronic obstructive pulmonary disease/SAHS, n (%)		5 (16.67%)
Neurologic condition, n (%)		3 (10.00%)
Diabetes mellitus, n (%)		2 (6.67%)
Hepatic condition, n (%)		2 (6.67%)
Immunosuppression, n (%)		1 (3.33%)
Clinical symptoms		
Fever at admission, n (%)		24 (80.00%)
Dyspnea at admission, n (%)		22 (73.33%)
Cough at admission, n (%)		17 (56.67%)
Asthenia at admission, n (%)		13 (43.33%)
Diarrhea at admission, n (%)		4 (13.33%)
Anosmia/Ageusia at admission, n (%)		4 (13.33%)
Nausea/Vomiting at admission, n (%)		3 (10.00%)
Temperature in Celsius at admission	Median (IQR)	36.5 (0.6)
	Min, Max	35.5, 38
Oxygen saturation at admission	Median (IQR)	88 (14.3)
	Min, Max	70, 99
Heart rate at admission	Median (IQR)	100 (25)
	Min, Max	70–141
Arrythmia, n (%)	Previously diagnosed	2 (6.67%)
	During hospitalization	6 (20%)
Department that requested the autopsy		
Anesthesiology department, n (%)		18 (60%)
Medical intensive care unit, n (%)		7 (23.33%)
Internal medicine department, n (%)		2 (6.67%)
Geriatrics department, n (%)		2 (6.67%)
Pneumology department, n (%)		1 (3.33%)

(Continued)

TABLE 1 | Continued

Demographics	Total	30 (100%)
Cause of death (according to autopsy report)		
Hypoxemia, n (%)		24 (80%)
Pancreatitis, n (%)		2 (6.67%)
Intestinal necrosis, n (%)		2 (6.67%)
Subarachnoid hemorrhage, n (%)		1 (3.33%)
Invasive aspergillosis, n (%)		1 (3.33%)
Laboratory test at admission (normal values)		
White cell count /μL (4–11 × 10^3)	Median (IQR)	11.1 (9.90)
	Min, Max	0.01, 21.9
% Neutrophils (45–75)	Median (IQR)	85.75 (20.28)
	Min, Max	18.2, 96.9
Lymphocytes/μL (1–4.5 × 10^3)	Median (IQR)	0.89 (0.47)
	Min, Max	0, 1.45
Creatinine mg/dL (0.3–1.3)	Median (IQR)	0.92 (0.37)
	Min, Max	0.48, 2.82
CRP mg/L (0–5)	Median (IQR)	188.20 (160.75)
	Min, Max	0, 0.8
Ferritin ng/mL (20–300)	Median (IQR)	1454.01 (1496.12)
	Min, Max	59.15, 5269.9
Lactate dehydrogenase U/L (140–240)	Median (IQR)	442 (274.25)
	Min, Max	333, 987
Platelets/μL (140–400 × 10^3)	Median (IQR)	195 (146.25)
	Min, Max	22.3, 599
Fibrinogen mg/dl (150–400)	Median (IQR)	740 (31.65)
	Min, Max	295.1,740
APTT% (76–128)	Median (IQR)	84.85 (21.25)
	Min, Max	16.1, 131.3
PT s (9.7–12, 6)	Median (IQR)	12.20 (1.18)
	Min, Max	10.2, 49.2
D-dimer ng/mL (0–500)	Median (IQR)	1,164 (2,098)
	Min, Max	152, 14,493.41
Troponin at admission ng/ml (0–0.1)	Median (IQR)	0.00 (0.00)
	Min, Max	0, 0.8
Highest troponin during hospitalization ng/ml (0–0.1)	Median (IQR)	0.00 (0.00)
	Min, Max	0, 10.4
Natriuretic peptide pg/mL (<100)	Median (IQR)	81.80 (125.30)
	Min, Max	0.4, 2,288
IL6 pg/mL (0)	Median (IQR)	62.15 (121.04)
	Min, Max	1.27, 589
IL10 pg/mL (0)	Median (IQR)	7.94 (6.79)
	Min, Max	0.5, 54.44
IL12 pg/mL (0)	Median (IQR)	1.19 (2.40)
	Min, Max	0, 6.66

Pathologic findings	Partial heart examination (n = 14)	Complete heart examination (n = 16)	Total (n = 30)
Heart			
Coronary artery atherosclerosis, n (%)	2 (14.29%)	6 (37.5%)	8 (26.67%)
Left ventricle hypertrophy, n (%)	3 (21.43%)	1 (6.25%)	4 (13.33%)
Chronic epicardial inflammation, n (%)	0	3 (18.75%)	3 (10%)
Myocarditis, n (%)	0	1 (6.25%)	1 (3.3%)

(Continued)

TABLE 1 | Continued

Pathologic findings	Partial heart examination (n = 14)	Complete heart examination (n = 16)	Total (n = 30)
Aspergillus myocarditis, n (%)	1 (7.14%)	0	1 (3.3%)
Senile amyloidosis, n (%)	1 (7.14%)	0	1 (3.3%)
Without significant alterations, n (%)	5 (35.71%)	8 (50%)	13 (43.33%)
Lung			
Patients with predominant pattern, n (%)	Normal lung		1 (3.3%)
	Exudative DAD		6 (20%)
	Proliferative/Organizing DAD		19 (63.3%)
	Fibrotic DAD		4 (13.3%)
Acute bronchopneumonia, n (%)			12 (40%)
Vascular thrombi, n (%)			20 (67%)
Endotheliitis, n (%)			13 (43%)

Diffuse alveolar damage (DAD).

For formalin-fixed-paraffin embedded (FFPE) samples, RNA was extracted from 10 sections of 5 μm obtained from paraffin blocks using RecoverAll Total Nucleic Acid Isolation Kit (Invitrogen), following the manufacturer's instructions. RNA quantity was measured fluorometrically with Qubit RNA high-sensitivity assay kit (Invitrogen, Waltham, MAS, USA).

Literature Review

We have performed a non-systematic PUBMED review of autopsy series published in English including 4 or more patients not previously reported in the reviews by Halushka and Vander Heide (11), Roshdy et al. (10) and Kawakami et al. (12).

RESULTS

Demographics

The main demographic, clinical and laboratory findings of the 30 patients are listed in **Table 1**. The median age of our cohort was 69.5 years (range 52–91). Twenty-three patients (76.6%) were male. The median time between admission and death was 29.5 days (range 3–102). The main comorbidities were arterial hypertension in 13 patients (43.3%), dyslipidemia in 11 patients (36.7%), cardiovascular conditions in 8 patients (26.7%), obesity in 8 patients (26.7%), and diabetes in 2 patients (6.67%). None of them were vaccinated.

Cardiovascular conditions included ischemic cardiopathy in 4 patients (13.3%), hypertrophic cardiomyopathy in 2 patients (6.7%) and mitral and aortic valve replacement and chronic heart failure in one patient each (3.3%). Two patients had a previous diagnosis of auricular flutter and auricular fibrillation, respectively. Six patients developed arrythmias during hospitalization, including supraventricular extrasystoles (6.7%), auricular flutter (3.3%), bundle branch block (3.3%), streaks of supraventricular tachycardia (3.3%), and self-limited periods of arrhythmias (3.3%).

Pathology

The main pathological findings of this series are presented in **Table 1**.

Cardiac Pathology

Macroscopic Findings

Mean post-fixation weight of the heart, in 16 (53.3%) patients in whom the complete organ was studied, was 474.2 g (range 310–720) (normal weight 365 ± 71 g). Regarding macroscopic findings, serous pericardial effusion was evidenced in 8 patients (26.6%), left ventricular hypertrophy (>1.5 cm in diameter) was present in 4 patients (13.3%), adipose myocardial replacement in 2 patients (6.6 %), and the presence of a macrothrombus in left atrium in one patient (3.3%). Two hearts showed post-surgical changes; one showed mitral and aortic valve replacement and another a coronary artery bypass grafting. In 14 patients (47%) no macroscopically relevant alterations were identified in the heart.

Histopathology

The most frequent histopathological finding was coronary artery atherosclerosis (8 patients, 26.7%). Three patients (10%) showed focal chronic epicardial inflammation, that consisted of a slight lymphocytic mononuclear inflammatory infiltrate associated with reactive mesothelium. This infiltrate was mainly composed of T lymphocytes (CD3+) with a predominant cytotoxic phenotype (CD8+) that exceed the CD3+/CD4+ population. One patient (3.3%) revealed myofibrils necrosis associated with abundant macrophage infiltration and occasional CD3+ lymphocytes in an area of ~1 cm^2 in the left ventricle, consistent with the diagnosis of myocarditis (**Figures 2A,B**).

In a 55-year-old male patient, without any comorbidity and 37 days of hospitalization, we observed the presence of ring-shaped fungal structures within the myocardium, associated to myofibrils necrosis and inflammation. This patient received corticosteroids and antibiotics, but no antifungal treatment. The fungal structures were positive for PAS and Grocott techniques (**Figures 2C–E**). They were also identified in lung and kidney parenchyma, where they were identified as *Aspergillus*

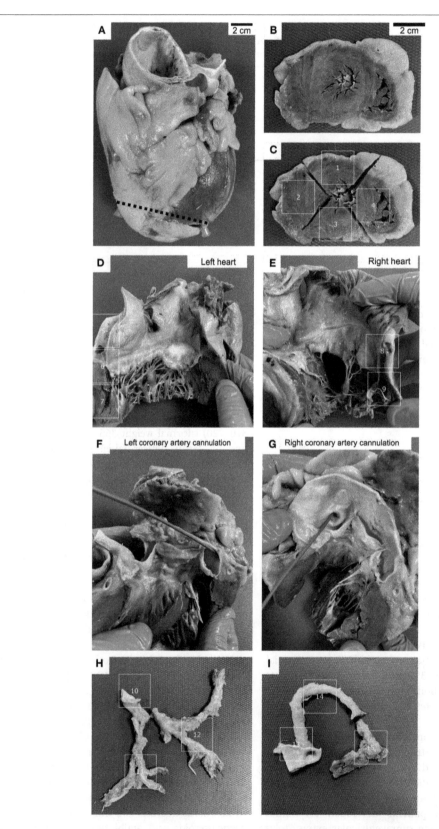

FIGURE 1 | Heart grossing protocol. **(A–C)** Apex sections. **(D)** Left atria and ventricle sections, including mitral valve. **(E)** Right atria and ventricle sections, including tricuspid valve. **(F–I)** Dissection of the coronary arteries. Cannulation of left **(F)** and right **(G)** coronary arteries. Left **(H)** and right **(I)** coronary arteries sections.

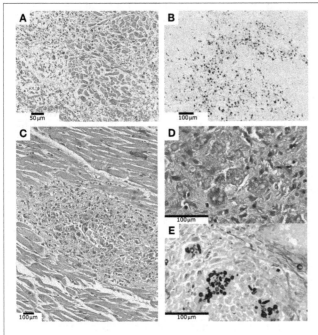

FIGURE 2 | (A) Myofibrils necrosis associated with abundant inflammatory infiltration. **(B)** Same case as **(A)**, showing CD68 positive macrophages infiltrating the myocardium. **(C)** Fungal structures within the myocardium, associated to myofibrils necrosis and inflammation. **(D)** Same case as **(C)**, PAS technique. **(E)** Same case as **(C)**, Grocott technique.

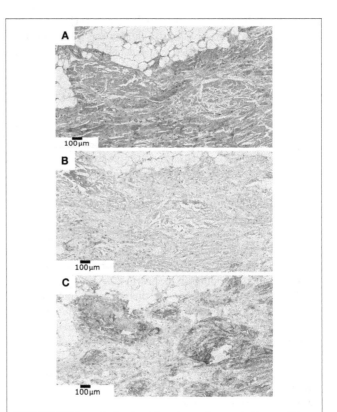

FIGURE 3 | (A) Deposit of eosinophilic and amorphous material compatible with amyloid within the myocardium. **(B)** Positive Congo Red histochemical stain. **(C)** Positive transthyretin immunohistochemistry.

fumigatus by postmortem microbiological culture and PCR. We did not observe intranuclear or intracytoplasmic inclusions in myocardial cells in none of our patients.

In a 90-year-old patient, suffering chronic cardiac failure, we evidenced a deposit of eosinophilic and amorphous material compatible with amyloid within the myocardium (**Figure 3**). This was confirmed with Congo red histochemical stain. This deposit was also identified in the cardiac and pulmonary vessels, pericardial adipose tissue, kidney and bone marrow. After performing immunohistochemical staining, the amyloid material was positive for transthyretin and negative for Kappa, Lambda and Amyloid AA, rendering the diagnosis of senile amyloidosis.

No histologically relevant alterations were found in 13 patients (43.3%), according to their age and clinical status.

Sars-Cov-2 RNA Analysis

All myocardial swabs except one [Cycle threshold (Ct) = 28] were negative for Sars-Cov2. The only positive case was also positive in the study of the FFPE tissue (Ct = 33), and Ct = 20 in nasopharyngeal sample obtained in the same autopsy. However, this patient did not show any relevant macroscopic or histopathological cardiac lesion. Interestingly, in spite of the absence of Sars-Cov-2 RNA in cardiac samples, all patients showed at least a positive result from the nasopharynx or lung in autopsy samples (manuscript in preparation).

Literature Review

Supplementary Table 1 compares the clinical and pathological findings reported by Halushka and Vander Heide (11) in their review of 293 cases and our review of 280 additional cases, including the 30 patients here reported.

DISCUSSION

In this study, we report the cardiovascular findings in the autopsies of 30 patients with severe COVID-19. Our results indicate a modest involvement of the heart in these patients, being the most frequent histopathological findings coronary artery atherosclerosis (8 patients, 26.7%), left ventricle hypertrophy (4 patients, 13.3%), chronic epicardial inflammation (3 patients, 10%), focal myocarditis (1 patient, 3.3%), and myocarditis due to Aspergillus (1 patient, 3.3%).

To the best of our knowledge, this is the autopsy series with the longest disease duration in which the heart has been histopathologically analyzed, and our results are in accordance with other studies with a shorter time of disease evolution.

Regarding duration of disease, in the review by Roshdy et al. (10), the median duration of prehospital symptoms ($n = 82$) and hospital stay ($n = 158$) were 5 (IQR, 2–7) and 6 days (IQR, 3–10), respectively. In total, the median duration from the onset of symptoms to death was 12 days (range, 0–52 days, $n = 98$).

In the review by Halushka and Vander Heide (11), the median number of days from diagnosis to fatality was 10 (range 1–51 days). In contrast, our series included patients with a median disease duration from symptoms onset to death of 36.5 and 29.5 days of hospitalization.

Pre-existing cardiovascular diseases are associated to a worse prognosis in patients with SARS-CoV-2 infection (6). In our series, eight patients had previous cardiac conditions, but the autopsy did not reveal other lesions than those related with the underlying disease. No differences were observed in the evolution of these cases in comparison to patients without previous cardiac conditions but presenting other comorbidity.

In addition to coronary atherosclerosis, the most frequent cardiac pathological finding was left ventricular hypertrophy in 4 patients. While two of them had a previous diagnosis of hypertrophic cardiomyopathy, the other two patients were not previously diagnosed of any cardiac disease. We did not find other pathological findings in the heart of these 4 patients.

We found focal and slight lymphocytic inflammatory infiltrates in the epicardium of 3 patients. However, the mere presence of these aggregates is not indicative of active pericarditis. They were mainly placed in the subepicardial adipose tissue and they were not associated with vessels. For this reason, we cannot argue in favor of a systemic endothelialitis involving epicardial lymphatic micro-vessels. Because in our series 26 of patients (86.7%) were treated with mechanical ventilation and we only found chronic pericarditis in 3 of them (10%), our data do not support an association between both facts. Although 8 patients showed different degrees of pericardial effusion, we related this finding to the common hemodynamic alterations in terminal ICU patients. Pericardial effusion has been reported in up to 94% of patients dying from COVID-19 without evidence of pericarditis (12). Although clinical studies have reported some cases of pericarditis secondary to SARS-CoV-2 (14–17), most autopsy studies have not found severe acute pericarditis.

One of the most controversial issue in COVID-19 cardiac pathology is to know if myocarditis is a common manifestation of the disease (7, 11, 18–20). In our series, only one patient (3.3%) showed focal myocarditis characterized by both myocyte necrosis and inflammation in absence of ischemic changes. The frequency of the diagnosis of myocarditis varies among series, probably due to different diagnostic criteria among authors. According to cardiac autopsy guidelines of the European Association of Cardiovascular Pathology (AECVP) (21), focal presence of myocardial inflammatory infiltrates in the myocardic tissue in the absence of myocyte necrosis is not enough evidence for diagnosis of myocarditis. It also maintains that small fibrosis foci have no pathological significance.

Following the mentioned restrictive criteria, it seems that myocarditis is not a frequent manifestation of severe COVID-19. Halushka and Vander Heide (11) reviewed 22 articles about cardiovascular findings in autopsies samples from COVID-19 patients and they concluded that although inflammatory infiltrates were present in the myocardium of 7% of the 277

patients, only 1.7% had complete histopathological evidence of myocarditis. In the partially overlapping review by Roshdy et al. (10) including 316 patients, clear myocarditis meeting the Dallas criteria was described in only five cases, whereas 35 additional patients had focal inflammatory infiltrates. In their review, Kawakami et al. (12) specifically discussed the role of myocarditis in COVID-19 patients. The authors reviewed literature findings (some series also reviewed by Halushka and Vander Heide (11) and by Roshdy et al. (10) and found that myocarditis was an uncommon pathologic diagnosis occurring in 4.5% of highly selected cases undergoing autopsy or endomyocardial biopsy. In their own series of 16 autopsied patients, the authors observed myocardial inflammatory infiltrates in 31% of the patients, which were not associated with myocardial necrosis. The authors concluded that given the extremely low frequency of myocarditis and the unclear therapeutic implications, the use of endomyocardial biopsy to diagnose myocarditis in the setting of COVID-19 is not recommended. A recent series (22), where 5% of the patients developed new onset myocarditis, confirms these results.

In our study, inflammatory infiltrates within the myocardium associated to myocyte necrosis were identified in only one patient (3.3%). In our review of 277 reported autopsied hearts (not included in previously reported reviews and including our 30 patients), 20 (7.2%) showed evidence of myocarditis; however, the frequency was highly variable, ranging from 0 out of 97 patients in the series reported by Bryce et al. (9), to 9 out of 9 patients in the series reported by del Nonno et al. (23).

The role of SARS-CoV-2 as the direct cause of viral myocarditis remains to be established, similarly as has been observed in other organs, such as the brain, in which no direct viral brain damage has been proven in large autopsy case series (24). In our study, myocardial PCR was performed in order to detect SARS-CoV-2 in the myocardium of all autopsies, but only one case became positive. However, all cases showed at least one positive result in samples taken during the autopsy from the nasopharynx or lungs. In the patient with the positive RT-PCR in cardiac samples, no relevant cardiac histological alterations were identified, whereas in the patient with focal myocarditis, no virus was detected. Several studies have investigated the presence of SARS-CoV-2 in the myocardium using different techniques. In the review by Roshdy et al. (10), 105 hearts were studied for the presence of SARS-CoV-2 and 50 (47%) were positive. In our review, which included 60 patients in whom the presence of SARS-CoV-2 in the myocardium was investigated, 17 (28%) had a positive result. Differences among series can be explain by the time of disease evolution. Thus, the median of hospital stay was 5 and 6 days in Roshdy's and our review, respectively, but 29.5 days in our series. In fact, the only positive patient in our series had an illness duration of 9 days from symptoms onset to death. According to these data, myocarditis as an immunologically mediated phenomena rather than direct viral damage cannot be excluded. In this sense, immune-mediated myocarditis has been reported as a rare complication of COVID-19 mRNA vaccines (25).

One patient in this series had lesions of focal myocarditis due to Aspergillus fumigatus. Pulmonary aspergillosis can develop in severe COVID-19 patients. A review of 15 COVID-19-associated pulmonary aspergillosis (CAPA) clinical case series in the ICU reported 158 CAPA cases among 1,702 COVID-19 patients (9.3%, range between 0 and 33%). Only in four cases, CAPA was proven, while the majority had a probable or putative diagnosis (26). In a systematic review of autopsy series, the authors found 8 CAPA cases among 677 decedents (1.2%) (27). Cardiac lesions occurring in the setting of disseminated aspergillosis, as occurred in our patient, seem to be very unusual. Hanley et al. (14) reported a patient with an acute fungal pericarditis without characterization of the fungus.

Regarding thrombotic phenomena, SARS-CoV-2 infection has been associated with an increased thrombotic risk (28–30) and the presence of both micro and macrothrombi. We identified a patient with an atrial thrombus, but no cases of microthrombosis were observed. However, macro and microthrombosis were frequent in the lungs, even though all but three patients were being treated with prophylactic anticoagulation treatment. Thrombosis in COVID-19 patients has been related to the expression of ACE2 in endothelial tissue, which binds with SARS-CoV-2 causing direct endothelial damage and favoring thrombotic phenomena. The presence of thrombi has also been associated with an exaggerated immune response that triggers endothelial dysfunction and dysregulation. The frequency of both micro and macrothrombi varies largely among series (**Supplementary Table 1**). Thus, Pellegrini et al. (30) reported that 35% of patients in their series had myocardial necrosis and the most common cause associated with necrosis was the presence of microthrombi in 64% of cases. Bois et al. (31) also reported the presence of small vessel thrombosis in 80% of their patients. In contrast, other studies, including the series reported by Bryce et al. (9), who studied 97 patients, did not find heart vascular thrombosis. Since cardiac vascular pathology seems to be more frequent during the initial stage of the diseases (32), differences among series could be related, at least in part, with the time of evolution of the infection.

Regarding other histological findings, one of our elderly patients showed the presence of amyloid deposit within the myocardium that was positive for transthyretin. Other studies have identified the presence of cardiac amyloidosis in patients with COVID-19 (14, 33). Although not all series performed immunohistochemical studies, most cases, as the patient here reported and those reported by Menter et al. (34), are probably examples of senile amyloidosis. The frequency of cardiac amyloidosis is highly variable among series, ranging from 0 to 26.7%. In the reviews by Halushka and Vander Heide (11)

and by Roshdy et al. (10) the frequency was 4 and 3.5%, respectively. In our own review, the frequency was 7.2%. Probably, differences among series were partially explained by the age of the patients included, since in our review the frequency of amyloidosis was high (14 to 26.7%) in the series in which the median age was 74 years or older but was low (0 to 7.3%) in those series with a median age lower than 70 years.

The limitations of our study include a relative low number of patients, who probably do not represent the complete spectrum of COVID-19 causes of dead. The use of two methods to study the hearts (partial and complete examination) is another limitation. However, we have not found differences between the pathological findings between both, except the presence of chronic epicardial inflammation, which has been more prevalent following the complete examination protocol. Finally, the lack of a control group of non-COVID-19 patients of similar age precludes any conclusion regarding if some lesions, such as collagen deposition, are increased in COVID-19 hearts.

Our series indicates that cardiac pathology is only modest in most patients and mainly consists of focal epicardial and myocardial inflammation, with little contribution of a direct effect of SARS-CoV-2. However, the frequency of these and other manifestations is highly variable among series suggesting that, in addition to biological variables, such as the time of evolution and methodological variables, like the extent of sampling, are responsible of these differences.

AUTHOR CONTRIBUTIONS

AF-G, HP-A, and JP contributed to conception and design of the study. AF-G, BP-M, and IR-C organized the database. IC-B, AN-C, DP, and JP wrote the first draft of the manuscript. RP, JZ, and JG wrote sections of the manuscript. All authors contributed to manuscript revision, read, and approved the submitted version.

ACKNOWLEDGMENTS

We want to thank all members of the MACROCOVID and Pathology Departments from Hospital Universitario Ramón y Cajal (Madrid, Spain) for their constant support to the COVID-19 Autopsy Project. To Hospital Universitario Ramón y Cajal-IRyCIS Biobank (Madrid, Spain), for the management of tissue samples.

REFERENCES

1. Zhou F, Yu T, Du R, Fan G, Liu Y, Liu Z, et al. Clinical course and risk factors for mortality of adult inpatients with COVID-19 in Wuhan, China: a retrospective cohort study. Lancet. (2020) 395:1054–62. doi: 10.1016/S0140-6736(20)30566-3

2. Falasca L, Nardacci R, Colombo D, Lalle E, Di Caro A, Nicastri E, et al. Postmortem findings in Italian patients with COVID-19: a descriptive full autopsy study of cases with and without comorbidities. J Infect Dis. (2020) 222:1807–15. doi: 10.1093/infdis/jiaa578

3. Yang X, Yu Y, Xu J, Shu H, Xia J, Liu H, et al. Clinical course and outcomes of critically ill patients with SARS-CoV-2 pneumonia in Wuhan, China: a

single-centered, retrospective, observational study. *Lancet Respir Med.* (2020) 8:475–81. doi: 10.1016/S2213-2600(20)30079-5

4. Huang C, Wang Y, Li X, Ren L, Zhao J, Hu Y, et al. Clinical features of patients infected with 2019 novel coronavirus in Wuhan, China. *Lancet.* (2020) 395:497–506. doi: 10.1016/S0140-6736(20)30183-5

5. Nguyen JL, Yang W, Ito K, Matte TD, Shaman J, Kinney PL. Seasonal influenza infections and cardiovascular disease mortality. *JAMA Cardiol.* (2016) 1:274–81. doi: 10.1001/jamacardio.2016.0433

6. Farshidfar F, Koleini N, Ardehali H. Cardiovascular complications of COVID-19. *JCI Insight.* (2021) 6:148980. doi: 10.1172/jci.insight.148980

7. Bansal M. Cardiovascular disease and COVID-19. *Diabetes Metab Syndr.* (2020) 14:247–50. doi: 10.1016/j.dsx.2020.03.013

8. Rozado J, Ayesta A, Morís C, Avanzas P. Fisiopatología de la enfermedad cardiovascular en pacientes con COVID-19. Isquemia, trombosis y disfunción cardiaca. *Rev Esp Cardiol.* (2020) 20:2–8. doi: 10.1016/S1131-3587(20)30028-5

9. Bryce C, Grimes Z, Pujadas E, Ahuja S, Beasley MB, Albrecht R, et al. Pathophysiology of SARS-CoV-2: the Mount Sinai COVID-19 autopsy experience. *Mod Pathol.* (2021) 34:1456–67. doi: 10.1038/s41379-021-00793-y

10. Roshdy A, Zaher S, Fayed H, Coghlan JG. COVID-19 and the heart: a systematic review of cardiac autopsies. *Front Cardiovasc Med.* (2021) 7:626975. doi: 10.3389/fcvm.2020.626975

11. Halushka MK, Vander Heide RS. Myocarditis is rare in COVID-19 autopsies: cardiovascular findings across 277 postmortem examinations. *Cardiovasc Pathol.* (2021) 50:107300. doi: 10.1016/j.carpath.2020.107300

12. Kawakami R, Sakamoto A, Kawai K, Gianatti A, Pellegrini D, Nasr A, et al. Pathological evidence for SARS-CoV-2 as a cause of myocarditis: JACC review topic of the week. *J Am Coll Cardiol.* (2021) 77:314–25. doi: 10.1016/j.jacc.2020.11.031

13. The COVID-19 Autopsy. The first COVID-19 autopsy in Spain performed during the early stages of the pandemic. *Rev Esp Patol.* (2020) 53:182–7. doi: 10.1016/j.patol.2020.05.004

14. Hanley B, Naresh KN, Roufosse C, Nicholson AG, Weir J, Cooke GS, et al. Histopathological findings and viral tropism in UK patients with severe fatal COVID-19: a post-mortem study. *Lancet Microbe.* (2020) 1:e245–53. doi: 10.1016/S2666-5247(20)30115-4

15. Sandino Pérez J, Aubert Girbal L, Caravaca-Fontán F, Polanco N, Sevillano Prieto Á, Andrés A. Pericarditis secundaria a infección por COVID-19 en un paciente trasplantado renal. *Nefrología.* (2021) 41:349–52. doi: 10.1016/j.nefro.2020.07.003

16. Eiros R, Barreiro-Perez M, Martin-Garcia A, Almeida J, Villacorta E, Perez-Pons A, et al. Pericarditis and myocarditis long after SARS-CoV-2 infection: a cross-sectional descriptive study in health-care workers. *medRxiv.* (2020) 2020.07.12.20151316. doi: 10.1101/2020.07.12.20151316

17. Blagojevic NR, Bosnjakovic D, Vukomanovic V, Arsenovic S, Lazic JS, Tadic M. Acute pericarditis and severe acute respiratory syndrome coronavirus 2: case report. *Int J Infect Dis.* (2020) 101:180–2. doi: 10.1016/j.ijid.2020.09.1440

18. Ho JS, Sia C-H, Chan MY, Lin W, Wong RC. Coronavirus-induced myocarditis: a meta-summary of cases. *Heart Lung J Crit Care.* (2020) 49:681–5. doi: 10.1016/j.hrtlng.2020.08.013

19. Hu H, Ma F, Wei X, Fang Y. Coronavirus fulminant myocarditis treated with glucocorticoid and human immunoglobulin. *Eur Heart J.* (2021) 42:206. doi: 10.1093/eurheartj/ehaa190

20. Sekhawat V, Green A, Mahadeva U. COVID-19 autopsies: conclusions from international studies. *Diagn Histopathol Oxf Engl.* (2021) 27:103–7. doi: 10.1016/j.mpdhp.2020.11.008

21. Basso C, Aguilera B, Banner J, Cohle S, d'Amati G, de Gouveia RH, et al. Guidelines for autopsy investigation of sudden cardiac death: 2017 update from the Association for European Cardiovascular Pathology. *Virchows Arch Int J Pathol.* (2017) 471:691–705. doi: 10.1007/s00428-017-2221-0

22. Buckley BJR, Harrison SL, Fazio-Eynullayeva E, Underhill P, Lane DA, Lip GYH. Prevalence and clinical outcomes of myocarditis and pericarditis in 718,365 COVID-19 patients. *Eur J Clin Invest.* (2021) 13:e13679. doi: 10.1111/eci.13679

23. del Nonno F, Frustaci A, Verardo R, Chimenti C, Nicastri E, Antinori A, et al. Virus-negative myopericarditis in human coronavirus infection. *Circ Heart Fail.* (2020) 13:e007636. doi: 10.1161/CIRCHEARTFAILURE.120.007636

24. Matschke J, Lütgehetmann M, Hagel C, Sperhake JP, Schröder AS, Edler C, et al. Neuropathology of patients with COVID-19 in Germany: a post-mortem case series. *Lancet Neurol.* (2020) 19:919–29. doi: 10.1016/S1474-4422(20)30308-2

25. Bozkurt B, Kamat I, Hotez PJ. Myocarditis with COVID-19 mRNA vaccines. *Circulation.* (2021) 144:471–84. doi: 10.1161/CIRCULATIONAHA.121.056135

26. Verweij PE, Brüggemann RJM, Azoulay E, Bassetti M, Blot S, Buil JB, et al. Taskforce report on the diagnosis and clinical management of COVID-19 associated pulmonary aspergillosis. *Intensive Care Med.* (2021) 47:819–34. doi: 10.1007/s00134-021-06449-4

27. Kula BE, Clancy CJ, Hong Nguyen M, Schwartz IS. Invasive mould disease in fatal COVID-19: a systematic review of autopsies. *Lancet Microbe.* (2021) 2:E405–14. doi: 10.1101/2021.01.13.21249761

28. Klok FA, Kruip MJHA, van der Meer NJM, Arbous MS, Gommers DAMPJ, Kant KM, et al. Incidence of thrombotic complications in critically ill ICU patients with COVID-19. *Thromb Res.* (2020) 191:145–7. doi: 10.1016/j.thromres.2020.04.013

29. Snell J. SARS-CoV-2 infection and its association with thrombosis and ischemic stroke: a review. *Am J Emerg Med.* (2021) 40:188–92. doi: 10.1016/j.ajem.2020.09.072

30. Pellegrini D, Kawakami R, Guagliumi G, Sakamoto A, Kawai K, Gianatti A, et al. Microthrombi as a major cause of cardiac injury in COVID-19: a pathologic study. *Circulation.* (2021) 143:1031–42. doi: 10.1161/CIRCULATIONAHA.120.051828

31. Bois MC, Boire NA, Layman AJ, Aubry M-C, Alexander MP, Roden AC, et al. COVID-19-associated nonocclusive fibrin microthrombi in the heart. *Circulation.* (2021) 143:230–43. doi: 10.1161/CIRCULATIONAHA.120.050754

32. Haslbauer JD, Tzankov A, Mertz KD, Schwab N, Nienhold R, Twerenbold R, et al. Characterization of cardiac pathology in 23 autopsies of lethal COVID-19. *J Pathol Clin Res.* (2021) 7:326–37. doi: 10.1002/cjp2.212

33. Bradley BT, Maioli H, Johnston R, Chaudhry I, Fink SL, Xu H, et al. Histopathology and ultrastructural findings of fatal COVID-19 infections in Washington State: a case series. *Lancet Lond Engl.* (2020) 396:320–32. doi: 10.1016/S0140-6736(20)31305-2

34. Menter T, Haslbauer JD, Nienhold R, Savic S, Hopfer H, Deigendesch N, et al. Postmortem examination of COVID-19 patients reveals diffuse alveolar damage with severe capillary congestion and variegated findings in lungs and other organs suggesting vascular dysfunction. *Histopathology.* (2020) 77:198–209. doi: 10.1111/his.14134

Smoking in Patients with Chronic Cardiovascular Disease During COVID-19 Lockdown

Frédéric Chagué[1,2*], Mathieu Boulin[3], Jean-Christophe Eicher[1], Florence Bichat[1], Maïlis Saint-Jalmes[1], Amélie Cransac[3], Agnès Soudry[4], Nicolas Danchin[5], Gabriel Laurent[1], Yves Cottin[1] and Marianne Zeller[2,6]

[1] Service de Cardiologie, Centre Hospitalier Universitaire, Dijon, France, [2] Réseau Français d'Excellence de Recherche sur le tabac, la nicotine et les produits connexes, Paris, France, [3] Département de Pharmacie, Centre Hospitalier Universitaire, Dijon, France, [4] Département de Recherche Clinique, Centre Hospitalier Universitaire, Dijon, France, [5] Service de Cardiologie, Hôpital Européen Georges Pompidou, Paris, France, [6] PEC2, EA 7460, Université Bourgogne Franche-Comté, Dijon, France

Correspondence:
Frédéric Chagué
frederic.chague@gmail.com

Objectives: This cross-sectional study aims to investigate health-related behaviors including tobacco consumption among patients with cardiovascular diseases (CVD), during the first COVID-19-related lockdown.

Methods: After 5 weeks of COVID-19 lockdown, 220 patients with chronic coronary syndromes (CCS) and 124 with congestive heart failure (CHF) answered a phone questionnaire.

Results: Among these 344 patients, 43 (12.5%) were current smokers, and none had quit during the lockdown. When compared with non-smokers, smokers were 15 years younger, more often diabetic, more likely to live in an urban than a rural lockdown location, and more often in the CCS cohort ($p = 0.011$). Smokers described greater psychological impairment, but their rates of decrease in physical activity and of increase in screen time were similar to non-smokers. More than one-third (13/43) increased their tobacco consumption, which was mainly related to stress or boredom, but not driven by media messages on a protective effect of nicotine.

Conclusions: During the first COVID-19 lockdown, we found a decrease in favorable lifestyle behaviors among patients with CVD. Strikingly, one-third of smokers with CCS or CHF increased their tobacco consumption. Given the major impact of persistent smoking in patients with CVD, this highlights the need for targeted prevention strategies, in particular during such periods.

Keywords: smoking, COVID-19, lockdown, chronic coronary syndrome, congestive heart failure (CHF)

INTRODUCTION

Cardiovascular disease (CVD), including congestive heart failure (CHF) and chronic coronary syndrome (CCS), and smoking are among the factors that can dramatically worsen prognosis in patients hospitalized for COVID-19 (1). Tobacco smoking is a major reversible risk factor for CVD, and cessation is a major target for prevention. Unfortunately, patients often do not quit smoking after an acute CVD event (2, 3). Although considered as less harmful than smoking, the cardiovascular impact of vaping is still debated (1).

Since the start of the current pandemic, the fear of severe acute respiratory syndrome coronavirus-2 (SARS-CoV2) infection and the strict lockdowns may have generated anxiety and stress, delayed access to care, and favored unhealthy behaviors, such as smoking increase, start or relapse. All of these factors can worsen a CVD patient's long-term prognosis (1, 3–5). On the other hand, the pandemic-related lockdowns were particular situations that may also have potentially favored smoking cessation through fear of illness, the lifting of social barriers, and enabling patients to focus on the health benefits of a healthier lifestyle (6, 7). At the same time, some media outlets spread the unconfirmed information that nicotine could confer a protective effect against COVID-19, thus potentially encouraging patients to smoke (6, 8). While the subject of smoking during the COVID-19 lockdowns has been addressed, investigations in CVD patients are paradoxically very scarce. We hypothesized that smoking rate and related health behaviors could have been modified in patients with CVD during the 2020 lockdown.

METHODS

CLEO-CD (COVID-19 Lockdown Effect On Chronic Diseases) is a cross-sectional study including more than 1200 outpatients with chronic disease from our university hospital in Dijon, France. Among them, 250 CCS subjects were randomly selected from the RICO (observatoire des Infarctus du myocarde de Côte d'Or) survey, which prospectively includes all patients hospitalized for acute myocardial infarction (AMI) in the coronary care unit of our hospital, as previously described (9). Only patients hospitalized for AMI in 2018 and 2019 were selected for inclusion. In addition, 150 CHF outpatients were randomly selected from the Heart Failure Clinic (10). This questionnaire was previously tested on 10 subjects (members of our research unit) as an internal procedure in order to assess compliance (understanding, coherence, reliability), leading to changes in the questions regarding medications and tobacco consumption. Then the questionnaire was tested by phone on eight CCS outpatients and eight CHF outpatients, all non-included in the randomly-selected patients and no changes were found to be necessary. A translated version of the questionnaire addressing tobacco consumption is available in **Supplementary File 1 - Questionnaire**. A smoker and a vaper were defined as a current tobacco smoker or electronic cigarette user (daily or occasional) at the time of the interview, and an ex-smoker and ex-vaper as having quit any time before the interview. Psychological distress was assessed by the Kessler 6 (K6) score (11). Residence during the lockdown was defined as rural when patients were living in areas with <2,000 inhabitants, and urban when in areas with 2,000 inhabitants or more, in agreement with French demographical definition (https://www.insee.fr/fr/metadonnees/definition/c1501) and as previously described (9). Informed consent was obtained from all of individual participants included in the study.

Because of the nature of the survey, patients were invited to participate and had to give their oral consent before the beginning of the interview.

TABLE 1 | Population characteristics according to cardiovascular disease.

		CCS	CHF	P-value
Population		**220 (64.0)**	**124 (36.0)**	
Female		66 (29.6)	49 (39.5)	0.08
Age (y)		67 (58–75)	70 (64–82)	0.01
Diagnosis ≥6 months		215 (97.7)	120 (96.8)	0.73
CCS				
History of revascularisation		184 (83.6)		
Medications	Antiplatelets agents	200 (91.7)		
	Betablockers	188 (87.0)		
	ACEI or ARB	181 (84.5)		
	Statins	188 (87.0)		
CHF				
Type of CHF	HFrEF		87 (70.2)	
	HFmrEF		12 (9.7)	
	HFpEF		25 (20.2)	
Etiology	DCM		50 (40.3)	
	Ischemic		23 (18.5)	
	Others		51 (41.2)	
NYHA Class	I		39 (31.5)	
	II		48 (38.7)	
	III		28 (22.6)	
	IV		9 (7.3)	

CCS, chronic coronary syndrome; ACEI, angiotensin converting enzyme inhibitor; ARB, angiotensin receptor blocker; CHF, congestive heart failure; IQR, interquartile range; HFrEF, heart failure with reduced ejection fraction; HFmrEF, heart failure with mildly-reduced ejection fraction; HFpEF, heart failure with preserved ejection fraction; DCM, dilated cardiomyopathy; NYHA, New York Heart Association.
n (%) or median (IQR).

The present study complied with the Declaration of Helsinki and was approved by the Ethics Committee of the Dijon University Hospital (NCT04390126).

Statistical Analysis

Continuous variables were expressed as medians and interquartile ranges (IQR) and dichotomous variables as n (%). Student t-tests or Mann-Whitney tests were used to compare continuous variables, and Pearson's Chi^2 or Fisher's tests to compare dichotomous data, as appropriate. Current smokers were compared with non-smokers.

RESULTS

Among the 400 selected patients, 56 declined the interview or were lost to follow-up and 344 questionnaires were finally analyzed, including 220 CCS and 124 CHF; patients with CCS were 3 years younger than those with CHF ($p = 0.01$). The rate of smoking was high ($n = 43$, 12.5%), and smokers were 15 years younger than non-smokers ($p < 0.001$). Population characteristics are summarized in **Tables 1**, **2**. Prevalence of smoking was higher in the CCS than in the CHF group ($p = 0.011$). Smokers were more frequently diabetic, single or divorced, and unemployed than non-smokers, and they were

TABLE 2 | Patient characteristics according to smoking status.

	Total N = 344	Non-smoker N = 301	Smoker N = 43	P-value*
Risk factors				
Age, years	70 (59–78)	71 (62–79)	56 (52–65)	<0.001
Men	229 (66.6)	197 (65.4)	32 (74.4)	0.243
Diabetes	81 (23.7) {342}	68 (22.7) {299}	13 (30.2)	0.028
BMI, kg/m²	27 (24-30) {319}	27 (24-30) {279}	28 (25-31) {40}	0.202
BMI ≥ 25 kg/m²	231 (72.4) {319}	200 (71.7) {279}	31 (77.5) {40}	0.442
BMI ≥ 30 kg/m²	86 (24.5) {319}	73 (26.2)	13 (32.5)	0.398
Type of CVD	{344}	{301}	{43}	0.011
CCS	220 (64.0)	185 (61.5)	35 (81.4)	
CHF	124 (36.0)	116 (38.5)	8 (18.6)	
History of depression	54 (16.0) {338}	46 (15.5) {297}	8 (19.5) {41}	0.510
COVID-19 screening (RT-PCR)	11 (3.2) {342}	7 (2.3) {299}	4 (9.3)	**0.037**
Socio-economic status				
Marital status	{336}	{296}	{40}	0.004
Single	35 (10.4)	26 (8.8)	9 (22.5)	
Divorced	28 (8.3)	22 (7.4)	6 (15.0)	
Married	225 (67.0)	203 (68.6)	22 (55)	
Widower	48 (14.3)	45 (15.2)	3 (7.5)	
Professional activity	{341}	{299}	{42}	<0.001
Current	69 (20.2)	55 (18.4)	14 (33.3)	
Retired	238 (69.8)	222 (74.2)	16 (38.1)	
Unemployed	13 (3.8)	7 (2.3)	6 (14.3)	
Other	21 (6.2)	15 (5.0)	6 (14.3)	
Education	{342}	{300}	{42}	0.112
≥High school diploma	106 (32.1)	97 (33.7)	9 (21.4)	0.133
Lockdown place				
Residence area				0.066
Urban	163 (45.3)	137 (45.5)	26 (60.5)	
Rural	181 (54.7)	164 (54.5)	17 (39.5)	
Type of accommodation				0.086
Flat without terrace/garden	47 (12.4)	37 (12.4)	10 (23.3)	
Flat with terrace/garden	66 (18.8)	56 (18.8)	10 (23.3)	
House with garden	228 (68.8)	205 (68.8)	23 (63.5)	
Alone in accommodation	83 (24.4) {340}	68 (22.9) {297}	15 (34.9)	0.087
Number of cohabitants	{340}	{297}	{43}	
Median (IQR)	1 (1–2)	1 (1–2)	1 (0–2)	0.864
Minimum/maximum	0/6	0/6	0/5	

IQR, interquartile range; BMI, Body Mass Index; CVD, cardiovascular disease; CCS, chronic coronary syndrome; CHF, congestive heart failure; RT-PCR, nasal Reverse Transcriptase-Polymerase Chain Reaction detection for SARS-CoV-2.
*p value comparison between smokers and non-smokers.
n (%) or median (IQR), {Number of answers}.

more often screened for COVID-19. In addition, smokers' place of residence during the lockdown tended to be more often urban and they were more likely to be living alone. Feeling and lifestyle behavior of patients according to their smoking status is summarized in **Table 3**. Among psychological factors, smokers were three times more likely to feel cramped and the psychological distress level (K6 ≥ 8) tended to be higher. Among the 43 current smokers, a high rate [n = 10 (30%)] increased their tobacco consumption during the lockdown period. Moreover,

during this period, one started to smoke and two had relapsed. Only six patients were vapers, and none was a dual user. Among the ex-smokers, none had quitted since the beginning of the lockdown.

Stress was the most commonly cited cause of smoking, followed by boredom. Lifestyle changes, including physical activity, alcohol consumption, and increase in screen time were similar for the two groups. In contrast, smokers had a much higher rate of weight variations, either for increase or for

TABLE 3 | Patients feeling and behavior according to smoking status during lockdown.

	Total N = 344	Non-smoker N = 301	Smoker N = 43	P-value*
Psychological factors				
Lockdown rules compliance	335 [97.7] {343}	294 [98.0] {300}	41 [95.3]	0.264
Feeling cramped	19 [5.6] {337}	13 [4.4] {294}	6 [14]	0.023
Sleep quality/duration change	83 [24.3] {342}	68 [22.7] {300}	15 [35.7] {42}	0.158
Currently feeling:	{342}	{300}	{42}	0.427
Bad	21 [6.1]	16 [5.3]	5 [11.9]	
Fairly good	75 (21.9)	67 (22.3)	8 (19.0)	
Well	175 (51.2)	154 (51.3)	21 (50.0)	
Very well	71 (20.8)	63 (21.0)	8 (19)	
Feeling less well (compared to before lockdown)	75 (21.9) {342}	65 (21.7) {300}	10 (32) {42}	0.743
Kessler score	2 (0–4) {337}	2 (0–4) {294}	2 (0–4)	0.633
K6 ≥ 8	37 (11.0)	29 (9.9)	8 (18.6)	0.079
Health behavior change				
Physical activity	{341}	{298}		0.466
Same	171 (50.1)	153 (51.3)	18 (41.9)	
Decreased	147 (43.1)	125 (41.9)	22 (51.2)	
Increased	23 (6.7)	20 (6.7)	3 (7.0)	
Alcohol intake	284	245	39	0.341
Same	242 (85.2)	210 (85.7)	32 (82.1)	
Decreased	27 (9.5)	24 (9.8)	3 (7.7)	
Increased	15 (6.7)	11 (4.5)	4 (10.3)	
Screen time increase	155 (45.3) {342}	131 (43.7) {300}	24 (57.1) {42}	0.10
Weight	{343}	{301}	{42}	0.01
Same	223 (65.0)	204 (67.8)	19 (45.2)	
Decreased	43 (12.5)	33 (11.0)	10 (23.8)	
Increased	77 (22.4)	64 (21.3)	13 (31)	
Tobacco consumption				
Same			21 (48.8)	
Decreased			9 (20.9)	
Increased (or started)			13 (30.2)	
Cause of increase/start smoking			{12}	
Stress	–	–	7 (58.3)	
Boredom	–	–	3 (25.0)	
Other			2 (16.7)	
Electronic cigarette	6 (1.8) {333}	6 (2.1) {290}	0 (0.0)	1
With nicotine	1 (20) {5}	1 (20) {5}	0	

IQR, interquartile range.
*p-value comparison between smokers and non-smokers.
n (%) or median (IQR), {Number of answers}.

decrease, when compared with non-smokers. At the time of the interview, 29 patients reported the use of telemedicine, 16 in the CCS group (7.3%) and 13 in CHF group (10.5%); the difference was non-significant (p = 0.317). As tobacco quitting may have been encouraged during these sessions, we assume that such advice may have been given in the same way in both groups.

Among the 344 patients, three patients developed conditions highly suggesting a COVID-19 (anosmia and/or ageusia associated with fever and cough) and underwent PCR testing (unknown timing according to the symptoms), of whom only one was positive. Eight other patients underwent PCR testing, of

whom all were negative. Among them, four had no symptoms, neither contact with any COVID-19 patient.

Among the patients with CCS, 13 declared an increase of symptoms of angina, of whom two were smokers. One of them did not report a change in smoking behavior, the other declared a reduction in tobacco consumption.

The subgroup analysis among smokers showed that the decrease in physical activity and the increase in screen time were more common in urban than in rural areas (61.5 vs. 35.3%, p = 0.092 and 69.2 vs. 37.5%, p = 0.044, respectively). Although not significant, tobacco consumption increased less frequently among rural vs. urban patients (17.6 and 38.5%, $p = 0.187$).

DISCUSSION

Smoking cessation is associated with major health benefits and some studies even suggest a favorable effect on biological age (12). Although smoking cessation is one of the key targets for secondary prevention in CVD, we found a high rate of current smokers (12.5%) among French CVD patients interviewed during the first lockdown (March-May 2020), consistent with smoking prevalence in CAD patients from contemporary European surveys (2, 13).

Relations between tobacco smoking and COVID-19 are controversial. Comorbidities including tobacco-induced diseases are associated with severe forms of COVID-19 and smokers are at higher risk of poor outcomes when infected (14, 15). Moreover, tobacco smoking up-regulates angiotensin-converting enzyme 2 (ACE2), receptor, binding site of Sars-Cov2 on membrane, promoting cell-invasion (16). The initial lower prevalence of smokers among patients with COVID-19 in early publications were not confirmed and could be related to selection bias, inadequate tobacco smoking definition and other confounding factors such as social habits (7, 16).

As expected, younger age and unemployment were more prevalent among smokers, which could interfere with other findings such as occupational characteristics.

Smokers also reported a higher rate of COVID-19 screening, which could be a result of respiratory symptoms mimicking COVID-19 symptoms, thus justifying the request for testing. In our population, diabetes was more prevalent among smokers than non-smokers, and the association of these factors exacerbates CV risk. This underlines the importance of implementing strategies for tobacco cessation in smokers with comorbidities (7, 17).

Although the lockdown period provided a potential opportunity for smoking cessation, none of our participants had quit, a third of patients had increased their tobacco consumption, one patient started smoking, and two patients relapsed (7). Psychological distress induced by social isolation and fear of the disease may have created conditions for smoking increase during the lockdown (1, 4). In addition, weight variations were more common among smokers than non-smokers. Whether it could relate to the influence of lockdown on mental health or to other factors such as variations in physical activity, or any confounding factors including socio-economic status is only speculative (6).

In a web-survey conducted in US dual users, 28.3 and 24.9% decreased their smoking and vaping consumption, but more subjects, 30.3 and 29.1%, respectively, had increased consumption since the beginning of the COVID-19 outbreak, and there was a positive correlation between the two products (18). In England, an analysis of monthly cross-sectional surveys demonstrated the stability of smoking prevalence and found an increase quitting since the lockdown, but they could not exclude an increase in uptake or relapse (19). In a german survey, almost 10% of smokers quit and 50% increased their tobacco

consumption. The increase was associated with COVID-19-related stress and living alone (20). To the best of our knowledge, our work is the first to specifically address smoking in CVD outpatients, who constitute a high-risk population.

In France during the first COVID-19-related lockdown, a nationwide web-based survey was conducted in 1,454 respondents aged 25–64 years, including some with CVD (21). When compared with our findings, they found a similar rate of smokers who decreased their tobacco consumption (22.6 vs. 20.9% respectively), but a higher rate of increased consumption (40.4 vs. 30.2%, respectively). A cross-sectional study in smokers from the general French population covering the same lockdown period yielded similar variations, including decreased tobacco consumption in 18.6% of and increased consumption in 26.7% (6). In this online survey, smoking increase was closely related with anxiety and overcrowded housing.

A large nationwide cross-sectional survey was conducted in USA smokers and e-cigarettes users during 2020 August; 21% of smokers had decreased their tobacco consumption in the 6 last months. Although they were aware of the amplified risk of COVID-19 related to tobacco smoking, 33% of smokers had increased their consumption; one the main reasons was stress; results were similar between only cigarettes users and dual-users. Moreover, 15% of the subjects who had quitted during the last 6 months relapsed. Conversely, 23% of vapers increased their e-cigarette consumption. However, 26% of smokers reported trying to quit, and this was associated with an increase risk perception of COVID-19 related to tobacco smoking (22). In California, an online survey did not find an increase in the number of smokers but tobacco consumption was higher among smokers likely related to a shift in time spent in smoke free places toward time spent at home (20). In an on-line survey in Pennsylvania, stress, more time to smoke and boredom were the main reasons to smoking increase (23).

A link between stress and unhealthy behaviors has been found in Australian subjects, of whom more than 50% suffered from chronic disease, mostly driven by a decrease in physical activity (almost 50%) (24).

In Netherlands, Van der Werf et al. observed some change in lifestyle behaviors among 1,004 adults who answered an online questionnaire after the first 3 months of COVID-19 pandemics, of whom 153 (15.2%) were smokers (25). A greater number of subjects declared healthier than unhealthier lifestyle behaviors (19.3 vs. 12.2%, respectively). Unhealthier lifestyle was associated to stress and was similar among smokers and non-smokers. Most of smokers did not change their tobacco consumption; however, 8.3% declared a decrease in tobacco consumption and only 3.7% an increase which is very different from findings from other surveys (18–24, 26). In Netherlands the lockdown rules were much less strict than in other countries including France, thus potentially influencing such findings.

Altogether, these data suggest that tobacco-smoking patterns evolution during lockdown were quite similar whatever CV health status. Although smoking has been associated with increased COVID-19 severity, studies have suggested that nicotine could be protective against SARS-COv2 infection (1, 8,

19). Our data suggest that smoking increase was not related to medical or media messages.

Smoking during lockdown was characterized by living alone, feeling cramped and urban environment. Both living alone and overcrowded housing have been associated with increased smoking, even if other socio-economic factors can interfere (6, 20). Living in a rural location during lockdown was associated with less tobacco use when compared with an urban area. Green spaces have been associated with better CV health, through reduced stress, and increased physical activity (27). However, socioeconomic factors may also influence these findings by selecting subjects with a psychological profile more prone to healthy lifestyle. An Irish study reported that increasing smoking was associated with increased alcohol intake and stress, but was not influenced by the type of residence (28). In a recent French survey, a rural residence was protective against increased screen time but not smoking (29).

Unfortunately, we did not evaluate the motivation of our patients to reduce their tobacco consumption or to quit. Among the patients with CCS, 13 declared an increase of symptoms of angina of whom two were smokers. One of them did not report a change in smoking behavior, the other declared a reduction of tobacco consumption; unfortunately, we did not assess if this reduction was related to worsening angina. These motivations have been studied among 659 smokers living in Hong-Kong. In this phone-call survey performed during the COVID-19 pandemic (while no stay-at-home orders were displayed), perceived susceptibility to COVID-19 and perceived severity of COVID-19 due to smoking were associated with likelihood of quit attempts; the authors suggested that the lower rate of perceived susceptibility than severity could be explained by medias misinformation (30, 31). Data addressing patients are however very scarce. Although not detailing their health conditions, Rigotti et al. conducted a survey enrolling post-hospitalized smokers wishing to quit; among these patients, 32% have increased their tobacco consumption since the beginning of the pandemic (mainly because of stress) and 31% have decreased or stopped; these latter behaviors were associated with increase in perceived risk of COVID-19 or developing severe infections (32). Interestingly, Gold et al. have evaluated motivations to reduce or quit smoking through an online survey. Among the 103 daily smokers, 88.3% declared one or more comorbidities - including cardiovascular diseases, known to be associated with severe COVID-19 patterns. The main reasons of reducing their tobacco consumption (68.9% of the subjects) were health concerns (33).

We acknowledge some limitations in our study. Our study was conducted at the beginning of the pandemic and thus the design was only exploratory and hypothesis-free, given the uniqueness and the previously unknown magnitude of the subsequent lockdown. However, given the consistency of our data, in agreement with current literature, we think our works provide contributory findings on this high health impact topic.

The present data were obtained by self-reporting, so we cannot exclude a reporting bias for the declaration of behaviors such as smoking and alcohol consumption, screentime, physical activity or weight. Some randomly-selected patients could not be included because they declined to participate in the study, could not be reached by phone or because of language barriers. However, the participation rate was high (86%) and the characteristics of the study population, consistent with contemporary data (13) suggest the representativeness of the study population.

Because of the small sample of smokers in our cohort, an extrapolation of our results to other population is only speculative. However, our findings are consistent with larger French general populations covering the same lockdown period, thus strongly suggesting the representativeness of our study population (6, 21).

As cardiovascular risk gradually increases with daily tobacco consumption even for one cigarette, we did not perform a quantitative evaluation of cigarette consumption (34).

Our study did not assess cardiovascular outcomes, which was out of our scope, thus we were not able to analyse the prognosis in subjects who increased their tobacco consumption.

In conclusion, CVD patients had a high rate of smoking during the 1st COVID-19 related lockdown; their behaviors were characterized by a triad of factors: psychological, socio-demographic and living environment. Moreover, the frequent increase in smoking (30%), mainly driven by stress, was particularly alarming in patients with diabetes, suggesting that more aggressive lifestyle management is needed. A longitudinal extension of this cross-sectional survey could provide relevant information regarding the duration of the behaviors described herein and their longer-term health consequences. If confirmed by large sample or experiment design, our findings may help to target tailored preventive strategies in this high-risk population.

AUTHOR CONTRIBUTIONS

FC, MB, J-CE, ND, YC, and MZ: conceptualization. MS-J, AS, and GL: methodology. YC: funding acquisition. FC, FB, and MS-J: data acquisition. J-CE, FB, AC, and AS: analysis. MB, AC, ND, and YC: project administration. FC and MZ: writing draft. FC, MB, ND, YC, and MZ: writing, review, and editing. All authors has approved the submitted version and agrees to be personally accountable for its own contribution.

ACKNOWLEDGMENTS

The authors thank Maud Maza for statistical assistance, Michèle Vourc'h for technical assistance, Lucie Vadot and the research assistant team for their involvement in the survey, Sylvie Mazencieux-Agobert and Jessica Massenot for editing assistance, and Suzanne Rankin for English reviewing.

REFERENCES

1. Münzel T, Hahad O, Kuntic M, Keaney JF, Deanfield JE, Daiber A. Effects of tobacco cigarettes, e-cigarettes, and waterpipe smoking on endothelial function and clinical outcomes. *Eur Heart J.* (2020) 41:4057–70. doi: 10.1093/eurheartj/ehaa460

2. Piepoli MF, Abreu A, Albus C, Ambrosetti M, Brotons C, Catapano AL, et al. Update on cardiovascular prevention in clinical practice: a position paper of the European Association of Preventive Cardiology of the European Society of Cardiology. *Eur J Prev Cardiol.* (2020) 27:181–205. doi: 10.1177/2047487319893035

3. Gaalema D, Pericot-Valverde I, Bunn JY, Villanti AC, Cepeda-Benito A, Doogan NJ, et al. Tobacco use in cardiac patients: perceptions, use, and changes after a recent myocardial infarction among US adults in the PATH study [2013-2015]. *Prev Med.* (2018) 117:76–82. doi: 10.1016/j.ypmed.2018.05.004

4. Duffy EY, Cainzos-Achirica M, Michos ED. Primary and secondary prevention of cardiovascular disease in the era of the coronavirus pandemic. *Circulation.* (2020) 141:1943–5. doi: 10.1161/CIRCULATIONAHA.120.047194

5. Lavie CJ, Ozemek C, Kachur S. Promoting physical activity in primary and secondary prevention. *Eur Heart J.* (2019) 40:3556–8. doi: 10.1093/eurheartj/ehz697

6. Guignard R, Andler R, Quatremère G, Pasquereau A, du Roscoät E, Arwidson P, et al. Changes in smoking and alcohol consumption during COVID-19-related lockdown: # cross-sectional study in France. *Eur J Public Health.* (2021) 31:ckab054. doi: 10.1093/eurpub/ckab054

7. Berlin I, Thomas D, Le Faou AL, Cornuz J. COVID-19 and smoking. *Nicotine Tob Res.* (2020) 22:1650–2. doi: 10.1093/ntr/ntaa059

8. Dautzenberg B, Levi A, Adler M, Gaillard R. Transdermal nicotine in non-smokers: a systematic review to design COVID-19 clinical trials. *Respir Med Res.* (2021) 80:100844. doi: 10.1016/j.resmer.2021.100844

9. Cransac-Miet A, Zeller M, Chagué F, Faure AS, Bichat F, Danchin N, et al. Impact of COVID-19 lockdown on lifestyle adherence in stay-at-home patients with chronic coronary syndromes: towards a time bomb. *Int J Cardiol.* (2021) 323:285–7. doi: 10.1016/j.ijcard.2020.08.094

10. Chagué F, Boulin M, Eicher JC, Bichat F, Saint Jalmes M, Cransac-Miet A, et al. Impact of lockdown on patients with congestive heart failure during the coronavirus disease 2019 pandemic. *ESC Heart Fail.* (2020) 7:4420–3. doi: 10.1002/ehf2.13016

11. Breslau J, Finucane ML, Locker AR, Baird MD, Roth EA, Collins RL. A longitudinal study of psychological distress in the United States before and during the COVID-19 pandemic. *Prev Med.* (2021) 143:106362. doi: 10.1016/j.ypmed.2020.106362

12. Lei MK, Beach SR, Dogan MV, Philibert RA. A pilot investigation of the impact of smoking cessation on biological age. *Am J Addict.* (2017) 26:129–35. doi: 10.1111/ajad.12502

13. De Bacquer D, Astin F, Kotseva K, Pogosova N, De Smedt D, De Backer G, et al. Poor adherence to lifestyle recommendations in patients with coronary heart disease: results from the EUROASPIRE surveys. *Eur J Prev Cardiol.* (2021) 55:zwab115. doi: 10.1093/eurjpc/zwab115

14. Guan WJ, Liang WH, Zhao Y, Liang HR, Chen ZS, Li YM, et al. Comorbidity and its impact on 1590 patients with COVID-19 in China: a nationwide analysis. *Eur Respir J.* (2020) 55:2000547. doi: 10.1183/13993003.00547-2020

15. Reddy RK, Charles WN, Sklavounos A, Dutt A, Seed PT, Khajuria A, et al. The effect of smoking on COVID-19 severity: a systematic review and meta-analysis. *J Med Virol.* (2021) 93:1045–56. doi: 10.1002/jmv.26389

16. Alla F, Berlin I, Nguyen-Thanh V, Guignard R, Pasquereau A, Quelet S, et al. Tobacco and COVID-19: a crisis within a crisis? *Can J Public Health.* (2020) 111:995–9. doi: 10.17269/s41997-020-00427-x

17. Campagna D, Alamo A, Di Pino A, Russo C, Calogero A.E, Purrello F, et al. Smoking and diabetes: dangerous liaisons and confusing relationships. *Diabetol Metab Syndr.* (2019) 11:85. doi: 10.1186/s13098-019-0482-2

18. Klemperer EM, West JC, Peasley-Miklus C, Villanti AC. Change in tobacco and electronic cigarette use and motivation to quit in response to COVID-19. *Nicotine Tob Res.* (2020) 22:1662–3. doi: 10.1093/ntr/ntaa072

19. Jackson SE, Garnett C, Shahab L, Oldham M, Brown J. Association of the COVID-19 lockdown with smoking, drinking and attempts to quit in England: an analysis of 2019-20 data. *Addiction.* (2021) 116:1233–44. doi: 10.1111/add.15295

20. Koopman A, Georgiadou E, Reinhard I, Müller A, Lemenager T, Kiefer F, et al. The effects of lockdown during the COVID-19 pandemic on alcohol and tobacco consumption behavior in Germany. *Eur Addict Res.* (2021) 27:242–56. doi: 10.1159/000515438

21. Rossinot H, Fantin R, Venne J. Behavioral changes during COVID-19 confinement in France: a web-based study. *Int J Env Res Public Health.* (2020) 17:8444. doi: 10.3390/ijerph17228444

22. Kalkhoran SM, Levy DE, Rigotti NA. Smoking and e-cigarette use among U.S. adults during the COVID-19 pandemic. *Am J Prev Med.* (2021) 6:2582. doi: 10.1101/2021.03.18.21253902

23. Yingst JM, Krebs NM, Bordner CR, Hobkirk AL, Allen SI, Foulds J. Tobacco use changes and perceived health risk among current tobacco users during the COVID-19 pandemic. *Int J Environ Res Public Health.* (2021) 18:1975. doi: 10.3390/ijerph18041795

24. Stanton R, To QG, Khalesi S, Williams SL, Alley SJ, Thwaite TL, et al. Depression, anxiety and stress during COVID-19: associations with changes in physical activity, sleep, tobacco and alcohol use in Australian adults. *Int J Environ Res Public Health.* (2020) 17:4065. doi: 10.3390/ijerph17114065

25. Van der Werf ET, Busch M, Jong MC, Rogier Hoenders HJ. Lifestyle changes during the first wave of the COVID-19 pandemic: a cross-sectional survey in the Netherlands. *BMC Public Health.* (2021) 21:1226. doi: 10.1186/s12889-021-11264-z

26. Gonzalez M, Epperson AE, Halpern-Felsher B, Halliday DM, Song AV. Smokers are more likely to smoke more after the COVID-19 California lockdown order. *Int J Environ Res Public Health.* (2021) 18:2582. doi: 10.3390/ijerph18052582

27. Yeager RA, Smith TR, Bhatnagar A. Green environments and cardiovascular health. *Trends Cardiovasc Med.* (2020) 30:241–6. doi: 10.1016/j.tcm.2019.06.005

28. Reynolds C, Purdy J, Rodriguez L, McAvoy H. Factors associated with changes in consumption among smokers and alcohol drinkers during the COVID-19 'lockdown' period. *Eur J Public Health.* (2021) 6:ckab050. doi: 10.1093/eurpub/ckab050

29. Rolland B, Haesebaert F, Zante E, Benyamina A, Haesebaert J, Franck N. Global changes and factors of increase in caloric/salty food intake, screen use, and substance use during the early COVID-19 containment phase in the general population in France: Survey study. *JMIR Public Health Surveill.* (2020) 6:e19630. doi: 10.2196/19630

30. Li Y, Luk TT, Wu Y, Cheung DYT, Li WHC, Tong HSC, et al. High perceived susceptibility to and severity of COVID-19 in smokers are associated with quitting-related behaviors. *Int J Environ Res Public Health.* (2021) 18:10894. doi: 10.3390/ijerph182010894

31. Luk TT, Zhao S, Weng X, Wong JY, Wu YS, Ho SY, et al. Exposure to health misinformation about COVID-19 and increased tobacco and alcohol use: a population-based survey in Hong Kong. *Tob Control.* (2021) 30:696–9. doi: 10.1136/tobaccocontrol-2020-055960

32. Rigotti NA, Chang Y, Regan S, Lee S, Kelley JHK, Davis E, et al. Cigarette smoking and risk perceptions during the COVID-19 pandemic reported by recently hospitalized participants in a smoking cessation trial. *J Gen Intern Med.* (2021) 36:3786–93. doi: 10.1007/s11606-021-06913-3

33. Gold AK, Hoyt DL, Milligan M, Hiserodt ML, Samora J, Leyro TM, et al. The role of fear of COVID-19 in motivation to quit smoking and reductions in cigarette smoking: a preliminary investigation of at-risk cigarette smokers. *Cogn Behav Ther.* (2021) 50:295–304. doi: 10.1080/16506073.2021.1877340

34. Teo KK, Ounpuu S, Hawken S, Pandey MR, Valentin V, Hunt D, et al. Tobacco use and risk of myocardial infarction in 52 countries in the INTERHEART study: a case-control study. *Lancet.* (2006) 368:647–58. doi: 10.1016/S0140-6736(06)69249-0

4

Impaired Myocardial Function is Prognostic for Severe Respiratory Failure in the Course of COVID-19 Infection

Alvaro Petersen-Uribe[1†], Alban Avdiu[1†], Peter Martus[2], Katja Witzel[1], Philippa Jaeger[1], Monika Zdanyte[1], David Heinzmann[1], Elli Tavlaki[1], Verena Warm[1], Tobias Geisler[1], Karin Müller[1], Meinrad Gawaz[1] and Dominik Rath[1*]

[1] Department of Cardiology and Angiology, University Hospital Tübingen, Eberhard Karls Universität Tübingen, Tübingen, Germany, [2] Institute for Clinical Epidemiology and Applied Biostatistics, University Hospital Tübingen, Eberhard Karls Universität Tübingen, Tübingen, Germany

*Correspondence:
Dominik Rath
dominik.rath@med.uni-tuebingen.de

† These authors have contributed equally to this work and share first authorship

COVID-19 may lead to severe acute respiratory distress syndrome (ARDS) resulting in increased morbidity and mortality. Heart failure and/or pre-existing cardiovascular disease may correlate with poor outcomes and thus require special attention from treating physicians. The present study sought to investigate a possible impact of impaired myocardial function as well as myocardial distress markers on mortality or ARDS with need for mechanical ventilation in 157 consecutive patients with confirmed SARS-CoV-2 infection. All patients were admitted and treated at the University Hospital of Tübingen, Germany, during the first wave of the pandemic. Electrocardiography, echocardiography, and routine blood sampling were performed at hospital admission. Impaired left-ventricular and right-ventricular function, tricuspid regurgitation > grade 1, and elevated RV-pressure as well as thrombotic and myocardial distress markers (D-dimers, NT-pro-BNP, and troponin-I) were associated with mechanical ventilation and/or all-cause mortality. Impaired cardiac function is more frequent amidst ARDS, leading to subsequent need for mechanical ventilation, and thus denotes a poor outcome in COVID-19. Since a causal treatment for SARS-CoV-2 infection is still lacking, guideline-compliant cardiovascular evaluation and treatment remains the best approach to improve outcomes in COVID-19 patients with cardiovascular comorbidities.

Keywords: COVID-19, mechanical ventilation, mortality, myocardial function, prognosis

INTRODUCTION

Severe acute respiratory syndrome coronavirus 2 (SARS-CoV-2) is an emerging cause of acute respiratory distress syndrome (ARDS) (1). Depending on the severity of ARDS, mechanical ventilation is the cornerstone for treatment of these critically ill patients (2). Patients in need for mechanical ventilation endure prolonged intra-hospital stay, neurological dysfunctions associated with concomitant anesthesia, and increased incidence of thrombosis and thromboembolism due to pro-thrombotic effects of SARS-CoV-2 and immobilization (3). Most importantly, severe respiratory failure is strongly associated with increased mortality in COVID-19 patients (4).

COVID-19 may cause severe acute myocardial injury or exacerbate an underlying chronic cardiovascular disease. Elevated levels of myocardial distress markers NT-pro-BNP and troponin are common findings in these patients (5). Moreover, pre-existing cardiovascular disease and compromised myocardial function have been associated with worse outcomes (6). Electrocardiography (ECG), echocardiography, and blood sampling for specific myocardial distress markers, e.g., troponin I and NT-pro-BNP, are essential for identifying COVID-19 patients with cardiovascular risk in order to improve management and consequently course of the disease. Since we currently lack a specific treatment for COVID-19, management of pre-existing or developing cardiac impairment is critical for improving outcomes in severely affected patients. Effects of impaired myocardial function on development of progressive respiratory failure and subsequent need for mechanical ventilation are unknown so far. Here, we report that markers of myocardial distress and impaired myocardial function are associated with progressive respiratory failure and increased mortality.

MATERIALS AND METHODS

Study Design and Participants

In March and April 2020, this prospective study enrolled 157 consecutive patients diagnosed with severe COVID-19-associated respiratory failure, including the first wave of COVID-19 infections at the University Hospital of Tübingen, Germany. The aim of the current study was to enroll all COVID-19-positive patients requiring hospital admission. Hence, a confirmed SARS-CoV-2 infection requiring hospital admission represented the only selection criterion. According to our official hospital database, 187 patients with confirmed SARS-CoV-2 infection were treated in our university hospital in March and April 2020. We managed to include 84.0% of these COVID-19 patients into the current study. Within 24 h after hospital admission, an extensive cardiovascular assessment including ECG, transthoracic echocardiography (TTE), and testing for myocardial distress biomarkers (e.g., pro-NT-BNP and troponin I) was performed. Written informed consent was obtained wherever possible ($n = 128$, 81.5%). We strongly assume that the remaining patients would not have refused to participate in the study since the cardiologic assessment was performed routinely and not purely study associated. In mechanically ventilated patients, the patient consent was obtained once invasive ventilation was discontinued or after discharge. In these patients, no study-associated measurements were performed but already existing clinical data was analyzed in accordance with the local ethics committee. The study was approved by the institutional ethics committee (238/2018BO2) and complies with the Declaration of Helsinki and good clinical practice guidelines (7–9).

Diagnosis of SARS-CoV-2 Infection and ARDS

SARS-CoV-2 was detected from nasopharyngeal secretions using real-time reverse transcriptase polymerase chain reaction. Severe

TABLE 1 | Baseline characteristics of the overall cohort ($n = 157$).

	All ($n = 157$)
Age, years (mean ± SD)	68 (±15)
Male, n (%)	99 (63.1)
Body mass index (mean ± SD)	29 (±5)
Cardiovascular risk factors, n (%)	
Arterial hypertension	110 (70.1)
Dyslipidemia	55 (36.2)
Diabetes mellitus	36 (23.1)
Current smokers	7 (4.6)
Obesity	39 (25.8)
Atrial fibrillation	36 (23.1)
Known CAD	34 (22.4)
Chronic kidney disease	20 (12.7)
Echocardiography	
Left ventricular function, % (mean ± SD)	57 (±7)
Left ventricular hypertrophy, n (%)	94 (69.1)
Visually estimated normal right ventricular function, n (%)	112 (82.4)
Visually estimated impaired right ventricular function, n (%)	17 (12.5)
Right ventricular dilatation, n (%)	51 (37.5)
TAPSE, mm (mean ± SD)	22 (±5)
RV pressure, mmHg (mean ± SD)	29 (±11)
Aortic stenosis >1, n (%)	5 (3.7)
Aortic regurgitation >1, n (%)	12 (8.8)
Mitral regurgitation >1, n (%)	31 (22.8)
Tricuspid regurgitation >1, n (%)	34 (25.0)
Pericardial effusion, n (%)	64 (47.1)
Electrocardiography	
Rate, bpm (mean ± SD)	84 (±22)
Sinus rhythm, n (%)	108 (81.2)
QRS, ms (mean ± SD)	93 (±20)
Regular R progression, n (%)	78 (58.6)
Right bundle branch block, n (%)	4 (3.0)
Left bundle branch block, n (%)	2 (1.5)
PQ segment, ms (mean ± SD)	170 (±87)
QTc, ms (mean ± SD)	437 (±65)
Negative T wave, n (%)	14 (10.5)
ST segment depression, n (%)	2 (1.5)
ST segment elevation, n (%)	0 (0.0)
Admission laboratory, median (25th percentile–75th percentile)	
Leucocytes, 1,000/µL	6.6 (4.8–9.5)
Lymphocytes, 1,000/µL	0.8 (0.6–1.1)
Creatinine, mg/dL	0.9 (0.7–1.3)
GFR, mL/m²	74 (48–92)
D-Dimer, µg/dL	1.3 (0.7–2.8)
C-reactive protein, mg/dL	8.2 (2.6–16.0)
Procalcitonin, ng/mL	0.14 (0.07–0.74)
Troponin I, ng/dL	17 (6–56)
NT pro-BNP, ng/L	458 (139–2827)
CK, U/L	149 (74–346)
AST, U/L	43 (27–70)
ALT, U/L	32 (21–47)
LDH, U/L	337 (232–446)
Medication at admission, n (%)	
Oral anticoagulation	21 (14.8)
ACEi/ARB	78 (54.9)
Aldosterone inhibitors	17 (12.0)
Diuretics	52 (36.6)
Calcium channel blockers	32 (22.5)
Beta blockers	58 (40.8)
Statins	51 (35.9)
ASA	36 (25.4)
P2Y12 blockers	3 (2.1)

TABLE 2 | Baseline characteristics stratified according to the combined endpoint.

	Combined endpoint		
	No (*n* = 85)	Yes (*n* = 72)	*p* value
Age, years (mean ± SD)	67 (±14)	68 (±16)	0.575
Male, *n* (%)	48 (56.5)	51 (70.8)	0.063
Body mass index (mean ± SD)	29 (±6)	29 (±5)	0.709
Cardiovascular risk factors, *n* (%)			
Arterial hypertension	53 (62.4)	57 (79.2)	**0.022**
Dyslipidemia	34 (40.0)	21 (29.2)	0.179
Diabetes mellitus	19 (22.4)	17 (23.6)	0.546
Current smokers	5 (5.9)	2 (2.8)	0.368
Obesity	21 (24.7)	18 (25.0)	0.870
Atrial fibrillation	15 (17.6)	21 (29.2)	0.095
Known CAD	14 (16.5)	20 (27.8)	0.311
Chronic kidney disease	9 (10.6)	11 (15.3)	0.380
Echocardiography			
Left ventricular function, % (mean ± SD)	59 (±4)	54 (±10)	**0.002**
Left ventricular hypertrophy, *n* (%)	57 (78.1)	37 (62.7)	0.514
Visually estimated normal right ventricular function, *n* (%)	71 (93.4)	41 (69.5)	**0.008**
Visually estimated impaired right ventricular function, *n* (%)	5 (6.6)	12 (20.3)	**0.008**
Right ventricular dilatation, *n* (%)	29 (39.7)	22 (37.3)	0.164
TAPSE, mm (mean ± SD)	22 (±5)	21 (±6)	0.441
RV pressure, mmHg (mean ± SD)	27 (±9)	32 (±12)	**0.045**
Aortic stenosis >1, *n* (%)	2 (2.7)	3 (5.1)	0.478
Aortic regurgitation >1, *n* (%)	7 (9.6)	5 (8.5)	0.989
Mitral regurgitation >1, *n* (%)	15 (20.5)	16 (27.1)	0.185
Tricuspid regurgitation >1, *n* (%)	13 (17.8)	21 (35.6)	**0.004**
Pericardial effusion, *n* (%)	32 (43.8)	30 (50.8)	0.180
Electrocardiography			
Rate, bpm (mean ± SD)	80 (±18)	88 (±26)	**0.029**
Sinus rhythm, *n* (%)	64 (84.2)	44 (77.2)	0.566
QRS, ms (mean ± SD)	93 (±23)	93 (±16)	0.931
Regular R progression, *n* (%)	47 (61.8)	31 (54.4)	0.385
Right bundle branch block, *n* (%)	2 (2.6)	2 (3.5)	0.877
Left bundle branch block, *n* (%)	2 (2.6)	0 (0.0)	0.243
PQ segment, ms (mean ± SD)	167 (±83)	173 (±93)	0.722
QTc, ms (mean ± SD)	427 (±81)	451 (±31)	**0.041**
Negative T wave, *n* (%)	4 (5.3)	10 (17.5)	**0.036**
ST segment depression, *n* (%)	1 (1.3)	1 (1.7)	0.821
ST segment elevation, *n* (%)	0 (0.0)	0 (0.0)	0.557
Admission laboratory, median (25th percentile–75th percentile)			
Leucocytes, 1,000/µL	5.7 (4.2–7.5)	7.7 (5-9–11.9)	**<0.001**
Lymphocytes, 1,000/µL	0.9 (0.7–1.2)	0.7 (0.5–1.0)	**0.005**
Creatinine, mg/dL	0.9 (0.7–1.2)	1.0 (0.8–1.6)	**0.027**
GFR, mL/m²	79.0 (58.9–97.2)	68.3 (37.5–91.6)	0.071
D-Dimer, µg/dL	0.8 (0.5–1.5)	2.4 (1.2–5.9)	**<0.001**
C-reactive protein, mg/dL	3.5 (1.3–8.7)	16.3 (9.2–27.4)	**<0.001**
Procalcitonin, ng/mL	0.08 (0.05–0.17)	0.58 (0.13–2.01)	**<0.001**

(Continued)

TABLE 2 | Continued

	Combined endpoint		
	No (*n* = 85)	Yes (*n* = 72)	*p* value
Troponin I, ng/dL	9 (4–18)	33 (18–124)	**<0.001**
NT pro-BNP, ng/L	310 (93–839)	1815 (401–6026)	**<0.001**
CK, U/L	121 (67–240)	273 (91–727)	**0.001**
AST, U/L	34 (20–47)	61 (39–102)	**<0.001**
ALT, U/L	28 (19–38)	41 (26–66)	**<0.001**
LDH, U/L	265 (207–361)	429 (337–494)	**<0.001**
Medication at admission, *n* (%)			
Oral anticoagulation	12 (14.1)	9 (12.5)	0.919
ACEi/ARB	44 (51.8)	34 (47.7)	0.640
Aldosterone inhibitors	9 (10.6)	8 (11.1)	0.642
Diuretics	29 (34.1)	23 (31.9)	0.701
Calcium channel blockers	19 (22.4)	13 (18.1)	0.843
Beta blockers	31 (36.5)	27 (37.6)	0.343
Statins	29 (34.1)	22 (370.6)	0.815
ASA	21 (24.7)	15 (20.8)	0.973
P2Y12 blockers	1 (1.2)	2 (2.8)	0.370

Bold values indicate statistical significance.

respiratory failure was defined according to the Berlin Definition of Acute Respiratory Distress Syndrome (10).

Twelve-Channel ECG and Laboratory Parameters

Twelve-channel ECG was registered according to standard procedure. Peripheral venous blood was drawn for routine laboratory parameters.

Transthoracic Echocardiography

TTE was performed by our Cardio-COVID-19 team. Left ventricular ejection fraction (LVEF) was assessed visually and measured using Simpson's method (11). Impaired LVEF was defined as an EF <50% (12). Impaired right ventricular function (RV-function) was evaluated combining visual assessment and measuring of tricuspid annular plane systolic excursion (TAPSE). TAPSE was assessed by placing an M-mode cursor through the lateral tricuspid valve annulus in the apical four-chamber view. Then, the total systolic excursion distance of the tricuspid annulus was measured. Impaired RV-function was defined by TAPSE < 20 mm (13). Mitral regurgitation was assessed based on regurgitant orifice area and width of vena contracta (14). Severity of aortic stenosis was defined based on valve area measured by continuity equation and planimetry (15). Jet/left ventricular outflow tract width ratio, pressure half time, as well as diastolic flow reversal in proximal descending aorta were used to quantify severity of aortic regurgitation (16). Central jet area and width of vena contracta were applied to determine tricuspid regurgitation (14). Right ventricular pressure was estimated using the simplified Bernoulli equitation [RVPsys = 4 × (Vmax)^2] (17) when tricuspid regurgitation was present (18). High probability of pulmonary hypertension was defined as RV-pressure > 35 mmHg (19). Finally, the presence of pericardial effusion (PE) was visually assessed (20).

Clinical Follow-Up

All patients were followed up for 30 days after study inclusion for the primary combined endpoint (poor outcome): mechanical ventilation and/or mortality. Secondary endpoint included all-cause mortality and mechanical ventilation.

Statistical Analysis

SPSS version 26.0 (SPSS Inc., Chicago, IL) and GraphPad Prism8.4.0 (GraphPad Software, San Diego, CA) were used for all statistical analyses. Student's t-test was applied for normally distributed data, whereas Mann–Whitney U-test served for analysis of non-normally distributed data. Accordingly, mean values are presented as mean ± standard deviation and median

values are presented as median and 25th/75th percentiles. Categorical endpoints were analyzed *via* cross-tabulations and Chi-square tests. Correlations of non-normally distributed were assessed using Spearman's rank correlation coefficient (rho). Kaplan–Meier curves with log rank tests were applied to compare survival between groups, whereas multiple Cox regression analyses were used to analyse independent associations between myocardial distress markers and the combined endpoint after adjustment for epidemiological factors. Regarding Cox regression analyses, LVEF, RV-pressure, and age were included as continuous variables, whereas RV-function (normal vs. impaired), significant TR, arterial hypertension, coronary artery disease, as well as diabetes mellitus (no vs. yes) were coded as binary variables. Discriminatory performance of myocardial distress markers and other clinical factors was evaluated using receiver operator curves (ROC) and expressed as c-statistics with 95% CI. Depending on the area under the curve (AUC), ROC 0.5 suggests no discrimination, ≥0.7–<0.8 acceptable,

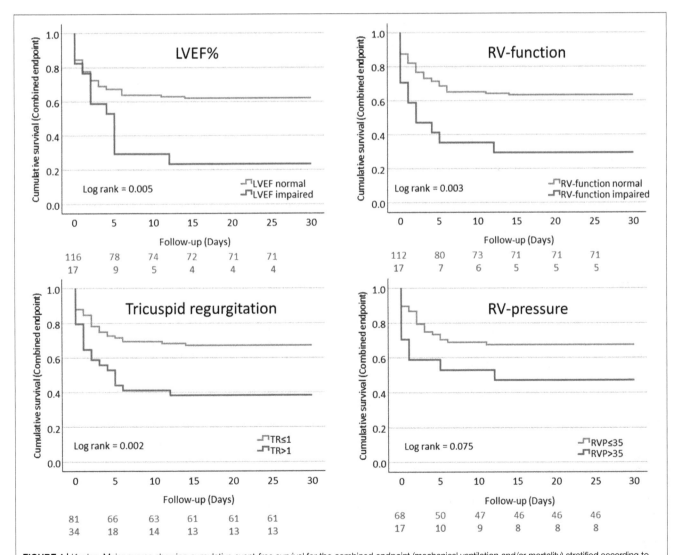

FIGURE 1 | Kaplan–Meier curves showing cumulative event-free survival for the combined endpoint (mechanical ventilation and/or mortality) stratified according to LVEF%, RV-function, tricuspid regurgitation, and RV-pressure.

TABLE 3 | Cox regression with markers of myocardial function as well as epidemiological factors as independent variables and the combined endpoint as dependent variables.

	p-value	HR	95% CI
Age	0.167	0.985	(0.964–1.006)
Arterial hypertension	0.321	1.456	(0.693–3.061)
Coronary artery disease	0.873	1.047	(0.594–1.845)
Diabetes mellitus	0.409	1.283	(0.709–2.321)
LVEF	**0.002**	0.955	(0.926–0.984)
Age	0.332	0.989	(0.969–1.011)
Arterial hypertension	0.292	1.496	(0.707–3.166)
Coronary artery disease	0.798	1.086	(0.579–2.037)
Diabetes mellitus	0.901	1.040	(0.563–1.922)
RV-Function	**0.010**	2.463	(1.239–4.895)
Age	0.062	0.977	(0.954–1.001)
Arterial hypertension	0.357	1.463	(0.651–3.288)
Coronary artery disease	0.335	1.312	(0.756–2.276)
Diabetes mellitus	0.505	1.233	(0.666–2.283)
Significant TR	**0.002**	2.851	(1.480–5.490)
Age	0.070	0.970	(0.939–1.002)
Arterial hypertension	0.074	3.085	(0.898–10.596)
Coronary artery disease	0.426	1.348	(0.647–2.808)
Diabetes mellitus	0.979	0.979	(0.451–2.170)
RV-pressure	**0.025**	1.040	(1.005–1.076)

Bold values indicate statistical significance.

≥0.8–<0.9 excellent, and ≥0.9 outstanding discrimination (21). ROC analyses using combinations of predictors were based on multiple logistic regression analysis with leaving one out correction. Ninety-five percent CIs of these areas are included in the figures. Course of biomarkers and respective associations with poor outcome were analyzed *via* linear mixed-models with random intercept.

RESULTS

A total of 157 patients were included, and their baseline characteristics are shown in **Table 1**. Stratification according to incidence of the combined endpoint is presented in **Table 2**. Routine blood sampling was performed in the whole collective; ECG and echocardiography were performed in 136 (86.6%) and 133 (84.7%) patients, respectively. Rate of mechanical ventilation within 30 days after hospital admission was 44.6% (*n* = 70). Twenty (12.7%) patients developed severe ARDS in the course of the hospital stay. Twenty-two (14.0%) patients were already mechanically ventilated at admission. Twenty-eight (17.8%) patients were intubated due to rapidly increasing respiratory failure and for airway protection. A total of 25 patients died (15.9%); two patients died without being mechanically ventilated (1.3%).

Patients with poor outcome displayed a significantly lower LVEF, worse RV-function, more severe tricuspid regurgitation, and increased RV pressure when compared to those with milder course of COVID-19 (**Table 2** and **Figure 1**).

Multivariable Cox-regression analysis revealed that impaired LVEF and RV-function as well as tricuspid regurgitation >1 and increased RV-pressure were independently associated with poor outcome (**Table 3**).

Amidst patients with poor outcome, leucocyte count, D-dimers, C-reactive protein, procalcitonin, troponin I, NT-pro-BNP, CK, AST, and LDH levels were significantly higher when compared to COVID-19 patients with a more favorable course of disease (**Table 2**).

Increased QTc interval and a higher heart rate, just as a larger proportion of T wave inversion, were more frequently observed in patients requiring ventilation in the course of disease (**Table 2**). The locations of inverted T waves were distributed as follows: Lead I: *n* = 6 (42.9%), lead II: *n* = 2 (14.3%), lead III: *n* = 5 (35.7%), lead aVR: *n* = 10 (71.4%), lead aVL: *n* = 6 (42.9%), lead aVF: *n* = 5 (35.7%), lead V$_1$: *n* = 6 (42.9%), lead V$_2$: *n* = 5 (35.7%), lead V$_3$: *n* = 7 (50.0%), lead V$_4$: *n* = 6 (42.9%), lead V$_5$: *n* = 4 (28.6%), and lead V$_6$: *n* = 3 (21.4%), respectively.

Mechanically ventilated patients showed significantly progressive D-dimer levels when compared to the remaining subjects (*p* = 0.043). Furthermore, non-survivors showed significantly progressive NT-pro-BNP and troponin-I levels when compared to survivors (*p* = 0.002 and *p* < 0.001, respectively) (**Table 4**, **Figure 2**).

LVEF correlated significantly with troponin I and NT-pro-BNP at admission (rho = −0.310, *p* < 0.001 and rho = −0.456, *p* < 0.001, respectively). TAPSE correlated significantly with troponin I (rho = −0.293, *p* = 0.003). Finally, RV-pressure was significantly associated with troponin I and NT-pro-BNP (rho = 0.310, *p* = 0.005 and rho = 0.511, *p* < 0.001, respectively) (**Figure 3**).

ROC analyses (combined endpoint) revealed an AUC of 0.588 for a multivariable model containing age, arterial hypertension, coronary artery disease, diabetes mellitus type II, and LVEF, 0.475 for a combination of age, arterial hypertension, coronary artery disease, diabetes mellitus type II, and RV-function, 0.520 for age, arterial hypertension, coronary artery disease, diabetes mellitus type II, and significant TR, and 0.590 for age, arterial hypertension, coronary artery disease, diabetes mellitus type II, and elevated RV-pressure. Cardiac biomarkers and D-dimer showed significantly better predictive performance (AUC 0.737 for D-dimers, 0.764 for NT-pro-BNP, and 0.735 for troponin-I). The best discrimination performance was achieved by a model including D-dimers, NT-pro-BNP, and troponin-I (AUC 0.788), whereas a combined model including age, arterial hypertension, coronary artery disease, diabetes mellitus type II, LVEF, RV-function, significant TR, and elevated RV-pressure performed poorly in predicting the combined endpoint (AUC 0.603) (**Figure 4**).

DISCUSSION

The major findings of this study are as follows: (1) Early impaired left and right ventricular systolic function, higher degree tricuspid regurgitation, and higher RV-pressure are more prevalent among COVID-19-positive patients with poor

TABLE 4 | D-dimer, troponin-I, and NT-pro-BNP levels at admission (1st sample), median of hospital stay (interval sample), and discharge/death (close-up sample) stratified according to mechanical ventilation, all-cause mortality, and the combined endpoint.

		1st sample	Interval sample	Close-up sample	p-value (int)	p-value (time)	p-value (group)
Mechanical ventilation							
D-dimers (±SD)	Ventilated	10.3 (±18.1) 0.5 (±0.6)	7.3 (±9.0) 0.6 (±0.4)	7.1 (±8.8) 0.6 (±0.4)	**0.043**	0.760	**<0.001**
	Non-ventilated	4.1 (±11.6) 0.1 (±0.5)	1.7 (±2.6) 0.0 (±0.4)	1.7 (±2.9) −0.2 (±0.4)			
Troponin-I (±SD)	Ventilated	167 (±412) 1.7 (±0.6)	351 (±1061) 1.8 (±0.7)	202 (±586) 1.6 (±0.7)	0.345	**0.023**	**<0.001**
	Non-ventilated	38 (±66) 1.1 (±0.6)	40 (±73) 1.2 (±0.6)	32 (±48) 1.1 (±0.6)			
NT pro-BNP (±SD)	Ventilated	6894 (±9695) 3.4 (±0.8)	9114 (±8691) 3.6 (±0.8)	11623 (±12862) 3.7 (±0.8)	0.985	**<0.001**	**<0.001**
	Non-ventilated	7818 (±39032) 2.6 (±0.9)	7352 (±36658) 2.8 (±0.8)	6550 (±29070) 2.9 (±0.7)			
All-cause mortality							
D-dimers (±SD)	Non-survivors	9.6 (±14.3) 0.5 (±0.7)	5.6 (±5.4) 0.6 (±0.3)	7.4 (±7.1) 0.7 (±0.4)	0.258	0.360	**<0.001**
	Survivors	6.7 (±15.7) 0.2 (±0.6)	4.5 (±7.7) 0.3 (±0.5)	3.8 (±6.9) 0.2 (±0.5)			
Troponin-I (±SD)	Non-survivors	244 (±535) 1.8 (±0.7)	141 (±253) 1.8 (±0.5)	352 (±816) 2.0 (±0.6)	**<0.001**	0.860	**0.002**
	Survivors	84 (±248) 1.4 (±0.6)	264 (±949) 1.5 (±0.8)	82 (±311) 1.2 (±0.7)			
NT pro-BNP (±SD)	Non-survivors	5064 (±6750) 3.3 (±0.7)	8931 (±5697) 3.8 (±0.4)	16023 (±15442) 4.1 (±0.3)	**0.002**	**<0.001**	**0.002**
	Survivors	7854 (±34447) 2.8 (±0.9)	7819 (±31940) 3.0 (±0.9)	7137 (±25882) 3.0 (±0.8)			
Combined endpoint (CE)							
D-dimers (±SD)	CE yes	10.3 (±18.0) 0.5 (±0.6)	7.2 (±9.0) 0.6 (±0.4)	7.1 (±8.7) 0.6 (±0.4)	0.070	0.779	**<0.001**
	CE no	4.0 (±11.7) 0.1 (±0.5)	1.7 (±2.6) 0.0 (±0.4)	1.7 (±3.0) −0.0 (±0.4)			
Troponin-I (±SD)	CE yes	167 (±412) 1.7 (±0.6)	352 (±1062) 1.8 (±0.7)	202 (±586) 1.6 (±0.7)	0.345	**0.023**	**<0.001**
	CE no	38 (±66) 1.2 (±0.6)	40 (±73) 1.2 (±0.6)	32 (±48) 1.1 (±0.6)			
NT pro-BNP (±SD)	CE yes	6894 (±9695) 3.4 (±0.8)	9114 (±8691) 3.6 (±0.8)	11623 (±12862) 3.7 (±0.8)	0.985	**<0.001**	**<0.001**
	CE no	7818 (±39032) 2.6 (±0.9)	7352 (±36658) 2.8 (±0.8)	6550 (±29070) 2.9 (±0.7)			

Both raw and logarithmic values are shown. P-values were calculated for logarithmic data. Int, interaction. Bold values indicate statistical significance.

outcome. (2) The course of the myocardial distress markers NT-pro-BNP and troponin-I may predict outcome in COVID-19 patients. (3) Troponin I and NT-pro-BNP correlate with LVEF, RV-function, and RV pressure at admission. (4) A combined model including D-dimers, troponin-I, and NT-pro-BNP may facilitate risk assessment in COVID-19 patients.

The current findings provide further evidence that an extensive cardiologic assessment of patients suffering from COVID-19 is required at the earliest time point before severe respiratory symptoms are evident.

Our current data and previous reports emphasize that myocardial injury represents a prevalent finding in COVID-19 patients with respiratory insufficiency. Severe respiratory failure

and ARDS are currently considered as the main cause of COVID-19-associated morbidity and mortality (22). Recently, Richardson and collaborators reported that 12.2% of hospitalized COVID-19 patients require mechanical ventilation (23). Among those, up to 20% developed cardiac injury, defined as an increase in troponin I (24). Interestingly, in our consecutive collective, ~45% of patients required mechanical ventilation, with 24% showing significant troponin I elevation. Susceptibility to SARS-CoV-2 infection seems to be higher in patients with pre-existing cardiovascular disease (25). Furthermore, these patients suffer from increased morbidity and mortality (26).

As the precise mechanisms leading to myocardial damage in COVID-19 await a thorough investigation, current research

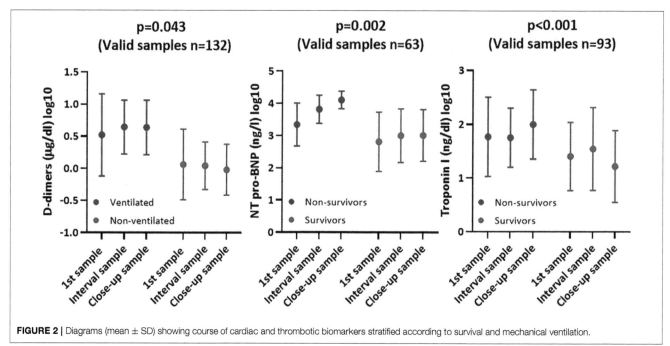

FIGURE 2 | Diagrams (mean ± SD) showing course of cardiac and thrombotic biomarkers stratified according to survival and mechanical ventilation.

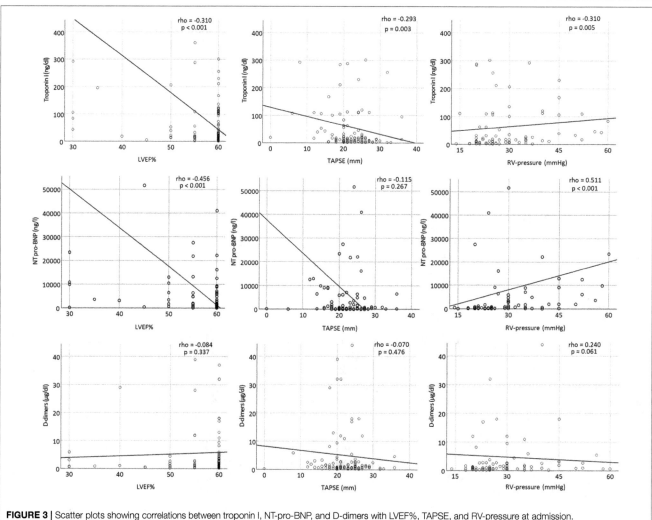

FIGURE 3 | Scatter plots showing correlations between troponin I, NT-pro-BNP, and D-dimers with LVEF%, TAPSE, and RV-pressure at admission.

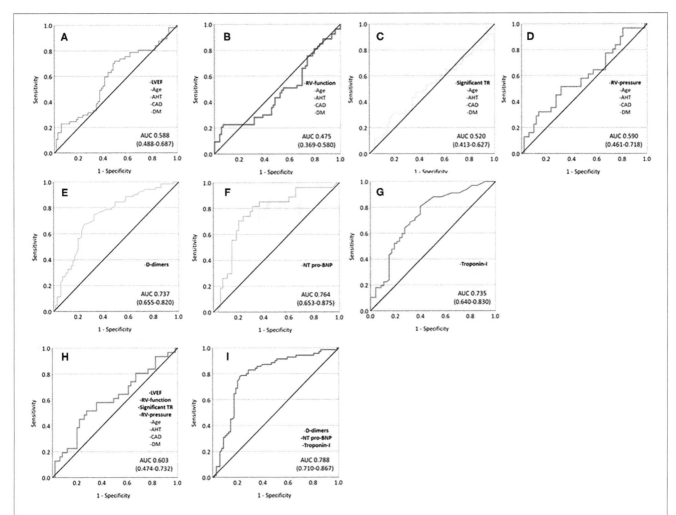

FIGURE 4 | ROC analyses showing predictive performance of different univariate and multivariable models. **(A)** Age, arterial hypertension, coronary artery disease, diabetes mellitus, and impaired LVEF; **(B)** age, arterial hypertension, coronary artery disease, diabetes mellitus, and impaired RV-function; **(C)** age, arterial hypertension, coronary artery disease, diabetes mellitus, and significant TR; **(D)** age, arterial hypertension, coronary artery disease, diabetes mellitus, and elevated RV-pressure; **(E)** D-dimers; **(F)** NT-pro-BNP; **(G)** troponin-I; **(H)** age, arterial hypertension, coronary artery disease, diabetes mellitus, impaired LVEF, impaired RV-function, significant TR, and elevated RV-pressure; and **(I)** D-dimers, NT-pro-BNP, and troponin-I.

suggests that myocardial damage may result from direct viral or inflammatory myocardial injury and may be augmented by systemic inflammatory response, which further promotes microcirculatory impairment or arrest (22). Diagnosing COVID-19-induced direct myocardial damage is a challenging process requiring myocardial biopsy as a gold standard, although SARS-CoV-2 genome could not be identified within the myocardium in biopsy and autopsy findings so far (27). Furthermore, cardiac MRI may help identify myocarditis as a cause of impaired LV-function. These two diagnostic modalities were, however, not applied in our department during the first COVID-19 wave due to patient overload and protection of clinic personnel.

According to available echocardiography findings prior to the diagnosis of SARS-CoV-2 infection, impaired systolic LV-function was commonly a chronic condition, whereas impaired RV-function tended to be a new finding in the current patient cohort. This suggests that elevated RV-pressure and

RV-dysfunction is an acute process caused by COVID-19-induced ARDS. Significantly elevated BNP and troponin-I levels found in mechanically ventilated COVID-19 patients in our cohort support the development of acute right ventricular failure, which is consistent with recent findings (28, 29). Furthermore, pulmonary distress could fittingly account for QRS prolongation and higher amount of abnormal T waves seen in our collective (30). Impaired LV-function at hospital admission may fasten this process by congestion caused by elevated LVEDP and thus raising pulmonary artery pressure. Our hypothesis of COVID-19-induced right ventricular failure as a result of major hemodynamic stress is presented in **Figure 5**.

CONCLUSION

As cardiovascular comorbidities and myocardial injury significantly contribute to mortality in COVID-19, early

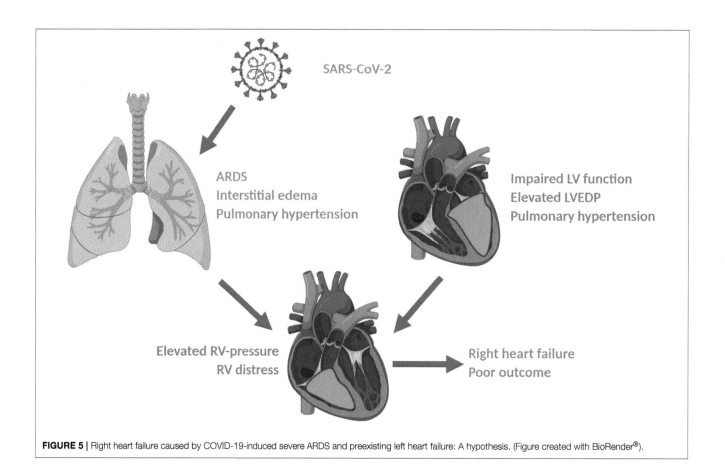

FIGURE 5 | Right heart failure caused by COVID-19-induced severe ARDS and preexisting left heart failure: A hypothesis. (Figure created with BioRender®).

cardiologic assessment and identification of high-risk patients is of critical importance to optimize the management and improve prognosis of COVID-19 patients.

Limitations

The current study offers several major limitations. First, we could not differentiate between COVID-19-induced and non-COVID-19-induced impairment of myocardial function, which may have affected outcome to an unknown degree. Second, the number of patients enrolled was low, rendering generation of risk prediction models difficult. Third, we were not able to include all COVID-19-positive patients admitted to our hospital during the first wave of the disease. Finally, biomarker levels were not available for all patients.

and good clinical practice guidelines. The patients/participants provided their written informed consent to participate in this study.

AUTHOR'S NOTE

We submitted this manuscript at the end of the first COVID-19 wave at the University Hospital Hospital of Tübingen. We have previously submitted an interimanalysis of COVID-19 positive patients to a different journal, which has been accepted

for publication onMay 28th (Rath et al., Clin Res Cardiol 2020 Jun 14:1-9). The endpoint differed however and the number of events was significantly lower. Fewer patients were enrolled. Finally, additional analyses were performed in the current manuscript.

AUTHOR CONTRIBUTIONS

AP-U and AA: data collection, data analysis, and drafting of the manuscript. PM: expert data analysis. KW, PJ, MZ, DH, ET, VW, TG, and KM: data collection and critical revision. MG: study concept and drafting of the manuscript. DR: data collection, and data analysis, drafting of the manuscript, and study concept. All authors contributed to the article and approved the submitted version.

ACKNOWLEDGMENTS

We thankfully acknowledge the work of Lydia Laptev for assisting us to isolate and process the blood samples. We acknowledge support by Open Access Publishing Fund of University of Tübingen.

REFERENCES

1. Lai CC, Shih TP, Ko WC, Tang HJ, Hsueh PR. Severe acute respiratory syndrome coronavirus 2 (SARS-CoV-2) and coronavirus disease-2019 (COVID-19): the epidemic and the challenges. *Int J Antimicrob Agents.* (2020) 55:105924. doi: 10.1016/j.ijantimicag.2020.105924

2. Aoyama H, Uchida K, Aoyama K, Pechlivanoglou P, Englesakis M, Yamada Y, et al. Assessment of therapeutic interventions and lung protective ventilation in patients with moderate to severe acute respiratory distress syndrome: a systematic review and network meta-analysis. *JAMA Netw Open.* (2019) 2:e198116. doi: 10.1001/jamanetworkopen.2019.8116

3. Fogarty H, Townsend L, Ni Cheallaigh C, Bergin C, Martin-Loeches I, Browne P, et al. More on COVID-19 coagulopathy in Caucasian patients. *Br J Haematol.* (2020) 189:1044–9. doi: 10.1111/bjh.16791

4. Grasselli G, Zangrillo A, Zanella A, Antonelli M, Cabrini L, Castelli A, et al. Baseline characteristics and outcomes of 1591 patients infected with SARS-CoV-2 admitted to ICUs of the Lombardy Region, Italy. *JAMA.* (2020) 323:1574–81. doi: 10.1001/jama.2020.5394

5. Zheng YY, Ma YT, Zhang JY, Xie X. COVID-19 and the cardiovascular system. *Nat Rev Cardiol.* (2020) 17:259–60. doi: 10.1038/s41569-020-0360-5

6. Bansal M. Cardiovascular disease and COVID-19. *Diabetes Metab Syndr.* (2020) 14:247–50. doi: 10.1016/j.dsx.2020.03.013

7. World Medical Association Declaration of Helsinki. Recommendations guiding physicians in biomedical research involving human subjects. *Cardiovasc Res.* (1997) 35:2–3.

8. ICH Harmonised Tripartite Guideline: Guideline for Good Clinical Practice. *J Postgrad Med.* (2001) 47:199–203.

9. Directive 2001/20/EC of the European Parliament and of the Council of 4 April 2001 on the approximation of the laws, regulations and administrative provisions of the member states relating to the implementation of good clinical practice in the conduct of clinical trials on medicinal products for human use. *Med Etika Bioet.* (2002) 9:12–9.

10. Force ADT, Ranieri VM, Rubenfeld GD, Thompson BT, Ferguson ND, Caldwell E, et al. Acute respiratory distress syndrome: the Berlin Definition. *JAMA.* (2012) 307:2526–33. doi: 10.1001/jama.2012.5669

11. Schiller NB, Shah PM, Crawford M, DeMaria A, Devereux R, Feigenbaum H, et al. Recommendations for quantitation of the left ventricle by two-dimensional echocardiography. American Society of Echocardiography Committee on Standards, Subcommittee on Quantitation of Two-Dimensional Echocardiograms. *J Am Soc Echocardiogr.* (1989) 2:358–67. doi: 10.1016/S0894-7317(89)80014-8

12. Ponikowski P, Voors AA, Anker SD, Bueno H, Cleland JGF, Coats AJS, et al. 2016 ESC Guidelines for the diagnosis and treatment of acute and chronic heart failure: the Task Force for the diagnosis and treatment of acute and chronic heart failure of the European Society of Cardiology (ESC)Developed with the special contribution of the Heart Failure Association (HFA) of the ESC. *Eur Heart J.* (2016) 37:2129–200. doi: 10.1093/eurheartj/ehw128

13. Lang RM, Badano LP, Mor-Avi V, Afilalo J, Armstrong A, Ernande L, et al. Recommendations for cardiac chamber quantification by echocardiography in adults: an update from the American Society of Echocardiography and the European Association of Cardiovascular Imaging. *J Am Soc Echocardiogr.* (2015) 28:1–39.e14. doi: 10.1016/j.echo.2014.10.003

14. Lancellotti P, Moura L, Pierard LA, Agricola E, Popescu BA, Tribouilloy C, et al. European Association of Echocardiography recommendations for the assessment of valvular regurgitation. Part 2: mitral and tricuspid regurgitation (native valve disease). *Eur J Echocardiogr.* (2010) 11:307–32. doi: 10.1093/ejechocard/jeq031

15. Nishimura RA, Otto CM, Bonow RO, Carabello BA, Erwin JP III, Guyton RA, et al. 2014 AHA/ACC guideline for the management of patients with valvular heart disease: executive summary: a report of the American College of Cardiology/American Heart Association Task Force on Practice Guidelines. *J Am Coll Cardiol.* (2014) 63:2438–88. doi: 10.1161/CIR.0000000000000029

16. Lancellotti P, Tribouilloy C, Hagendorff A, Moura L, Popescu BA, Agricola E, et al. European Association of Echocardiography recommendations for the assessment of valvular regurgitation. Part 1: aortic and pulmonary regurgitation (native valve disease). *Eur J Echocardiogr.* (2010) 11:223–44. doi: 10.1093/ejechocard/jeq030

17. Yock PG, Popp RL. Noninvasive estimation of right ventricular systolic pressure by Doppler ultrasound in patients with tricuspid regurgitation. *Circulation.* (1984) 70:657–62. doi: 10.1161/01.CIR.70.4.657

18. Parasuraman S, Walker S, Loudon BL, Gollop ND, Wilson AM, Lowery C, et al. Assessment of pulmonary artery pressure by echocardiography-a comprehensive review. *Int J Cardiol Heart Vasc.* (2016) 12:45–51. doi: 10.1016/j.ijcha.2016.05.011

19. Galie N, Humbert M, Vachiery JL, Gibbs S, Lang I, Torbicki A, et al. 2015 ESC/ERS Guidelines for the diagnosis and treatment of pulmonary hypertension: The Joint Task Force for the Diagnosis and Treatment of Pulmonary Hypertension of the European Society of Cardiology (ESC) and the European Respiratory Society (ERS): Endorsed by: Association for European Paediatric and Congenital Cardiology (AEPC), International Society for Heart and Lung Transplantation (ISHLT). *Eur Heart J.* (2016) 37:67–119. doi: 10.1093/eurheartj/ehv317

20. Pepi M, Muratori M. Echocardiography in the diagnosis and management of pericardial disease. *J Cardiovasc Med.* (2006) 7:533–44. doi: 10.2459/01.JCM.0000234772.73454.57

21. Hosmer David W. Lemeshow S. *Model-Building Strategies and Methods for Logistic Regression. Applied Logistic Regression.* (2000). p. 91–142. doi: 10.1002/0471722146

22. Yuki K, Fujiogi M, Koutsogiannaki S. COVID-19 pathophysiology: a review. *Clin Immunol.* (2020) 215:108427. doi: 10.1016/j.clim.2020.108427

23. Richardson S, Hirsch JS, Narasimhan M, Crawford JM, McGinn T, Davidson KW, et al. Presenting characteristics, comorbidities, and outcomes among 5700 patients hospitalized with COVID-19 in the New York City Area. *JAMA.* (2020) 323:2052–9. doi: 10.1001/jama.2020.6775

24. Shi S, Qin M, Shen B, Cai Y, Liu T, Yang F, et al. Association of cardiac injury with mortality in hospitalized patients with COVID-19 in Wuhan, China. *JAMA Cardiol.* (2020) 5:802–10. doi: 10.1001/jamacardio.2020.0950

25. Yang J, Zheng Y, Gou X, Pu K, Chen Z, Guo Q, et al. Prevalence of comorbidities and its effects in patients infected with SARS-CoV-2: a systematic review and meta-analysis. *Int J Infect Dis.* (2020) 94:91–5. doi: 10.1016/j.ijid.2020.03.017

26. Santoso A, Pranata R, Wibowo A, Al-Farabi MJ, Huang I, Antariksa B. Cardiac injury is associated with mortality and critically ill pneumonia in COVID-19: a meta-analysis. *Am J Emerg Med.* (2020). doi: 10.1016/j.ajem.2020.04.052. [Epub ahead of print].

27. Ho JS, Sia CH, Chan MY, Lin W, Wong RC. Coronavirus-induced myocarditis: a meta-summary of cases. *Heart Lung.* (2020) 49:681–5. doi: 10.1016/j.hrtlng.2020.08.013

28. Sandoval Y, Januzzi JL, Jr., Jaffe AS. Cardiac troponin for assessment of myocardial injury in COVID-19: JACC review topic of the week. *J Am Coll Cardiol.* (2020) 76:1244–58. doi: 10.1016/j.jacc.2020.06.068

29. Deng Q, Hu B, Zhang Y, Wang H, Zhou X, Hu W, et al. Suspected myocardial injury in patients with COVID-19: evidence from front-line clinical observation in Wuhan, China. *Int J Cardiol.* (2020) 311:116–21. doi: 10.1016/j.ijcard.2020.03.087

30. Stein PD, Matta F, Ekkah M, Saleh T, Janjua M, Patel YR, et al. Electrocardiogram in pneumonia. *Am J Cardiol.* (2012) 110:1836–40. doi: 10.1016/j.amjcard.2012.08.019

5

The Role of MSC Therapy in Attenuating the Damaging Effects of the Cytokine Storm Induced by COVID-19 on the Heart and Cardiovascular System

Georgina M. Ellison-Hughes[1]*, Liam Colley[2], Katie A. O'Brien[3], Kirsty A. Roberts[4], Thomas A. Agbaedeng[5] and Mark D. Ross[6]

[1] Faculty of Life Sciences & Medicine, Centre for Human and Applied Physiological Sciences, School of Basic and Medical Biosciences, King's College London Guy's Campus, London, United Kingdom, [2] School of Sport, Health, and Exercise Sciences, Bangor University, Bangor, United Kingdom, [3] Department of Physiology, Development, and Neuroscience, University of Cambridge, Cambridge, United Kingdom, [4] Research Institute for Sport and Exercise Sciences, Liverpool John Moores University, Liverpool, United Kingdom, [5] Faculty of Health & Medical Sciences, Centre for Heart Rhythm Disorders, School of Medicine, The University of Adelaide, Adelaide, SA, Australia, [6] School of Applied Sciences, Edinburgh Napier University, Edinburgh, United Kingdom

*Correspondence:
Georgina M. Ellison-Hughes
georgina.ellison@kcl.ac.uk

The global pandemic of severe acute respiratory syndrome coronavirus 2 (SARS-CoV-2) that causes coronavirus disease 2019 (COVID-19) has led to 47 m infected cases and 1. 2 m (2.6%) deaths. A hallmark of more severe cases of SARS-CoV-2 in patients with acute respiratory distress syndrome (ARDS) appears to be a virally-induced over-activation or unregulated response of the immune system, termed a "cytokine storm," featuring elevated levels of pro-inflammatory cytokines such as IL-2, IL-6, IL-7, IL-22, CXCL10, and TNFα. Whilst the lungs are the primary site of infection for SARS-CoV-2, in more severe cases its effects can be detected in multiple organ systems. Indeed, many COVID-19 positive patients develop cardiovascular complications, such as myocardial injury, myocarditis, cardiac arrhythmia, and thromboembolism, which are associated with higher mortality. Drug and cell therapies targeting immunosuppression have been suggested to help combat the cytokine storm. In particular, mesenchymal stromal cells (MSCs), owing to their powerful immunomodulatory ability, have shown promise in early clinical studies to avoid, prevent or attenuate the cytokine storm. In this review, we will discuss the mechanistic underpinnings of the cytokine storm on the cardiovascular system, and how MSCs potentially attenuate the damage caused by the cytokine storm induced by COVID-19. We will also address how MSC transplantation could alleviate the long-term complications seen in some COVID-19 patients, such as improving tissue repair and regeneration.

Keywords: COVID-19, mesenchymal stem cells, cytokine storm, cardiovascular, regeneration and repair

INTRODUCTION

As of 3rd November 2020, there are >47 million cases of the coronavirus 19 or severe acute respiratory syndrome coronavirus 2 (SARS-CoV-2) that causes coronavirus disease 2019 (COVID-19) in the World. There have been >1.2 million reported deaths due to COVID-19, and >34 million infected cases have recovered. As it stands, the infection and death rate due to COVID-19 is below that of previous pandemics. For example, the 1918 Spanish flu outbreak saw 500 million people infected throughout the World and 17–50 million people died over a 2 year span; with up to 25 million deaths in the first 25 weeks (1). Prior to the 1918 flu pandemic, influenza outbreaks had only killed juveniles and the elderly or already weakened patients. However, the Spanish flu was killing completely healthy young adults, while leaving children and those with weaker immune systems still alive (2). This high mortality was attributed to malnourishment, overcrowded medical camps and hospitals, and poor hygiene, all exacerbated by the recent war which promoted bacterial superinfection (3). The outcome of the COVID-19 pandemic is impossible to predict, however history shows that past pandemics have reshaped societies in profound ways. It is clear that COVID-19 has already changed the World and the way we live and work forever.

SARS-CoV-2 gains entry to human cells through the angiotensin-converting enzyme 2, or ACE2 receptor (4). ACE2-mediated viral entry is facilitated by serine proteases, most notably transmembrane protease serine 2 (TMPRSS2), which primes the SARS-CoV-2 spike glycoprotein (5). Initial infection of lung epithelia or alveoli allows SARS-CoV-2 to access the otherwise enclosed systemic circulation, subsequently predisposing multiple organs to potential infection. Multiple organs and tissues, such as the lungs, heart, kidneys, liver, and the vasculature, contain cells which co-express ACE2 and TMPRSS2, or other serine proteases (cathepsin B and cathepsin L1) (6–9).

Similar to other diseases caused by coronaviruses, the main transmission route of SARS-CoV-2 is *via* respiratory droplets and aerosolised particles (10) that are propelled into the air when a person speaks, coughs, shouts, sings, sneezes, or laughs. At the onset of the COVID-19 pandemic, the main symptoms were fever (98%), cough (76%), and myalgia or fatigue (44%) (11). Then, loss of sense of taste and smell, termed anosmia, became a symptom in March 2020 (12), with a large proportion of those reporting anosmia presenting with mild symptoms. Patients can then develop breathing difficulty within 1 week and the severely ill patients soon developed acute respiratory distress syndrome (ARDS), acute cardiac injury, secondary infections, or a combination, resulting in hospital admission and severe cases requiring mechanical ventilation in the ICU (11). Such patients typically exhibit an exaggerated immune response, or cytokine storm, that has become a hallmark of severe SARS-CoV-2 infection. Suppressing the pro-inflammatory nature of the disease is critical to improving patient morbidity and mortality rates and, therefore, developing and identifying viable therapeutic strategies is of urgent scientific importance. Transplantation of mesenchymal stem/stromal cells (MSCs) is one such potential therapy to combat COVID-19 induced inflammation and regeneration of damaged tissues.

The merits of MSCs are that they are multipotent stromal cells that can differentiate into a variety of cell types, including osteoblasts, chondrocytes, myocytes, and adipocytes that have their own characteristic structures and functions of specific tissues. They are typically found in the bone marrow, but have also been characterized in the adipose tissue, dental pulp, umbilical cord tissue, amniotic fluid, and heart (13). Mesenchymal stromal cells are easily accessible from various tissues, are free from ethical issues and have demonstrated no adverse outcomes in clinical trials. They have high proliferation rates, can be systemically administered, and possess key stem cell properties, such as multipotency (14, 15), in addition to being effective immunomodulators, collectively making MSCs a promising therapy in improving COVID-19 morbidity and mortality.

Old Age, Being Male and CVD Co-morbidity—Significant Risk Factors for Mortality

Severity and high mortality from COVID-19 has been linked to old age, being male, cardiovascular disease (CVD), hypertension, and cardiometabolic disease including diabetes and obesity. A retrospective, multicentre cohort study by Zhou et al. (16) examined 191 patients, of whom 137 were discharged and 54 died in hospital. Of these patients, 91 (48%) had a comorbidity, with hypertension being the most common [58 (30%) patients], followed by diabetes [36 (19%) patients] and coronary heart disease [15 (8%) patients]. Multivariable regression analysis showed increasing odds of in-hospital death associated with older age [odds ratio (OR) 1.10, 95% CI 1.03–1.17, per year increase; $p = 0.0043$], higher Sequential Organ Failure Assessment (SOFA) score (5.65, 2.61–12.23; $p < 0.0001$), and D-dimer >1 µg/mL (18.42, 2.64–128.55; $p = 0.0033$) on admission. In univariable analysis, odds of in-hospital death was higher in patients with diabetes or coronary heart disease. Age, lymphopenia, leucocytosis, and elevated ALT, lactate dehydrogenase, high-sensitivity cardiac troponin I, creatine kinase, D-dimer, serum ferritin, IL-6, prothrombin time, creatinine, and procalcitonin were also associated with death (16).

In a retrospective case series involving 1,591 critically ill COVID-19 patients admitted from February 20 to March 18, 2020 in Lombardy, Italy, who required treatment in the ICU, the median (IQR) age was 63 (56–70) years and 1,304 (82%) were male. Of the 1,043 patients with available data, 709 (68%) had at least one comorbidity and 509 (49%) had hypertension. The second most common comorbidities were CVD [223 patients, 21% (95% CI, 19–24)] and hypercholesterolemia [188 patients, 18% (95% CI, 16–20%)]. ICU mortality was higher in those who were older (≥64 years). The prevalence of hypertension was higher among patients who died in the ICU (63%, 195 of 309 patients) compared with those discharged from the ICU (40%, 84 of 212 patients) [difference, 23% (95% CI, 15–32); $P < 0.001$] (17).

Emerging evidence strongly implicates COVID-19 as a vascular disease, with many COVID-19 positive patients purportedly developing cardiovascular complications, such as myocardial injury (18), cardiac arrhythmia (19) and thromboembolism (20, 21). Interestingly, cardiovascular complications have also been reported in patients with no underlying pathology, for instance with acute viral myocarditis (22, 23). Cardiovascular (CV) system involvement is associated with higher mortality rates and is largely indicated by elevated inflammatory biomarkers, including D-dimer, cardiac troponin (cTn), ferritin, and interleukin (IL)-6 (24). For further insight, readers are directed to our review on Vascular Manifestations of COVID-19 (25) in this series.

Myocardial Damage: The Role of Cardiac Troponin and Other Relevant Markers

A number of studies show that a high proportion of COVID-19 patients exhibit elevated levels of cardiac damage biomarkers, such as cTn, with reports of up to 38% of patients testing positive for COVID-19 displaying high circulating levels of cTn (26). In comparison to COVID-19 patients with low cTn, those exhibiting high levels of cTn are hospitalized for longer requiring mechanical ventilation and admission to ICU, are at a significantly greater risk of developing ARDS and cardiac arrhythmias, and ultimately have a higher risk of mortality (27). In a study comparing clinical characteristics between survivors of COVID-19, and those who succumbed to the disease, researchers found that elevated levels of cTn were found in 77% of patients who subsequently died, compared to only 14% of patients who had survived (28). In addition, Guo et al. (29) showed that myocardial injury (elevated cTnT levels) was associated with worse outcome. Patients with underlying CVD are more likely to present with high cTn levels, with the poor prognosis for those with elevated levels further compounded if the patient had underlying CVD, compared to those without underlying CVD (69.4 vs. 37.5% mortality rate, respectively) (29). In the study by Zhou et al. (16) the highest OR for mortality in COVID-19 patients ($n = 191$) was for elevated cTn (>28 pg/mL, OR: 80.1) compared to other biomarkers, including circulating lymphocyte count (OR: 0.02) and D-dimer (OR: 20.04). It is also evident that throughout hospitalization, levels of cTn rise, and importantly, survivors showed no rise in this biomarker during the hospital stay, whereas patients with COVID-19 who died from complications, showed a steady upward rise in cTn until death (16). In another study, a significant predictor of mortality due to COVID-19 was the peak cTn during hospitalization, not the level measured upon admission (26), suggestive that risk stratification should include serial cTn measurements.

Besides cTn, other biomarkers, such as creatine kinase (CK), electrocardiographic (ECG) changes, and imaging might also reveal cardiac pathology in COVID-19 patients. Data acquired from multi-centers showed plasma lactate dehydrogenase and CK levels were correlated with COVID-19 severity and ICU admissions, reaching 26.1 and 70.5%, respectively (30). CK isoenzyme-MB (CK-MB), myohaemoglobin (MYO), and N-terminal pro-brain natriuretic peptide (NT-proBNP) are elevated above normal ranges in 3.7, 10.6, and 12.4% confirmed cases, respectively (31). When stratified by disease severity, patients with abnormal CK-MB, MYO, and NT-proBNP increased to 6.7, 26.7, and 33.3% respectively in the critical cases, underscoring underlying ischaemia and cardiac dysfunction. This is further supported by ECG findings characteristic of ischaemia, such as T-wave depression and inversion, ST depression, and presence of Q waves (18). In a case report, the presence of acute pulmonary embolism in COVID-19 was associated with right ventricular dilatation and dyskinesis on echocardiography, indicating that some patients develop ventricular hypertrophy (32).

Immune Response to COVID-19: Healthy vs. Hyperactive

The immune response to COVID-19 can be split into a healthy antiviral immune response or a defective/overactive immune response. The latter has been linked to damage to the lungs and other organs, resulting in onset of severe illness. Initially, SARS-CoV-2 infection and destruction of lung cells switches on antiviral defenses triggering a local immune response. This includes recruitment of macrophages and monocytes to respond to the infection, interferons and release of cytokines and chemokines and primed adaptive T and B cell immune responses. In most cases, this process is capable of resolving the infection. However, in some cases, a dysfunctional immune response occurs, resulting in severe lung and multi-system damage, and possible failure (33).

In the healthy immune response, the innate antiviral defenses fight against the virus and virus-specific T cells can later eliminate the infected cells before the virus spreads. Neutralizing antibodies in these individuals can block viral infection, and phagocytic cells such as alveolar macrophages recognize neutralized viruses and apoptotic cells and clear them by phagocytosis. Altogether, these processes lead to clearance of the virus with minimal lung and multi-system damage, resulting in recovery (33).

In a defective immune response, there is a hyperactivation of the immune cells, with excessive infiltration of monocytes, macrophages and T cells, in the lungs. This causes overproduction of pro-inflammatory cytokines, the so-called "cytokine storm" or "cytokine release syndrome," which eventually can lead to lung damage, pulmonary oedema and pneumonia. The resulting cytokine storm leads to widespread inflammation circulating to other organs, leading to multiple organ damage (33). Elucidating the mechanisms underlying the immune response to COVID-19 and the causes for the hyperactivation of the immune response are at the forefront of this exciting research area. Recently, Merad and Martin (34) reviewed how activated monocyte-derived macrophages leading to a dysregulated macrophage response contribute to the COVID-19 cytokine storm by releasing massive amounts of pro-inflammatory cytokines (34). Moreover, the biological and clinical consequences of the so-called cytokine storm are still largely unknown.

CYTOKINE STORM IN COVID-19

The term cytokine storm was first employed in describing the events modulating the onset of graft-vs.-host disease (35). Cytokine storms characterize a wide spectrum of infectious and non-infectious diseases. Since 2005, it was associated to the avian H5N1 influenza virus infection (36) and then infections with MERS and SARS, with an inflammatory milieu containing IL-1β, IL-6, and TNF-α being associated with worse disease outcomes (37). Now, severe COVID-19 disease caused by SARS-CoV-2 infection is also associated with a dysregulated and hyperactive systemic inflammatory response; a cytokine storm (38).

It was first reported that several pro-inflammatory cytokines and chemokines, including IL-2, IL-7, IL-10, CXCL10 (IP-10), CXCL8, CCL2 (MCP1), TNFα, and IFNγ were higher in the plasma of COVID-19 patients as compared to healthy controls. More importantly, among infected patients, IL-2, IL-7, IL-10, granulocyte colony- stimulating factor (G-CSF), macrophage inflammatory protein 1α (MIP1α), CXCL10, CCL2, and TNFα circulating concentrations (but not those of IFNγ) were found to be significantly higher in patients requiring admission to ICU and mechanical ventilation, compared to patients experiencing a less severe clinical course (11).

Chen et al. (39) characterized the immunological features of COVID-19 patients presenting with differing disease severity. Eleven patients with severe disease displayed significantly higher serum levels of IL-6, IL-10, and TNF-α and lower absolute numbers of T lymphocytes, CD4$^+$T cells, and CD8$^+$T cells as compared with 10 patients with moderate disease. Of note, severe cases were characterized by a lower expression of IFN-γ by CD4$^+$T cells as compared with moderate cases (39). Likewise, analysis from Liu et al. (40) demonstrated significant decreases in the counts of T cells, especially CD8$^+$ T cells, as well as increases in IL-6, IL-10, IL-2, and IFN-γ levels in the peripheral blood in the severe COVID-19 cases ($n = 13$) compared to those in the mild cases ($n = 27$), suggesting that disease severity is associated with significant lymphopenia and hyperinflammation.

Del Valle et al. (41) used a multiplex cytokine assay to measure serum IL-6, IL-8, TNF-α, and IL-1β in hospitalized COVID-19 patients ($n = 1,484$) upon admission to the Mount Sinai Health System in New York, USA. They showed that serum IL-6, IL-8, and TNFα levels at the time of hospitalization were strong and independent predictors of patient outcomes, with elevated inflammatory profile associated with reduced survival. Importantly, when adjusting for disease severity score, common laboratory inflammation markers, hypoxia and other vitals, demographics, and a range of comorbidities, IL-6 and TNF-α serum levels remained independent and significant predictors of disease severity and death (41).

In an elegant study, Lucas et al. (42) have identified that development of a maladaptive immune response profile was associated with severe COVID-19 outcome, and early immune signatures correlated with divergent disease trajectories. Through serially analyzing immune responses in peripheral blood in 113 COVID-19 patients with moderate (non-ICU) and severe (ICU) disease, they revealed an association between early, elevated cytokines and worse disease outcomes. Indeed, they observed

a "core COVID-19 signature" shared by both moderate and severe groups of patients defined by the following inflammatory cytokines that positively correlated with each other; these included: IL-1α, IL-1β, IL-17A, IL-12 p70, and IFN-α. In severe patients, they observed an additional inflammatory cluster defined by: thyroid peroxidase (TPO), IL-33, IL-16, IL-21, IL-23, IFN-λ, eotaxin, and eotaxin 3. Interestingly, most of the cytokines linked to cytokine release syndrome, such as IL-1α, IL-1β, IL-6, IL-10, IL-18, and TNF-α, showed increased positive associations in severe patients. After day 10, in patients with moderate disease, these markers steadily declined. In contrast, severe patients maintained elevated levels of these core signature makers. Notably, additional correlations between cytokines emerged in patients with severe disease following day 10. Therefore, there were sharp differences in the expression of inflammatory markers along disease progression between patients who exhibit moderate vs. severe COVID-19 symptoms. Altogether, data showed a broad elevation of type-1, type-2, and type-3 signatures in severe cases of COVID-19, with distinct temporal dynamics and quantities between severe and moderate patients. Unsupervised clustering analysis of plasma and peripheral blood leukocyte data identified four immune signatures, representing (A) tissue repair growth factors, (B) type-2/3 cytokines, (C) mixed type-1/2/3 cytokines, and (D) chemokines involved in leukocyte trafficking that correlated with three distinct disease trajectories of patients. The immune profile of patients who recovered with moderate disease was enriched in tissue reparative growth factor signature (A), while the profile for those with worsened disease trajectory had elevated levels of all four signatures. Overall, results suggested that a multi-faceted inflammatory response is associated with late COVID-19 severity, which raises the possibility that early immunological interventions that target inflammatory markers predictive of worse disease outcome are preferred to blocking late-appearing cytokines.

Supporting the work of Lucas et al. (42) a recently published article has identified a core peripheral blood immune signature across 63 hospital-treated patients in London, UK with COVID-19. Specifically, among several changes in immune cells expressed at unusual levels in the blood of patients, the work identified a triad of IP-10 (CXCL10), IL-10, and IL-6 to correlate strongly with disease severity. Indeed, patients with COVID-19 who displayed measurably higher levels of IP-10 (CXCL10), IL-10, and IL-6 when first admitted to hospital went on to become more severely ill. The triad of cytokines was found to be a rigorous predictor of disease severity than commonly-used clinical indicators, including CRP, D-dimer, and ferritin (43).

As the COVID-19 cytokine storm is a multi-faceted inflammatory response, therapies that target this as a whole and those that enhance tissue repair (i.e. mesenchymal stem/stromal cells; MSCs) should be considered. Indeed, Lucas et al. (42) found IL-6 to be highly enriched in patients with severe disease. In fact, all ICU patients in their study, including the ones who succumbed to the disease, received Tocilizumab, an IL-6R blocking antibody. Positive outcomes have been reported with Tocilizumab treatment, including a reduction in an inflammatory-monocyte population associated with worse outcomes (44). However, as patients still succumbed to COVID-19, this highlights the need for combination therapy to block other cytokines highly represented in severe COVID-19 cases, including inflammasome-dependent cytokines and type-2 cytokines (42).

THE EFFECTS OF THE COVID-19 CYTOKINE STORM

On the Lungs Leading to Acute Respiratory Distress Syndrome (ARDS)

Acute respiratory distress syndrome (ARDS) is a form of hypoxaemic respiratory failure that is characterized by severe impairment of gas exchange and lung mechanics, with a high case fatality rate. Acute respiratory distress syndrome can come about through the severe widespread inflammatory injury present throughout the lungs, leading to a loss of vascular barrier integrity and likely promoting pulmonary oedema, thereby causing inflammation of endothelial cells (endothelialitis). Acute respiratory distress syndrome is a prominent feature in patients with severe COVID-19 infection (45, 46) and is the leading cause of mortality (47).

The precise pathophysiological mechanisms underlying ARDS in COVID-19 patients are not fully understood. However, alveolar macrophages are central to mediating the inflammation associated with ARDS (48), with the initial inflammatory stage involving alveolar macrophages interacting with lymphocytes (49) and epithelial cells (50), thereby augmenting the inflammatory response and accentuating tissue damage (51). Following initial stimulation, neutrophils and circulating macrophages are recruited to the lungs (activated by the pro-inflammatory cytokines), thereby triggering further inflammatory responses (52) equating to a positive feedback loop. These cells may disrupt the air–blood barrier by causing collateral tissue damage, particularly to airway epithelial cells and vascular endothelial cells, which express the ACE2 entry receptor for SARS-CoV-2; the damage of vascular endothelial cells may account for thrombotic microangiopathies (53). Furthermore, severe infection of the lung alveoli allows the SARS-CoV-2 virus and pro-inflammatory cytokine overload to enter the systemic circulation where it can infiltrate multiple organs, particularly since cells in many of them co-express ACE2 and TMPRSS2 (7, 8, 54).

In addition to the marked lung damage observed in COVID-19 infection, clinical cohort studies have revealed involvement of the kidneys (11, 16, 19, 30, 55, 56), liver (11, 30, 57, 58), gastrointestinal tract (11, 30, 59, 60), central nervous system (61, 62), and CV system (16, 18, 19, 63).

Mitochondrial-Related Mechanisms

Mitochondria are essential for meeting the rise in energy demand required to fuel the immune system response and also for inducing immunomodulatory mechanisms, serving as a platform for host defense against RNA viruses such as SARS-CoV-2 (64, 65). The effects of SARS-CoV-2 infection upon mitochondrial respiratory capacity is a key consideration in the context of the host cytokine response. Mitochondrial respiratory capacity has been suggested to account for 10–30% of the variance in circulating leukocyte immune reaction across individuals, influencing the cytokine signature produced by leukocytes in response to lipopolysaccharide (LPS) administration (66). In particular, complex IV activity was positively correlated with LPS-stimulated IL-6 release (66). This is of particular interest in relation to SARS-CoV-2, whereby blood IL-6 has been identified as a predictor of patient fatality (47).

Aside from respiration, mitochondria are essential in host cell detection of RNA via pattern recognition receptors (PPRs), including cytosolic sensors retinoic acid-inducible gene 1 (RIG-1) and melanoma differentiation-associated protein 5 (MDA5) (67). These utilize the mitochondrial signaling protein MAVS (mitochondrial antiviral signaling protein), which recruits the E3 ligases TNF receptor associated factor 3 (TRAF3) and TRAF6, facilitating activation of interferon regulatory factors (IRFs) and NF-κB to induce antiviral genes. In this manner, MAVS activity coordinates the activation of a dominant antiviral mechanism, the type 1 interferon (IFN) pathway (64). SARS-CoV-2 open reading frame (Orf) 9b targets the translocase of outer mitochondrial membrane protein 70 (TOMM70), linking mitochondrial signaling to induction of the IFN pathway (68). The Orf9b of SARS-CoV-2 also localizes to the outer mitochondrial membrane, disrupting the MAVS signalosome (69) and impairing the host IFN response (69, 70). Other mitochondrial factors that may impact the IFN response include mitochondrial stress, whereby release of mtDNA into the cytosol is detected by the DNA sensor cGAS, which promotes STING-IRF3 signaling, potentiating IFN pathway signaling (71).

Inflammasomes, the multiprotein complexes providing a platform for the activation of pro-inflammatory caspase-1 culminating in cytokine release, are also mitochondrial-dependent. An example is NLRX1, a target of SARS-CoV-2 Orf9c (68). NLRX1 interacts with mitochondrial complex III, stimulating reactive oxygen species (ROS) production (72). ROS production from mitochondrial complexes I and III is known to mediate both innate and adaptive viral immune responses (73), impacting both MAVS and NF-κB signaling (72).

Pro-inflammatory cytokines are known to elicit metabolic alterations, with NF-κB and interleukin signaling impacting glucose control and glycolytic function. For instance, development of insulin resistance has been linked to IL-1 and IL-6 signaling in the context of type 2 diabetes mellitus (74). This is a key consideration in SARS-CoV-2, whereby poor blood glucose control has been associated with higher mortality in diabetic patients (75) and high glucose levels associated with viral replication in monocytes, with enhanced glycolytic capacity coinciding with raised IL-1β (76).

NF-κB mediated metabolic re-programming has been demonstrated in acute viral myocarditis (VM) (77, 78), a condition characterized by viral induced leukocyte infiltration and cardiac dysfunction. Case studies of acute VM have been reported in female COVID-19 patients (ages 21 and 43), resulting in substantial disruption to cardiac function in the absence of coronary artery disease (22, 23). Viral fulminant myocarditis, a syndrome on the clinical spectrum of acute myocarditis, has also been associated with death in SARS-CoV-2 patients suffering from cardiac injury (79).

In human and mouse models of VM, cardiac inflammation indicated through cytokine mediated NF-κB activation was linked to impaired expression of genes related to oxidative metabolism. This included downregulation of genes encoding mitochondrial regulatory proteins associated with biogenesis (PGC-1α, PGC1-1β, Tfam, and NRF-1) alongside regulators of β-oxidation (e.g., PPAR-α), tricarboxylic acid cycle and electron transport chain (ETC) function. This coincided with a fall in high energy phosphates and NAD levels and a shift toward anaerobic glycolysis, indicated through increased expression of glucose and lactate transporters and glycolytic enzymes (77). Together, this indicates that the inflammatory response associated with acute VM initiates reprogramming of cardiomyocyte energy metabolism away from oxidative metabolism and toward glycolysis. This culminated in an energy-starved status of the heart, the extent to which likely contributed to impaired cardiac function. NF-κB signaling has also been linked to impaired insulin signaling by stimulating phosphorylation of insulin receptor substrate-1, in turn inducing insulin resistance and cardiac dysfunction associated with VM (78). The metabolic implications of VM onset and resulting impairment of myocardial function are thus vital considerations in the pathophysiology of SARS-CoV-2 infection.

On the Cardiovascular System

A number of case reports have demonstrated cardiac abnormalities in patients with COVID-19, including myocarditis, myo-pericarditis, electrocardiographic complications, cardiogenic shock, decompensated heart failure, and other histological/imaging complications, such as reduced left ventricular ejection fraction (LVEF) (80–85). Moreover, and as described previously, cross-sectional studies have consistently reported elevations in cardiac injury markers, such as cTn, NT-proBNP, and creatine kinase myocardial band (CK-MB) concentrations, with patients presenting with cardiac injury being at a higher risk of mortality, even after being adjusted for confounding variables such as age, pre-existing CVD, and ARDS (18). These data give strong evidence for cardiac complications associated with COVID-19, however, the mechanisms for these complications may not be solely the result of a direct viral infection of cardiac cells.

The CV system is also at high-risk as a result of indirect mechanisms, such as the cytokine storm. The cytokine storm is likely to induce cardiovascular damage through mechanisms related to endothelial dysfunction, atherosclerotic plaque instability/rupture, cardiomyocyte death, and myocarditis. The mechanisms of endothelial dysfunction within the COVID-19 population are not limited to elevations in pro-inflammatory cytokine concentrations and include direct viral infection of endothelial cells, angiotensin II (Ang II) hyperactivity, complement activation, and other elements of immune dysregulation, such as neutrophil extracellular trap (NET) formation. Indeed, evidence of SARS-CoV-2 viral structures have been observed in endothelial cells in various tissue beds (63), which may promote an imbalance between ACE2 and

Ang II. Liu et al. (86) support this notion by demonstrating elevated plasma Ang II concentrations in patients with COVID-19. For a more in depth review of direct viral infection of endothelial cells, including Ang II hyperactivity, readers are directed to our recent review on the vascular manifestations of COVID-19 (25). Complement activation has been associated with microthrombosis in a small number of patients with COVID-19 (87) and NET formation has been correlated with COVID-19-associated ARDS (88). Both complement activation and NET formation are associated with pro-inflammatory responses. The complement system detects viral pathogens, thus contributing to the innate immune response to viral infections (89), whilst NETs have the ability to induce IL-1β secretion from macrophages and play a role in the development of atherosclerosis, causing endothelial damage and dysfunction (90, 91). Moreover, endothelial cells undergoing apoptosis have been shown to activate the complement system (92), which may further exacerbate cytokine secretion and promote microthrombosis. Therefore, it should be acknowledged that direct viral infection of endothelial cells, subsequent Ang II hyperactivity and the pro-inflammatory effects of complement activation and NET formation promote both direct and indirect perturbations to the cardiovascular system, whilst exacerbating the cytokine storm. Moving forward, the predominant focus of this section is to discuss the potential effects of the cytokine storm upon the cardiovascular system.

The cytokine storm is not only one of the predominant pathophysiological mechanisms of fulminant myocarditis (without evidence of viral infiltration) (93), which has been reported in patients with COVID-19, but inflammatory infiltration into endothelial cells has also been reported in histological studies (63, 94). Inflammatory infiltration into endothelial cells promotes endothelialitis, perturbing endothelial cell membrane function, loosening inter-endothelial junctions, and causing cell swelling (94, 95). Indeed, Varga et al. (63) showed endothelial cell death and dysfunction in patients infected with SARS-CoV-2, which facilitated the induction of endothelialitis in several organs, including cardiac tissue, as a direct consequence of viral involvement and of the host inflammatory response.

The presence of endothelialitis demonstrates the activation of endothelial cells, promoting the expression of cell-surface adhesion molecules and thus the binding of inflammatory cells to the endothelium (96, 97). These pathophysiological consequences promote vascular hyperpermeability. Disruption of inter-endothelial junctions cause endothelial cells to be "pulled apart," thus resulting in inter-endothelial gaps (95, 98), denoting cytoskeletal alterations to the endothelium. Moreover, this cytokine storm-induced endothelial dysfunction pre-disposes the CV system to a pro-coagulant state, promoting thromboembolic events, which has been linked to higher disease severity, and higher instances of mortality (99). Interestingly thrombin exposure, coupled with an elevation in the influx of Ca^{2+} promotes elevations in endothelial cell permeability which can be induced by an increase in TNF-α expression (100, 101).

Elevations in cytosolic Ca^{2+} influx into endothelial cells is a pivotal step in the disruption to inter-endothelial junctions and thus the progression to increased vascular permeability

(101, 102). A determinant of this increased Ca^{2+} influx is the upregulation of transient receptor potential channels, which is induced *via* TNF-α (100), causing a destabilization of microtubules (103). Evidence supports the notion of a cytokine-induced hyperpermeability response of the vasculature, with Tinsley et al. (104) demonstrating the role of cytokine (TNF-α, IL-1β, and IL-6) induced-vascular hyperpermeability through a protein kinase C (PKC) and myosin light chain kinase (MLCK) dependent mechanism in cultured rat heart microvascular endothelial cells. Moreover, the authors replicated these findings *in vivo* using a coronary ischemia/reperfusion (I/R) rodent model of heart failure, demonstrating TNF-α increases endothelial permeability in a PKC and MLCK dependent manner (104). Therefore, translating this to COVID-19 pathophysiology, cytokine storm induced Ca^{2+} influx into endothelial cells may be a contributing mechanism underpinning the disruption to inter-endothelial junctions and the promotion of vascular permeability. Furthermore, the cytokine-induced stimulation of PKC and MLCK may promote direct damage to cardiac tissue, which may pose significant deleterious effects upon patients with pre-existing CVD, a common comorbidity in the more severe COVID-19 population (105).

Histological studies in pulmonary vasculature have indicated endothelialitis, with unexpected observations of intussuseptive angiogenesis. In this study (94), the degree of intussuseptive angiogenesis was associated with the duration of hospitalization. Whilst hypoxia may be a contributing mechanism, the authors concluded the predominant mechanism was likely the presence of endothelialitis and thrombosis (94). Intussuseptive angiogenesis is the formation of intravascular vessel formation, through non-sprouting mechanisms, commonly observed as "pillar" formation within the vasculature (106), which can significantly alter the microcirculation, and can be triggered by extraluminal processes, including inflammation (107). Inflammatory-mediated intussuseptive angiogenesis has been demonstrated previously in murine models of colitis, suggesting this is an adaptive response to prolonged inflammation (108). This provides further evidence of the perturbations to the vasculature caused by the cytokine storm in COVID-19. The promotion of intussuseptive angiogenesis as an adaptive response to vascular damage, has also been shown to accelerate fibrotic neovascularisation (109).

Inflammatory environments also promote the generation of ROS which can result in damage and dysfunction of the vasculature. ROS act as signaling molecules to defend against oxidative stress by promoting the upregulation of antioxidant mechanisms, however, high concentrations of ROS can activate endothelial cells and inhibit normal endothelial functioning. Cytokines, such as TNF-α, have been shown to interact with the ETC and stimulate the release of mitochondrial-derived ROS, such as hydrogen peroxide (110) and superoxide (111). Moreover, in response to infections, inflammatory cytokines, such as TNF-α and IL-1β, coming into contact with endothelial cells induce NAD(P)H oxidase-derived ROS (112, 113). The generation of excessive ROS elevates superoxide anion production, which can degrade nitric oxide (NO), lead to the formation of other free radicals, such as peroxynitrite, and thus result in endothelial cell dysfunction and apoptosis (96, 114, 115). Therefore, it is likely that the cytokine storm experienced in patients with COVID-19 will promote the elevation in ROS and result in oxidative stress, which is a key mechanism of endothelial dysfunction in hypertension (116) and CVD (117). Elevations in ROS also act as secondary inflammatory signals, which has been shown to induce the secretion of pro-inflammatory cytokines, such as IL-1β, TNF-α, and IL-6 (118). Therefore, this creates a vicious cycle of cytokine-induced oxidative stress and ROS-induced pro-inflammatory cytokine signaling, secondary to the COVID-19 hyper-activation of the immune response.

Inflammatory cytokines do not just alter endothelial structure and function. Cytokines such as TNF-α, IL-1β, and IL-6 promote vascular smooth muscle cell (VSMC) proliferation from the media to the intima of the vasculature, which results in the secretion of extracellular matrix proteins within, and thus expanding the intima in pathological conditions, such as atherosclerosis (119). Moreover, in human coronary VSMCs, IL-1β has been shown to stimulate an upregulation in Rho-kinase, *via* a PKC-dependent mechanism, which may contribute to medial thickening and the atherogenic environment (120). Interestingly, this can also be stimulated by an upregulation in angiotensin II, which has been noted within the COVID-19 literature if infected cells experience a downregulation of ACE2 expression (121), which will also contribute to the pro-inflammatory environment experienced in patients with COVID-19. Activation of RhoA can also be stimulated by TNF-α which has been shown to promote endothelial cell permeability in cultured human umbilical vein endothelial cells (HUVECs) (122). These pathophysiological processes are shared with thrombosis, which is a common manifestation in patients with severe COVID-19 (99). Combined with damage to endothelial cells contributing to the apparent "COVID-19 coagulopathy" (123), VSMC proliferation, stimulated by various cytokines, may contribute to the high instance of coagulation derangements and thromboembolic events observed in patients with severe COVID-19.

Whilst the COVID-19 induced cytokine storm can predispose the CV system to damage and progression of pre-existing cardiovascular comorbidities, perturbations to vascular cells may also contribute to the overexpression of pro-inflammatory cytokines. Both endothelial cells and VSMCs secrete pro-inflammatory cytokines when either damaged or undergoing apoptosis. Expression of cell-surface adhesion molecules and certain cytokines, such as IL-8, on the surface of endothelial cells induce a pro-inflammatory phenotype and the recruitment of blood monocytes which induce the secretion of pro-inflammatory cytokines, such as TNF-α and IL-1β (124). Moreover, under atherogenic conditions, VSMCs have been shown to also adopt a pro-inflammatory phenotype, promoting the secretion of IL-6 and IL-8, along with cell-surface adhesion molecules, such as vascular cell adhesion molecule 1 (124, 125). Therefore, both endothelial cells and VSMCs, once damaged, may switch to a pro-inflammatory phenotype and thus propagate the expression of pro-inflammatory cytokines.

Whilst there is a plethora of evidence which suggests that the cytokine storm experienced in COVID-19 patients may promote damage to the vasculature, sustained inflammation directly contributes to progressive cardiomyocyte apoptosis. Elevated TNF-α levels seen in a variety of clinical conditions including COVID-19, drives cardiomyocytes to apoptosis (126, 127). TNF-α can induce cardiomyocyte apoptosis directly, *via* the TNF receptor, or indirectly, through stimulation of NO production or ROS, which in turn is induced by pro-inflammatory cytokines such as IL-1, IL-6, TNF-α, and IFN-7 (128). High levels of cTn are reflective of cardiomyocyte death and injury, and as stated earlier, are associated with COVID-19 disease severity and mortality (16).

In the heart, the acute inflammatory response can expand tissue damage and prolonged inflammation leads to accentuated adverse remodeling. Indeed, pro-inflammatory cytokines and upregulated monocytes/macrophages can inhibit cardiac repair, which is dependent on timely suppression and resolution of pro-inflammatory signaling. Activation of IL-1 signaling induces cytokine expression, promotes matrix-degrading properties, suppresses fibroblast proliferation and inhibits transdifferentiation of fibroblasts into myofibroblasts, altogether delaying activation of a reparative response (129). Moreover, a severe or prolonged reparative response is associated with pathological scarring and fibrosis (130).

The full extent of cardiovascular cell dysfunction and death, induced by the cytokine storm in COVID-19, is yet to be fully elucidated. This section provides evidence of the potential effects and mechanisms of the COVID-19 cytokine storm on the cardiovascular system. It is likely that cardiomyocyte and vascular cell damage and dysfunction, as well as mitochondrial-related mechanisms play a role in the progression of COVID-19 and in the pathogenesis of cardiovascular injury in COVID-19. The induction of ROS generation and the ensuing oxidative stress, coupled with vascular cell secretion of pro-inflammatory cytokines further propagates the inflammatory environment and exaggerated immune response in patients with COVID-19, promoting disease progression and multi-organ dysfunction. Moreover, cardiac and vascular cell dysfunction pre-disposes the CV system to a pro-inflammatory and pro-atherogenic state and thus increases the risk of serious cardiac events. Therefore, suppression of the cytokine storm, is key for improving patient outcomes with COVID-19, whilst also protecting the CV system. One such therapy is transplantation of mesenchymal stem/stromal cells (MSCs).

MSCs AS A THERAPY FOR SEVERE COVID-19 PATIENTS

Immunomodulatory Role of MSCs

An important function of MSCs is that they have powerful immunomodulatory properties, possessing natural abilities to detect changes in their environment such as inflammation. Mesenchymal stromal cells can both directly and indirectly stimulate immunomodulation by interacting with immune cells and releasing various anti-inflammatory cytokines *via* paracrine effects, respectively (131). Functional alterations to dendritic cells, monocytes, macrophages, regulatory T-cells (Tregs), and B-cells underpin MSCs' immunomodulatory capacity, whilst also through cell-to-cell interaction mechanisms (13). Once systemically administered, a significant portion of MSCs accumulate within the lungs, which can promote anti-inflammatory effects, thus improving the lung microenvironment and potentially restoring vascular barrier integrity and reducing oedema; whilst also promoting endogenous repair and regeneration mechanisms to reduce (or prevent further) fibrosis of the lung (132, 133).

Animal models of ARDS lung injury due to influenza virus have shown that infection by this and related viruses causes ion channel transporter abnormalities which causes fluid secretion, a major cause of the pulmonary oedema in the lungs of infected individuals. In such animal models, MSCs prevent or reduce the secretory effect of influenza virus on lung alveolar cell ion channels, and when administered intravenously in aged animals have resulted in increased oxygenation, improved respiration, reduction in pro-inflammatory cytokines, and an increase in survival (134).

Mesenchymal stromal cells are well-known to respond to the inflammatory environment with multimodal activity resulting in sustained anti-inflammatory effects; conversion of Th17 cells to anti-inflammatory FOXP3 Treg cells by MSC-secreted transforming growth factor (TGF) $\beta 1$ and the essential presence of CCL18 producing type-2 anti-inflammatory macrophages from differentiated pro-inflammatory monocytes (135). They are known to dampen the innate immune response to insult (such as acute lung injury, burn injuries) or infection *via* preventing neutrophil infiltration into injured/infected sites (136–139) or *via* shifting the phenotype of macrophages from an M1 to M2 anti-inflammatory phenotype (140). Specifically the MSCs appear to reduce inflammation *via* reducing macrophage secretion of neutrophil chemoattractant proteins CXCL1, CXCL2 (137, 141) as a result of activation of phosphorylation of p38 MAPK (141) and greater IL-10 release (137), dampened production of IL-6 and TNF-α (137, 138), and suppression of reactive oxygen species production by neutrophils (142, 143). Together this contributes toward a shift from a pro- to an anti-inflammatory environment and is an essential part of the immunomodulatory function of MSCs as this helps prevent against autoimmunity (13), as demonstrated in MSC-treated graft vs. host disease (144).

Mesenchymal stromal cells can also induce local and systemic immunomodulatory responses independently of the cytokine storm. For instance, MSCs can prevent the infiltration of cells of the innate immune system, thereby indirectly reducing the secretion of inflammatory cytokines. In a murine model, BM-MSCs reduced CD45$^+$ cells and neutrophil populations in the mucosa *via* release of tumor necrosis factor-induced protein 6 (TSG-6) (145). Both MSCs and TSG-6 induced the expansion of regulatory macrophages, expressing IL-10 and inducible nitric oxide synthase (NOS), and increased the population of FOXP3CD45$^+$ cells. Interestingly, TSG-6 was associated with MSC-mediated depletion of corneal, splenic, and peripheral blood CD11b$^+$ monocytes/macrophages in a model of inflammatory corneal neovascularization (146). In addition to TSG-6, MSCs can also release other bioactive molecules that promote protective responses in innate immune cells, including kynurenic acid (147), spermine (148, 149), and lactate (150). Adaptive immune cells, such as T and B cells, are also direct targets of MSCs. Following transplantation, MSCs form aggregates with B and T cells, stimulating the production of FOXP3 and IL-10 (145). Mesenchymal stromal cells directly inhibit the activation of cytotoxic $CD8^+$ T-cells *via* downregulation of CD25, CD38, and CD69 (151). In B cells, MSCs downregulate chemotactic properties, with no effect on costimulatory molecules or cytokine production (152). Mesenchymal stromal cell-mediated indoleamine 2,3-dioxygenase signaling promotes the survival and proliferation of $CD5^+$ Bregs (153). There are also data to suggest that MSCs could act *via* extracellular vesicles and exosomes to modulate innate and adaptive immunity (154, 155). The immunoregulatory mechanisms of mesenchymal stem and stromal cells in inflammatory disease are reviewed in (156).

Consequently, on the basis of these and other studies with MSCs in animal models, clinical investigators have postulated that human MSCs should be effective in the pathology of human ARDS (157). Indeed in a report of allogeneic MSCs in ARDS patients, a single low dose of cells (2 million cells/kg/BW) achieved rapid reduction in inflammatory cytokines and efficacy in influenza-related ARDS which was otherwise refractory to conventional supportive therapy (158). For further insight on the therapeutic potential of cell therapy to treat ARDS readers are directed too (159, 160).

The systemic redistribution of MSCs have the ability to target other organs that are damaged. As multi-organ damage is a common manifestation in patients with severe COVID-19, this makes MSCs an attractive therapy to combat not only lung damage, but also damage observed in other organs, such as the heart. Therefore, the use of MSCs to modulate the immune response, avoiding, preventing or attenuating the cytokine storm leading to multi-organ failure may be the key for the treatment of COVID-19 infected patients.

Use of MSCs to Treat COVID-19

Table 1 summarizes the published clinical studies thus far using MSCs as a therapy to treat COVID-19. **Table 2** summarizes the ongoing, registered clinical trials using MSCs as a therapy to treat COVID-19. For review articles on the rationale and treatment of COVID-19-related ARDS using MSCs, readers are directed to Moll et al. (165) and Can and Coskun (166).

The first clinical study undertaken in China, showed that for seven patients with COVID-19-related pneumonia, transplantation of 1×10^6 MSCs/Kg/BW allogeneic MSCs was effective by restoring the balance of the immune system resulting in significant resolution of signs and symptoms of pulmonary disease (133). Before the transplantation, all patients had COVID-19-related pneumonia with symptoms of high fever, weakness, shortness of breath, and low oxygen saturation. Results showed that all symptoms had disappeared by 2–4 days after the transplantation. The oxygen saturations rose to $\geq$ 95% at rest, without or with oxygen treatment. This was not the case in the three placebo control patients. Among the MSC-treated patients, one severe and two mild patients were able to make a recovery and be discharged 10 days after treatment. The study

found improvement was particularly dramatic for an elderly male patient in a severe critical condition (133). The improved recovery time with MSC treatment would lead to decreased hospitalization which would be vital for overwhelmed hospital wards and ICUs.

The transplanted MSCs significantly elevated IL-10 and reduced TNF-α concentrations in seven MSC transplanted patients with COVID-19-pneumonia compared to the three patients in the placebo control group receiving standard care. In the severe ($n = 4$) and critically severe ($n = 1$) patients, a significant elevation in Tregs and dendritic cells were observed after MSC administration, compared with the mild and control patients. Specifically, there was a switch from pro-inflammatory cytokine producing $CXCR3^+CD4^+$ T cells, $CXCR3^+CD8^+$ T cells, and $CXCR3^+$ NK cells to $CD14^+CD11c^+CD11b$ mid regulatory dendritic cell (DCreg) population, indicating improvement in immunomodulatory function. Furthermore, in the critically severe patient an over activation of T-cells and natural killer (NK) cells were evident, however, after MSC treatment, T-cells and NK cells were almost eradicated, with the CD14+CD11c+CD11b mid DCregs restored to normal levels (133). These findings demonstrate the ability of MSCs to induce their immunomodulatory benefits in a set of patients with COVID-19, restoring the balance of the immune response by attenuating the cytokine storm.

These findings have been further supported within the literature with a case study by Zhang et al. (162) demonstrating a regression of COVID-19 symptoms between 2 and 7 days post-Wharton's Jelly derived human umbilical cord MSCs administration, with a reduction in ground glass opacity and pneumonia infiltration within the lungs 6 days post-transplantation. Moreover, $CD3^+$, $CD4^+$, and $CD8^+$ T-cells were increased and CRP, IL-6, and TNF-α concentrations were reduced. Another case report of a patient with severe COVID-19 who experienced two cytokine storms, was treated with a synergistic use of convalescent plasma and umbilical cord MSCs. Treatment resulted in lymphocyte counts returning to normal after the fourth day following convalescent plasma administration and a reduction in inflammatory markers, with a steady elevation in PaO_2 following the administration of umbilical cord MSCs (167).

One limitation to MSC therapies for treating COVID-19 may be the expression of ACE2 and the predominant serine protease responsible for priming the SARS-CoV-2 spike glycoprotein, TMPRSS2, which may promote SARS-CoV-2 infection of transplanted cells and thus promote further spread and progression of COVID-19. However, Leng et al. (133) after performing 10x single cell RNA sequencing analysis, demonstrated transplanted MSCs are ACE2-negative and TMPRSS2-negative.

Taken together, *via* their immunomodulatory and reparative role these studies provide support to the rationale for MSC transplantation as a therapy to treat COVID-19. Moreover, whilst these studies demonstrate evidence for their use against lung damage, the suppression of pro-inflammatory markers will provide protection against damage or further damage to other organs. For example, with COVID-19 leading

TABLE 1 | Summarisation of clinical studies and ongoing clinical trials assessing the therapeutic benefit of MSC transplantation in patients with COVID-19, including studies assessing the therapeutic potential of MSCs in patients with acute respiratory distress syndrome (ARDS), without COVID-19.

Citation	N	Subjects	MSC source and dose	MSC timing	Recipient site	Results
Leng et al. (133)	MSC transplant: $n = 7$; CON: $n = 3$	COVID-19 pneumonia	Clinical grade ACE2$^-$ MSCs at 1×10^6 cells/kg	The time when symptoms and/or signs were still getting worse, even as the expectant treatments were being conducted	Systemic	- ↑ IL-10 vs. CON - ↓ TNF-α vs. CON - ↔ IP-10 - Trend for ↑ VEGF vs. CON - Inflammation, AAT, MYO and CK reduced in critically severe patient with a reduction in ground-glass opacity and pneumonia infiltration
Liang et al. (161)	Case study	Critical COVID-19	Allogenic hUCMSCs at 5×10^7 cells 3 times	Admitted 2 days after symptoms onset and MSCs were transplanted on the 9, 12, and 15th days after admission. In combination with antibiotics and thymosin α1	Systemic	No side effects were observed. After 2nd administration: - ↓ Bilirubin, WBC and neutrophil count, CRP and ALT/AST - ↑ lymphocyte count - ↑ CD3$^+$, CD4$^+$, and CD8$^+$ T cells - Trachea cannula removed After 3rd administration: - Pneumonia relieved - Removed from ICU 2 days following - Negative throat swab
Zhang et al. (162)	Case study	COVID-19 pneumonia - History of diabetes	Wharton's jelly-derived hUCMSCs at 1×10^6 cells/kg	Admitted 5 days after symptoms onset and MSCs were transplanted on the 17th day of admission	Systemic	Post-transplant: - COVID-19 symptoms disappeared 2 to 7 days - Ground glass opacity and pneumonia infiltration day 6 - ↑ CD3$^+$, CD4$^+$ & CD8$^+$ T cells - ↓ CRP, IL-6 & TNF-α
Chen et al. (163)	MSC transplant: $n = 17$; CON: $n = 44$	H7N9-induced ARDS	Allogenic menstrual-blood-derived MSCs at 1×10^6 cells/kg	3 patients treated with 3 infusion at the early stage of infection; 6 patients were treated with 3 infusions at the late stage of infection; 8 patients accepted 4 infusions of at late stage of infection	Systemic	At admission: - No differences, except ↓ PCT vs. CON At discharge: - ↑ mortality rate of CON - ↓ PCT, ALT, sCr, CK, PT, and D-dimer vs. CON At follow-up (5 year; $n = 4$): - ↑ Hb - ↓ PT
Sengupta et al. (164)	$N = 23$	COVID-19: cohort a (mild COVID-19): $n = 1$; cohort b (hypoxaemia and COVID-19): $n = 20$; cohort c (intubated COVID-19): $n = 3$	Bone-marrow derived MSCs exosome agent—ExoFlow —15 mL	Not specified	Systemic	- 71% patients recovered and/or were discharged after 5.6 days post-infusion - 13% remained critically ill - 16% died - 80% improved PaO$_2$/FiO$_2$ ratio within 3 days - ↓ CRP, ferritin and D-dimer on day 5 - ↑ CD3$^+$, CD4$^+$, and CD8$^+$ T cells on day 5

CON, control; ACE2, Angiotensin converting enzyme 2; IL-10, Interleukin-10; TNF-α, Tumor necrosis factor α; IP-10, Interferon gamma-induced protein 10; VEGF, Vascular endothelial growth factor; AST, Aspartate amino transferase; MYO, Myoglobin; CK, Creatine kinase; hUCMSC, human umbilical cord mesenchymal stem cells; WBC, white blood cell; CRP, C-reactive protein; ALT, Alanine aminotransferase; ICU, intensive care unit; ARDS, Acute respiratory distress syndrome; PCT, Procalcitonin; sCr, serum creatinine; PT, Prothrombin time.

TABLE 2 | List of registered, ongoing, clinical trials using mesenchymal stem/stromal cells (MSCs) as a therapy to treat COVID-19.

Clinical trials number	Participants	MSC source	Outcomes
NCT04371393 (USA)	Target: $N = 300$	MSCs (Remestemcel-L) at 2×10^6 cells/kg administered twice during first week (second infusion 4 days following first) plus standard care vs. placebo (Plasma-Lyte) (second infusion 4 days following first) plus standard care	- All-cause mortality - SAEs - No. of days off mechanical ventilation - Resolution/improvement of ARDS - Length of stay - Clinical improvement scale - Hs-CRP, IL-6, IL-8, TNF-α
NCT03042143 (Northern Ireland)—REALIST trial	Target: $N = 75$	Single infusion of human umbilical cord derived CD362 enriched MSCs at maximum tolerable dose from phase I (dose escalation pilot study) plus standard care vs. placebo (Plasma-Lyte) plus standard care	- Oxygenation index - SAEs - SOFA - Respiratory compliance - P/F ratio - Driving pressure - Extubation and reintubation - Ventilation free days - Length of ICU/hospital stay - Mortality
NCT04444271 (Pakistan)	Target: $N = 20$	Bone marrow derived MSCs at 2×10^6 cells/kg on day 1 and 7 plus standard care vs. saline injection plus standard care	- Survival - No. oxygen support days - Time to negative nCoV test - CT scan - No. days to discharge
NCT04416139 (Mexico)	Target: $N = 10$	Umbilical cord derived MSCs from De bank Laboratory at 1×10^6 cells/kg (no control group—data compared to controls treated in a previous trial)	- PaO$_2$/FiO$_2$ ratio - HR and RR - Body temperature - Leukocyte, lymphocyte, and platelet counts - PCT, fibrinogen, D-dimer, ferritin - CRP, TNF-α, IL-1, IL-10, IL-6, IL-17 - VEGF - T-cell analysis (CD4$^+$ and CD8$^+$) - NK and dendritic cells - SAEs - CT scan - nCoV-test
NCT04429763 (Colombia)—CELMA	Target: $N = 30$	Umbilical cord derived MSCs at 1×10^6 cells/kg plus standard care vs. placebo (not stated) plus standard care control	- NEWS scale - Time to hospital discharge - Respiratory function - Inflammatory markers - Hematological and renal assessments
NCT04315987 (Brazil)	Target: $N = 90$	NestaCell MSCs at 2×10^7 cells/kg on days 1, 3, 5, and 7 plus standard care vs. placebo (not stated) on days 1, 3, 5, and 7 plus standard care	- Change in clinical condition - Mortality - SpO$_2$ - PaO$_2$/FiO$_2$ ratio - T-cell analysis (CD4$^+$ and CD8$^+$) - SAEs - Blood count and cardiac, hepatic, and renal profiles
NCT04366323 (Spain)	Target: $N = 26$	Allogenic and expanded adipose tissue derived MSCs at 8×10^6 cells $\times$ 2 (no control group)	- Safety of administration (SAEs) - Efficacy of administration
NCT04456361 (Mexico)	Target: $N = 9$	Wharton's jelly derived MSCs at 1×10^8 cells/kg (no control group)	- SpO$_2$ - PaO$_2$/FiO$_2$ ratio - Ground glass opacity and pneumonia infiltration - LDH, CRP, D-dimer, and Ferritin
NCT04366271 (Spain)	Target: $N = 106$	Undifferentiated allogenic umbilical cord MSCs (dose not stated) vs. standard care	- Mortality due to lung involvement - All-cause mortality - Days without mechanical ventilation - Days without vasopressors - Negative nCoV-test - SAEs

(Continued)

TABLE 2 | Continued

Clinical trials number	Participants	MSC source	Outcomes
NCT04252118 (China)	Target: $N = 20$	MSCs (source not stated) at 3×10^7 cells at day 0, 3, and 6 vs. standard care	- CT scan - SAEs - Pneumonia evaluation - Mortality - T-cell analysis (CD4$^+$ and CD8$^+$) - AAT, CRP, and CK
NCT04313322 (Jordan)	Target: $N = 5$	Wharton's jelly derived MSCs at 1×10^6 cells/kg for 3 doses, spaced 3 days apart (No control group)	- Alleviations of symptoms - CT scan - Negative nCoV-test
NCT04336254 (China)	Target: $N = 20$	Allogenic human dental pulp MSCs at 3×10^7 cells at day 1, 4, and 7 vs. saline control at day 1, 4, and 7	- TTCI - CT scan - Immune function markers - Time for negative nCoV-test - Blood count and classification - SpO$_2$ - RR - Body temperature - SAEs - CRP
NCT04346368 (China)	Target: $N = 20$	Bone marrow derived MSCs at 1×10^6 cells/kg at day 1 vs. standard care	- PaO$_2$/FiO$_2$ ratio - SAEs - Clinical outcome - No. days in hospital - CT scan - Changes in viral load - T-cell analysis (CD4$^+$ and CD8$^+$) - Mortality - CRP
NCT04288102 (China)	Target: $N = 100$	Umbilical cord derived MSCs at 4×10^7 at day 0, 3, and 6 vs. saline control at day 0, 3, and 6	- Pneumonia evaluation - Time to clinical improvement - PaO$_2$/FiO$_2$ ratio - Days on oxygen therapy - SpO$_2$ - 6-min walk test - Lymphocyte counts - Cytokine/chemokine assessment - SAEs - All-course mortality
NCT04273646 (China)	Target: $N = 48$	Umbilical cord derived MSCs at 0.5×10^6 cells/kg at day 1, 3, 5, and 7 plus standard care vs. saline control at day 1, 3, 5, and 7 plus standard care	- Pneumonia evaluation - SAEs - Survival - Organ failure assessment - CRP and Procalcitonin - Lymphocyte count - T-cell analysis (CD3$^+$, CD4$^+$, and CD8$^+$) - CD4$^+$/CD8$^+$ ratio
NCT04339660 (China)	Target: $N = 30$	Umbilical cord derived MSCs at 1×10^6 cells/kg vs. saline control	- TNF-α, IL-1β, IL-6, TGF-β, IL-8, PCT, CRP - SpO$_2$ - Mortality - CT scan - Blood count recovery time - Duration of respiratory symptoms - Negative nCoV-test
NCT04382547 (Belarus)	Target: $N = 40$	Allogenic pooled olfactory mucosa derived MSCs (dose not stated) vs. standard care control	- nCoV-test - SAEs
NCT04457609 (Indonesia)	Target: $N = 40$	Umbilical cord derived MSCs at 1×10^6 cells/kg with Oseltamivir and Azithromycin vs. standard care with Oseltamivir and Azithromycin	- Clinical improvement markers - General laboratory outcomes - PCT, bilirubin, D-dimer, and fibrinogen - Troponin and NT-proBNP - LIF, IL-6, IL-10, ferritin, CXCR3 - T-cell analysis (CD4$^+$, CD8$^+$, and CD56$^+$)

(Continued)

TABLE 2 | Continued

Clinical trials number	Participants	MSC source	Outcomes
NCT04352803 (USA)	Target: $N = 20$	Autologous adipose derived MSCs at 0.5×10^6 cells/kg vs. standard care control	- VEGF - CT scan - SAEs - Progression and time to/on mechanical ventilation - Length of hospital stay - All-cause mortality
NCT04490486 (USA)	Target: $N = 21$	Umbilical cord derived MSCs at 1×10^8 cells on day 0 and 3 vs. 1% human serum albumin in Plasmalyte A on day 0 and 3	- SAEs - Inflammatory markers - COVID-19 viral load - SOFA score - Electrolyte levels - LDH - No. ICU discharges - Vasoactive agent use - Mortality - Immune markers - CT scan
NCT04522986 (Japan)	Target: $N = 6$	Adipose derived MSCs at 1×10^8 cells once a week for 4 weeks (no control group)	- SAEs
NCT04461925 (Ukraine)	Target: $N = 30$	Placenta derived MSCs at 1×10^6 cells/kg once every 3 days for 3 infusions vs. standard care control	- PaO$_2$/FiO$_2$ ratio - Length of hospital stay - Mortality - CRP - CT scan - Duration of respiratory symptoms - Blood count recovery time
NCT04362189 (USA)	Target: $N = 100$	Allogenic adipose tissue derived MSCs (Hope Biosciences) at 1×10^6 cells/dose at day 0, 3, 7, and 10 vs. saline control at day 0, 3, 7, and 10	- IL-6, CRP, TNF-α, and IL-10 - Oxygenation - RTRA - ECG assessment - Routine blood assessments - Cardiac, hepatic, and renal assessment - Blood count - Platelets, Prothrombin time, D-dimer, and INR - Immune markers - SAEs - Chest X-ray - CT scan - Negative nCoV-test
NCT04371601 (China)	Target: $N = 60$	Umbilical cord derived MSCs at 1×10^6 cells/kg once every 4 days for 4 infusions vs. standard care control	- PaO$_2$/FiO$_2$ ratio - TNF-α and IL-6 - Immune markers - CRP and calcitonin
NCT04348461 (Spain)	Target: $N = 100$	Allogenic expanded adipose tissue derived MSCs at 1.5×10^6 cells/kg vs. standard care control	- Efficacy of administration of MSCs - SAEs
NCT04452097 (USA)	Target: $N = 9$	Umbilical cord derived MSCs (3 groups): - Low dose: 0.5×10^6 cells/kg - Middle dose: 1×10^6 cells/kg - High dose: 1.5×10^6 cells/kg	- SAEs - TEAEs - Selection of appropriate dose for Phase II trial
NCT04494386 (USA)	Target: $N = 60$	Umbilical cord lining derived MSCs at 1×10^6 cells/dose vs. saline control—either a single dose or 2 doses separated by 48 h	- DLT - SAEs - Berlin definition of ARDS - SpO$_2$ and PaO$_2$/FiO$_2$ ratio - No. of VFDs - Blood count - Routine blood assessments - BUN and urinalysis - AAT
NCT04345601 (USA)	Target: $N = 30$	MSCs (source not specified) at 1×10^8 cells vs. standard care control	- SAEs - Change to clinical status

(Continued)

TABLE 2 | Continued

Clinical trials number	Participants	MSC source	Outcomes
NCT04377334 (Germany)	Target: $N = 40$	Allogenic bone marrow derived MSCs (dose not stated) vs. standard care control	- Lung injury score - D-dimer - Pro-resolving lipid mediators - Phenotype of immune cells - Cytokine and chemokine analysis - Survival - Extubation - Lymphocyte subpopulation - Complement molecules - SARS-CoV-2 specific antibody
NCT04390139 (Spain)	Target: $N = 30$	Wharton's jelly derived MSCs at 1×10^6 cells/kg on day 1 and 3 vs. placebo (not stated) on day 1 and 3	- All-cause mortality - SAEs - Need for mechanical ventilation - No. of VFDs - PaO_2/FiO_2 ratio - SOFA index - APACHE II score - Duration of hospitalization - Immune response - Feasibility of MSCs - nCoV-test - LDH, D-dimer, and ferritin - Subpopulations of lymphocytes and immunoglobins - *In vitro* response of receptor lymphocytes
NCT04392778 (Turkey)	Target: $N = 30$	MSCs (source not stated) at 3×10^6 cells/kg on day 0, 3, and 6 to COVID-19 patients with a ventilator vs. saline control on day 0, 3, and 6 to COVID-19 patients with a ventilator vs. standard care control to COVID-19 patients without a ventilator	- Clinical improvement - CT scan - Negative nCoV-test - Blood tests
NCT04467047 (Brazil)	Target: $N = 10$	MSCs (source not stated) at 1×10^6 cells/kg (safety and feasibility study)	- Survival - CRP - Length of hospital stay - PaO_2/FiO_2 ratio - Liao's score (2020) - CT scan - Negative nCoV-test
NCT04398303 (USA)	Target: $N = 70$	Allogenic umbilical cord derived MSCs at 1×10^6 cells/kg vs. MSC conditioned media at 100 ml vs. placebo (MEM-α) at 100 ml	- Mortality - No. of VFDs - No. of days on O_2 therapy - No. of ICU-free days - Pulmonary function - Berlin criteria score
NCT04437823 (USA)	Target: $N = 20$	Umbilical cord derived MSCs at 0.5×10^6 cells/kg on day 1, 3, and 5 vs. standard care control	- SAEs - CT scan - Negative nCoV-test - SOFA score - Mortality - Clinical respiratory changes
NCT04269525 (China)	Target: $N = 16$	Umbilical cord derived MSCs at 3.3×10^7 cells on day 1, 3, 5, and 7	- PaO_2/FiO_2 ratio - Mortality - Length of hospital stay - nCoV PCR and antibody-test - Lung imaging - WBC and lymphocyte count - PCT - IL-2, IL-4, IL-4, IL-6, IL-10, TNF-α, γ-IFN, and CRP - NK cells - T-cell analysis (CD4$^+$, CD8$^+$)

(Continued)

TABLE 2 | Continued

Clinical trials number	Participants	MSC source	Outcomes
NCT04447833 (Sweden)	Target: $N = 9$	Allogenic bone marrow derived MSCs at 1×10^6 cells/kg ($n = 3$) and 2×10^6 cells/kg ($n = 6$)	- SAEs - All-cause mortality - Leucocytes and thrombocytes - CRP - Prothrombin - Creatinine - AST and AAT - NT-proBNP - Blood pressure - Body temperature - Efficacy for MSC use - Lung function - 6-min walk test - Quality of life assessment - Blood biomarkers - Sensitisation test
NCT04491240 (Russia)	Target: $N = 90$	Inhalation of MSC exosomes at $0.5–2 \times 10^{10}$ nanoparticles for COVID-19 patients ($n = 30$) and SARS-CoV-2 pneumonia patients ($n = 30$) vs. inhalation of solution free placebo ($n = 30$)—inhalation twice a day for 10 days	- SAEs - TTCI - Blood gases - SpO$_2$ - Chest imaging
NCT04333368 (France)	Target: $N = 40$	Umbilical cord Wharton's jelly derived MSCs at 1×10^6 cells/kg at day 1, 3, and 5 vs. placebo (NaCl) control at day 1, 3, and 5	- PaO$_2$/FiO$_2$ ratio - Lung injury score - Mortality - No. of VFDs - Use of sedatives - Use of neuromuscular blocking agent - ICU-acquired weakness - SAEs - Quality of life at 1 year - Cytokine analysis - Anti-HLA antibodies
NCT04466098 (USA)	Target: $N = 30$	Thawed product containing MSCs (source not stated) at 300×10^6 cells 3 times separated by 48 h vs. placebo (dextran and human serum albumin) control 3 times separated by 48 h	- SAEs - Inflammatory markers - PaO$_2$/FiO$_2$ ratio - Mean airway, peak and plateau pressure - PEEP - Mortality - No. of ICU free days - No. of VFDs - Acute lung injury score - No. of days off O$_2$ therapy
NCT04445220 (USA)	Target: $N = 22$	Allogenic human MSCs at 2.5×10^6 cells (low dose) and 7.5×10^6 cells (high dose) vs. standard care control—patients with COVID-19 and acute kidney injury	- Safety and tolerability - SAEs
NCT04276987 (China)	Target: $N = 30$	Allogenic adipose tissue derived MSC exosomes inhaled at 2×10^8 nano-vesicles on 5 consecutive days	- SAEs - TTCI - No. of patients weaning from mechanical ventilation - Vasoactive agent use - No. of days on mechanical ventilation - Mortality - SOFA score - Lymphocyte count - CRP, LDH, and D-dimer - NT-proBNP - IL-1β, IL-2R, IL-6, and IL-8 - Chest imaging - Negative nCoV-test

(Continued)

TABLE 2 | Continued

Clinical trials number	Participants	MSC source	Outcomes
IRCT20140528017891N8 (Iran)	Target: $N = 10$	Umbilical cord derived MSCs at 0.5–1 million cells/kg at 1st, 3rd, and 6th day vs. saline injection at 1st, 3rd, and 6th day plus standard care	- Mortality - Pneumonia severity index and CT scan - SpO_2 supply - CRP and PCT - Lymphocyte count - T-cell analysis ($CD3^+$, $CD4^+$, and $CD8^+$)
NCT04355728 (USA)	Target: $N = 24$	Umbilical cord derived vs. standard care control	- Adverse events - 90 day survival post-infusion - No. of VFDs - Change in oxygenation index and plat-PEEP - SOFA and SIT scores - TnI, CRP, and D-dimer - WBC and platelet count - AA/EPA ratio - 25-Hydroxyl Vitamin D - Alloantibody levels
CHICTR2000030224 (China)	Target: $N = NA$	MSCs (source unknown): critical and severe group injected with MSCs vs. critical and severe control group injected with saline	- SpO_2 - CT scan - Temperature - Routine blood markers - Inflammatory markers - Hepatic and renal function
ChiCTR2000030173 (China)	Target: $N = NA$	Umbilical cord derived vs. standard care control	- Pulmonary function - nCoV pneumonic nucleic acid test - Pulmonary CT and chest radiography
CHICTR2000030138 (China)	Target: $N = NA$	Umbilical cord derived vs. standard care plus saline injection control	- Clinical index
ChiCTR2000030088 (China)	Target: $N = NA$	Umbilical cord Wharton's jelly derived MSCs at 1×10^6 cells/kg vs. standard care and saline injection control	- nCoV pneumonic nucleic acid test - CT scan of ground glass shadow
CHICTR2000029990; TARGET $N = NA$ (China)	Target: $N = NA$	MSCs (source unknown) vs. standard care and saline injection control	- Respiratory system function (O_2 saturation) recovery time
ChiCTR2000029817 (NA)	Target: $N = NA$	Umbilical cord derived MSCs and NK cells: - High dose group: NK cells and MSCs at $> 5 \times 10^9$; Once every 2 days, five times - Conventional dose group: NK cells and MSCs at $> 3 \times 10^9$; once every 2 days, three times - Preventive dose group: NK cells and MSCs at $> 3 \times 10^9$; one infusion	- Time to disease recovery and time to negative nCoV test - Clearance rate and time of main symptoms - Transfer to ICU time - Routine blood tests - Biochemical indicators - Immune indices
CHICTR2000029816 (NA)	Target: $N = NA$	Umbilical cord derived MSCs (dose not stated) vs. standard care control	- Time to disease recovery and time to negative nCoV test - Clearance rate and time of main symptoms - Transfer to ICU time - Routine blood tests - Biochemical indicators - Immune indices
ChiCTR2000029580 (China)	Target: $N = NA$	Ruxolitinib and MSCs (source and dose not stated) vs. standard care control	- Safety
CHICTR2000029569 (China)	Target: $N = NA$	Umbilical cord derived blood mononuclear cells conditioned medium vs. standard care control	- PSI, CT, and X-Ray - Arterial blood gas - Assisted breathing time - Mortality - Disease evolution - Hospitalization days - Safety outcome index
EUCTR2020-001450-22-ES (Spain)	Target: $N = NA$	Allogenic umbilical cord derived MSCs (dose not stated)	- Mortality - Mechanical ventilation incidence - Need for vasopressors - Safety profile of MSCs - Neutrophils, monocytes and NK cells

(Continued)

TABLE 2 | Continued

Clinical trials number	Participants	MSC source	Outcomes
			PCT, ferritin, D-dimer and hs-troponin - PCR test - B and T lymphocytes - Interleukins, Th1, 2&17, NLRP3, and HMGB1
IRCT20200421047150N1 (Iran)	Target: N = NA	Umbilical card Wharton's jelly derived: three injections at 0.5–1 million cells/kg at 1st, 3rd, and 6th day. Control receiving standard care plus saline injection at 1st, 3rd, and 6th day	- Not stated
ACTRN12620000612910 (Australia)	Target: N = NA	Mesenchymoangioblast derived MSCs (CYP-001) at 2×10^6 cells/kg twice vs. ICU standard care control	- Not stated
NCT04361942 (Spain)	Target: N = 24	Allogenic MSCs (source unknown) vs. placebo (not stated)	- Withdrawal of invasive mechanical ventilation - Mortality - Patients achieving a clinical response - Patients achieving a radiological response
EUCTR2020-001266-11-ES (Spain)	Target: N = 100	Allogenic adipose tissue MSCs	- Efficacy and safety of administration of MSCs - Survival - Temperature - Withdrawal of mechanical ventilation - Patients transitioning to O_2 therapy from mechanical ventilation - O_2 therapy duration - Days in ICU - Duration of hospitalization - PaO_2/FiO_2 - Chest radiology - Routine blood markers - Inflammatory markers - Coagulation markers - Immune markers

Source: https://clinicaltrials.gov/ct2/home and https://trialstreamer.robotreviewer.net/.

hs-CRP, high sensitivity C-reactive protein; IL-, Interleukin-; TNF-α, Tumor necrosis factor-α; SAE, Serious adverse event; HR, Heart rate; RR, Respiratory rate; PCT, Procalcitonin; VEGF, Vascular endothelial growth factor; RTRA, Return to room air; INR, International normalized ratio of blood coagulation; TEAE, treatment emergent serious adverse events; DLT, Dose limiting toxicity; VFD, Ventilator free days; BUN, Blood urea nitrogen; APACHE, Acute physiology and chronic health disease classification; AST, Aspartate aminotransferase; NEWS, National early warning score; LDH, Lactate dehydrogenase; AAT, Alanine aminotransferase; CK, Creatine kinase; TTCl, Time to clinical improvement; LIF, Leukemia inhibiting factor; PEEP, Positive end-expiratory pressure; SOFA, Sequential organ failure assessment; SIT, Small identification test; TnI, Troponin I; AA, Arachidonic acid; EPA, Eicosapentaenoic acid; nCoV, novel coronavirus; Polymerase chain reaction; NK, Natural killer; Th, T helper; NLRP3, NLR Family Pyrin Domain Containing 3; HMGB1, High mobility group box 1.

to myocardial injury, MSC transplantation could offer a cardioprotective role.

MSC TRANSPLANTATION COULD ATTENUATE DAMAGE AND FACILITATE REPAIR OF THE CARDIOVASCULAR SYSTEM SEEN WITH COVID-19

In addition to the potential for MSCs to modulate the immune response and subsequent tissue damage in COVID-19, there is prospect for MSCs to treat the cardiac and cardiovascular effects of the SARS-CoV-2 virus, which may be long-lasting (**Figure 1**). As previously discussed, in a large proportion of patients there is evidence of myocardial injury, as suggested by elevated cTnI and cTnT levels (16, 19, 168, 169), and ventricular dysfunction indicated by raised circulating NT-proBNP (29, 31). Elevated cardiac biomarkers are associated with more severe prognosis and mortality in COVID-19 patients (18, 26, 29, 169, 170), suggesting the cardiac effects of the virus can drive worsening prognosis for the patient. Moreover, there are a number of studies

detailing the severe cardiac effects of the virus, such as the development of heart failure (HF) (28), as well as incidences of acute coronary syndromes (ACS) (171, 172), ischaemic stroke (173) and myocardial infarction (MI) (171, 172). Given the significant deleterious effect of the virus on the myocardium, treatment options to minimize or to alleviate the cardiovascular side effects of the infection and disease are needed.

Treatment with MSCs may offer a clinical benefit to patients due to their regenerative and reparative potential if there is significant myocardial injury and myocardial cell death. There have been a number of studies investigating the use of autologous (174–180) or allogeneic MSCs (178, 181–184) for the treatment of cardiomyopathies and post-MI. Although the use of MSCs to treat cardiovascular dysfunction and damage in COVID-19 patients has yet to be fully elucidated, the studies over the past decade provide good preliminary evidence for researchers and clinicians alike to further investigate the use of this cellular therapy in COVID-19 patient cohorts.

Several studies in pig, rat and mouse models of MI showed significant reduction in infarct size or fibrosis (185–194), and improvements in cardiac function (185–187, 189, 190, 195, 196).

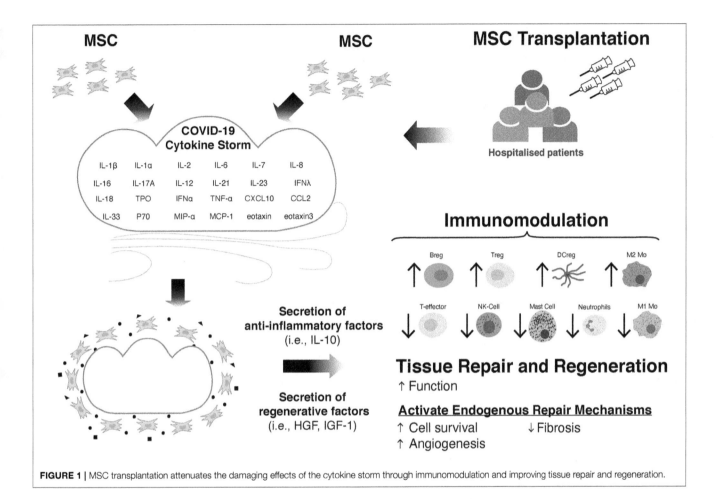

FIGURE 1 | MSC transplantation attenuates the damaging effects of the cytokine storm through immunomodulation and improving tissue repair and regeneration.

A meta-analysis of 52 pre-clinical animal studies of cell therapy for ischaemic heart disease reported that MSC therapy is safe and associated with significant ∼7.5% improvements in LVEF (197). In order to elicit increased efficacy, cell combination therapy has been investigated. In swine models of MI, human bone marrow-derived MSCs and cardiac-derived stromal MSC stem/progenitor cells from autologous or allogeneic sources were co-injected into the border zone of the infarct. Results showed that by combining the cell types there was greater therapeutic efficacy, improving cardiac repair/regeneration and LV functional recovery without adverse immunologic reaction (198, 199).

These promising findings have been followed by a number of human clinical trials. In a number of these human studies, the infusion and transplantation of MSCs have been deemed safe for treating MI patients (179, 200) as well as having been successful in improving some cardiac functional measures post-MI, such as LVEF (175, 177, 200–204), and improving global longitudinal strain measures (201). Penn et al. (204) showed in a phase I clinical trial in patients with first ST-elevation–myocardial infarction (STEMI), delivery of MSCs (MultiStem) using a coronary adventitial delivery system was well-tolerated and safe. In patients who exhibited significant myocardial damage, the delivery of ≥50 million MultiStem resulted in improved EF and

stroke volume 4 months later (204). However, some of these studies, and others, found no difference between MSC treatment and no treatment/placebo on infarct size or perfusion changes in the months following the enrolment to the study (177, 205, 206). Additionally, several human studies fail to observe any clinical benefit for patients (179, 184, 205, 207). Inconsistent findings are likely due to the number and phenotype of MSCs being transplanted, their source, as well as mode and location of administration (myocardial, epicardial, or endocardial injection; systemic transplantation).

Despite mixed findings on the efficacy for improving cardiac function, MSCs can offer potential as regenerative cells for the CV system, where through a paracrine mechanism they activate endogenous repair mechanisms leading to blood vessel growth *via* angiogenesis, improved cardiomyocyte survival, reduced cardiomyocyte reactive hypertrophy, and fibrosis (**Figure 1**). We have clonally derived (from a single cell) a population of stromal cells with multipotent stem/progenitor cell properties from the adult mammalian heart, including human (208–210). These cells produce a repertoire of pro-survival and cardiovascular regenerative growth factors. We administered these cells intracoronary at differential doses (5×10^6, 5×10^7, and 1×10^8) in three groups of white Yorkshire female pigs with MI, 30 min after coronary reperfusion. Pig serum was injected to six control pigs after MI. We found a high degree of cell engraftment in the damaged pig myocardium. By 3 weeks after MI and cell transplantation, there was increased new cardiomyocyte and capillary formation, which was not evident in the control hearts (194). Moreover, cell treatment preserved myocardial wall structure and attenuated remodeling by reducing cardiomyocyte hypertrophy, apoptosis, and scar formation (fibrosis) (211).

In mouse, rat and *in vitro* cell model studies, MSCs have been found to be potently angiogenic (192, 212–221). As outlined previously, MSCs most likely promote angiogenesis *via* paracrine means, such as secretion of angiogenic factors; vascular endothelial growth factor (VEGF), basic fibroblast growth factor (bFGF), transforming growth factor beta (TGF-β), and platelet-derived growth factor (PDGF) (222, 223), which are promoted under hypoxic conditions (224). Proteomic analysis of secreted exosomes, which carry lipids, proteins and genetic material to target tissues, from MSCs reveal several target pathways (225). These include inflammation and angiogenesis, of which, the angiogenesis pathway revealed specific interaction with NF-κ-B signaling. When these exosomes were cultured with HUVECs, a significant increase in endothelial tube formation was detected in a dose-dependent fashion (225). Zhang et al. (226) investigated the potential for MSC-derived exosomes to promote angiogenesis and cardiac repair post-MI in rats. Firstly, they observed that exosomes isolated from MSCs promoted tube formation of cardiac stem/progenitor cells *in vitro*. They subsequently transplanted cardiac stem/progenitor cells internalized with these exosomes into a rat model of MI, and observed an increased capillary density, which was followed by an improvement in LVEF, and reduction in fibrosis after 28 days post-implantation. Interestingly, the source of MSCs can significantly alter their pro-angiogenic potential. Du et al. (219) isolated MSCs from bone marrow, adipose tissue, umbilical cord and placenta and assessed their pro-angiogenic capacity using *in vitro* tube formation assays, as well as endothelial cell proliferation and assessment of angiogenic gene expression by RT-PCR. They found that MSCs isolated from the bone marrow and the placenta promoted angiogenesis *in vitro* to a greater extent than MSCs from adipose tissue and umbilical cord. In addition, they found that MSCs from these sources had a greater expression of VEGF mRNA and protein (219).

As well as promoting angiogenesis, MSCs may promote recovery from cardiac injury/insult by differentiating into mature cardiomyocytes, or by promoting resident cardiomyocyte proliferation. Mesenchymal stromal cells have a broad differentiation capacity, and have been shown to be able to differentiate into osteoblasts (227), neuronal cells (228) as well as upregulate cardiomyocyte markers, such as cardiac myosin heavy chain (229) and troponin T (229, 230). However, several studies have failed to observe significant trans-differentiation of MSCs into either endothelial cells or functional cardiomyocytes (189, 231, 232). Otherwise, MSCs have been found to promote cardiomyocyte DNA synthesis and proliferation, and signal cardiomyocyte gene upregulation (including VEGF, cyclin A2, and TGF-β2) (194, 233). Through their paracrine activity,

they also prevent cardiomyocyte cell apoptosis (188, 221, 234–236) with several studies observing a reduced activation of the caspase-3 pathway in cardiomyocytes exposed to either MSC-derived exosomes (236) or conditioned media (237).

Other methods to maximize cellular function of cell therapies include "priming" which involves promoting expression of certain receptors, proteins and cytokines in the cells prior to transplantation or infusion. Mesenchymal stromal cells primed *in vitro*, prior to *in vivo* administration may offer opportunity to improve the efficacy of MSC treatment. Several studies have shown that by priming these cells *in vitro*, for example to highly express GATA-4 (MSC^{GATA-4}) (238), or CXCR4 (MSC^{CXCR4}) (233, 239) may improve the angiogenic paracrine activity of these cells. Mesenchymal stromal cells which were overexpressing GATA-4 contained more VEGF and IGF-1 protein, which, when blocked with neutralizing antibodies, attenuated the pro-angiogenic activity of MSC^{GATA-4} (238). Moreover, cardiac-derived stem/progenitor cells that express high levels of GATA-4 have shown to foster cardiomyocyte survival through IGF-1 paracrine signaling (240). MSC^{CXCR4} cells themselves were found to be highly angiogenic compared to un-primed MSCs, with greater expression of VEGF, which may partly explain the greater *in vitro* tube formation observed in a study by Zhang et al. (239). CXCR4 over-expression may be beneficial in promoting cell migration to ischaemic tissue due to the ligand stromal-derived factor-1 (SDF-1) (241), which is released in ischaemic tissue (242, 243). Thus, by selecting CXCR4⁺ MSCs, or promoting CXCR4 expression *in vitro*, MSC migration to target infarct or damaged areas may be improved, subsequently allowing the cells to stimulate repair in the area required more efficiently.

Heart tissue damage post-MI, although largely due to ischaemic tissue injury and insult and associated cardiomyocyte loss, is also due to inflammation associated in the hours and days post-MI (244, 245). This inflammatory response is associated with further cardiac tissue damage and injury, as indicated by sustained and continual increases in cTnI and cTnT (246). Indeed MSC exosomes can regulate T-cell proliferation (215) as well as alter the balance between M1 and M2 macrophages in the infarcted heart (191), and the number of neutrophils and NK cells post-MI in the cardiac tissue (244) suggesting strong anti-inflammatory properties of the MSCs. In fact, a study by Luger et al. (244) found that MSC exosomes were able to reduce the number of NK cells in cardiac tissue post-MI, followed by a separate experiment whereby depleting NK cells 24 h prior to MI in mice, reduced the resulting infarct size. These findings infer that NK cells are involved in causing, or significantly contributing to, the cardiac damage resulting from an ischaemic challenge, and that MSCs could attenuate this inflammation. Taken together, it appears that MSCs also promote cardiac recovery *via* attenuating the ongoing inflammatory response, which is also a likely pathway for COVID-19-associated myocardial injury.

Although there is significant promise in the use of MSCs for cellular therapy to treat cardiovascular conditions, their efficacy for use in treating COVID-19-related cardiac dysfunction and injury is yet to be determined.

MSC TRANSPLANTATION IN COVID-19 PATIENTS COULD ALLEVIATE PULMONARY FIBROSIS

Fibrotic disorders in the lung, such as idiopathic pulmonary fibrosis (IPF), share similar comorbidities with COVID-19. Both conditions are progressive in nature, often because of worsening lung injury and fibrosis of alveolar walls. This underscores a common anti-fibrotic strategy.

Clinical trials with anti-fibrotic agents have shown promise in reversing progression of pulmonary fibrosis, as evidenced with nintedanib (247) and pirfenidone (248), which were approved by the FDA more than 6 years ago (249). This is supported by findings from pre-clinical animal models. An animal model of IPF with increased fibrosis and defective clearance of fibrocytes and myofibroblasts, was improved upon treatment with nintedanib (250). However, whether these agents will have clinical efficacy in COVID-19 remains unknown. Notably, commercial anti-fibrotic drugs, such as nintedanib and pirfenidone, are only available for oral delivery. This limits their use in COVID-19 patients, given that the population with fibrotic lung damage are usually hospitalized and intubated. Moreover, the hepatoxic side effects of both drugs and the contraindication of pirfenidone in renal dysfunction further limit their use, especially noting that SARS-CoV-2 is associated with development of both liver and kidney dysfunctions (58, 251). This highlights the need for better therapeutic strategies for lung fibrosis. Novel treatment options, such as cell-based therapy for replenishing lost functional capacity of resident stromal cells, have great potential for patients with COVID-19.

Cell-based therapy has been keenly investigated in the pre-clinical models using bleomycin-induced pulmonary fibrosis. Bleomycin-induced lung injury is a well-characterized model of human pulmonary fibrosis, with an initial phase of inflammatory activation and consequent fibrosis. In mice, intravenous injection of the primary human amniotic epithelial cells (hAECs) reduced lung inflammation and expression of the pro-fibrotic ligand TGF-β1 (252). Human amniotic epithelial cells transplantation also reduced the Ashcroft score, a validated marker of severity of lung fibrosis (253), likely due to increased degradation by matrix metalloproteinase (MMP)-2 and reduced expressions of tissue inhibitors of MMPs (TIMP)-1 and 2 (252). A pooled analysis of pre-clinical evidence demonstrated significantly better results on Ashcroft score and collagen contents for hAECs compared to placebo (254). Much akin to hAECs, MSCs have been shown to ameliorate pulmonary injury induced by bleomycin in experimental models (255). This has been demonstrated for bone marrow, umbilical cord, and amniotic fluid derived MSCs, respectively. The therapeutic efficacy of MSCs is also reported in other models of lung fibrosis. For example, adipose tissue-derived MSCs significantly attenuated lung function and fibrosis in a rodent model of silica-induced lung fibrosis (256). In summary, these data show that MSC-based therapy is a promising tool to address the pathophysiological consequences of COVID-19 in the lung. However, clinical translation would require more refined understanding of the anti-fibrotic mechanisms of MSCs.

Cumulative data show that MSCs protect against fibrosis via hepatocyte growth factor (HGF)-mediated mechanisms. Hepatocyte growth factor was originally identified as a mitogen for hepatocytes. It has now been shown to mediate mitogenic, anti-inflammatory, anti-apoptotic, and regenerative effects during tissue repair. In models of I/R lung injury, transplanted HGF-overexpressed MSCs resulted in lessened oxidative stress, inflammation, and attenuated lung injury (257). Hepatocyte growth factor also prolonged the survival of engrafted MSCs via increased expression of the anti-apoptotic protein Bcl-2 and repression of caspase-3 activation. In the context of fibrosis, there is evidence to suggest that HGF modulates pro-fibrotic pathways. For instance, microvesicles from human Wharton's Jelly MSCs inhibited apoptosis, fibrosis in pulmonary tissues, and activation of PI3K/AKT/mTOR pathway (258). These effects were blocked by using HGF-mRNA-deficient microvesicles or PI3K inhibitor. Hepatocyte growth factor also inhibits alveolar epithelial-to-mesenchymal transition and production of TGF-β1 independent of MSCs (259).

Other pathways have also been implicated in mediating the anti-fibrotic role of MSCs, including the activation of MMP-9 (260), programmed death (PD)-1/PD-L1 (261), and anti-apoptotic Bcl-2 (256, 257). MMP-9 is said to promote the degradation of collagen deposits, thereby facilitating the repair process following lung injury. On the other hand, MSC transplantation has been associated with repressed TGF-β1/SMAD3 (255), Wnt/β-catenin signaling (262), MyD88/TGF-β1 signaling (263), and N-methyl-d-aspartate receptor activity (264). Inhibition of Wnt/β-catenin signaling has a two-fold function. Firstly, it prevents downstream activation of pro-fibrotic genes and development of fibrosis; and, secondly, it rescues lung resident MSCs from differentiating to myofibroblasts (265).

Whether similar benefits will be seen in COVID-19 patients remains to be established. A single center, non-randomized, dose-escalation phase 1b trial of eight patients with moderate-to-severe IPF treated with intravenous bone marrow-derived MSC showed a good short-term safety profile (266). CT fibrosis score did not change 6 months after administration compared to baseline; however, there was no further worsening of fibrosis during follow-up. Similar findings were noted in a larger (randomized) trial of 20 IPF patients treated with high-dose bone marrow-derived MSCs (267). Subsequently, a trial of 61 patients with influenza A (H7N9)-induced ARDS showed significant reduction in the inflammatory marker CRP following menstrual-blood-derived MSC treatment, compared to placebo (163). While treated patients showed linear fibrosis, ground-glass opacity, and pleural thickening on chest CT at baseline, there was improvement in all patients after 24 weeks and up to 1 year after MSC treatment.

Our current understanding of the mechanisms of MSC-mediated improvement in lung (fibrotic) injury is incomplete, especially in the context of COVID-19. There are other important questions that will need to be addressed, too. For instance, would the MSCs need to be primed for improved efficacy? Previous studies have shown that pre-conditioning of MSCs with oncostatin M (268, 269), low-dose TGF-β1 (270), IL-6

(269), or ischaemia (271) improves the survival and therapeutic benefits. Obtaining the best MSCs for transplantation in terms of optimum immunomodulatory capacity and availability should be considered in COVID-19 studies. Primary MSCs, such as those obtained from bone marrow, umbilical cord, or adipose tissue, are limited by lack of available donors, many lack standardized preparations, with variations in quality, limited regenerative capacity, and finite lifespans. To overcome these limitations, a recent study investigated a novel hESC-derived MSC-like cell population, termed Immunity-and Matrix-Regulatory Cells (IMRCs) (272). Produced to good manufacturing standards, IMRCs demonstrated excellent safety and efficacy profiles in *in vivo* models of mice and monkeys. Additionally, IMRCs demonstrated superior immunomodulatory effects compared to umbilical cord-derived MSCs and the anti-fibrotic agent, pirfenidone (272).

CONCLUSION

Evidence now supports severe COVID-19 being associated with a dysregulated and hyperactive inflammatory systemic response; a cytokine storm. Older people (>60 years) and people with co-morbidities are more likely to develop a dysfunctional immune response, and resultant cytokine storm, that causes pathology and fails to successfully eradicate the pathogen. The exact reasons for this are unclear, although one reason may be a decline in immune function with age and chronic sterile inflammation due

to the build-up of senescent cells and immunosenescence in aging humans (273).

The manifestations of elevated pro-inflammatory, sustained circulating factors due to the cytokine storm are not just confined to the lungs, with significant damage to the CV system and multi-organ damage and dysfunction. Interventions that target single cytokines (i.e., Tocilizumab targeting IL-6) do not seem efficacious in reducing mortality. Mesenchymal stromal cells owing to their powerful immunomodulatory function can holistically target and suppress the cytokine storm. At the same time, MSC transplantation is safe and has proven effective at activating endogenous repair mechanisms, leading to improved cardiac function, tissue regeneration and decreased fibrosis. Therefore, attenuating persistent organ dysfunction. Further mechanistic studies are required to investigate if MSC therapy can alleviate the cardiovascular consequences of COVID-19, and thus reduce cardiovascular risk in these patients. Work should also focus on determining the optimal dose, timing of injections (multiple dosing at different stages of the disease), systemic distribution of transplanted cells, type of MSCs used or use of exosomes, and the anti-viral effects of MSC transplantation.

AUTHOR CONTRIBUTIONS

LC put together the tables. TA put together the figure. GE-H oversaw the completion of the article. All authors contributed to writing the article.

REFERENCES

1. Rosenwald SM. History's deadliest pandemics, from ancient Rome to modern America | The Spokesman-Review. *The Spokesman-Review.* (2020) Available online at: https://www.spokesman.com/stories/2020/apr/15/historys-deadliest-pandemics-from-ancient-rome-to-/ (accessed August 23, 2020).

2. Gagnon A, Miller MS, Hallman SA, Bourbeau R, Herring DA, Earn DJD, et al. Age-specific mortality during the 1918 influenza pandemic: unravelling the mystery of high young adult mortality. *PLoS ONE.* (2013) 8:e69586. doi: 10.1371/journal.pone.0069586

3. Morens DM, Fauci AS. The 1918 influenza pandemic: insights for the 21st century. *J Infect Dis.* (2007) 195:1018–28. doi: 10.1086/511989

4. Yan R, Zhang Y, Li Y, Xia L, Guo Y, Zhou Q. Structural basis for the recognition of SARS-CoV-2 by full-length human ACE2. *Science.* (2020) 367:1444–8. doi: 10.1126/science.abb2762

5. Hoffmann M, Kleine-Weber H, Schroeder S, Mü MA, Drosten C, Pö S. SARS-CoV-2 cell entry depends on ACE2 and TMPRSS2 and is blocked by a clinically proven protease inhibitor. *Cell.* (2020) 181:271–80.e8. doi: 10.1016/j.cell.2020.02.052

6. Aimes TR, Zijlstra A, Hooper DJ, Ogbourne MS, Sit M-L, Fuchs S, et al. Endothelial cell serine proteases expressed during vascular morphogenesis and angiogenesis. *Thombosis Haemost.* (2003) 89:561–72. doi: 10.1055/s-0037-1613388

7. Pan X-W, Xu D, Zhang H, Zhou W, Wang L-H, Cui X-G. Identification of a potential mechanism of acute kidney injury during the COVID-19 outbreak: a study based on single-cell transcriptome analysis. *Intensive Care Med.* (2020) 46:1114–6. doi: 10.1007/s00134-020-06026-1

8. Sungnak W, Huang N, Bécavin C, Berg M, Queen R, Litvinukova M, et al. SARS-CoV-2 entry factors are highly expressed in nasal epithelial cells together with innate immune genes. *Nat Med.* (2020) 26:681–7. doi: 10.1038/s41591-020-0868-6

9. Chen L, Li X, Chen M, Feng Y, Xiong C. The ACE2 expression in human heart indicates new potential mechanism of heart injury among patients infected with SARS-CoV-2. *Eur Soc Cardiol.* (2020) 116:1097–100. doi: 10.1093/cvr/cvaa078

10. Meselson M. Droplets and aerosols in the transmission of SARS-CoV-2. *N Engl J Med.* (2020) 382:2063. doi: 10.1056/NEJMc2009324

11. Huang C, Wang Y, Li X, Ren L, Zhao J, Hu Y, et al. Clinical features of patients infected with 2019 novel coronavirus in Wuhan, China. *Lancet.* (2020) 395:497–506. doi: 10.1016/S0140-6736(20)30183-5

12. Kaye R, Chang CWD, Kazahaya K, Brereton J, Denneny JC. COVID-19 anosmia reporting tool: initial findings. *Otolaryngol Head Neck Surg (United States).* (2020) 163:132–4. doi: 10.1177/0194599820922992

13. Weiss ARR, Dahlke MH. Immunomodulation by mesenchymal stem cells (MSCs): mechanisms of action of living, apoptotic, and dead MSCs. *Front Immunol.* (2019) 10:1191. doi: 10.3389/fimmu.2019.01191

14. Golchin A, Seyedjafari E, Ardeshirylajimi A. Mesenchymal stem cell therapy for COVID-19: present or future. *Stem Cell Rev Rep.* (2020) 16:427–33. doi: 10.1007/s12015-020-09973-w

15. Golchin A, Farahany TZ, Khojasteh A, Soleimanifar F, Ardeshirylajimi A. The clinical trials of mesenchymal stem cell therapy in skin diseases: an update and concise review. *Curr Stem Cell Res Ther.* (2018) 14:22–33. doi: 10.2174/1574888x13666180913123424

16. Zhou F, Yu T, Du R, Fan G, Liu Y, Liu Z, et al. Clinical course and risk factors for mortality of adult inpatients with COVID-19 in Wuhan, China: a retrospective cohort study. *Lancet.* (2020) 395:1054–62. doi: 10.1016/S0140-6736(20)30566-3

17. Grasselli G, Zangrillo A, Zanella A, Antonelli M, Cabrini L, Castelli A, et al. Baseline characteristics and outcomes of 1591 patients infected with SARS-CoV-2 admitted to ICUs of the Lombardy Region, Italy. *JAMA.* (2020) 323:1574–81. doi: 10.1001/jama.2020.5394

18. Shi S, Qin M, Shen B, Cai Y, Liu T, Yang F, et al. Association of cardiac injury with mortality in hospitalized patients with COVID-19 in

Wuhan, China. *JAMA Cardiol.* (2020) 5:802–10. doi: 10.1001/jamacardio.2020.0950

19. Wang D, Hu B, Hu C, Zhu F, Liu X, Zhang J, et al. Clinical characteristics of 138 hospitalized patients with 2019 novel coronavirus-infected pneumonia in Wuhan, China. *JAMA.* (2020) 323:1061–9. doi: 10.1001/jama.2020.1585

20. Léonard-Lorant I, Delabranche X, Séverac F, Helms J, Pauzet C, Collange O, et al. Acute pulmonary embolism in patients with COVID-19 at CT angiography and relationship to d-Dimer levels. *Radiology.* (2020) 296:E189–91. doi: 10.1148/radiol.2020201561

21. Poissy J, Goutay J, Caplan M, Parmentier E, Duburcq T, Lassalle F, et al. Pulmonary embolism in patients with COVID-19: awareness of an increased prevalence. *Circulation.* (2020) 142:184–6. doi: 10.1161/CIRCULATIONAHA.120.047430

22. Sala S, Peretto G, Gramegna M, Palmisano A, Villatore A, Vignale D, et al. Acute myocarditis presenting as a reverse Tako-Tsubo syndrome in a patient with SARS-CoV-2 respiratory infection. *Eur Heart J.* (2020) 41:1861–2. doi: 10.1093/eurheartj/ehaa286

23. Kim IC, Kim JY, Kim HA, Han S. COVID-19-related myocarditis in a 21-year-old female patient. *Eur Heart J.* (2020) 41:1859. doi: 10.1093/eurheartj/ehaa288

24. Clerkin KJ, Fried JA, Raikhelkar J, Sayer G, Griffin JM, Masoumi A, et al. COVID-19 and cardiovascular disease. *Circulation.* (2020) 141:1648–55. doi: 10.1161/CIRCULATIONAHA.120.046941

25. Roberts KA, Colley L, Agbaedeng TA, Ellison-Hughes GM, Ross MD. Vascular manifestations of COVID-19—thromboembolism and microvascular dysfunction. *Front Cardiovasc Med.* (2020) 7:598400. doi: 10.3389/fcvm.2020.598400

26. Deng Q, Hu B, Zhang Y, Wang H, Zhou X, Hu W, et al. Suspected myocardial injury in patients with COVID-19: evidence from front-line clinical observation in Wuhan, China. *Int J Cardiol.* (2020) 311:116–21. doi: 10.1016/j.ijcard.2020.03.087

27. Santoso A, Pranata R, Wibowo A, Al-Farabi MJ, Huang I, Antariksa B. Cardiac injury is associated with mortality and critically ill pneumonia in COVID-19: a meta-analysis. *Am J Emerg Med.* (in press). doi: 10.1016/j.ajem.2020.04.052

28. Chen T, Wu D, Chen H, Yan W, Yang D, Chen G, et al. Clinical characteristics of 113 deceased patients with coronavirus disease 2019: retrospective study. *BMJ.* (2020) 368:m1091. doi: 10.1136/bmj.m1091

29. Guo T, Fan Y, Chen M, Wu X, Zhang L, He T, et al. Cardiovascular implications of fatal outcomes of patients with coronavirus disease 2019 (COVID-19). *JAMA Cardiol.* (2020) 5:811–8. doi: 10.1001/jamacardio.2020.1017

30. Guan W, Ni Z, Hu Y, Liang W, Ou C, He J, et al. Clinical characteristics of coronavirus disease 2019 in China. *N Engl J Med.* (2020) 382:1708–20. doi: 10.1056/NEJMoa2002032

31. Han H, Xie L, Liu R, Yang J, Liu F, Wu K, et al. Analysis of heart injury laboratory parameters in 273 COVID-19 patients in one hospital in Wuhan, China. *J Med Virol.* (2020) 92:819–23. doi: 10.1002/jmv.25809

32. Danzi GB, Loffi M, Galeazzi G, Gherbesi E. Acute pulmonary embolism and COVID-19 pneumonia: a random association? *Eur Heart J.* (2020) 41:1858. doi: 10.1093/eurheartj/ehaa254

33. Tay MZ, Poh CM, Rénia L, MacAry PA, Ng LFP. The trinity of COVID-19: immunity, inflammation and intervention. *Nat Rev Immunol.* (2020) 20:363–74. doi: 10.1038/s41577-020-0311-8

34. Merad M, Martin JC. Pathological inflammation in patients with COVID-19: a key role for monocytes and macrophages. *Nat Rev Immunol.* (2020) 20:355–62. doi: 10.1038/s41577-020-0331-4

35. Ferrara JLM, Abhyankar S, Gilliland DG. Cytokine storm of graft-versus-host disease: a critical effector role for interleukin-1. *Transpl Proc.* (1993) 56:1518–23. doi: 10.1097/00007890-199312000-00045

36. Yuen K, Wong S. Human infection by avian influenza A H5N1. *Hong Kong Med.* (2005) 11:189–199.

37. Noroozi R, Branicki W, Pyrc K, Łabaj PP, Pospiech E, Taheri M, et al. Altered cytokine levels and immune responses in patients with SARS-CoV-2 infection and related conditions. *Cytokine.* (2020) 133:155143. doi: 10.1016/j.cyto.2020.155143

38. Blanco-Melo D, Nilsson-Payant BE, Liu W-C, Lim JK, Albrecht RA, Tenoever BR. Imbalanced host response to SARS-CoV-2 drives development of COVID-19. *Cell.* (2020) 181:1036–45. doi: 10.1016/j.cell.2020.04.026

39. Chen G, Wu D, Guo W, Cao Y, Huang D, Wang H, et al. Clinical and immunological features of severe and moderate coronavirus disease 2019. *J Clin Invest.* (2020) 130:2620–9. doi: 10.1172/JCI137244

40. Liu J, Li S, Liu J, Liang B, Wang X, Wang H, et al. Longitudinal characteristics of lymphocyte responses and cytokine profiles in the peripheral blood of SARS-CoV-2 infected patients. *EBioMedicine.* (2020) 55:102763. doi: 10.1016/j.ebiom.2020.102763

41. Del Valle DM, Kim-Schulze S, Hsin-Hui H, Beckmann ND, Nirenberg S, Wang B, et al. An inflammatory cytokine signature helps predict COVID-19 severity and death. *medRxiv Prepr Serv Heal Sci. [Preprint]* (2020). doi: 10.1101/2020.05.28.20115758

42. Lucas C, Wong P, Klein J, Castro TBR, Silva J, Sundaram M, et al. Longitudinal analyses reveal immunological misfiring in severe COVID-19. *Nature.* (2020) 584:463. doi: 10.1038/s41586-020-2588-y

43. Laing AG, Lorenc A, Del Molino Del Barrio I, Das A, Fish M, Monin L, et al. A dynamic COVID-19 immune signature includes associations with poor prognosis. *Nat Med.* (2020) 26:1–13. doi: 10.1038/s41591-020-1038-6

44. Guo C, Li B, Ma H, Wang X, Cai P, Yu Q, et al. Single-cell analysis of two severe COVID-19 patients reveals a monocyte-associated and tocilizumab-responding cytokine storm. *Nat Commun.* (2020) 11:1–11. doi: 10.1038/s41467-020-17834-w

45. Mehta P, McAuley DF, Brown M, Sanchez E, Tattersall RS, Manson JJ. COVID-19: consider cytokine storm syndromes and immunosuppression. *Lancet.* (2020) 395:1033–4. doi: 10.1016/S0140-6736(20)30628-0

46. Pedersen SF, Ho YC. SARS-CoV-2: a storm is raging. *J Clin Invest.* (2020) 130:2202–5. doi: 10.1172/JCI137647

47. Ruan Q, Yang K, Wang W, Jiang L, Song J. Clinical predictors of mortality due to COVID-19 based on an analysis of data of 150 patients from Wuhan, China. *Intensive Care Med.* (2020) 46:846–8. doi: 10.1007/s00134-020-05991-x

48. Aggarwal NR, King LS, D'Alessio FR. Diverse macrophage populations mediate acute lung inflammation and resolution. *Am J Physiol Lung Cell Mol Physiol.* (2014) 306:709–25. doi: 10.1152/ajplung.00341.2013

49. D'Alessio FR, Tsushima K, Aggarwal NR, West EE, Willett MH, Britos MF, et al. CD4$^+$CD25$^+$Foxp3$^+$ tregs resolve experimental lung injury in mice and are present in humans with acute lung injury. *J Clin Invest.* (2009) 119:2898–913. doi: 10.1172/JCI36498

50. Geiser T, Atabai K, Jarreau P-H, Ware BL, Pugin JR, Matthay AM. Pulmonary edema fluid from patients with acute lung injury augments *in vitro* alveolar epithelial repair by an IL-1b-dependent mechanism. *Am J Respir Crit Care Med.* (2001) 163:1384–8. doi: 10.1164/ajrccm.163.6.2006131

51. Han S, Mallampalli RK. The acute respiratory distress syndrome: from mechanism to translation. *J Immunol.* (2015) 194:855–60. doi: 10.4049/jimmunol.1402513

52. Hu X, Chakravarty SD, Ivashkiv LB. Regulation of interferon and toll-like receptor signaling during macrophage activation by opposing feedforward and feedback inhibition mechanisms. *Immunol Rev.* (2008) 226:41–56. doi: 10.1111/j.1600-065X.2008.00707.x

53. Risitano AM, Mastellos DC, Huber-Lang M, Yancopoulou D, Garlanda C, Ciceri F, et al. Complement as a target in COVID-19? *Nat Rev Immunol.* (2020) 20:343–4. doi: 10.1038/s41577-020-0320-7

54. Xu H, Zhong L, Deng J, Peng J, Dan H, Zeng X, et al. High expression of ACE2 receptor of 2019-nCoV on the epithelial cells of oral mucosa. *Int J Oral Sci.* (2020) 12:1–5. doi: 10.1038/s41368-020-0074-x

55. Arentz M, Yim E, Klaff L, Lokhandwala S, Riedo FX, Chong M, et al. Characteristics and outcomes of 21 critically ill patients with COVID-19 in Washington State. *JAMA.* (2020) 323:1612–4. doi: 10.1001/jama.2020.4326

56. Chen N, Zhou M, Dong X, Qu J, Gong F, Han Y, et al. Epidemiological and clinical characteristics of 99 cases of 2019 novel coronavirus pneumonia in Wuhan, China: a descriptive study. *Lancet.* (2020) 395:507–13. doi: 10.1016/S0140-6736(20)30211-7

57. Wong SH, Lui RNS, Sung JJY. Covid-19 and the digestive system. *J Gastroenterol Hepatol.* (2020) 35:744–8. doi: 10.1111/jgh.15047

58. Zhang C, Shi L, Wang FS. Liver injury in COVID-19: management and challenges. *Lancet Gastroenterol Hepatol.* (2020) 5:428–30. doi: 10.1016/S2468-1253(20)30057-1

59. Jin X, Lian JS, Hu JH, Gao J, Zheng L, Zhang YM, et al. Epidemiological, clinical and virological characteristics of 74 cases of coronavirus-infected disease 2019 (COVID-19) with gastrointestinal symptoms. *Gut.* (2020) 69:1002–9. doi: 10.1136/gutjnl-2020-320926

60. Zhou Z, Zhao N, Shu Y, Han S, Chen B, Shu X. Effect of gastrointestinal symptoms in patients with COVID-19. *Gastroenterology.* (2020) 158:2294–7. doi: 10.1053/j.gastro.2020.03.020

61. Mao L, Jin H, Wang M, Hu Y, Chen S, He Q, et al. Neurologic manifestations of hospitalized patients with coronavirus disease 2019 in Wuhan, China. *JAMA Neurol.* (2020) 77:683–90. doi: 10.1001/jamaneurol.2020.1127

62. Varatharaj A, Thomas N, Ellul M, Davies NW, Pollak T, Tenorio EL, et al. UK-wide surveillance of neurological and neuropsychiatric complications of COVID-19: the first 153 patients. *SSRN Electron J [Preprint].* (2020). doi: 10.2139/ssrn.3601761

63. Varga Z, Flammer AJ, Steiger P, Haberecker M, Andermatt R, Zinkernagel AS, et al. Endothelial cell infection and endotheliitis in COVID-19. *Lancet.* (2020) 395:1417–8. doi: 10.1016/S0140-6736(20)30937-5

64. Jacobs JL, Coyne CB. Mechanisms of MAVS regulation at the mitochondrial membrane. *J Mol Biol.* (2013) 425:5009–19. doi: 10.1016/j.jmb.2013.10.007

65. Rongvaux A. Innate immunity and tolerance toward mitochondria. *Mitochondrion.* (2018) 41:14–20. doi: 10.1016/j.mito.2017.10.007

66. Karan KR, Trumpff C, McGill MA, Thomas JE, Sturm G, Lauriola V, et al. Mitochondrial respiratory capacity modulates LPS-induced inflammatory signatures in human blood. *Brain Behav Immun Heal.* (2020) 5:1–12. doi: 10.1016/j.bbih.2020.100080

67. Kawai T, Akira S. Antiviral signaling through pattern recognition receptors. *J Biochem.* (2007) 141:137–45. doi: 10.1093/jb/mvm032

68. Gordon DE, Jang GM, Bouhaddou M, Xu J, Obernier K, White KM, et al. A SARS-CoV-2 protein interaction map reveals targets for drug repurposing. *Nature.* (2020) 583:459–68. doi: 10.1038/s41586-020-2286-9

69. Shi C-S, Qi H-Y, Boularan C, Huang N-N, Abu-Asab M, Shelhamer JH, et al. SARS-coronavirus open reading frame-9b suppresses innate immunity by targeting mitochondria and the MAVS/TRAF3/TRAF6 signalosome. *J Immunol.* (2014) 193:3080–9. doi: 10.4049/jimmunol.1303196

70. Spiegel M, Pichlmair A, Martínez-Sobrido L, Cros J, García-Sastre A, Haller O, et al. Inhibition of beta interferon induction by severe acute respiratory syndrome coronavirus suggests a two-step model for activation of interferon regulatory factor 3. *J Virol.* (2005) 79:2079–86. doi: 10.1128/jvi.79.4.2079-2086.2005

71. West AP, Khoury-Hanold W, Staron M, Tal MC, Pineda CM, Lang SM, et al. Mitochondrial DNA stress primes the antiviral innate immune response. *Nature.* (2015) 520:553–7. doi: 10.1038/nature14156

72. Arnoult D, Soares F, Tattoli I, Castanier C, Philipott D, Girardi ES. An N-terminal addressing sequence targets NLRX1 to the mitochondrial matrix. *J Cell Sci.* (2009) 122:3161–8. doi: 10.1242/jcs.051193

73. Breda CN de S, Davanzo GG, Basso PJ, Saraiva Câmara NO, Moraes-Vieira PMM. Mitochondria as central hub of the immune system. *Redox Biol.* (2019) 26:101255. doi: 10.1016/j.redox.2019.101255

74. Fève B, Bastard J-P. The role of interleukins in insulin resistance and type 2 diabetes mellitus. *Nat Rev Endocrinol.* (2009) 5:305–11. doi: 10.1038/nrendo.2009.62

75. Zhu L, She ZG, Cheng X, Qin JJ, Zhang XJ, Cai J, et al. Association of blood glucose control and outcomes in patients with COVID-19 and pre-existing type 2 diabetes. *Cell Metab.* (2020) 31:1068–77.e3. doi: 10.1016/j.cmet.2020.04.021

76. Codo AC, Davanzo GG, Monteiro L de B, de Souza GF, Muraro SP, Virgilio-da-Silva JV, et al. Elevated glucose levels favor SARS-CoV-2 infection and monocyte response through a HIF-1α/glycolysis-dependent axis. *Cell Metab.* (2020) 32:437–46.e5. doi: 10.1016/j.cmet.2020.07.007

77. Remels AHV, Derks WJA, Cillero-Pastor B, Verhees KJP, Kelders MC, Heggermont W, et al. NF-κB-mediated metabolic remodelling in the inflamed heart in acute viral myocarditis. *Biochim Biophys Acta Mol Basis Dis.* (2018) 1864:2579–89. doi: 10.1016/j.bbadis.2018.04.022

78. Al-Huseini I, Harada M, Nishi K, Nguyen-Tien D, Kimura T, Ashida N. Improvement of insulin signalling rescues inflammatory cardiac dysfunction. *Sci Rep.* (2019) 9:1–13. doi: 10.1038/s41598-019-51304-8

79. Chen C, Zhou Y, Wang DW. SARS-CoV-2: a potential novel etiology of fulminant myocarditis. *Herz.* (2020) 45:230–2. doi: 10.1007/s00059-020-04909-z

80. Fried JA, Ramasubbu K, Bhatt R, Topkara VK, Clerkin KJ, Horn E, et al. The variety of cardiovascular presentations of COVID-19. *Circulation.* (2020) 141:1930–6. doi: 10.1161/CIRCULATIONAHA.120.047164

81. He J, Wu B, Chen Y, Tang J, Liu Q, Zhou S, et al. Characteristic electrocardiographic manifestations in patients with COVID-19. *Can J Cardiol.* (2020) 36:966.e1–e4. doi: 10.1016/j.cjca.2020.03.028

82. Hu H, Ma F, Wei X, Fang Y. Coronavirus fulminant myocarditis treated with glucocorticoid and human immunoglobulin. *Eur Heart J.* (2020) ehaa190. doi: 10.1093/eurheartj/ehaa190

83. Hua A, O'gallagher K, Sado D, Byrne J. Life-threatening cardiac tamponade complicating myo-pericarditis in COVID-19. *Eur Heart J.* (2020) 41:2130. doi: 10.1093/eurheartj/ehaa253

84. Inciardi RM, Lupi L, Zaccone G, Italia L, Raffo M, Tomasoni D, et al. Cardiac involvement in a patient with coronavirus disease 2019 (COVID-19). *JAMA Cardiol.* (2020) 5:819–24. doi: 10.1001/jamacardio.2020.1096

85. Tavazzi G, Pellegrini C, Maurelli M, Belliato M, Sciutti F, Bottazzi A, et al. Myocardial localization of coronavirus in COVID-19 cardiogenic shock. *Eur J Heart Fail.* (2020) 22:911–5. doi: 10.1002/ejhf.1828

86. Liu Y, Yang Y, Zhang C, Huang F, Wang F, Yuan J, et al. Clinical and biochemical indexes from 2019-nCoV infected patients linked to viral loads and lung injury. *Sci China Life Sci.* (2020) 63:364–74. doi: 10.1007/s11427-020-1643-8

87. Magro C, Mulvey JJ, Berlin D, Nuovo G, Salvatore S, Harp J, et al. Complement associated microvascular injury and thrombosis in the pathogenesis of severe COVID-19 infection: a report of five cases. *Transl Res.* (2020) 220:1–13. doi: 10.1016/j.trsl.2020.04.007

88. Middleton EA, He XY, Denorme F, Campbell RA, Ng D, Salvatore SP, et al. Neutrophil extracellular traps contribute to immunothrombosis in COVID-19 acute respiratory distress syndrome. *Blood.* (2020) 136:1169–79. doi: 10.1182/blood.2020007008

89. Li G, Fan Y, Lai Y, Han T, Li Z, Zhou P, et al. Coronavirus infections and immune responses. *J Med Virol.* (2020) 92:424–32. doi: 10.1002/jmv.25685

90. Warnatsch A, Ioannou M, Wang Q, Papayannopoulos V. Neutrophil extracellular traps license macrophages for cytokine production in atherosclerosis. *Science.* (2015) 349:316–20. doi: 10.1126/science.aaa8064

91. Barnes BJ, Adrover JM, Baxter-Stoltzfus A, Borczuk A, Cools-Lartigue J, Crawford JM, et al. Targeting potential drivers of COVID-19: neutrophil extracellular traps. *J Exp Med.* (2020) 217:e20200652. doi: 10.1084/jem.20200652

92. Mold C, Morris CA. Complement activation by apoptotic endothelial cells following hypoxia/reoxygenation. *Immunology.* (2001) 102:359–64. doi: 10.1046/j.1365-2567.2001.01192.x

93. Irabien-Ortiz Á, Carreras-Mora J, Sionis A, Pàmies J, Montiel J, Tauron M. Fulminant myocarditis due to COVID-19. *Rev Española Cardiol (English Ed).* (2020) 73:503–4. doi: 10.1016/j.rec.2020.04.005

94. Ackermann M, Verleden SE, Kuehnel M, Haverich A, Welte T, Laenger F, et al. Pulmonary vascular endothelialitis, thrombosis, and angiogenesis in Covid-19. *N Engl J Med.* (2020) 383:120–8. doi: 10.1056/NEJMoa2015432

95. Teuwen L-A, Geldhof V, Pasut A, Carmeliet P. COVID-19: the vasculature unleashed. *Nat Rev Immunol.* (2020) 20:389–91. doi: 10.1038/s41577-020-0343-0

96. Incalza MA, Perrini S. Oxidative stress and reactive oxygen species in endothelial dysfunction associated with cardiovascular and metabolic diseases. *Vascul Pharmacol.* (2017) 100:1–19. doi: 10.1016/j.vph.2017.05.005

97. Liu PP, Blet A, Smyth D, Li H. The science underlying COVID-19 implications for the cardiovascular system. *Circulation.* (2020) 142:68–78. doi: 10.1161/CIRCULATIONAHA.120.047549

98. Pober JS, Sessa WC. Evolving functions of endothelial cells in inflammation. *Nat Rev Immunol.* (2007) 7:803–15. doi: 10.1038/nri2171

99. Tang N, Bai H, Chen X, Gong J, Li D, Sun Z. Anticoagulant treatment is associated with decreased mortality in severe coronavirus disease

2019 patients with coagulopathy. *J Thromb Haemost.* (2020) 18:1094–9. doi: 10.1111/jth.14817

100. Paria BC, Vogel SM, Ahmmed GU, Alamgir S, Shroff J, Malik AB, et al. Tumor necrosis factor-α-induced TRPC1 expression amplifies store-operated Ca2+ influx and endothelial permeability. *Am J Physiol Lung Cell Mol Physiol.* (2004) 287:1303–13. doi: 10.1152/ajplung.00240.2004

101. Vandenbroucke E, Mehta D, Minshall R, Malik AB. Regulation of endothelial junctional permeability. *Ann N Y Acad Sci.* (2008) 1123:134–45. doi: 10.1196/annals.1420.016

102. Sandoval R, Malik AB, Minshall RD, Kouklis P, Ellis CA, Tiruppathi C. Ca2+ signalling and PKCα activate increased endothelial permeability by disassembly of VE-cadherin junctions. *J Physiol.* (2001) 533:433–45. doi: 10.1111/j.1469-7793.2001.0433a.x

103. Petrache I, Birukova A, Ramirez SI, Garcia JGN, Verin AD. The role of the microtubules in tumor necrosis factor-induced endothelial cell permeability. *Am J Respir Cell Mol Biol.* (2003) 28:574–81. doi: 10.1165/rcmb.2002-0075OC

104. Tinsley JH, Hunter FA, Childs EW. PKC and MLCK-dependent, cytokine-induced rat coronary endothelial dysfunction. *J Surg Res.* (2009) 152:76–83. doi: 10.1016/j.jss.2008.02.022

105. Wu Z, McGoogan JM. Characteristics of and important lessons from the coronavirus disease 2019 (COVID-19) outbreak in China: summary of a report of 72314 cases from the Chinese center for disease control and prevention. *JAMA.* (2020) 323:1239–42. doi: 10.1001/jama.2020.2648

106. Styp-Rekowska B, Hlushchuk R, Pries AR, Djonov V. Intussusceptive angiogenesis: pillars against the blood flow. *Acta Physiol.* (2011) 202:213–23. doi: 10.1111/j.1748-1716.2011.02321.x

107. Mentzer, SJ, Konerding, MA. Intussusceptive angiogenesis: expansion and remodeling of microvascular networks. *Angiogenesis* (2014) 17:499–509. doi: 10.1007/s10456-014-9428-3

108. Konerding MA, Turhan A, Ravnic DJ, Lin M, Fuchs C, Secomb TW, et al. Inflammation-induced intussusceptive angiogenesis in murine colitis. *Anat Rec.* (2010) 293:849–57. doi: 10.1002/ar.21110

109. Ackermann M, Stark H, Neubert L, Schubert S, Borchert P, Linz F, et al. Morphomolecular motifs of pulmonary neoangiogenesis in interstitial lung diseases. *Eur Respir J.* (2020) 55:1900933. doi: 10.1183/13993003.00933-2019

110. García-Ruiz C, Colell A, Marí M, Morales A, Fernández-Checa JC. Direct effect of ceramide on the mitochondrial electron transport chain leads to generation of reactive oxygen species: role of mitochondrial glutathione. *J Biol Chem.* (1997) 272:11369–77. doi: 10.1074/jbc.272.17.11369

111. Zhang D, Yi F-X, Zou A-P, Li P-L. Role of ceramide in TNF-α-induced impairment of endothelium-dependent vasorelaxation in coronary arteries. *Am J Physiol Circ Physiol.* (2002) 283:H1785–94. doi: 10.1152/ajpheart.00318.2002

112. Frey RS, Rahman A, Kefer JC, Minshall RD, Malik AB. PKCζ regulates TNF-α-induced activation of NADPH oxidase in endothelial cells. *Circ Res.* (2002) 90:1012–9. doi: 10.1161/01.RES.0000017631.28815.8E

113. Wu F, Schuster DP, Tyml K, Wilson JX. Ascorbate inhibits NADPH oxidase subunit p47phox expression in microvascular endothelial cells. *Free Radic Biol Med.* (2007) 42:124–31. doi: 10.1016/j.freeradbiomed.2006.10.033

114. Liaudet L, Vassalli G, Pacher P. Role of peroxynitrite in the redox regulation of cell signal transduction pathways. *Front Biosci.* (2009) 14:4809–14. doi: 10.2741/3569

115. Radi R. *Nitric Oxide, Oxidants, and Protein Tyrosine Nitration.* (2004). Available online at: www.pnas.orgcgidoi10.1073pnas.0307446101 (accessed August 5, 2020).

116. Schulz E, Gori T, Münzel T. Oxidative stress and endothelial dysfunction in hypertension. *Hypertens Res.* (2011) 34:665–73. doi: 10.1038/hr.2011.39

117. Landmesser U, Spiekermann S, Dikalov S, Tatge H, Wilke R, Kohler C, et al. Vascular oxidative stress and endothelial dysfunction in patients with chronic heart failure. *Circulation.* (2002) 106:3073–8. doi: 10.1161/01.CIR.0000041431.57222.AF

118. Naik E, Dixit VM. Mitochondrial reactive oxygen species drive proinflammatory cytokine production. *J Exp Med.* (2011) 208:417–20. doi: 10.1084/jem.20110367

119. Browner NC, Sellak H, Lincoln TM. Downregulation of cGMP-dependent protein kinase expression by inflammatory cytokines in vascular smooth muscle cells. *Am J Physiol Cell Physiol.* (2004) 287:88–96. doi: 10.1152/ajpcell.00039.2004.-NO

120. Hiroki J, Shimokawa H, Higashi M, Morikawa K, Kandabashi T, Kawamura N, et al. Inflammatory stimuli upregulate Rho-kinase in human coronary vascular smooth muscle cells. *J Mol Cell Cardiol.* (2004) 37:537–46. doi: 10.1016/j.yjmcc.2004.05.008

121. Cheng H, Wang Y, Wang G. Organ-protective effect of angiotensin-converting enzyme 2 and its effect on the prognosis of COVID-19. *J Med Virol.* (2020) 92:726–30. doi: 10.1002/jmv.25785

122. Yan C, Yu H, Huang M, Li J, Zhang X, Han Y. Tumor necrosis factor-α promote permeability of human umbilical vein endothelial cells *via* activating RhoA-ERK1/2 pathway. *Zhonghua Xin Xue Guan Bing Za Zhi.* (2011) 39:531–7.

123. Goshua G, Pine AB, Meizlish ML, Chang C, Zhang H, Bahel P, et al. Articles Endotheliopathy in COVID-19-associated coagulopathy: evidence from a single-centre, cross-sectional study. *Lancet Haematol.* (2020) 3026:1–8. doi: 10.1016/S2352-3026(20)30216-7

124. Orr AW, Hastings NE, Blackman BR, Wamhoff BR. Complex regulation and function of the inflammatory smooth muscle cell phenotype in atherosclerosis. *J Vasc Res.* (2010) 47:168–80. doi: 10.1159/000250095

125. Jung YD, Fan F, McConkey DJ, Jean ME, Liu W, Reinmuth N, et al. Role of P38 MAPK, AP-1, and NF-κb in interleukin-1β-induced IL-8 expression in human vascular smooth muscle cells. *Cytokine.* (2002) 18:206–13. doi: 10.1006/cyto.2002.1034

126. Krown KA, Page MT, Nguyen C, Zechner D, Gutierrez V, Comstock KL, et al. Tumor necrosis factor alpha-induced apoptosis in cardiac myocytes: involvement of the sphingolipid signaling cascade in cardiac cell death. *J Clin Invest.* (1996) 98:2854–65. doi: 10.1172/JCI119114

127. Haudek SB, Taffet GE, Schneider MD, Mann DL. TNF provokes cardiomyocyte apoptosis and cardiac remodeling through activation of multiple cell death pathways. *J Clin Invest.* (2007) 117:2692–701. doi: 10.1172/JCI29134

128. Pulkki KJ. Cytokines and cardiomyocyte death. *Ann Med.* (1997) 29:339–43. doi: 10.3109/07853899708999358

129. Frangogiannis NG. Inflammation in cardiac injury, repair and regeneration. *Curr Opin Cardiol.* (2015) 30:240–5. doi: 10.1097/HCO.0000000000000158

130. Prabhu SD, Frangogiannis NG. The biological basis for cardiac repair after myocardial infarction. *Circ Res.* (2016) 119:91–112. doi: 10.1161/CIRCRESAHA.116.303577

131. Bernardo ME, Fibbe WE. Mesenchymal stromal cells: sensors and switchers of inflammation. *Cell Stem Cell.* (2013) 13:392–402. doi: 10.1016/j.stem.2013.09.006

132. de Witte SFH, Luk F, Sierra Parraga JM, Gargesha M, Merino A, Korevaar SS, et al. Immunomodulation by therapeutic mesenchymal stromal cells (MSC) is triggered through phagocytosis of MSC by monocytic cells. *Stem Cells.* (2018) 36:602–15. doi: 10.1002/stem.2779

133. Leng Z, Zhu R, Hou W, Feng Y, Yang Y, Han Q, et al. Transplantation of ACE2- mesenchymal stem cells improves the outcome of patients with covid-19 pneumonia. *Aging Dis.* (2020) 11:216–28. doi: 10.14336/AD.2020.0228

134. Chan MCW, Kuok DIT, Leung CYH, Hui KPY, Valkenburg SA, Lau EHY, et al. Human mesenchymal stromal cells reduce influenza A H5N1-associated acute lung injury *in vitro* and *in vivo*. *Proc Natl Acad Sci USA.* (2016) 113:3621–6. doi: 10.1073/pnas.1601911113

135. Melief SM, Schrama E, Brugman MH, Tiemessen MM, Hoogduijn MJ, Fibbe WE, et al. Multipotent stromal cells induce human regulatory T cells through a novel pathway involving skewing of monocytes toward anti-inflammatory macrophages. *Stem Cells.* (2013) 31:1980–91. doi: 10.1002/stem.1432

136. Huh JW, Kim WY, Park YY, Lim CM, Koh Y, Kim MJ, et al. Anti-inflammatory role of mesenchymal stem cells in an acute lung injury mouse model. *Acute Crit Care.* (2018) 33:154–61. doi: 10.4266/acc.2018.00619

137. Asami T, Ishii M, Namkoong H, Yagi K, Tasaka S, Asakura T, et al. Anti-inflammatory roles of mesenchymal stromal cells during acute Streptococcus pneumoniae pulmonary infection in mice. *Cytotherapy.* (2018) 20:302–13. doi: 10.1016/j.jcyt.2018.01.003

138. Lee SH, Jang AS, Kim YE, Cha JY, Kim TH, Jung S, et al. Modulation of cytokine and nitric oxide by mesenchymal stem cell transfer in lung injury/fibrosis. *Respir Res.* (2010) 11:16. doi: 10.1186/1465-9921-11-16

139. Khedoe PPSJ, de Kleijn S, van Oeveren-Rietdijk AM, Plomp JJ, de Boer HC, van Pel M, et al. Acute and chronic effects of treatment with mesenchymal stromal cells on LPS-induced pulmonary inflammation, emphysema and atherosclerosis development. *PLoS ONE.* (2017) 12:e0183741. doi: 10.1371/journal.pone.0183741

140. Geng Y, Zhang L, Fu B, Zhang J, Hong Q, Hu J, et al. Mesenchymal stem cells ameliorate rhabdomyolysis-induced acute kidney injury *via* the activation of M2 macrophages. *Stem Cell Res Ther.* (2014) 5:80. doi: 10.1186/scrt469

141. Li S, Zheng X, Li H, Zheng J, Chen X, Liu W, et al. Mesenchymal stem cells ameliorate hepatic ischemia/reperfusion injury *via* inhibition of neutrophil recruitment. *J Immunol Res.* (2018) 2018:1–10. doi: 10.1155/2018/7283703

142. Espinosa G, Plaza A, Schenffeldt A, Alarcón P, Gajardo G, Uberti B, et al. Equine bone marrow-derived mesenchymal stromal cells inhibit reactive oxygen species production by neutrophils. *Vet Immunol Immunopathol.* (2020) 221:109975. doi: 10.1016/j.vetimm.2019.109975

143. Jiang D, Muschhammer J, Qi Y, Kügler A, de Vries JC, Saffarzadeh M, et al. Suppression of neutrophil-mediated tissue damage-a novel skill of mesenchymal stem cells. *Stem Cells.* (2016) 34:2393–406. doi: 10.1002/stem.2417

144. Hashmi S, Ahmed M, Murad MH, Litzow MR, Adams RH, Ball LM, et al. Survival after mesenchymal stromal cell therapy in steroid-refractory acute graft-versus-host disease: systematic review and meta-analysis. *Lancet Haematol.* (2016) 3:e45–52. doi: 10.1016/S2352-3026(15)00224-0

145. Sala E, Genua M, Petti L, Anselmo A, Arena V, Cibella J, et al. Mesenchymal stem cells reduce colitis in mice *via* release of TSG6, independently of their localization to the intestine. *Gastroenterology.* (2015) 149:163–76.e20. doi: 10.1053/j.gastro.2015.03.013

146. Song HB, Park SY, Ko JH, Park JW, Yoon CH, Kim DH, et al. Mesenchymal stromal cells inhibit inflammatory lymphangiogenesis in the cornea by suppressing macrophage in a TSG-6-dependent manner. *Mol Ther.* (2018) 26:162–72. doi: 10.1016/j.ymthe.2017.09.026

147. Wang G, Cao K, Liu K, Xue Y, Roberts AI, Li F, et al. Kynurenic acid, an IDO metabolite, controls TSG-6-mediated immunosuppression of human mesenchymal stem cells. *Cell Death Differ.* (2018) 25:1209–23. doi: 10.1038/s41418-017-0006-2

148. Tjabringa GS, Zandieh-Doulabi B, Helder MN, Knippenberg M, Wuisman PIJM, Klein-Nulend J. The polymine spermine regulates osteogenic differentiation in adipose stem cells. *J Cell Mol Med.* (2008) 12:1710–7. doi: 10.1111/j.1582-4934.2008.00224.x

149. Yang Q, Zheng C, Cao J, Cao G, Shou P, Lin L, et al. Spermidine alleviates experimental autoimmune encephalomyelitis through inducing inhibitory macrophages. *Cell Death Differ.* (2016) 23:1850–61. doi: 10.1038/cdd.2016.71

150. Selleri S, Bifsha P, Civini S, Pacelli C, Dieng MM, Lemieux W, et al. Human mesenchymal stromal cell-secreted lactate induces M2-macrophage differentiation by metabolic reprogramming. *Oncotarget.* (2016) 7:30193–210. doi: 10.18632/oncotarget.8623

151. Groh ME, Maitra B, Szekely E, Koç ON. Human mesenchymal stem cells require monocyte-mediated activation to suppress alloreactive T cells. *Exp Hematol.* (2005) 33:928–34. doi: 10.1016/j.exphem.2005.05.002

152. Corcione A, Benvenuto F, Ferretti E, Giunti D, Cappiello V, Cazzanti F, et al. Human mesenchymal stem cells modulate B-cell functions. *Blood.* (2006) 107:367–72. doi: 10.1182/blood-2005-07-2657

153. Peng Y, Chen X, Liu Q, Zhang X, Huang K, Liu L, et al. Mesenchymal stromal cells infusions improve refractory chronic graft versus host disease through an increase of CD5[+] regulatory B cells producing interleukin 10. *Leukemia.* (2015) 29:636–46. doi: 10.1038/leu.2014.225

154. Zhu Y, Wang Y, Zhao B, Niu X, Hu B, Li Q, et al. Comparison of exosomes secreted by induced pluripotent stem cell-derived mesenchymal stem cells and synovial membrane-derived mesenchymal stem cells for the treatment of osteoarthritis. *Stem Cell Res The.r.* (2017) 8:64. doi: 10.1186/s13287-017-0510-9

155. Dabrowska S, Andrzejewska A, Strzemecki D, Muraca M, Janowski M, Lukomska B. Human bone marrow mesenchymal stem cell-derived extracellular vesicles attenuate neuroinflammation evoked by focal brain injury in rats. *J Neuroinflammation.* (2019) 16:1–15. doi: 10.1186/s12974-019-1602-5

156. Shi Y, Wang Y, Li Q, Liu K, Hou J, Shao C, et al. Immunoregulatory mechanisms of mesenchymal stem and stromal cells in inflammatory diseases. *Nat Rev Nephrol.* (2018) 14:493–507. doi: 10.1038/s41581-018-0023-5

157. Huppert LA, Matthay MA. Alveolar fluid clearance in pathologically relevant conditions: *in vitro* and *in vivo* models of acute respiratory distress syndrome. *Front Immunol.* (2017) 8:371. doi: 10.3389/fimmu.2017.00371

158. Simonson OE, Mougiakakos D, Heldring N, Bassi G, Johansson HJ, Dalén M, et al. *In vivo* effects of mesenchymal stromal cells in two patients with severe acute respiratory distress syndrome. *Stem Cells Transl Med.* (2015) 4:1199–213. doi: 10.5966/sctm.2015-0021

159. Horie S, Gonzalez HE, Laffey JG, Masterson CH. Cell therapy in acute respiratory distress syndrome. *J Thorac Dis.* (2018) 10:5607–20. doi: 10.21037/jtd.2018.08.28

160. Xiao K, Hou F, Huang X, Li B, Qian ZR, Xie L. Mesenchymal stem cells: current clinical progress in ARDS and COVID-19. *Stem Cell Res Ther.* (2020) 11:305. doi: 10.1186/s13287-020-01804-6

161. Liang B, Chen J, Li T, Wu H, Yang W, Li Y, Li J, Yu C, Nie F, Ma Z, et al. Clinical remission of a critically ill COVID-19 patient treated by human umbilical cord mesenchymal stem cells. *Medicine.* (2020) 99:e21429. doi: 10.1097/MD.0000000000021429

162. Zhang Y, Ding J, Ren S, Wang W, Yang Y, Li S, et al. Intravenous infusion of human umbilical cord Wharton's jelly-derived mesenchymal stem cells as a potential treatment for patients with COVID-19 pneumonia. *Stem Cell Res Ther.* (2020) 11:207. doi: 10.1186/s13287-020-01725-4

163. Chen J, Hu C, Chen L, Tang L, Zhu Y, Xu X, et al. Clinical study of mesenchymal stem cell treatment for acute respiratory distress syndrome induced by epidemic influenza A (H7N9) infection: a hint for COVID-19 treatment. *Engineering.* (in press). doi: 10.1016/j.eng.2020.02.006

164. Sengupta V, Sengupta S, Lazo A, Woods P, Nolan A, Bremer N. Exosomes derived from bone marrow mesenchymal stem cells as treatment for severe COVID-19. *Stem Cells Dev.* (2020) 29:747–54. doi: 10.1089/scd.2020.0080

165. Moll G, Drzeniek N, Kamhieh-Milz J, Geissler S, Volk H-D, Reinke P. MSC therapies for COVID-19: importance of patient coagulopathy, thromboprophylaxis, cell product quality and mode of delivery for treatment safety and efficacy. *Front Immunol.* (2020) 11:1091. doi: 10.3389/fimmu.2020.01091

166. Can A, Coskun H. The rationale of using mesenchymal stem cells in patients with COVID-19-related acute respiratory distress syndrome: what to expect. *Stem Cells Transl Med.* (2020) 9:sctm.20-0164. doi: 10.1002/sctm.20-0164

167. Peng H, Gong T, Huang X, Sun X, Luo H, Wang W, et al. A synergistic role of convalescent plasma and mesenchymal stem cells in the treatment of severely ill COVID-19 patients: a clinical case report. *Stem Cell Res Ther.* (2020) 291:1–6. doi: 10.1186/s13287-020-01802-8

168. Lippi G, Lavie CJ, Sanchis-Gomar F. Cardiac troponin I in patients with coronavirus disease 2019 (COVID-19): evidence from a meta-analysis. *Prog Cardiovasc Dis.* (2020) 63:390–1. doi: 10.1016/j.pcad.2020.03.001

169. Wei JF, Huang FY, Xiong TY, Liu Q, Chen H, Wang H, et al. Acute myocardial injury is common in patients with COVID-19 and impairs their prognosis. *Heart.* (2020) 106:1154–9. doi: 10.1136/heartjnl-2020-317007

170. Du RH, Liang LR, Yang CQ, Wang W, Cao TZ, Li M, et al. Predictors of mortality for patients with COVID-19 pneumonia caused by SARSCoV- 2: a prospective cohort study. *Eur Respir J.* (2020) 55:2000524. doi: 10.1183/13993003.00524-2020

171. Bangalore S, Sharma A, Slotwiner A, Yatskar L, Harari R, Shah B, et al. ST-segment elevation in patients with covid-19—a case series. *N Engl J Med.* (2020) 382:2478–80. doi: 10.1056/NEJMc2009020

172. Lodigiani C, Iapichino G, Carenzo L, Cecconi M, Ferrazzi P, Sebastian T, et al. Venous and arterial thromboembolic complications in COVID-19 patients admitted to an academic hospital in Milan, Italy. *Thromb Res.* (2020) 191:9–14. doi: 10.1016/j.thromres.2020.04.024

173. Klok FA, Kruip MJHA, van der Meer NJM, Arbous MS, Gommers DAMPJ, Kant KM, et al. Incidence of thrombotic complications in critically ill ICU patients with COVID-19. *Thromb Res.* (2020) 191:145–7. doi: 10.1016/j.thromres.2020.04.013

174. Zhu H, Song X, Jin LY, Jin P, Guan R, Liu X, et al. Comparison of intra-coronary cell transplantation after myocardial infarction: autologous skeletal myoblasts versus bone marrow mesenchymal stem cells. *J Int Med Res.* (2009) 37:298–307. doi: 10.1177/147323000903700203

175. Chen SL, Fang WW, Ye F, Liu YH, Qian J, Shan SJ, et al. Effect on left ventricular function of intracoronary transplantation of autologous bone marrow mesenchymal stem cell in patients with acute myocardial infarction. *Am J Cardio.l.* (2004) 94:92–5. doi: 10.1016/j.amjcard.2004.03.034

176. Chin SP, Poey AC, Wong CY, Chang SK, Tan CS, Ng MT, et al. Intramyocardial and intracoronary autologous bone marrow-derived mesenchymal stromal cell treatment in chronic severe dilated cardiomyopathy. *Cytotherapy.* (2011) 13:814–21. doi: 10.3109/14653249.2011.574118

177. Lu M, Liu S, Zheng Z, Yin G, Song L, Chen H, et al. A pilot trial of autologous bone marrow mononuclear cell transplantation through grafting artery: a sub-study focused on segmental left ventricular function recovery and scar reduction. *Int J Cardiol.* (2013) 168:2221–7. doi: 10.1016/j.ijcard.2013.01.217

178. Premer C, Blum A, Bellio MA, Schulman IH, Hurwitz BE, Parker M, et al. Allogeneic mesenchymal stem cells restore endothelial function in heart failure by stimulating endothelial progenitor cells. *EBioMedicine.* (2015) 2:467–75. doi: 10.1016/j.ebiom.2015.03.020

179. Rodrigo SF, Van Ramshorst J, Hoogslag GE, Boden H, Velders MA, Cannegieter SC, et al. Intramyocardial injection of autologous bone marrow-derived *Ex vivo* expanded mesenchymal stem cells in acute myocardial infarction patients is feasible and safe up to 5 years of follow-up. *J Cardiovasc Transl Res.* (2013) 6:816–25. doi: 10.1007/s12265-013-9507-7

180. Heldman AW, DiFede DL, Fishman JE, Zambrano JP, Trachtenberg BH, Karantalis V, et al. Transendocardial mesenchymal stem cells and mononuclear bone marrow cells for ischemic cardiomyopathy: the TAC-HFT randomized trial. *JAMA.* (2014) 311:62–73. doi: 10.1001/jama.2013.282909

181. Anastasiadis K, Antonitsis P, Westaby S, Reginald A, Sultan S, Doumas A, et al. Implantation of a novel allogeneic mesenchymal precursor cell type in patients with ischemic cardiomyopathy undergoing coronary artery bypass grafting: an open label phase iia trial. *J Cardiovasc Transl Res.* (2016) 9:202–13. doi: 10.1007/s12265-016-9686-0

182. Florea V, Rieger AC, DiFede DL, El-Khorazaty J, Natsumeda M, Banerjee MN, et al. Dose comparison study of allogeneic mesenchymal stem cells in patients with ischemic cardiomyopathy (The TRIDENT study). *Circ Res.* (2017) 121:1279–90. doi: 10.1161/CIRCRESAHA.117.311827

183. Chullikana A, Majumdar A Sen, Gottipamula S, Krishnamurthy S, Kumar AS, Prakash VS, et al. Randomized, double-blind, phase I/II study of intravenous allogeneic mesenchymal stromal cells in acute myocardial infarction. *Cytotherapy.* (2015) 17:250–61. doi: 10.1016/j.jcyt.2014.10.009

184. Hare JM, Traverse JH, Henry TD, Dib N, Strumpf RK, Schulman SP, et al. A randomized, double-blind, placebo-controlled, dose-escalation study of intravenous adult human mesenchymal stem cells (prochymal) after acute myocardial infarction. *J Am Coll Cardiol.* (2009) 54:2277–86. doi: 10.1016/j.jacc.2009.06.055

185. Cai B, Wang G, Chen N, Liu Y, Yin K, Ning C, et al. Bone marrow mesenchymal stem cells protected post-infarcted myocardium against arrhythmias *via* reversing potassium channels remodelling. *J Cell Mol Med.* (2014) 18:1407–16. doi: 10.1111/jcmm.12287

186. Zhang S, Ge J, Sun A, Xu D, Qian J, Lin J, al. Comparison of various kinds of bone marrow stem cells for the repair of infarcted myocardium: single clonally purified non-hematopoietic mesenchymal stem cells serve as a superior source. *J Cell Biochem.* (2006) 99:1132–47. doi: 10.1002/jcb.20949

187. Haider HK, Jiang S, Idris NM, Ashraf M. IGF-1-overexpressing mesenchymal stem cells accelerate bone marrow stem cell mobilization *via* paracrine activation of SDF-1α/CXCR4 signaling to promote myocardial repair. *Circ Res.* (2008) 103:1300–8. doi: 10.1161/CIRCRESAHA.108.186742

188. Herrmann JL, Abarbanell AM, Weil BR, Wang Y, Poynter JA, Manukyan MC, et al. Postinfarct intramyocardial injection of mesenchymal stem cells pretreated with TGF-α improves acute myocardial function. *Am J Physiol Integr Comp Physiol.* (2010) 299:R371–8. doi: 10.1152/ajpregu.00084.2010

189. Beitnes JO, Øie E, Shahdadfar A, Karlsen T, Müller RMB, Aakhus S, et al. Intramyocardial injections of human mesenchymal stem cells following acute myocardial infarction modulate scar formation and improve left ventricular function. *Cell Transplant.* (2012) 21:1697–709. doi: 10.3727/096368911X627462

190. Chen L, Zhang Y, Tao L, Yang Z, Wang L. Mesenchymal stem cells with eNOS over-expression enhance cardiac repair in rats with myocardial infarction. *Cardiovasc Diagn Ther.* (2017) 31:9–18. doi: 10.1007/s10557-016-6704-z

191. Czapla J, Matuszczak S, Wiśniewska E, Jarosz-Biej M, Smolarczyk R, Cichoń T, et al. Human cardiac mesenchymal stromal cells with CD105+ CD34− phenotype enhance the function of post-infarction heart in mice. *PLoS ONE.* (2016) 11:e0158745. doi: 10.1371/journal.pone.0158745

192. Shyu K-G, Wang B-W, Hung H-F, Chang C-C, Tzu-Bi Shih D. Mesenchymal stem cells are superior to angiogenic growth factor genes for improving myocardial performance in the mouse model of acute myocardial infarction. *J Biomed Sci.* (2006) 13:47–58. doi: 10.1007/s11373-005-9038-6

193. Zhang J, Wu Y, Chen A, Zhao Q. Mesenchymal stem cells promote cardiac muscle repair *via* enhanced neovascularization. *Cell Physiol Biochem.* (2015) 35:1219–29. doi: 10.1159/000373945

194. Ellison GM, Nadal-Ginard B, Torella D. Optimizing cardiac repair and regeneration through activation of the endogenous cardiac stem cell compartment. *J Cardiovasc Transl Res.* (2012) 5:667–77. doi: 10.1007/s12265-012-9384-5

195. Dai W, Hale SL, Kloner RA. Role of a paracrine action of mesenchymal stem cells in the improvement of left ventricular function after coronary artery occlusion in rats. *Regen Med.* (2007) 2:63–8. doi: 10.2217/17460751.2.1.63

196. De Macedo Braga LMG, Lacchini S, Schaan BDA, Rodrigues B, Rosa K, De Angelis K, et al. *In situ* delivery of bone marrow cells and mesenchymal stem cells improves cardiovascular function in hypertensive rats submitted to myocardial infarction. *J Biomed Sci.* (2008) 15:365–74. doi: 10.1007/s11373-008-9237-z

197. Van Der Spoel TIG, Jansen Of Lorkeers SJ, Agostoni P, Van Belle E, Gyongyosi M, Sluijter JPG, et al. Human relevance of pre-clinical studies in stem cell therapy: systematic review and meta-analysis of large animal models of ischaemic heart disease. *Cardiovasc Res.* (2011) 91:649–58. doi: 10.1093/cvr/cvr113

198. Natsumeda M, Florea V, Rieger AC, Tompkins BA, Banerjee MN, Golpanian S, et al. A combination of allogeneic stem cells promotes cardiac regeneration. *J Am Coll Cardiol.* (2017) 70:2504–15. doi: 10.1016/j.jacc.2017.09.036

199. Karantalis V, Suncion-Loescher VY, Bagno L, Golpanian S, Wolf A, Sanina C, et al. Synergistic effects of combined cell therapy for chronic ischemic cardiomyopathy. *J Am Coll Cardiol.* (2015) 66:1990–9. doi: 10.1016/j.jacc.2015.08.879

200. Lee JW, Lee SH, Youn YJ, Ahn MS, Kim JY, Yoo BS, et al. A randomized, open-label, multicenter trial for the safety and efficacy of adult mesenchymal stem cells after acute myocardial infarction. *J Korean Med Sci.* (2014) 29:23–31. doi: 10.3346/jkms.2014.29.1.23

201. Qi Z, Duan F, Liu S, Lv X, Wang H, Gao Y, et al. Effects of bone marrow mononuclear cells delivered through a graft vessel for patients with previous myocardial infarction and chronic heart failure: an echocardiographic study of left ventricular function. *Echocardiography.* (2015) 32:937–46. doi: 10.1111/echo.12787

202. Kim SH, Cho JH, Lee YH, Lee JH, Kim SS, Kim MY, et al. Improvement in left ventricular function with intracoronary mesenchymal stem cell therapy in a patient with anterior wall ST-segment elevation myocardial infarction. *Cardiovasc Drugs Ther.* (2018) 32:329–38. doi: 10.1007/s10557-018-6804-z

203. Chen S, Fang W, Qian J, YE F, Liu Y, Shan S, et al. Improvement of cardiac function after transplantation of autologous bone marrow mesenchymal stem cells in patients with acute myocardial infarction. *Chin Med J (Engl).* (2004) 117:1443–8.

204. Penn MS, Ellis S, Gandhi S, Greenbaum A, Hodes Z, Mendelsohn FO, et al. Adventitial delivery of an allogeneic bone marrow-derived adherent stem cell in acute myocardial infarction: phase i clinical study. *Circ Res.* (2012) 110:304–11. doi: 10.1161/CIRCRESAHA.111.253427

205. Wang X, Xi W-C, Wang F. The beneficial effects of intracoronary autologous bone marrow stem cell transfer as an adjunct to percutaneous coronary intervention in patients with acute myocardial infarction. *Biotechnol Lett.* (2014) 36:2163–8. doi: 10.1007/s10529-014-1589-z

206. Gao LR, Pei XT, Ding QA, Chen Y, Zhang NK, Chen HY, et al. A critical challenge: dosage-related efficacy and acute complication intracoronary injection of autologous bone marrow mesenchymal stem

cells in acute myocardial infarction. *Int J Cardiol.* (2013) 168:3191–9. doi: 10.1016/j.ijcard.2013.04.112

207. Yang Z, Zhang F, Ma W, Chen B, Zhou F, Xu Z, et al. A novel approach to transplanting bone marrow stem cells to repair human myocardial infarction: delivery *via* a noninfarct-relative artery. *Cardiovasc Ther.* (2010) 28:380–5. doi: 10.1111/j.1755-5922.2009.00116.x

208. Scalise M, Torella M, Marino F, Ravo M, Giurato G, Vicinanza C, et al. Atrial myxomas arise from multipotent cardiac stem cells. *Eur Heart J.* (2020) ehaa156. doi: 10.1093/eurheartj/ehaa156

209. Vicinanza C, Aquila I, Scalise M, Cristiano F, Marino F, Cianflone E, et al. Adult cardiac stem cells are multipotent and robustly myogenic: C-kit expression is necessary but not sufficient for their identification. *Cell Death Differ.* (2017) 24:2101–16. doi: 10.1038/cdd.2017.130

210. Lewis-McDougall FC, Ruchaya PJ, Domenjo-Vila E, Shin Teoh T, Prata L, Cottle BJ, et al. Aged-senescent cells contribute to impaired heart regeneration. *Aging Cell.* (2019) 18:1–15. doi: 10.1111/acel.12931

211. Ellison-Hughes GM, Madeddu P. Exploring pericyte and cardiac stem cell secretome unveils new tactics for drug discovery. *Pharmacol Ther.* (2017) 171:1–12. doi: 10.1016/j.pharmthera.2016.11.007

212. Zhu M, Chu Y, Shang Q, Zheng Z, Li Y, Cao L, et al. Mesenchymal stromal cells pretreated with pro-inflammatory cytokines promote skin wound healing through VEGFC-mediated angiogenesis. *Stem Cells Transl Med.* (2020) 9:1218–32. doi: 10.1002/sctm.19-0241

213. Miyahara Y, Nagaya N, Kataoka M, Yanagawa B, Tanaka K, Hao H, et al. Monolayered mesenchymal stem cells repair scarred myocardium after myocardial infarction. *Nat Med.* (2006) 12:459–65. doi: 10.1038/nm1391

214. Qian D, Gong J, He Z, Hua J, Lin S, Xu C, et al. Bone marrow-derived mesenchymal stem cells repair necrotic pancreatic tissue and promote angiogenesis by secreting cellular growth factors involved in the SDF-1 /CXCR4 axis in rats. *Stem Cells Int.* (2015) 2015:1–20. doi: 10.1155/2015/306836

215. Teng X, Chen L, Chen W, Yang J, Yang Z, Shen Z. Mesenchymal stem cell-derived exosomes improve the microenvironment of infarcted myocardium contributing to angiogenesis and anti-inflammation. *Cell Physiol Biochem.* (2015) 37:2415–24. doi: 10.1159/000438594

216. Huang NF, Lam A, Fang Q, Sievers RE, Li S, Lee RJ. Bone marrow-derived mesenchymal stem cells in fibrin augment angiogenesis in the chronically infarcted myocardium. *Regen Med.* (2009) 4:527–38. doi: 10.2217/rme.09.32

217. Cai M, Ren L, Xiaoqin Y, Guo Z, Li Y, He T, et al. PET monitoring angiogenesis of infarcted myocardium after treatment with vascular endothelial growth factor and bone marrow mesenchymal stem cells. *Amino Acids.* (2016) 48:811–20. doi: 10.1007/s00726-015-2129-4

218. Carrion B, Kong YP, Kaigler D, Putnam AJ. Bone marrow-derived mesenchymal stem cells enhance angiogenesis *via* their α6β1 integrin receptor. *Exp Cell Res.* (2013) 319:2964–76. doi: 10.1016/j.yexcr.2013.09.007

219. Du WJ, Chi Y, Yang ZX, Li ZJ, Cui JJ, Song BQ, et al. Heterogeneity of proangiogenic features in mesenchymal stem cells derived from bone marrow, adipose tissue, umbilical cord, and placenta. *Stem Cell Res Ther.* (2016) 7:1–11. doi: 10.1186/s13287-016-0418-9

220. Gangadaran P, Rajendran RL, Lee HW, Kalimuthu S, Hong CM, Jeong SY, et al. Extracellular vesicles from mesenchymal stem cells activates VEGF receptors and accelerates recovery of hindlimb ischemia. *J Control Release.* (2017) 264:112–26. doi: 10.1016/j.jconrel.2017.08.022

221. Huang B, Qian J, Ma J, Huang Z, Shen Y, Chen X, et al. Myocardial transfection of hypoxia-inducible factor-1α and co-transplantation of mesenchymal stem cells enhance cardiac repair in rats with experimental myocardial infarction. *Stem Cell Res Ther.* (2014) 5:22. doi: 10.1186/scrt410

222. Kwon HM, Hur SM, Park KY, Kim CK, Kim YM, Kim HS, et al. Multiple paracrine factors secreted by mesenchymal stem cells contribute to angiogenesis. *Vascul Pharmacol.* (2014) 63:19–28. doi: 10.1016/j.vph.2014.06.004

223. Kehl D, Generali M, Mallone A, Heller M, Uldry AC, Cheng P, et al. Proteomic analysis of human mesenchymal stromal cell secretomes: a systematic comparison of the angiogenic potential. *npj Regen Med.* (2019) 4:1–13. doi: 10.1038/s41536-019-0070-y

224. Liu L, Gao J, Yuan Y, Chang Q, Liao Y, Lu F. Hypoxia preconditioned human adipose derived mesenchymal stem cells enhance angiogenic potential *via*

secretion of increased VEGF and bFGF. *Cell Biol Int.* (2013) 37:551–60. doi: 10.1002/cbin.10097

225. Anderson JD, Johansson HJ, Graham CS, Vesterlund M, Pham MT, Bramlett CS, et al. Comprehensive proteomic analysis of mesenchymal stem cell exosomes reveals modulation of angiogenesis *via* nuclear factor-kappaB signaling. *Stem Cells.* (2016) 34:601–13. doi: 10.1002/stem.2298

226. Zhang Z, Yang J, Yan W, Li Y, Shen Z, Asahara T. Pretreatment of cardiac stem cells with exosomes derived from mesenchymal stem cells enhances myocardial repair. *J Am Heart Assoc.* (2016) 5:e002856. doi: 10.1161/JAHA.115.002856

227. Hanna H, Mir LM, Andre FM. *In vitro* osteoblastic differentiation of mesenchymal stem cells generates cell layers with distinct properties. *Stem Cell Res Ther.* (2018) 9:203. doi: 10.1186/s13287-018-0942-x

228. Takeda YS, Xu Q. Neuronal differentiation of human mesenchymal stem cells using exosomes derived from differentiating neuronal cells. *PLoS ONE.* (2015) 10:e0135111. doi: 10.1371/journal.pone.0135111

229. Xie X, Wang J, Cao J, Zhang X. Differentiation of bone marrow mesenchymal stem cells induced by myocardial medium under hypoxic conditions. *Acta Pharmacol Sin.* (2006) 27:1153–8. doi: 10.1111/j.1745-7254.2006.00436.x

230. Choi J-W, Kim K-E, Lee CY, Lee J, Seo H-H, Lim KH, et al. Alterations in cardiomyocyte differentiation-related proteins in rat mesenchymal stem cells exposed to hypoxia. *Cell Physiol Biochem.* (2016) 39:1595–607. doi: 10.1159/000447861

231. Noiseux N, Gnecchi M, Lopez-Ilasaca M, Zhang L, Solomon SD, Deb A, et al. Mesenchymal stem cells overexpressing Akt dramatically repair infarcted myocardium and improve cardiac function despite infrequent cellular fusion or differentiation. *Mol Ther.* (2006) 14:840–50. doi: 10.1016/j.ymthe.2006.05.016

232. Derval N, Barandon L, Dufourcq P, Leroux L, Lamazière J-MD, Daret D, et al. Epicardial deposition of endothelial progenitor and mesenchymal stem cells in a coated muscle patch after myocardial infarction in a murine model. *Eur J Cardio-Thoracic Surg.* (2008) 34:248–54. doi: 10.1016/j.ejcts.2008.03.058

233. Wu S-Z, Li Y-L, Huang W, Cai W-F, Liang J, Paul C, et al. Paracrine effect of CXCR4-overexpressing mesenchymal stem cells on ischemic heart injury. *Cell Biochem Funct.* (2017) 35:113–23. doi: 10.1002/cbf.3254

234. Yao Z, Liu H, Yang M, Bai Y, Zhang B, Wang C, et al. Bone marrow mesenchymal stem cell-derived endothelial cells increase capillary density and accelerate angiogenesis in mouse hindlimb ischemia model. *Stem Cell Res Ther.* (2020) 11:221. doi: 10.1186/s13287-020-01710-x

235. Nascimento DS, Mosqueira D, Sousa LM, Teixeira M, Filipe M, Resende TP, et al. Human umbilical cord tissue-derived mesenchymal stromal cells attenuate remodeling after myocardial infarction by proangiogenic, antiapoptotic, and endogenous cell-activation mechanisms. *Stem Cell Res The.r.* (2014) 5:1–14. doi: 10.1186/scrt394

236. Kang K, Ma R, Cai W, Huang W, Paul C, Liang J, et al. Exosomes secreted from CXCR4 overexpressing mesenchymal stem cells promote cardioprotection *via* akt signaling pathway following myocardial infarction. *Stem Cells Int.* (2015) 2015:1–14. doi: 10.1155/2015/659890

237. Li X, Xie X, Yu Z, Chen Y, Qu G, Yu H, et al. Bone marrow mesenchymal stem cells-derived conditioned medium protects cardiomyocytes from hypoxia/reoxygenation-induced injury through Notch2/mTOR/autophagy signaling. *J Cell Physiol.* (2019) 234:18906–16. doi: 10.1002/jcp.28530

238. Li H, Zuo S, He Z, Yang Y, Pasha Z, Wang Y, et al. Paracrine factors released by GATA-4 overexpressed mesenchymal stem cells increase angiogenesis and cell survival. *Am J Physiol Hear Circ Physiol.* (2010) 299:1772–81. doi: 10.1152/ajpheart.00557.2010.-Transplanted

239. Zhang D, Fan GC, Zhou X, Zhao T, Pasha Z, Xu M, et al. Over-expression of CXCR4 on mesenchymal stem cells augments myoangiogenesis in the infarcted myocardium. *J Mol Cell Cardiol.* (2008) 44:281–92. doi: 10.1016/j.yjmcc.2007.11.010

240. Kawaguchi N, Smith AJ, Waring CD, Hasan K, Miyamoto S, Matsuoka R, et al. c-kit pos GATA-4 high rat cardiac stem cells foster adult cardiomyocyte survival through IGF-1 paracrine signalling. *PLoS ONE.* (2010) 5:e14297. doi: 10.1371/journal.pone.0014297

241. Yamaguchi J-i, Kusano KF, Masuo O, Kawamoto A, Silver M, Murasawa S, et al. Stromal cell-derived factor-1 effects on *ex vivo* expanded endothelial progenitor cell recruitment for ischemic neovascularization. *Circulation.* (2003) 107:1322–8. doi: 10.1161/01.CIR.0000055313.77510.22

The Role of MSC Therapy in Attenuating the Damaging Effects of the Cytokine Storm Induced by COVID-19...
67

242. Ceradini DJ, Kulkarni AR, Callaghan MJ, Tepper OM, Bastidas N, Kleinman ME, et al. Progenitor cell trafficking is regulated by hypoxic gradients through HIF-1 induction of SDF-1. *Nat Med.* (2004) 10:858–64. doi: 10.1038/nm1075

243. De Falco E, Porcelli D, Torella AR, Straino S, Iachininoto MG, Orlandi A, et al. SDF-1 involvement in endothelial phenotype and ischemia-induced recruitment of bone marrow progenitor cells. *Blood.* (2004) 104:3472–82. doi: 10.1182/blood-2003-12-4423

244. Luger D, Lipinski MJ, Westman PC, Glover DK, Dimastromatteo J, Frias JC, et al. Intravenously delivered mesenchymal stem cells. *Circ Res.* (2017) 120:1598–613. doi: 10.1161/CIRCRESAHA.117.310599

245. Yan X, Anzai A, Katsumata Y, Matsuhashi T, Ito K, Endo J, et al. Temporal dynamics of cardiac immune cell accumulation following acute myocardial infarction. *J Mol Cell Cardiol.* (2013) 62:24–35. doi: 10.1016/j.yjmcc.2013.04.023

246. Park KC, Gaze DC, Collinson PO, Marber MS. Cardiac troponins: from myocardial infarction to chronic disease. *Cardiovasc Res.* (2017) 113:1708–18. doi: 10.1093/cvr/cvx183

247. Richeldi L, du Bois RM, Raghu G, Azuma A, Brown KK, Costabel U, et al. Efficacy and safety of nintedanib in idiopathic pulmonary fibrosis. *N Engl J Med.* (2014) 370:2071–82. doi: 10.1056/NEJMoa1402584

248. King TE, Bradford WZ, Castro-Bernardini S, Fagan EA, Glaspole I, Glassberg MK, et al. A phase 3 trial of pirfenidone in patients with idiopathic pulmonary fibrosis. *N Engl J Med.* (2014) 370:2083–92. doi: 10.1056/NEJMoa1402582

249. Karimi-Shah BA, Chowdhury BA. Forced vital capacity in idiopathic pulmonary fibrosis—FDA review of pirfenidone and nintedanib. *N Engl J Med.* (2015) 372:1189–91. doi: 10.1056/NEJMp1500526

250. Kasam RK, Reddy GB, Jegga AG, Madala SK. Dysregulation of mesenchymal cell survival pathways in severe fibrotic lung disease: the effect of nintedanib therapy. *Front Pharmacol.* (2019) 10:532. doi: 10.3389/fphar.2019.00532

251. Su H, Yang M, Wan C, Yi LX, Tang F, Zhu HY, et al. Renal histopathological analysis of 26 postmortem findings of patients with COVID-19 in China. *Kidney Int.* (2020) 98:219–27. doi: 10.1016/j.kint.2020.04.003

252. Moodley Y, Ilancheran S, Samuel C, Vaghjiani V, Atienza D, Williams ED, et al. Human amnion epithelial cell transplantation abrogates lung fibrosis and augments repair. *Am J Respir Crit Care Med.* (2010) 182:643–51. doi: 10.1164/rccm.201001-0014OC

253. Ashcroft T, Simpson JM, Timbrell V. Simple method of estimating severity of pulmonary fibrosis on a numerical scale. *J Clin Pathol.* (1988) 41:467–70. doi: 10.1136/jcp.41.4.467

254. He F, Zhou A, Feng S. Use of human amniotic epithelial cells in mouse models of bleomycin-induced lung fibrosis: a systematic review and meta-analysis. *PLoS ONE.* (2018) 13:1–17. doi: 10.1371/journal.pone.0197658

255. Gad ES, Salama AAA, El-Shafie MF, Arafa HMM, Abdelsalam RM, Khattab M. The anti-fibrotic and anti-inflammatory potential of bone marrow–derived mesenchymal stem cells and nintedanib in bleomycin-induced lung fibrosis in rats. *Inflammation.* (2020) 43:123–34. doi: 10.1007/s10753-019-01101-2

256. Chen S, Cui G, Peng C, Lavin MF, Sun X, Zhang E, et al. Transplantation of adipose-derived mesenchymal stem cells attenuates pulmonary fibrosis of silicosis *via* anti-inflammatory and anti-apoptosis effects in rats. *Stem Cell Res Ther.* (2018) 9:110. doi: 10.1186/s13287-018-0846-9

257. Chen S, Chen X, Wu X, Wei S, Han W, Lin J, et al. Hepatocyte growth factor-modified mesenchymal stem cells improve ischemia/reperfusion-induced acute lung injury in rats. *Gene Ther.* (2017) 24:3–11. doi: 10.1038/gt.2016.64

258. Chen W, Wang S, Xiang H, Liu J, Zhang Y, Zhou S, et al. Microvesicles derived from human Wharton's Jelly mesenchymal stem cells ameliorate acute lung injury partly mediated by hepatocyte growth factor. *Int J Biochem Cell Biol.* (2019) 112:114–22. doi: 10.1016/j.biocel.2019.05.010

259. Gazdhar A, Temuri A, Knudsen L, Gugger M, Schmid RA, Ochs M, et al. Targeted gene transfer of hepatocyte growth factor to alveolar type II epithelial cells reduces lung fibrosis in rats. *Hum Gene Ther.* (2013) 24:105–16. doi: 10.1089/hum.2012.098

260. Zhao Y, Lan X, Wang Y, Xu X, Lu S, Li X, et al. Human endometrial regenerative cells attenuate bleomycin-induced pulmonary fibrosis in mice. *Stem Cells Int.* (2018) 2018:1–13. doi: 10.1155/2018/3475137

261. Ni K, Liu M, Zheng J, Wen L, Chen Q, Xiang Z, et al. PD-1/PD-L1 pathway mediates the alleviation of pulmonary fibrosis by human mesenchymal stem cells in humanized mice. *Am J Respir Cell Mol Biol.* (2018) 58:684–95. doi: 10.1165/rcmb.2017-0326OC

262. Zhang E, Yang Y, Chen S, Peng C, Lavin MF, Yeo AJ, al. Bone marrow mesenchymal stromal cells attenuate silica-induced pulmonary fibrosis potentially by attenuating Wnt/β-catenin signaling in rats. *Stem Cell Res Ther.* (2018) 9:1–14. doi: 10.1186/s13287-018-1045-4

263. Li F, Han F, Li H, Zhang J, Qiao X, Shi J, et al. Human placental mesenchymal stem cells of fetal origins-alleviated inflammation and fibrosis by attenuating MyD88 signaling in bleomycin-induced pulmonary fibrosis mice. *Mol Immunol.* (2017) 90:11–21. doi: 10.1016/j.molimm.2017.06.032

264. Li X, Li C, Tang Y, Huang Y, Cheng Q, Huang X, et al. NMDA receptor activation inhibits the antifibrotic effect of BM-MSCs on bleomycin-induced pulmonary fibrosis. *Am J Physiol Lung Cell Mol Physiol.* (2018) 315:404–21. doi: 10.1152/ajplung.00002.2018.-Endogenous

265. Cao H, Wang C, Chen X, Hou J, Xiang Z, Shen Y, et al. Inhibition of Wnt/β-catenin signaling suppresses myofibroblast differentiation of lung resident mesenchymal stem cells and pulmonary fibrosis. *Sci Rep.* (2018) 8:13644. doi: 10.1038/s41598-018-28968-9

266. Chambers DC, Enever D, Ilic N, Sparks L, Whitelaw K, Ayres J, et al. A phase 1b study of placenta-derived mesenchymal stromal cells in patients with idiopathic pulmonary fibrosis. *Respirology.* (2014) 19:1013–18. doi: 10.1111/resp.12343

267. Averyanov A, Koroleva I, Konoplyannikov M, Revkova V, Lesnyak V, Kalsin V, et al. First-in-human high-cumulative-dose stem cell therapy in idiopathic pulmonary fibrosis with rapid lung function decline. *Stem Cells Transl Med.* (2020) 9:6–16. doi: 10.1002/sctm.19-0037

268. Lan Y-W, Theng S-M, Huang T-T, Choo K-B, Chen C-M, Kuo H-P, et al. Oncostatin M-preconditioned mesenchymal stem cells alleviate bleomycin-induced pulmonary fibrosis through paracrine effects of the hepatocyte growth factor. *Stem Cells Transl Med.* (2017) 6:1006–17. doi: 10.5966/sctm.2016-0054

269. Ayaub EA, Dubey A, Imani J, Botelho F, Kolb MRJ, Richards CD, et al. Overexpression of OSM and IL-6 impacts the polarization of pro-fibrotic macrophages and the development of bleomycin-induced lung fibrosis OPEN. *Sci Rep.* (2017) 7:1–16. doi: 10.1038/s41598-017-13511-z

270. Li D, Liu Q, Qi L, Dai X, Liu H, Wang Y. Low levels of TGF-β1 enhance human umbilical cord-derived mesenchymal stem cell fibronectin production and extend survival time in a rat model of lipopolysaccharide-induced acute lung injury. *Mol Med Rep.* (2016) 14:1681–92. doi: 10.3892/mmr.2016.5416

271. Chen S, Chen L, Wu X, Lin J, Fang J, Chen X, et al. Ischemia postconditioning and mesenchymal stem cells engraftment synergistically attenuate ischemia reperfusion-induced lung injury in rats. *J Surg Res.* (2012) 178:81–91. doi: 10.1016/j.jss.2012.01.039

272. Wu J, Song D, Li Z, Guo B, Xiao Y, Liu W, et al. Immunity-and-matrix-regulatory cells derived from human embryonic stem cells safely and effectively treat mouse lung injury and fibrosis. *Cell Res.* (2020) 30:1–16. doi: 10.1038/s41422-020-0354-1

273. Cunha LL, Perazzio SF, Azzi J, Cravedi P, Riella LV. Remodeling of the immune response with aging: immunosenescence and its potential impact on COVID-19 immune response. *Front Immunol.* (2020) 11:1748. doi: 10.3389/fimmu.2020.01748

6

Application of Machine Learning in Diagnosis of COVID-19 Through X-Ray and CT Images

Hossein Mohammad-Rahimi[1], Mohadeseh Nadimi[2,3], Azadeh Ghalyanchi-Langeroudi[2,3], Mohammad Taheri[4*] and Soudeh Ghafouri-Fard[5*]

[1] Dental Research Center, Research Institute of Dental Sciences, Shahid Beheshti University of Medical Sciences, Tehran, Iran, [2] Department of Medical Physics and Biomedical Engineering, Tehran University of Medical Sciences (TUMS), Tehran, Iran, [3] Research Center for Biomedical Technologies and Robotics (RCBTR), Tehran, Iran, [4] Urology and Nephrology Research Center, Shahid Beheshti University of Medical Sciences, Tehran, Iran, [5] Department of Medical Genetics, Shahid Beheshti University of Medical Sciences, Tehran, Iran

*Correspondence:
Mohammad Taheri
mohammad_823@yahoo.com
Soudeh Ghafouri-Fard
s.ghafourifard@sbmu.ac.ir

Coronavirus disease, first detected in late 2019 (COVID-19), has spread fast throughout the world, leading to high mortality. This condition can be diagnosed using RT-PCR technique on nasopharyngeal and throat swabs with sensitivity values ranging from 30 to 70%. However, chest CT scans and X-ray images have been reported to have sensitivity values of 98 and 69%, respectively. The application of machine learning methods on CT and X-ray images has facilitated the accurate diagnosis of COVID-19. In this study, we reviewed studies which used machine and deep learning methods on chest X-ray images and CT scans for COVID-19 diagnosis and compared their performance. The accuracy of these methods ranged from 76% to more than 99%, indicating the applicability of machine and deep learning methods in the clinical diagnosis of COVID-19.

Keywords: COVID-19, machine learning, detection, biomarker, X-ray image

INTRODUCTION

First identified in Wuhan, China, severe pneumonia caused by Severe Acute Respiratory Syndrome Coronavirus 2 (SARS-CoV-2) quickly spread all over the world. The resultant disorder was named coronavirus disease (COVID-19) (1, 2). COVID-19 has various clinical symptoms, including fever, cough, dyspnea, fatigue, myalgia, headache, and gastrointestinal complications (3–5). Diagnosis of COVID-19 infection through RT-PCR on nasopharyngeal and throat swab samples has been reported to yield positive results in 30–70% of cases (6, 7). On the other hand, chest CT scans and X-ray images have been reported to have sensitivity values of 98 and 69%, respectively (7–9). The most typical radiological signs in these patients include multifocal and bilateral ground-glass opacities and consolidations, particularly in the peripheral and basal sites (10). However, interpretation of the results of these imaging techniques by expert radiologists might encounter some problems leading to reduced sensitivity (11). Artificial intelligence has recently gained the attention of both clinicians and researchers for the appropriate management of the COVID-19 pandemic (12). As an accurate method, artificial intelligence is able to identify abnormal patterns of CT and X-ray images. Using this method, it is possible to assess certain segment regions and take precise structures in chest CT images facilitating diagnostic purposes. Artificial intelligence methods have been shown to detect COVID-19 and distinguish this condition from other pulmonary disorders and community-acquired pneumonia (13). Both deep learning and machine learning approaches have been used to predict different aspects of the COVID-19 outbreak. Support vector and random forest are among the most applied machine learning methods, while Convolutional Neural Network (CNN), Long Short-Term Memory (LSTM), Generative Adversarial Networks (GAN), and Residual Neural network are among the deep learning methods used in this regard (14). In this study, we reviewed studies which used machine and deep learning methods on chest X-ray images and CT scans for the purpose of COVID-19 diagnosis and compared their performance.

METHODS

Search Strategy

The research question was: "What are the applications of machine learning techniques and their performances in COVID-19 diagnosis using X-ray images?". The search of the present review was based on the PICO elements, which were as follows:

- **P (Problem/Patient/Population):** Patients' CT scans and Chest X-rays.
- **I (Intervention/Indicator):** Machine/deep learning models for diagnosis of Covid-19 patients
- **C (Comparison):** Ground truth or reference standards
- **O (Outcome):** Performance measurements including accuracy, AUC score, sensitivity, and specificity.

In other words, we were looking for publications that evaluated the performance of any machine learning or deep learning approaches based on inclusion and exclusion criteria. Studies that used other types of medical image modalities (e.g., ultrasound images) were excluded. An electronic search was conducted on PubMed, Google Scholar, Scopus, Embase, arXiv, and medRxiv for finding the relevant literature. Duplicate studies were removed. Studies that were cited within the retrieved papers were reviewed for finding missing studies. For identifying proper journal papers and conference proceedings, investigators screened the title and abstracts based on inclusion and exclusion criteria independently. Finally, considering the inclusion and exclusion criteria, investigators identified the eligible publications in this stage independently.

Inclusion Criteria

The following inclusion criteria were used in the selection of the articles: (1) Studies that applied machine learning or deep learning algorithms, (2) Studies that evaluated the measurement of model outcomes in comparison with ground truth or gold standards, and (3) Studies that used algorithms to analyze radiographic images (CT scan, Chest X-ray, etc.).

Exclusion Criteria

The following studies were excluded: (1) Studies that used any machine learning or deep learning approaches for problems not directly related to the COVID-19 imaging, (2) Studies that used other artificial intelligence techniques or classic computer vision approaches, (3) Studies that did not provide a clear explanation of the machine learning or deep learning model

that was used to solve their problem, and (4) Review studies. The latter were excluded as we did not aim to review the data on an original level without any second-hand interpretations (summation, inferences, etc.).

Figure 1 shows the flowchart of the study design.

RESULTS

We obtained 105 studies that used machine or deep learning methods to assess chest images of COVID-19 patients. These studies have used different analytical methods. For instance, Ardakani et al. (15) have assessed radiological features of CT images obtained from patients with COVID-19 and non-COVID-19 pneumonia. They used decision tree, K-nearest neighbor, naïve Bayes, support vector machine, and ensemble classifiers to find the computer-aided diagnosis system with the best performance in distinguishing COVID-19 patients from non-COVID-19 pneumonia. They reported that site and distribution of pulmonary involvement, the quantity of the pulmonary lesions, ground-glass opacity, and crazy-paving as the most important characteristics for differentiation of these two sets of patients. Their computer-aided diagnosis method yielded the accuracy of 91.94%, using an ensemble (COVIDiag) classifier. Alazab et al. (16) have developed an artificial-intelligence method based on a deep CNN to evaluate chest X-ray images and detection of COVID-19 patients. Their method yielded an F-measure ranging from 95 to 99%. Notably, three predicting strategies could forecast the numbers of COVID-19 confirmations, recoveries, and mortalities over the upcoming week. The average accuracy of the prediction models were 94.80 and 88.43% in two different countries. Albahli has applied deep learning-based models on CT images of COVID-19 patients. He has demonstrated a high performance of a Deep Neural Network model in detecting COVID-19 patients and has offered an efficient assessment of chest-related disorders according to age and sex. His proposed model has yielded 89% accuracy in terms of GAN-based synthetic data (17). Automatic detection of COVID-19 based on X-ray images has been executed through the application of three deep learning models, including Inception ResNetV2, InceptionNetV3, and NASNetLarge. The best results have been obtained from InceptionNetV3, which yielded the accuracy levels of 98.63 and 99.02% with and without application of data augmentation in model training, respectively (18). Alsharman et al. (19) have used the CNN method to detect COVID-19 based on chest CT images in the early stages of disease course. Authors have reported high accuracy of GoogleNet CNN architecture for diagnosis of COVID-19. Altan et al. (20) have used a hybrid model comprising two-dimensional curvelet transformation, chaotic salp swarm algorithm, and deep learning methods for distinguishing COVID-19 from other pneumonia cases. Application of their proposed model on chest X-ray images has led to accurate diagnosis of COVID-19 patients (Accuracy = 99.69%, Sensitivity = 99.44% and Specificity = 99.81%). Apostolopoulos et al. (21) have used a certain CNN strategy, namely MobileNet on X-Ray images of COVID-19 patients. This method has yielded more than 99% accuracy

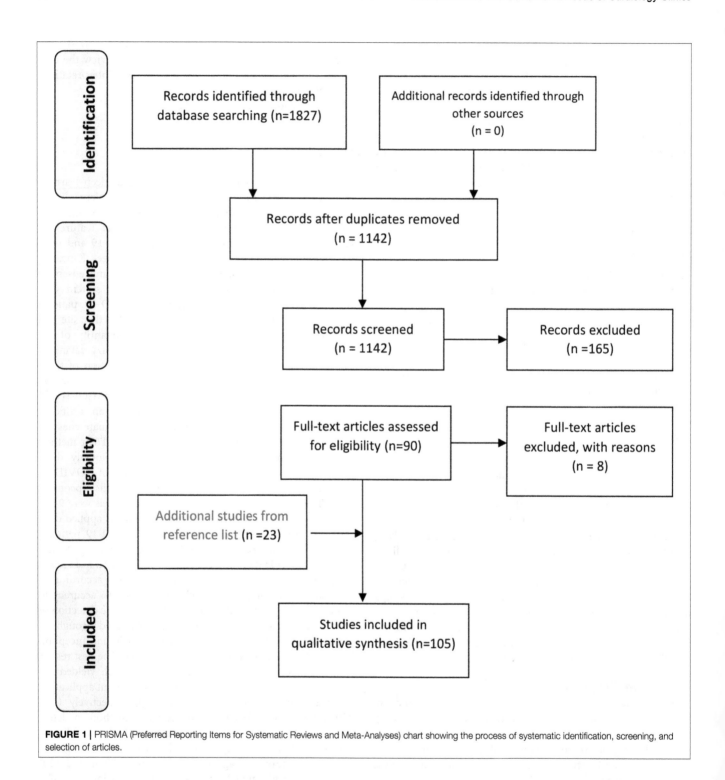

FIGURE 1 | PRISMA (Preferred Reporting Items for Systematic Reviews and Meta-Analyses) chart showing the process of systematic identification, screening, and selection of articles.

in the diagnosis of COVID-19. In another study, Ardakani et al. (22) used 10 CNN strategies, namely AlexNet, VGG-16, VGG-19, SqueezeNet, GoogleNet, MobileNet-V2, ResNet-18, ResNet-50, ResNet-101, and Xception, to differentiate COVID-19 cases from non-COVID-19 patients. They have demonstrated the best diagnostic values for ResNet-101 and Xception, both of them having area under curve (AUC) values higher than 0.99 which is superior to the performance of the radiologist. Das et al. (23) have used the CNN model Truncated InceptionNet to diagnose COVID-19 from other non-COVID and/or healthy cases based on chest X-ray. Their suggested model yielded AUC of 1.0 in distinguishing COVID-19 patients from combined Pneumonia and healthy subjects. **Tables 1, 2** summarize the features of studies which adopted machine learning methods in CT images and chest X-ray of COVID-19 patients, respectively.

TABLE 1 | Characteristics of papers that used CT images or a combination of X-ray and CT images.

Author, year	Data source	Data structure and size	Data preprocessing	Best model structure(s)	Performance measurements (on the best model)				References
					Accuracy	AUC score	Sensitivity	Specificity	
Abbasian et al. (2020)	Iran University of Medical Sciences (IUMS)	306 COVID-19 patients; 306 COVID-19 pneumonia (CT images)	Extracting 20 features of CT images	Ensemble	91.94%	0.965	93.54%	90.32%	(15)
Alsharman et al. (2020)	"COVID-CT-dataset"	CT images	Binarization (the separation of the object and background is known as Binarization); Converting input image from 2D Grayscale to 3D Color	GoogleNet CNN	82.14%				(19)
Ardakani et al. (2020)	Private dataset	108 COVID-19 patients; 86 viral pneumonia diseases (CT images)	Converted to the gray-scale Cropped and resized to 60 * 60 pixels	ResNet-101 Xception	Resnet: 99.51% Xception: 99.02% (compared to 86.7% in human)	Resnet: 0.994 Xception: 0.994% (compared to 0.873 in human)	Resnet: 100% Xception: 98.04% (compared to 89.21% in human)	Resnet: 99.02% Xception: 100% (compared to 83.33% in human)	(22)
Aswathy et al. (2020)	"National Cancer Institute and the Cancer Image Archive"	1,763 normal patients; 63 pneumonia patients	Thresholding; Texture-based feature extractionwith a wrapper	CNN	99%	–	–	–	(24)
Bai et al. (2020)	Private dataset	521 COVID-19 patients; 665 other pulmonary diseases (CT images)	Lung segmentation; Generate an 8-bit image for each axial slice by applying Lung windowing to the Hounsfield units	EfficientNet B4	96% (compared to 85% in human)	0.95	95% (compared to 79% in human)	96% (compared to 88% in human)	(11)
Bridge et al. (2020)	"Toy dataset," "Italian Society of Radiology," "Shenzhen Hospital X-Ray dataset," "ChestX-Ray8," "COVID-CT-Dataset"	129 COVID-19 patients; 62,267 normal patients; 5,689 pneumonia patients (X-ray images) 30 COVID-19 patients; 1,919 normal patients (CT images)	Using the GEV activation function for unbalanced data	Inception V3	100%	–	100%	100%	(25)
Butt et al. (2020)	Not mentioned	219 images from 110 COVID-19 patients; 399 normal patients (CT images)	Image processing method base on HU values	3D CNN	–	0.996	98.2%	92.2%	(26)

(Continued)

TABLE 1 | Continued

Author, year	Data source	Data structure and size	Data preprocessing	Best model structure(s)	Performance measurements (on the best model)				References
					Accuracy	AUC score	Sensitivity	Specificity	
Dey et al. (2020)	"COVID-19 CT segmentation dataset," "Chest X-rays (Radiopaedia)"	200 COVID-19 patients; 200 normal patients (grayscale lung CTI images)	Segmenting lung area related to pneumonia infection; Extracting CWT, DWT, EWT features from original image and Haralick, Hu moments from binary segmented area Feature selection based on statistical tests	KNN	87.75%	–	89.00%	86.50%	(27)
El Asnaoui et al. (2020)	COVID-19 X-ray image database developed by Cohen JP; Kermany et al. (28)	2,780 Bacterial pneumonia patients; 1,493 Coronavirus patients; 231 COVID-19 patients; 1,583 normal patients (X-ray and CT images)	Intensity Normalization; Contrast Limited Adaptive Histogram Equalization	Inception ResNetV2; Densnet201	Inception-ResNetV2: 92.18% Densnet201: 88.09%	Inception-ResNetV2: 0.920 Densnet201: 0.879	Inception-ResNetV2: 92.11% Densnet201: 87.99%	Inception-ResNetV2: 96.6% Densnet201: 94.00%	(29)
Han et al. (2020)	"COVID-19 hospitals in Shandong Province"	79 COVID-19 patients; 100 pneumonia patients; 130 normal patients (CT images)	Data augmentation	AD3D-MIL	97.9%	0.99	97.9%	97.9%	(30)
Harmon et al. (2020)	Private dataset	386 COVID-19 patients; 1,011 negative COVID-19 patients (CT images)	Lung segmentation; clipping images to HU range (−1,000, 500); Data augmentation (flipping, rotation, image intensity and contrast adjustment, adding random Gaussian noise);	Hybrid 3D based on Densnet-121	90.8%	–	84%	93%	(31)
Hasan et al. (2020)	"Radiopaedia and the cancer imaging archive websites"	118 COVID-19 patients; 96 pneumonia patients; 107 normal patients (CT images)	Histogram Thresholding; Dilation; Hole Filling	LSTM	99.68%	–	100%	–	(32)

(Continued)

TABLE 1 | Continued

Author, year	Data source	Data structure and size	Data preprocessing	Best model structure(s)	Performance measurements (on the best model)				References
					Accuracy	AUC score	Sensitivity	Specificity	
Hu et al. (2020)	"Hospital of Wuhan Red Cross Society;" "Shenzhen Hospital;" "TCIA dataset;" "Cancer Centre Archive (TCIA) Public Access;" "MD Anderson Cancer Centre;" "Memorial Sloan-Kettering Cancer Center;" "MAASTRO clinic"	150 COVID-19 patients; 150 pneumonia patients; 150 normal patients (CT images)	Data augmentation	CNN	96.2%	0.970	94.5%	95.3%	(33)
Jaiswal et al. (2020)	"The SARS-CoV-2 CT scan dataset"	1,262 COVID-19 patients; 1,230 non-COVID-19 patients (CT images)	Data augmentation (rotation up to 15, slant-angle of 0.2, horizontal flipping, filling new pixels as "nearest" for better robustness)	DenseNet201	96.25%	0.97	96.29%	96.21%	(34)
Kang et al. (2020)	"Tongji Hospital of Huazhong University of Science and Technology;" "China-Japan Union Hospital of Jilin University;" "Rujin Hospital ofShanghai Jiao Tong University"	1,495 COVID-19 patients; 1,027 community-acquired pneumonia (CAP) patients (CT images)	Normalization; Standardization	NN	93.90%	–	94.60%	91.70%	(35)
Lessmann et al. (2020)	"Emergency wards of an Academic center and teaching hospital in the Netherlands in March and April 2020"	237 COVID-19 patients; 606 normal patients (CT images)	Resampling; Normalization	CORADS-AI	–	0.95	85.7%	89.8%	(36)
Li et al. (2020)	Private	1,296 COVID-19 patients; 1,325—patients; 1,735 community-acquired (CT images)	Segmenting lung area with U-net	COVNet (ResNet-50)	–	0.96	90%	96%	(13)

(Continued)

TABLE 1 | Continued

Author, year	Data source	Data structure and size	Data preprocessing	Best model structure(s)	Performance measurements (on the best model)				References
					Accuracy	AUC score	Sensitivity	Specificity	
Li et al. (2020)	More than 10 medical centers between Nov. 11th, 2010 and Feb. 9th, 2020	305 images from 251 COVID-19 patients; 872 images from 869 pneumonia patients; 1,498 images from 1,475 non-pneumonia patients (CT images)	DL-based algorithm Image processing method base on HU values; Data augmentation	3D ResNet-18	Recall = 88% Precision = 89.6% F1 score = 87.8%				(37)
Liu et al. (2020)	Private	73 COVID-19 patients; 27 general pneumonia patients (CT images)	ROI delineation based on ground-glass opacities (GGOs); 13 gray level co-occurrence matrix (GLCM) features, 15 gray level-gradient co-occurrence matrix (GLGCM) features, and six histogram features were extracted; Feature selection by ReliefF;	An ensemble of bagged tree (EBT)	94.16%	0.99	88.62%	100%	(38)
Mei et al. (2020)	Private	419 COVID-19 patients; 486 non-COVID-19 patients (CT images)	Selecting pertinent slices by image segmentation to detect parenchymal tissue; Segmenting lung in CT images;	ResNet-18	79.6%	0.86	83.6%	75.9%	(39)
Panwar et al. (2020)	"COVID-chest X-ray;" "SARS-COV-2 CT-scan;" "Chest X-Ray Images (Pneumonia);"	206 COVID-19 patients; 364 Pneumonia patients (X-ray and CT images)	–	VGG-19	95.61% (COVID-19 vs. Pneumonia)	–	96.55% (COVID-19 vs. Pneumonia)	95.29% (COVID-19 vs. Pneumonia)	(40)
Pathak et al. (2020)	2 different COVID-19 datasets of chest-CT images	CT images	–	Deep bidirectional long short-term memory network with mixture density network (DBM)	96.19% (multi-class)	0.96 (multi-class)	96.22% (multi-class)	96.16% (multi-class)	(41)
Pathak et al. (2020)	"COVID-19 open datasets of chest CT images"	413 COVID-19 patients; 439 normal or pneumonia infected patients (CT images)	–	ResNet-50	93.01%	–	91.45%	94.77%	(41)
Peng et al. (2020)	Collected from PMC	606 COVID-19 patients; 222 Influenza; 397 Normal or other disease patients (CT images)	–	DenseNet121	–	0.87	72.3%	85.2%	(42)

(Continued)

TABLE 1 | Continued

Author, year	Data source	Data structure and size	Data preprocessing	Best model structure(s)	Performance measurements (on the best model)				References
					Accuracy	**AUC score**	**Sensitivity**	**Specificity**	
Pu et al. (2020)	Private	498 COVID-19 patients; 497 community-acquired pneumonia (CAP) (CT images)	Data augmentation [rotation, translation, vertical/horizontal flips, Hounsfield Unit (HU) shift, smoothing (blurring) operation, Gaussian noise]	3D CNNs	99%	0.7	–	–	(43)
Raajan et al. (2020)	X-ray images on public medical Github repositories; Kaggle chest X-ray database	349 images from 216 COVID-19 patients; 1,341 Normal patients (CT images)	Normalization	ResNet-16	95.09%	–	100%	81.89%	(44)
Rajaraman et al. (2020)	"Pediatric CXR dataset;" "RSNA CXR dataset;" "Twitter COVID-19 CXR dataset;" "Montreal COVID-19 CXR dataset"	313 COVID-19 patients; 7,595 pneumonia of unknown type patients; 2,780 bacterial pneumonia; 7,595 Normal patients (X-ray images)	Median filtering; Normalization; Standardization	Inception-V3	99.01%	0.997	98.4%	–	(45)
Sakagianni et al. (2020)	COVID-19 articles on medRxiv and bioRxiv	349 COVID-19 patients; 397 non-COVID-19 patients (CT images)	–	AutoML Cloud Vision	–	0.94	88.31%	–	(46)
Sharma (2020)	Dataset from Italian Society of Medical and Interventional Radiology; COVID-CT available in GitHub; Dataset from hospitals in Moscow, Russia; Dataset from SAL Hospital, Ahmedabad, India;	800 COVID-19 patients; 600 Viral Pneumonia; 800 normal patients (CT images)	Ground-glass opacities (GGO), consolidation and pleural effusion are the features	ResNet	91%	–	92.1%	90.29%	(47)
Singh et al. (2020)	Not mentioned	CT images	–	Multi-objective differential evolution (MODE) based CNN	90.22%	–	91.17%	89.23%	(48)
Song et al. (2020)	Private (two hospitals in China);	98 COVID-19 patients; 103 non-COVID-19 pneumonia (CT images)	–	BigBiGAN	–	0.972	92%	91%	(49)

(Continued)

TABLE 1 | Continued

Author, year	Data source	Data structure and size	Data preprocessing	Best model structure(s)	Performance measurements (on the best model)				References
					Accuracy	AUC score	Sensitivity	Specificity	
Wang et al. (2020)	Private	1,315 COVID-19 patients; 2,406 ILD patients; 936 Normal patients (CT images)	Lobe Segmentation by 3D-Unet; Converting CT numbers to grayscale	PA-66 model	93.3%	0.973	97.6%	–	(50)
Wang et al. (2020)	COVID-19 dataset (private); CT-epidermal growth factor receptor (CT-EGFR) dataset (private); *The CT-EGFR dataset was used for auxiliary training of the DL system	754 COVID-19 patients; 271 bacterial pneumonia 29 viral pneumonia; 42 Other pneumonia (CT images)	Lung segmentation; Using a fully automatic DL model (DenseNet121-FPN); suppress the intensities of non-lung areas inside the lung ROI;	COVID-19Net (DenseNet-like architecture)	Test-set1: 78.32% Test-set2: 80.12%	Test-set1: 0.87 Test-set2: 0.88	Test-set1: 80.39% Test-set2: 79.35%	Test-set1: 76.61% Test-set2: 81.16%	(51)
Warman et al. (2020)	"Public sources"	606 COVID-19 patients; 224 viral pneumonias patients; 74 Normal patients	Data augmentation	YOLOv3 model	96.80%	0.966	98.33%	94.95%	(52)
Wu et al. (2020)	Private	368 COVID-19 patients; 127 other pneumonia (CT images)	Lung region in each axial, coronal and sagittal CT slices were segmented using threshold segmentation and morphological optimization algorithms; The slice with the most pixels in the segmented lung area from each of the axial, coronal and sagittal views was selected as the inputs of the deep learning network;	Multi-view fusion ResNet50 architecture	76%	0.819	81.1%	61.5%	(53)
Xu et al. (2020)	Private "Hospitals in Zhejiang Province, China."	219 images from 110 COVID-19 patients; 224 Influenza-A viral pneumonia patients; 175 Normal patients (CT images)	Image processing method base on HU values	3D CNN segmentation model	86.7%	–	86.7%	–	(54)

(Continued)

TABLE 1 | Continued

Author, year	Data source	Data structure and size	Data preprocessing	Best model structure(s)	Performance measurements (on the best model)				References
					Accuracy	AUC score	Sensitivity	Specificity	
Xu et al. (2020)	Private	432 COVID-19 patients; 76 other viral pneumonia; 350 bacterial pneumonia; 418 normal patients (CT images)	Sampling 5 subsets of CT slices from all sequential images of one CT case to picture the infected lung regions.	3D-Densenet	–	0.98	97.5% (differentiating COVID-19 from three types of non-COVID-19 cases) (compared to 79% in human)	89.4% (differentiating COVID-19 from three types of non-COVID-19 cases) (compared to 90% in human)	(55)
Yan et al. (2020)	Private	416 images from 206 COVID-19 patients; 412 common pneumonia patients (CT images)	Transferring image slices to JPG; Normalization	MSCNN	97.7%	0.962	99.5%	95.6%	(56)
Yang et al. (2020)	Private	146 COVID-19 patients; 149 normal patients (CT images)	For patients, images containing round-glasses opacity (GGO), GGO with consolidation was selected; for healthy control, every 3 slices containing pulmonary parenchyma were selected; Lung windowing is performed over all image slices;	DenseNet	92% (compared to 95% in human)	0.98	97% (compared to 94% in human)	87% (compared to 96% in human)	(57)
Yu et al. (2020)	Private	202 COVID-19 patients (CT images)	–	DenseNet-201 with the cubic SVM model	95.2%	0.99	91.87%	96.87%	(58)
Al-Karawi et al. (2020)	"COVID-CT-Dataset"	275 COVID-19 patients; 195 normal patients (CT images)	Adaptive winner filter followed by inversion; Feature extraction by the FFT-spectrum	SVM	95.37%	–	95.99%	94.76%	(59)
Alom et al. (2020)	Publicly available datasets; "Kaggle repository"	3,875 pneumonia patients; 1,341 normal patients (X-Ray images) 178 COVID-19 patients; 247 normal patients (CT images)	Data augmentation; Adaptive Thresholding Approach	IRRCNN model; NABLA-3 network model	X-ray images: 84.67% CT images: 98.78%	0.93	–	–	(60)
Barstugan et al. (2020)	From the Italian Society of Medical and Interventional Radiology	150 COVID-19 patients (CT images)	13 features were extracted by Gray Level Size Zone Matrix (GLSZM)	SVM	98.77%	–	97.72%	99.67%	(61)

(Continued)

TABLE 1 | Continued

Author, year	Data source	Data structure and size	Data preprocessing	Best model structure(s)	Performance measurements (on the best model)				References
					Accuracy	AUC score	Sensitivity	Specificity	
Chen et al. (2020)	Private dataset	25,989 images from 51 COVID-19 patients; 20,107 images from 55 normal patients (retrospective dataset); 13,911 images from 27 consecutive patients (prospective dataset) (CT images)	Filtering	Deep learning model	Retrospective dataset: 95.24%; Prospective dataset: 92.59% (per patient)	–	Retrospective dataset: 100%; Prospective dataset: 100% (per patient)	Retrospective dataset:93.55%; Prospective dataset: 81.82% (per patient)	(62)
Farid et al. (2020)	Kaggle database	51 COVID-19 patients (CT images)	Feature extraction (MPEG7 Histogram Filter, Gabor Image Filter, Pyramid of Rotation-Invariant Local Binary Pattern, Fuzzy 64-bin Histogram Image Filter); Feature selection by composite hybrid feature selection	CHFS-Stacked (Irip, RF) with Naïve Bayes classifier	96.07%	–	–	–	(63)
Gozes et al. (2020)	Dataset1:ChainZ; Dataset2: Private; Dataset3: ChainZ;	50 suspicious COVID-19 patients from dataset1 used for training; 56 COVID-19 patients; 51 normal patients (CT images) used for testing	Data augmentation (rotation, horizontal flips and cropping)	Resnet-50-2D	–	0.996	98.2%	92.2%	(64)
Jin et al. (2020)	Three centers in China; "LIDC-IDRI;" "Tianchi-Alibaba;" "CC-CCII"	2,529 images from 1,502 COVID-19 patients; 1,338 images from 1,334 CAP patients; 135 images from 83 influenza-A/B patients; 258 images from 258 normal patients (CT images)	–	CNN	–	0.977	90.19%	95.76%	(65)
Jin et al. (2020)	Data from three different centers in Wuhan; Data from three publicly available databases, LIDC-IDRI26, Tianchi-Alibaba27, and CC-CCII18;	1,502 COVID-19 patients; 83 influenza-A/B patients; 1,334 CAP patients except for influenza; 258 healthy subjects (CT images)	Segmenting lung area with U-net	ResNet152	–	0.971	90.19%	95.76%	(66)

(Continued)

TABLE 1 | Continued

Author, year	Data source	Data structure and size	Data preprocessing	Best model structure(s)	Performance measurements (on the best model)				References
					Accuracy	AUC score	Sensitivity	Specificity	
Hosseinzadeh Kassani et al. (2020)	COVID-19 X-ray image database developed by Cohen JP; "Kaggle chest X-ray database," "Kaggle RSNA Pneumonia Detection dataset"	117 COVID-19 patients; 117 normal patients (X-Ray images); 20 COVID-19 patients; 20 normal patients (CT images)	Normalization	DenseNet121 with Bagging tree classifier	99%	–	96%	–	(67)
Ozkaya et al. (2020)	From the Italian Society of Medical and Interventional Radiology	53 COVID-19 patients (CT images)	Feature vectors obtained from Pre-trained VGG-16, GoogleNet and ResNet-50 networks and fusion method; Feature ranking by t-test method	SVM	98.27%	–	98.93%	97.60%	(68)
Shi et al. (2020)	From Tongji Hospital, Shanghai Public Health Clinical Center, and China-Japan Union Hospital (all in China)	183 COVID-19 patients; 5,521 Pneumonia patients (CT images)	Segmentation by a deep learning network (VB-Net)	Infection size-aware random forest	87.9%	0.942	90.7%	83.3%	(69)
Song et al. (2020)	From the Renmin Hospital of Wuhan University	88 COVID-19 patients (CT images)	We extracted the main regions of lungs and filled the blank of lung segmentation with the lung itself	Details Relation Extraction neural network	86%	0.96	96%	–	(3)
Wang et al. (2020)	Private dataset	44 COVID-19 patients; 55 Pneumonia patients (CT images)	Random selection of ROI; Feature extraction using Transfer Learning	Fully connected network and combination of Decision tree and Adaboost	82.9%	0.90	81%	84%	(6)
Zheng et al. (2020)	Private dataset	313 COVID-19 patients; 229 non-COVID-19 patients (CT images)	Data augmentation; Producing lung masks by a trained UNet	3D deep convolutional neural network	90.8%	0.959	–	–	(70)

Data Source: The source(s) that images were acquired from, Data Structure and Size: Number of images, image modalities, sample groups, Data Preprocessing: cleaning, Instance selection, normalization, transformation, feature extraction, selection, etc. The product of data preprocessing is the final training set, Best Model Structure(s): Best machine algorithm or deep learning model reported in the selected paper based on its performance, Performance Measurements (on the best model): The measurement of the model's output performance based on accuracy, sensitivity, specificity, and AUC score.

TABLE 2 | Characteristics of papers that used X-ray images.

Author, year	Data source	Data structure and size	Data preprocessing	Best model structure(s)	Performance measurements (on the best model)				References
					Accuracy	AUC score	Sensitivity	Specificity	
Alazab et al. (2020)	Kaggle database	70 COVID-19 patients; 28 normal patients (X-ray images)	Augmented to 1,000 images	VGG-16		F1 Score: 0.99			(16)
Albahli et al. (2020)	"ChestX-ray8" combined with the few samples of rare classes from the Kaggle challenge	108,948 X-ray images of 32,717 unique patients. Including 15 kinds of chest disease	Data augmentation (rotation, height shift, zoom, horizontal flip)	ResNet	89%	–	–	–	(17)
Albahli et al. (2020)	Open source COVIDx dataset	850 COVID-19 patients; 500 non-COVID-19 pneumonia cases; 915 normal patients (X-ray images)	Data augmentation	InceptionNetV3	99.02%	–	–	–	(18)
Altan et al. (2020)	Not mentioned	7,980 chest X-ray image (2,905 real raw X-ray images 5,075 synthetic chests X-ray images)	Data augmentation; The feature matrix is formed by 2D Curvelet transformation Coefficients; Optimizing the coefficients in the feature matrix with the CSSA	Hybrid model	99.69%	–	99.44%	99.81%	(20)
Apostolopoulos et al. (2020)	COVID-19 X-ray image database developed by Cohen JP; Common Bacterial and Viral Pneumonia X-ray Images by Kermany et al.; Public datasets (Radiological Society of North America, Radiopaedia, and the Italian Society of Medical and Interventional Radiology); "NIH Chest X-ray Dataset"	455 COVID-19 patients; 910 viral pneumonia; 2,540 other pulmonary diseases (X-ray images)	Data augmentation (randomly rotated by a maximum of 10° and randomly shifted horizontally or vertically by a maximum of 20 pixels toward any direction)	MobileNet v2	99.18%	–	97.36%	99.42%	(21)
Apostolopoulos et al. (2020)	X-ray images on public medical Github repositories; "Radiological Society of North America;" "Radiopaedia, and Italian Society of Medicine and Interventional Radiology"	Dataset 1: 224 COVID-19 patients; 700 bacterial pneumonia patients; 504 normal patients (X-ray images) Dataset 2: 224 Covid-19 patients; 714 bacterial and viral pneumonia patients; 504 normal patients (X-ray images)	–	MobileNet v2	96.78%	–	98.66%	96.46%	(71)
Brunese et al. (2020)	COVID-19 image data collection; COVID-19 X-ray image database developed by Cohen JP; "ChestX-ray8;" "NIH Chest X-ray Dataset"	250 COVID-19 patients; 2,753 other pulmonary diseases; 3,520 normal patients (X-Ray images)	Data augmentation (15 degrees rotation clockwise or counterclockwise)	VGG-16	96% (comparison between COVID-19 and other pulmonary diseases)	–	87% 96%	94% 98%	(72)

(Continued)

TABLE 2 | Continued

Author, year	Data source	Data structure and size	Data preprocessing	Best model structure(s)	Performance measurements (on the best model)				References
					Accuracy	AUC score	Sensitivity	Specificity	
Chowdhury et al. (2020)	Kaggle chest X-ray database; "Italian Society of Medical and Interventional Radiology COVID-19 database;" "Novel Corona Virus 2019 Dataset;" GitHub database; "COVID-19 Chest imaging at thread reader," "RSNA-Pneumonia-Detection-Challenge"	423 COVID-19 patients; 1,485 viral pneumonia patients; 1,579 normal patients (X-ray images)	Data augmentation	CNN	99.7%	—	99.7%	99.55%	(73)
Civit-Masot et al. (2020)	COVID-19 and Pneumonia Scans Dataset	132 COVID-19 patients; 132 normal patients; 132 Pneumonia patients (X-ray images)	Histogram equalization	VGG16	85%	—	85%	92%	(74)
Das et al. (2020)	COVID-19 collection; "Kaggle CXR collection;" "Tuberculosis collections;" "U.S. National Library of Medicine;" "National Institutes of Health;" Pneumonia collections	162 COVID-19 patients; 1,583 normal patients	Histogram matching	Truncated Inception Net	100% (Pneumonia collections)	1.0	100%	100%	(23)
Elaziz et al. (2020)	COVID-19 X-ray image database developed by Cohen JP; "Chest X-Ray Images Pneumonia;" Italian Society of Medical and Interventional Radiology COVID-19 DATABASE;	219 COVID-19 patients; 1,341 negative COVID-19 patients (X-ray images)	Feature extraction by Fractional Multichannel Exponent Moments (FrMEMs); Feature selection by modified Manta-Ray Foraging Optimization based on differential evolution	KNN	98.09	—	98.91	—	(75)
Hassantabar et al. (2020)	"COVID-CT-Dataset"	315 COVID-19 patients; 367 non-COVID-19 patients (X-ray images)	—	CNN	93.2%	—	96.1%	99.71%	(76)
Islam et al. (2020)	"GitHub;" "Radiopaedia;" "Cancer Imaging Archive;" "Italian Society of Radiology;" "Kaggle repository;" NIH dataset	1,525 COVID-19 patients; 1,525 pneumonia patients; 1,525 normal patients (X-ray images)	Normalization	CNN-LSTM	99.4%	0.999	99.3%	99.2%	(77)
Khan et al. (2020)	"Covid-chestxray-dataset" "Chest X-Ray Images (Pneumonia)"	284 COVID-19 patients; 330 Pneumonia Bacterial 327 Pneumonia Viral; 310 normal patients (X-ray images)	Random under-sampling (to overcome the unbalanced data problem)	CoroNet (based on Xception)	89.6%	—	89.92%	96.4%	(78)

(Continued)

TABLE 2 | Continued

Author, year	Data source	Data structure and size	Data preprocessing	Best model structure(s)	Performance measurements (on the best model)				References
					Accuracy	AUC score	Sensitivity	Specificity	
Khuzani et al. (2020)	"GitHub"	140 COVID-19 patients; 140 non-COVID-19 pneumonia patients; 140 normal patients (X-ray images)	PCA method; Min-Max Normalization; Adaptive Histogram Equalization	ML	94%	0.91	100%	–	(79)
Ko et al. (2020)	Private; Italian Society of Medical and Interventional Radiology COVID-19 DATABASE;	1,194 COVID-19 patients; 1,442 non-pneumonia patients; 1,357 Pneumonia patients (X-ray images)	Data augmentation (rotation, zoom)	FCONet (ResNet-50)	99.58%	–	99.58%	100%	(80)
Loey et al. (2020)	COVID-19 X-ray image database developed by Cohen JP	69 COVID-19 patients; 79 pneumonia bacterial patients; 79	Data augmentation	Googlenet	80.56% (Four classes)	–	80.56%	–	(81)
Mahmud et al. (2020)	Private	1,583 normal patients; 1,493 non-COVID viral pneumonia; 2,780 bacterial pneumonia; 305 COVID-19 patients (X-ray images)	–	CovXNet (CNN based architecture)	90.2% (multi-class)	0.911 (multi-class)	89.9% (multi-class)	89.1% (multi-class)	(82)
Martinez et al. (2020)	COVID-19 X-ray image database developed by Cohen JP	120 COVID-19 patients; 120 normal patients (X-ray images)	Data augmentation; Normalization	NASNet-type convolutional	97%	–	97%	97%	(83)
Minaee et al. (2020)	COVID-19 X-ray image database developed by Cohen JP; "ChexPert dataset"	40 COVID-19 patients; 3,000 normal patients (X-ray images)	Regularization	SqueezeNet	97%	–	97.5%	97.8%	(84)
Narayan Das et al. (2020)	COVID-19 X-ray image database developed by Cohen JP; "ChestX-ray8"	125 COVID-19 patients; 500 pneumonia patients; 500 normal patients (X-ray images)	–	Xception	97.4%	0.986	97.09%	97.29%	(85)
Nour et al. (2020)	"Public COVID-19 radiology database;" "Italian Society of Medical and Interventional Radiology;" "COVID-19 Database;" "Novel Corona Virus 2019 Dataset;" "COVID-19 positive chest X-ray images from different articles;"	219 COVID-19 patients; 1,345 Viral Pneumonia patients; 1,341 Normal patients (X-ray images)	Data augmentation	CNN	97.14%	0.995	94.61%	98.29%	(86)
Novitasari et al. (2020)	GitHub and Kaggle	102 COVID-19 patients; 204 Pneumonia and Normal patients (X-ray images)	Feature extraction by Googlenet, Resnet18, Resnet50, Resnet101; Feature selection by PCA, Relief;	SVM	97.33% (multi class)	–	96%	98%	(87)

(Continued)

TABLE 2 | Continued

Author, year	Data source	Data structure and size	Data preprocessing	Best model structure(s)	Performance measurements (on the best model)				References
					Accuracy	AUC score	Sensitivity	Specificity	
Oh et al. (2020)	"Japanese Society of Radiological Technology;" "SCR database;" "U.S. National Library of Medicine"	180 COVID-19 patients; 20 Viral Pneumonia patients; 54 pneumonia bacterial patients; 57 Tuberculosis patients; 191 Normal patients (X-ray images)	Data normalization; Data type casting; Histogram equalization; Gamma correction	(FC)-DenseNet103	88.9%	–	85.9%	96.4%	(88)
Ozturk et al. (2020)	COVID-19 X-ray image database developed by Cohen JP; "ChestX-ray8;"	(X-ray images)		DarkCovidNet inspired by the DarkNet architecture	87.02%	–	85.35%	92.18%	(89)
Pandit et al. (2020)	COVID-19 X-ray image database developed by Cohen JP; Kaggle chest X-ray database	224 COVID-19 patients; 700 pneumonia bacterial patients; 504 Normal patients (X-ray images)	Data augmentation	VGG-16	92.53% (Three class output)	–	86.7%	95.1%	(90)
Panwar et al. (2020)	COVID-19 X-ray image database developed by Cohen JP; Radiopedia.org website; Kaggle chest X-ray database	142 COVID-19 patients; 142 other ("Normal" "Bacterial Pneumonia" and "Viral Pneumonia") (X-ray images)	Data augmentation	nCOVnet	88.10%	0.880	97.62%	78.57%	(40)
Pereira et al. (2020)	"RYDLS-20;" Radiopedia Encyclopedia "Chest X-ray14"	90 COVID-19 patients; 1,000 Normal patients; 10 MERS patients; 11 SARS patients; 10 Varicella patients; 12 Streptococcus patients; 11 Pneumocystis patients (X-ray images)	Resampling algorithms; Fusion techniques;	Pre-trained CNN	F1 score = 89%				(91)
Rahaman et al. (2020)	COVID-19 X-ray image database developed by Cohen JP; "Chest X-Ray Images (pneumonia)"	260 COVID-19 patients; 300 Pneumonia; 300 Normal patients (X-ray images)	Data augmentation (rotate, shift, shear, zoom, horizontal and vertical flip)	VGG19	89.3%	–	89%	–	(92)
Rahimzadeh et al. (2020)	"Covid chestxray dataset;" "RSNA pneumonia detection challenge"	180 COVID-19 patients; 6,054 Pneumocystis patients; 8,851 Normal patients (X-ray images)	Data augmentation	Xception ResNet50V2 concatenated	91.4%	–	80.53%	99.56%	(93)
Rajaraman et al. (2020)	Pediatric CXR dataset; RSNA CXR dataset; CheXpert CXR dataset; NIH CXR-14 dataset; Twitter COVID-19 CXR dataset; Montreal COVID-19 CXR dataset;	4,683 Bacterial Pneumonia; 3,883 Viral Pneumonia (X-Ray images)	Segmenting lung area with dilated dropout U-Net; Image thresholding to remove very bright pixels; In-painting missing pixels using the surrounding pixel values; Using median-filter to remove noise and preserve edges;	VGG-16	94.05%	0.96	98.77%	86.24%	(45)

(Continued)

TABLE 2 | Continued

Author, year	Data source	Data structure and size	Data preprocessing	Best model structure(s)	Performance measurements (on the best model)				References
					Accuracy	AUC score	Sensitivity	Specificity	
Rajaraman et al. (2020)	"Pediatric CXR dataset;" "RSNA CXR dataset;" "Twitter COVID-19 CXR dataset;" "Montreal COVID-19 CXR dataset"	313 COVID-19 patients; 7,595 pneumonia of unknown type patients; 2,780 bacterial pneumonia; 7,595 Normal patients (X-ray images)	Median Filtering; Normalization; Standardization	Inception-V3	99.01%	0.997	98.4%	–	(45)
Sethy et al. (2020)	X-ray images on public medical Github repositories; Kaggle chest X-ray database	127 COVID-19 patients; 127 Pneumonia patients; 127 Normal patients (X-ray images)	–	ResNet50 plus SVM	98.66%	–	95.33%	–	(94)
Shibly et al. (2020)	COVID-19 X-ray image database developed by Cohen JP; "RSNA pneumonia detection challenge dataset;" Kaggle chest X-ray database; "COVIDx"	183 COVID-19 patients; 5,551 Pneumonia patients; 8,066 Normal patients (X-ray images)	–	Faster R-CNN	97.36%	–	97.65%	–	(95)
Toğaçar et al. (2020)	COVID-19 X-ray image database developed by Cohen JP; Kaggle COVID-19 dataset created by a team of researchers from Qatar University, medical doctors from Bangladesh, and collaborators from Pakistan and Malaysia.	295 COVID-19 patients; 98 Pneumonia; 65 normal patients (X-ray images)	Restructuring images using the Fuzzy Color technique and stacking them with the original images; Feature extracting using deep learning models (MobileNetV2, SqueezeNet) using the Social Mimic optimization method;	SVM	100%	–	100%	100%	(96)
Toraman et al. (2020)	COVID-19 X-ray image database developed by Cohen JP	231 COVID-19 patients; 1,050 Pneumonia patients; 1,050 Normal patients (X-ray images)	Data augmentation;	Convolutional capsnet	97.24% (Binary class)	–	97.42%	97.04%	(97)

(Continued)

TABLE 2 | Continued

Author, year	Data source	Data structure and size	Data preprocessing	Best model structure(s)	Performance measurements (on the best model)				References
					Accuracy	AUC score	Sensitivity	Specificity	
Tsiknakis et al. (2020)	COVID-19 X-ray image database developed by Cohen JP; Dataset originated from the QUIBIM imagingcovid19 platform database and various public repositories, including RSNA, IEEE, RadioGyan and the British Society of Thoracic Imaging; Publicly available X-ray dataset of patients with pneumonia;	137 COVID-19 patients; 150 Virus Pneumonia; 150 Bacteria Pneumonia; 150 normal patients (X-ray images)	Data augmentation (rotation, shear, zoom)	Inception V3	76% (multi-class)	0.93 (multi-class)	93% (multi-class)	91.8% (multi-class)	(98)
Tuncer et al. (2020)	GitHub website; Kaggle chest X-ray database	87 COVID-19 patients; 234 Normal patients (X-ray images)	Converting X-ray image to grayscale; ResExLBP and IRF based method	SVM	100%	–	98.29%	100%	(99)
Ucar et al. (2020)	"COVID chest X-ray dataset;" "Kaggle chest X-ray pneumonia dataset;"	403 COVID-19 patients; 721 normal patients (X-ray images)	Data augmentation (noise, shear, brightness increase, brightness decrease)	Bayes-SqueezeNet	98.26% (multi-class)	–	–	99.13% (multi-class)	(100)
Vaid et al. (2020)	Set of lately published articles; NIH dataset	181 COVID-19 patients; 364 Normal patients (X-ray images)	Normalization	VGG-19	96.3%	–	97.1%	–	(101)
Waheed et al. (2020)	"IEEE Covid Chest X-ray dataset;" "COVID-19 Radiography Database" "COVID-19 Chest X-ray Dataset;"	403 COVID-19 patients; 721 normal patients (X-ray images)	Data augmentation using CovidGAN	VGG16	95%	–	90%	97%	(102)
Yildirim et al. (2020)	"COVID-19 Chest X-Ray dataset;" Kaggle chest X-ray database	136 COVID-19 patients; 162 Pneumonia patients; 245 Normal patients (X-ray images)	–	Hybrid model	96.30%	–	96.30%	98.73%	(103)
Yoo et al. (2020)	"COVID-Chest XrayDataset;" Eastern Asian Hospital; Shenzen data;	162 COVID-19 Patients; 162 TB patients; 162 Non-TB patients (X-ray images)	Data augmentation (rotated, translated, and horizontally flipped)	ResNet18	95% Average of (COVID-19/TB) and (COVID-19/non-TB)	0.95 Average of (COVID-19/TB) and (COVID-19/non-TB)	97% Average of (COVID-19/TB) and (COVID-19/non-TB)	93% Average of (COVID-19/TB) and (COVID-19/non-TB)	(104)
Ghoshal et al. (2020)	COVID-19 X-ray image database developed by Cohen JP; "Kaggle chest X-ray database"	68 COVID-19 patients; 2,786 Bacterial Pneumonia patients; 1,504 Viral Pneumonia patients; 1,583 normal patients (X-Ray images)	Standardization; Data augmentation	Bayesian ResNet50V2 model	89.82%	–	–	–	(105)

(Continued)

TABLE 2 | Continued

Author, year	Data source	Data structure and size	Data preprocessing	Best model structure(s)	Performance measurements (on the best model)				References
					Accuracy	AUC score	Sensitivity	Specificity	
Hall et al. (2020)	"X-ray images on public medical Github repositories;" "Radiopaedia;" "Italian Society of Medical and Interventional Radiology (SIRM)"	135 COVID-19 patients; 320 Viral and Bacterial Pneumonia patients (X-Ray images)	Data augmentation	Resnet50 and VGG16 plus CNN	91.24%	0.94	–	–	(106)
Hammoudi et al. (2020)	"Chest XRay Images (Pneumonia) dataset;" COVID-19 X-ray image database developed by Cohen JP;	148 Bacterial pneumonia; 148 Viral pneumonia; 148 Normal patients (X-Ray Images)	–	DenseNet169	95.72%	–	–	–	(107)
El-Din Hemdan et al. (2020)	COVID-19 X-ray image database developed by Cohen JP; COVID-19 X-ray image database by Dr. Adrian Rosebrock	25 COVID-19 patients; 25 normal patients (X-Ray images)	Scaling to 224*224 pixels; One-hot encoding	COVIDX-Net (VGG19 and DenseNet201 models)	VGG19 = 90%; DenseNet201 = 90%	VGG19 = 0.90; DenseNet201 = 0.90	VGG19 = 100%; DenseNet201 = 100%	–	(108)
Jain et al. (2020)	"Chest XRay Images (Pneumonia) dataset;" COVID-19 X-ray image database developed by Cohen JP;	250 COVID-19 patients; 300 Bacterial pneumonia; 350 Viral pneumonia; 315 Normal patients (X-Ray Images)	Normalize images according to the images in the ImageNet database; Data augmentation (rotation and Gaussian blur);	ResNet50	97.77%	–	97.14%	–	(109)
Luz et al. (2020)	"COVIDx dataset;" "RSNA Pneumonia Detection Challenge dataset;" "COVID-19 image data collection"	183 COVID-19 patients; 5,521 Pneumonia patients; 8,066 normal patients (X-Ray images)	Intensity normalization; Data augmentation	EfficientNet B3	93.9%	–	96.8%	–	(110)
Ozkaya et al. (2020)	From the Italian Society of Medical and Interventional Radiology	53 COVID-19 patients (CT images)	Feature vectors obtained from Pre-trained VGG-16, GoogleNet and ResNet-50 networks and fusion method; Feature ranking by t-test method	SVM	98.27%	–	98.93%	97.60%	(68)

(Continued)

TABLE 2 | Continued

Author, year	Data source	Data structure and size	Data preprocessing	Best model structure(s)	Performance measurements (on the best model)				References
					Accuracy	AUC score	Sensitivity	Specificity	
Ozturk et al. (2020)	"covid-chestxray-dataset available at: https://github. com/ieee8023/covid-chestxray-dataset"	4 ARds images, 101 COVID images, 2 No finding images, 2 pneumocystis-pneumonia images, 11 Sars images, and 6 streptococcus (X-Ray images)	Data augmentation; SMOTE oversampling; creating feature vectors with sAE and PCA; feature extraction by feature vectors, Gray Level Co-occurrence Matrix, Local Binary Gray Level Co-occurrence Matrix, Gray Level Run Length Matrix, and Segmentation-based Fractal Texture Analysis	SVM	94.23%	0.99	91.88%	98.54%	(111)
Wang et al. (2020)	COVIDx dataset	266 COVID-19 patients; 5,536 Pneumonia patients; 8,066 normal patients (X-Ray images)	–	COVID-Net Network Architecture using a "lightweight residual projection-expansion-projection-extension design pattern" (Customized CNN)	93.3%		91.0%	–	(1)
Zhang et al. (2020)	X-COVID, OpenCOVID	599 COVID-19 patients; 2,107 non-COVID-19 patients (non-viral pneumonia and healthy) (X-Ray images)	Data augmentation; Feature extraction using EfficientNet	Confidence-aware anomaly detection	78.57%	0.844	77.13%	78.97%	(112)

Data Source: The source(s) that images were acquired from, Data Structure and Size: Number of images, image modalities, sample groups, Data Preprocessing: cleaning, Instance selection, normalization, transformation, feature extraction, selection, etc. The product of data preprocessing is the final training set, Best Model Structure(s): Best machine algorithm or deep learning model reported in the selected paper based on its performance, Performance Measurements (on the best model): The measurement of the model's output performance based on accuracy, sensitivity, specificity, and AUC score.

DISCUSSION

Machine and deep learning methods have been proven as valuable strategies to assess massive high-dimensional characteristics of medical images. CT or X-Ray findings of COVID-19 patients have similarities with other atypical and viral pneumonia diseases. Therefore, machine and deep learning methods might facilitate automatic discrimination of COVID-19 from other pneumonia conditions. The differential diagnosis of COVID also includes drug-induced diseases or immune pneumonitis. However, most of the studies reviewed here lack these kinds of samples. This point is the limitation of these studies. Different methods, such as Ensemble, VGG-16, ResNet, InceptionNetV3, MobileNet v2, Xception, CNN, VGG16, Truncated Inception Net, and KNN, have been used for the purpose of assessment of chest images of COVID-19 patients. Notably, the application of these methods on X-rays has offered promising results. Such a finding is particularly important since X-rays are easily accessible and low cost. These methods not only can diagnose COVID-19 patients from non-COVID pneumonia cases, but can also predict the severity of COVID-19 pneumonia and the risk of short-term mortality. In spite of the low expense of X-ray compared with CT images, the numbers of studies that assessed these two types of imaging using machine/deep learning methods are not meaningfully different. However, few studies have used these methods on both types of imaging (25, 29, 40). CNN-based methods have achieved accuracy values above 99% in classifying COVID-19 patients from other cases of pneumonia or related disorders, as reported by several independent studies, suggesting these strategies as screening methods for initial evaluation of COVID-19 cases.

Although both deep learning and machine learning strategies can be used for the mentioned purpose, they differ in some respects. For instance, deep learning methods usually need a large amount of labeled training data to make a concise conclusion. However, machine learning can apply a small amount of data delivered by users. Moreover, deep learning methods need high-performance hardware. Machine learning, on the other hand, needs features to be precisely branded by users, deep learning generates novel features by itself, thus requires more time to train. Machine learning classifies tasks into small fragments and subsequently combines obtained results into one conclusion, whereas deep learning resolves the problems using end-to-end principles.

Several studies have diagnosed COVID-19 patients through the application of machine learning methods rather than using deep learning methods by retrieving the features from the images. These studies have yielded high recognition outcomes and have the advantage of high learning speed (12). Pre-processing is an essential step for reducing the impacts of intensity variations in CT slices and getting rid of noise. Subsequent thresholding and morphological operations have also enhanced the analytical performance. Data augmentation and histogram equalization are among the most applied preprocessing methods.

One of the most promising approaches used in the included studies was transfer learning. Transfer learning is defined as using model knowledge on a huge dataset (which is referred to as the "pre-trained model") and transferring it to use on a new problem. This is very useful in settings like medical imaging, where there is a limited number of labeled data (113). Previous studies showed favorable outcomes of the transfer learning approaches in medical imaging tasks (114, 115). Among the included studies, Bridge et al. (25) even reached 100% classification accuracy on COVID-19 using the pre-trained InceptionV3.

The availability of public databases of CT and X-ray images of patients with COVID-19 has facilitated the application of machine learning methods on large quantities of clinical images and execution of training and verification steps. However, since these images have come from various institutes using different scanners, preprocessing of the obtained data is necessary to make them uniform and facilitate further analysis (12). Appraisal of demographic and clinical data of COVID-19 patients and their association with CT/ X-ray images features as well as the accuracy of machine learning prediction methods would provide more valuable information in the stratification of COVID-19 patients. Moreover, one of the major challenges of deep learning models in medical applications is its unexplainable features due to its black-box nature, which should be solved (116). Future studies can focus on approaches that provide interpretation besides black-box predictions.

CONCLUSION

Deep and machine learning methods have high accuracy in the differentiation of COVID-19 from non-COVID-19 pneumonia based on chest images. These techniques have facilitated the automatic evaluation of these images. However, deep learning methods suffer from the absence of transparency and interpretability, as it is not possible to identify the exact imaging feature that has been applied to define the output (13). As no single strategy has the capacity to distinguish all pulmonary disorders based merely on the imaging presentation on chest CT scans, the application of multidisciplinary approaches is suggested for overcoming diagnostic problems (13).

AUTHOR CONTRIBUTIONS

HM-R, MN, and AG-L collected the data and designed the tables. MT and SG-F designed the study, wrote the draft, and revised it. All the authors read the draft and approved the submitted version.

REFERENCES

1. Wang L, Wong A. COVID-Net: a tailored deep convolutional neural network design for detection of covid-19 cases from chest X-ray images. *arXiv.* (2020) Preprint arXiv:200309871. doi: 10.1038/s41598-020-76550-z

2. Ghafouri-Fard S, Noroozi R, Vafaee R, Branicki W, Pośpiech E, Pyrc K, et al. Effects of host genetic variations on response to, susceptibility and severity of respiratory infections. *Biomed Pharmacother.* (2020) 128:110296. doi: 10.1016/j.biopha.2020.110296

3. Song Y, Zheng S, Li L, Zhang X, Zhang X, Huang Z, et al. Deep learning enables accurate diagnosis of novel coronavirus (COVID-19) with CT images. *medRxiv.* (2020).

4. Samsami M, Mehravaran E, Tabarsi P, Javadi A, Arsang-Jang S, Komaki A, et al. Clinical and demographic characteristics of patients with COVID-19 infection: statistics from a single hospital in Iran. *Human Antibodies.* (2020) 1–6. doi: 10.3233/HAB-200428

5. Ghafouri-Fard S, Noroozi R, Omrani MD, Branicki W, Pośpiech E, Sayad A, et al. Angiotensin converting enzyme: a review on expression profile and its association with human disorders with special focus on SARS-CoV-2 infection. *Vascular Pharmacol.* (2020) 130:106680. doi: 10.1016/j.vph.2020.106680

6. Wang S, Kang B, Ma J, Zeng X, Xiao M, Guo J, et al. A deep learning algorithm using CT images to screen for Corona Virus Disease (COVID-19). *medRxiv.* (2020) 14:1–9. doi: 10.1101/2020.02.14.20023028

7. Fang Y, Zhang H, Xie J, Lin M, Ying L, Pang P, et al. Sensitivity of chest CT for COVID-19: comparison to RT-PCR. *Radiology.* (2020) 296:1–2. doi: 10.1148/radiol.2020200432

8. Zhang J, Tian S, Lou J, Chen Y. Familial cluster of COVID-19 infection from an asymptomatic. *Crit Care.* (2020) 24:1–3. doi: 10.1186/s13054-020-2817-7

9. Lei Y, Zhang H-W, Yu J, Patlas MN. *COVID-19 Infection: Early Lessons.* Los Angeles, CA: Sage (2020).

10. Rousan LA, Elobeid E, Karrar M, Khader Y. Chest x-ray findings and temporal lung changes in patients with COVID-19 pneumonia. *BMC Pulmonary Med.* (2020) 20:1–9. doi: 10.1186/s12890-020-01286-5

11. Bai HX, Hsieh B, Xiong Z, Halsey K, Choi JW, Tran TML, et al. Performance of radiologists in differentiating COVID-19 from viral pneumonia on chest CT. *Radiology.* (2020) 296:1–8. doi: 10.1148/radiol.2020200823

12. Ozsahin I, Sekeroglu B, Musa MS, Mustapha MT, Uzun Ozsahin D. Review on diagnosis of COVID-19 from chest CT images using artificial intelligence. *Comput Math Methods Med.* (2020) 2020:1–10. doi: 10.1155/2020/9756518

13. Li L, Qin L, Xu Z, Yin Y, Wang X, Kong B, et al. Using artificial intelligence to detect COVID-19 and community-acquired pneumonia based on pulmonary CT: evaluation of the diagnostic accuracy. *Radiology.* (2020) 296:E65–71. doi: 10.1148/radiol.2020200905

14. rekha Hanumanthu S. Role of intelligent computing in COVID-19 prognosis: a state-of-the-art review. *Chaos Solitons Fractals.* (2020) 138:109947. doi: 10.1016/j.chaos.2020.109947

15. Abbasian Ardakani A, Acharya UR, Habibollahi S, Mohammadi A. COVIDiag: a clinical CAD system to diagnose COVID-19 pneumonia based on CT findings. *Eur Radiol.* (2020) 31:1–10. doi: 10.1007/s00330-020-07087-y

16. Alazab M, Awajan A, Mesleh A, Abraham A, Jatana V, Alhyari S. COVID-19 prediction and detection using deep learning. *Int J Comput Information Syst Indus Manage Appl.* (2020) 12:168–81. doi: 10.1016/j.chaos.2020.110338

17. Albahli S. Efficient GAN-based Chest Radiographs (CXR) augmentation to diagnose coronavirus disease pneumonia. *Int J Med Sci.* (2020) 17:1439–48. doi: 10.7150/ijms.46684

18. Albahli S, Albattah W. Detection of coronavirus disease from X-ray images using deep learning and transfer learning algorithms. *J Xray Sci Technol.* (2020) 28:841–50. doi: 10.3233/XST-200720

19. Alsharman N, Jawarneh I. GoogleNet CNN neural network towards chest CT-coronavirus medical image classification. *J Comput Sci.* (2020) 16:620–5 doi: 10.3844/jcssp.2020.620.625

20. Altan A, Karasu S. Recognition of COVID-19 disease from X-ray images by hybrid model consisting of 2D curvelet transform, chaotic salp swarm algorithm and deep learning technique. *Chaos Solitons Fractals.* (2020) 140:110071. doi: 10.1016/j.chaos.2020.110071

21. Apostolopoulos ID, Aznaouridis SI, Tzani MA. Extracting possibly representative COVID-19 biomarkers from X-ray images with deep learning approach and image data related to pulmonary diseases. *J Med Biol Eng.* (2020) 40:1–8. doi: 10.1007/s40846-020-00529-4

22. Ardakani AA, Kanafi AR, Acharya UR, Khadem N, Mohammadi A. Application of deep learning technique to manage COVID-19 in routine clinical practice using CT images: results of 10 convolutional neural networks. *Comput Biol Med.* (2020) 121:103795. doi: 10.1016/j.compbiomed.2020.103795

23. Das D, Santosh KC, Pal U. Truncated inception net: COVID-19 outbreak screening using chest X-rays. *Phys Eng Sci Med.* (2020) 43:1–11. doi: 10.21203/rs.3.rs-20795/v1

24. Aswathy SU, Jarin T, Mathews R, Nair LM, Rroan M. CAD systems for automatic detection and classification of COVID-19 in nano CT lung image by using machine learning technique. *Int J Pharm Res.* (2020) 12:1865–70. doi: 10.31838/ijpr/2020.12.02.247

25. Bridge J, Meng Y, Zhao Y, Du Y, Zhao M, Sun R, et al. Introducing the GEV activation function for highly unbalanced data to develop COVID-19 diagnostic models. *IEEE J Biomed Health Inform.* (2020) 24:1–10. doi: 10.1109/JBHI.2020.3012383

26. Butt C, Gill J, Chun D, Babu BA. Deep learning system to screen coronavirus disease 2019 pneumonia. *Appl Intell.* (2020) 6:1–7. doi: 10.1007/s10489-020-01714-3

27. Dey N, Rajinikanth V, Fong SJ, Kaiser MS, Mahmud M. Social group optimization-assisted Kapur's entropy and morphological segmentation for automated detection of COVID-19 infection from computed tomography images. *Cognit Comput.* (2020) 12:1–13. doi: 10.20944/preprints202005.0052.v1

28. Kermany D, Zhang K, Goldbaum M. Labeled optical coherence tomography (OCT) and Chest X-Ray images for classification. *Mendeley Data.* (2018) 2. doi: 10.17632/RSCBJBR9SJ.2

29. El Asnaoui K, Chawki Y. Using X-ray images and deep learning for automated detection of coronavirus disease. *J Biomol Struct Dyn.* (2020) 1–12. doi: 10.1080/07391102.2020.1767212

30. Han Z, Wei B, Hong Y, Li T, Cong J, Zhu X, et al. Accurate screening of COVID-19 using attention-based deep 3D multiple instance learning. *IEEE Trans Med Imaging.* (2020) 39:2584–94. doi: 10.1109/TMI.2020.2996256

31. Harmon SA, Sanford TH, Xu S, Turkbey EB, Roth H, Xu Z, et al. Artificial intelligence for the detection of COVID-19 pneumonia on chest CT using multinational datasets. *Nat Commun.* (2020) 11:4080. doi: 10.1038/s41467-020-17971-2

32. Hasan AM, Al-Jawad MM, Jalab HA, Shaiba H, Ibrahim RW, Al-Shamasneh AR. Classification of Covid-19 coronavirus, pneumonia and healthy lungs in CT scans using Q-deformed entropy and deep learning features. *Entropy.* (2020) 22:517. doi: 10.3390/e22050517

33. Hu S, Gao Y, Niu Z, Jiang Y, Li L, Xiao X, et al. Weakly supervised deep learning for COVID-19 infection detection and classification from CT images. *IEEE Access.* (2020) 8:118869–83. doi: 10.1109/ACCESS.2020.3005510

34. Jaiswal A, Gianchandani N, Singh D, Kumar V, Kaur M. Classification of the COVID-19 infected patients using DenseNet201 based deep transfer learning. *J Biomol Struct Dyn.* (2020) 1–8. doi: 10.1080/07391102.2020.1788642

35. Kang H, Xia L, Yan F, Wan Z, Shi F, Yuan H, et al. Diagnosis of coronavirus disease 2019 (COVID-19) with structured latent multi-view representation learning. *IEEE Trans Med Imaging.* (2020) 39:2606–14. doi: 10.1109/TMI.2020.2992546

36. Lessmann N, Sánchez CI, Beenen L, Boulogne LH, Brink M, Calli E, et al. Automated assessment of CO-RADS and chest CT severity scores in patients with suspected COVID-19 using artificial intelligence. *Radiology.* (2020) 202439.

37. Li Y, Dong W, Chen J, Cao S, Zhou H, Zhu Y, et al. Efficient and effective training of COVID-19 classification networks with self-supervised dual-track learning to rank. *IEEE J Biomed Health Inform.* (2020) 24:1–10. doi: 10.1109/JBHI.2020.3018181

38. Liu C, Wang X, Liu C, Sun Q, Peng W. Differentiating novel coronavirus pneumonia from general pneumonia based

on machine learning. *Biomed Eng Online.* (2020) 19:66. doi: 10.1186/s12938-020-00809-9

39. Mei X, Lee HC, Diao KY, Huang M, Lin B, Liu C, et al. Artificial intelligence-enabled rapid diagnosis of patients with COVID-19. *Nat Med.* (2020) 26:1224–8. doi: 10.1038/s41591-020-0931-3

40. Panwar H, Gupta PK, Siddiqui MK, Morales-Menendez R, Singh V. Application of deep learning for fast detection of COVID-19 in X-Rays using nCOVnet. *Chaos Solitons Fractals.* (2020) 138:109944. doi: 10.1016/j.chaos.2020.109944

41. Pathak Y, Shukla PK, Tiwari A, Stalin S, Singh S, Shukla PK. Deep transfer learning based classification model for COVID-19 disease. *Ing Rech Biomed.* (2020) 1–6. doi: 10.1016/j.irbm.2020.05.003

42. Peng Y, Tang YX, Lee S, Zhu Y, Summers RM, Lu Z. COVID-19-CT-CXR: a freely accessible and weakly labeled chest X-ray and CT image collection on COVID-19 from biomedical literature. *ArXiv.* (2020). doi: 10.1109/TBDATA.2020.3035935

43. Pu J, Leader J, Bandos A, Shi J, Du P, Yu J, et al. Any unique image biomarkers associated with COVID-19? *Eur Radiol.* (2020) 30:1–7. doi: 10.1007/s00330-020-06956-w

44. Raajan NR, Lakshmi VSR, Prabaharan N. Non-invasive technique-based novel corona (COVID-19) virus detection using CNN. *Natl Acad Sci Lett.* (2020) 1–4. doi: 10.1007/s40009-020-01009-8

45. Rajaraman S, Siegelman J, Alderson PO, Folio LS, Folio LR, Antani SK. Iteratively pruned deep learning ensembles for COVID-19 detection in chest X-rays. *IEEE Access.* (2020) 8:115041–50. doi: 10.1109/ACCESS.2020.3003810

46. Sakagianni A, Feretzakis G, Kalles D, Koufopoulou C, Kaldis V. Setting up an easy-to-use machine learning pipeline for medical decision support: a case study for COVID-19 diagnosis based on deep learning with CT scans. *Stud Health Technol Inform.* (2020) 272:13–6. doi: 10.3233/SHTI200481

47. Sharma S. Drawing insights from COVID-19-infected patients using CT scan images and machine learning techniques: a study on 200 patients. *Environ Sci Pollut Res Int.* (2020) 27:1–9. doi: 10.21203/rs.3.rs-23863/v1

48. Singh D, Kumar V, Vaishali, Kaur M. Classification of COVID-19 patients from chest CT images using multi-objective differential evolution-based convolutional neural networks. *Eur J Clin Microbiol Infect Dis.* (2020) 39:1379–89. doi: 10.1007/s10096-020-03901-z

49. Song J, Wang H, Liu Y, Wu W, Dai G, Wu Z, et al. End-to-end automatic differentiation of the coronavirus disease 2019 (COVID-19) from viral pneumonia based on chest CT. *Eur J Nucl Med Mol Imaging.* (2020) 47:1–9. doi: 10.1007/s00259-020-04929-1

50. Wang J, Bao Y, Wen Y, Lu H, Luo H, Xiang Y, et al. Prior-attention residual learning for more discriminative COVID-19 screening in CT images. *IEEE Trans Med Imaging.* (2020) 39:2572–83. doi: 10.1109/TMI.2020.2994908

51. Wang S, Zha Y, Li W, Wu Q, Li X, Niu M, et al. A fully automatic deep learning system for COVID-19 diagnostic and prognostic analysis. *Eur Respir J.* (2020) 56:2000775. doi: 10.1183/13993003.00775-2020

52. Warman A, Warman P, Sharma A, Parikh P, Warman R, Viswanadhan N, et al. Interpretable artificial intelligence for COVID-19 diagnosis from chest CT reveals specificity of ground-glass opacities. *medRxiv.* (2020) 1–13. doi: 10.1101/2020.05.16.20103408

53. Wu X, Hui H, Niu M, Li L, Wang L, He B, et al. Deep learning-based multi-view fusion model for screening 2019 novel coronavirus pneumonia: a multicentre study. *Eur J Radiol.* (2020) 128:109041. doi: 10.1016/j.ejrad.2020.109041

54. Xu X, Jiang X, Ma C, Du P, Li X, Lv S, et al. A deep learning system to screen novel coronavirus disease 2019 pneumonia. *Engineering.* (2020) 6:1–7. doi: 10.1016/j.eng.2020.04.010

55. Xu Y, Ma L, Yang F, Chen Y, Ma K, Yang J, et al. A collaborative online AI engine for CT-based COVID-19 diagnosis. *medRxiv.* (2020). doi: 10.1101/2020.05.10.20096073

56. Yan T, Wong PK, Ren H, Wang H, Wang J, Li Y. Automatic distinction between COVID-19 and common pneumonia using multi-scale convolutional neural network on chest CT scans. *Chaos Solitons Fractals.* (2020) 140:110153. doi: 10.1016/j.chaos.2020.110153

57. Yang S, Jiang L, Cao Z, Wang L, Cao J, Feng R, et al. Deep learning for detecting corona virus disease 2019 (COVID-19) on high-resolution computed tomography: a pilot study. *Ann Transl Med.* (2020) 8:450. doi: 10.21037/atm.2020.03.132

58. Yu Z, Li X, Sun H, Wang J, Zhao T, Chen H, et al. Rapid identification of COVID-19 severity in CT scans through classification of deep features. *Biomed Eng Online.* (2020) 19:63. doi: 10.1186/s12938-020-00807-x

59. Al-Karawi D, Al-Zaidi S, Polus N, Jassim S. Machine learning analysis of chest CT scan images as a complementary digital test of coronavirus (COVID-19) patients. *medRxiv.* (2020) 1–8. doi: 10.1101/2020.04.13.20063479

60. Alom MZ, Rahman M, Nasrin MS, Taha TM, Asari VK. COVID_MTNet: COVID-19 detection with multi-task deep learning approaches. *arXiv.* (2020) Preprint arXiv:200403747.

61. Barstugan M, Ozkaya U, Ozturk S. Coronavirus (covid-19) classification using ct images by machine learning methods. *arXiv.* (2020) Preprint arXiv:200309424.

62. Chen J, Wu L, Zhang J, Zhang L, Gong D, Zhao Y, et al. Deep learning-based model for detecting 2019 novel coronavirus pneumonia on high-resolution computed tomography. *Sci Rep.* (2020) 10:1–11. doi: 10.1101/2020.02.25.20021568

63. Farid AA, Selim GI, Awad H, Khater A. A novel approach of CT images feature analysis and prediction to screen for corona virus disease (COVID-19). *Int J Sci Eng Res.* (2020) 11:1–9. doi: 10.14299/ijser.2020.03.02

64. Gozes O, Frid-Adar M, Greenspan H, Browning PD, Zhang H, Ji W, et al. Rapid ai development cycle for the coronavirus (covid-19) pandemic: initial results for automated detection & patient monitoring using deep learning CT image analysis. *arXiv.* (2020) Preprint arXiv:200305037.

65. Jin C, Chen W, Cao Y, Xu Z, Zhang X, Deng L, et al. Development and evaluation of an AI system for COVID-19 diagnosis. *medRxiv.* (2020) 11:1–14. doi: 10.1101/2020.03.20.20039834

66. Jin S, Wang B, Xu H, Luo C, Wei L, Zhao W, et al. AI-assisted CT imaging analysis for COVID-19 screening: building and deploying a medical AI system in four weeks. *medRxiv.* (2020). doi: 10.1101/2020.03.19.20039354

67. Kassani SH, Kassasni PH, Wesolowski MJ, Schneider KA, Deters R. Automatic detection of coronavirus disease (COVID-19) in X-ray and CT images: a machine learning-based approach. *arXiv.* (2020) Preprint arXiv:200410641.

68. Ozkaya U, Ozturk S, Barstugan M. Coronavirus (COVID-19) classification using deep features fusion and ranking technique. *arXiv.* (2020) Preprint arXiv:200403698. doi: 10.1007/978-3-030-55258-9_17

69. Shi F, Xia L, Shan F, Wu D, Wei Y, Yuan H, et al. Large-scale screening of covid-19 from community acquired pneumonia using infection size-aware classification. *arXiv.* (2020) Preprint arXiv:200309860. doi: 10.1088/1361-6560/abe838

70. Zheng C, Deng X, Fu Q, Zhou Q, Feng J, Ma H, et al. Deep learning-based detection for COVID-19 from chest CT using weak label. *medRxiv.* (2020) 1–13. doi: 10.1101/2020.03.12.20027185

71. Apostolopoulos ID, Mpesiana TA. Covid-19: automatic detection from X-ray images utilizing transfer learning with convolutional neural networks. *Phys Eng Sci Med.* (2020) 43:635–40. doi: 10.1007/s13246-020-00865-4

72. Brunese L, Mercaldo F, Reginelli A, Santone A. Explainable deep learning for pulmonary disease and coronavirus COVID-19 detection from X-rays. *Comput Methods Programs Biomed.* (2020) 196:105608. doi: 10.1016/j.cmpb.2020.105608

73. Chowdhury MEH, Rahman T, Khandakar A, Mazhar R, Kadir MA, Mahbub ZB, et al. Can AI help in screening viral and COVID-19 pneumonia? *IEEE Access.* (2020) 8:132665–76. doi: 10.1109/ACCESS.2020.3010287

74. Civit-Masot J, Luna-Perejón F, Morales MD, Civit A. Deep learning system for COVID-19 diagnosis aid using X-ray pulmonary images. *Appl Sci.* (2020) 10:4640. doi: 10.3390/app10134640

75. Elaziz MA, Hosny KM, Salah A, Darwish MM, Lu S, Sahlol AT. New machine learning method for image-based diagnosis of COVID-19. *PLoS ONE.* (2020) 15:e0235187. doi: 10.1371/journal.pone.0235187

76. Hassantabar S, Ahmadi M, Sharifi A. Diagnosis and detection of infected tissue of COVID-19 patients based on lung x-ray image using

convolutional neural network approaches. *Chaos Solitons Fractals*. (2020) 140:110170. doi: 10.1016/j.chaos.2020.110170

77. Islam MZ, Islam MM, Asraf A. A combined deep CNN-LSTM network for the detection of novel coronavirus (COVID-19) using X-ray images. *Inform Med Unlocked*. (2020) 20:100412. doi: 10.1016/j.imu.2020.100412

78. Khan AI, Shah JL, Bhat MM. CoroNet: a deep neural network for detection and diagnosis of COVID-19 from chest x-ray images. *Comput Methods Programs Biomed*. (2020) 196:105581. doi: 10.1016/j.cmpb.2020.105581

79. Khuzani AZ, Heidari M, Shariati SA. COVID-Classifier: an automated machine learning model to assist in the diagnosis of COVID-19 infection in chest x-ray images. *medRxiv*. (2020).

80. Ko H, Chung H, Kang WS, Kim KW, Shin Y, Kang SJ, et al. COVID-19 pneumonia diagnosis using a simple 2D deep learning framework with a single chest CT image: model development and validation. *J Med Internet Res*. (2020) 22:e19569. doi: 10.2196/19569

81. Loey M, Smarandache F, Khalifa NEM. Within the lack of chest COVID-19 X-ray dataset: a novel detection model based on GAN and deep transfer learning. *Symmetry*. (2020) 12:651. doi: 10.3390/sym12040651

82. Mahmud T, Rahman MA, Fattah SA. CovXNet: a multi-dilation convolutional neural network for automatic COVID-19 and other pneumonia detection from chest X-ray images with transferable multi-receptive feature optimization. *Comput Biol Med*. (2020) 122:103869. doi: 10.1016/j.compbiomed.2020.103869

83. Martínez F, Martínez F, Jacinto E. Performance evaluation of the NASnet convolutional network in the automatic identification of COVID-19. *Int J Adv Sci Engin Information Technol*. (2020) 10:662–7. doi: 10.18517/ijaseit.10.2.11446

84. Minaee S, Kafieh R, Sonka M, Yazdani S, Jamalipour Soufi G. Deep-COVID: predicting COVID-19 from chest X-ray images using deep transfer learning. *Med Image Anal*. (2020) 65:101794. doi: 10.1016/j.media.2020.101794

85. Narayan Das N, Kumar N, Kaur M, Kumar V, Singh D. Automated deep transfer learning-based approach for detection of COVID-19 infection in chest X-rays. *Ing Rech Biomed*. (2020) 1–7. doi: 10.1016/j.irbm.2020.07.001

86. Nour M, Cömert Z, Polat K. A novel medical diagnosis model for COVID-19 infection detection based on deep features and Bayesian optimization. *Appl Soft Comput*. (2020) 97:1–14. doi: 10.1016/j.asoc.2020.106580

87. Novitasari DCR, Hendradi R, Caraka RE, Rachmawati Y, Fanani NZ, Syarifudin A, et al. Detection of COVID-19 chest x-ray using support vector machine and convolutional neural network. *Commun Math Biol Neurosci*. (2020) 2020:1–19. doi: 10.28919/cmbn/4765

88. Oh Y, Park S, Ye JC. Deep Learning COVID-19 Features on CXR using limited training data sets. *IEEE Trans Med Imaging*. (2020) 39:2688–700. doi: 10.1109/TMI.2020.2993291

89. Ozturk T, Talo M, Yildirim EA, Baloglu UB, Yildirim O, Rajendra Acharya U. Automated detection of COVID-19 cases using deep neural networks with X-ray images. *Comput Biol Med*. (2020) 121:103792. doi: 10.1016/j.compbiomed.2020.103792

90. Pandit MK, Banday SA. SARS n-CoV2-19 detection from chest x-ray images using deep neural networks. *Int J Pervasive Comput Commun*. (2020) 16:1–9. doi: 10.1108/IJPCC-06-2020-0060

91. Pereira RM, Bertolini D, Teixeira LO, Silla CN, Jr., Costa YMG. COVID-19 identification in chest X-ray images on flat and hierarchical classification scenarios. *Comput Methods Programs Biomed*. (2020) 194:105532. doi: 10.1016/j.cmpb.2020.105532

92. Rahaman MM, Li C, Yao Y, Kulwa F, Rahman MA, Wang Q, et al. Identification of COVID-19 samples from chest X-Ray images using deep learning: a comparison of transfer learning approaches. *J Xray Sci Technol*. (2020) 28:1–19. doi: 10.3233/XST-200715

93. Rahimzadeh M, Attar A. A modified deep convolutional neural network for detecting COVID-19 and pneumonia from chest X-ray images based on the concatenation of Xception and ResNet50V2. *Inform Med Unlocked*. (2020) 19:100360. doi: 10.1016/j.imu.2020.100360

94. Sethy PK, Behera SK, Ratha PK, Biswas P. Detection of coronavirus disease (COVID-19) based on deep features and support vector machine. *Int J Math Eng Manage Sci*. (2020) 5:643–51. doi: 10.33889/IJMEMS.2020.5.4.052

95. Shibly KH, Dey SK, Islam MT, Rahman MM. COVID faster R-CNN: a novel framework to diagnose novel coronavirus disease (COVID-19) in X-ray images. *Inform Med Unlocked*. (2020) 20:100405. doi: 10.1016/j.imu.2020.100405

96. Togaçar M, Ergen B, Cömert Z. COVID-19 detection using deep learning models to exploit social mimic optimization and structured chest X-ray images using fuzzy color and stacking approaches. *Comput Biol Med*. (2020) 121:103805. doi: 10.1016/j.compbiomed.2020.103805

97. Toraman S, Alakus TB, Turkoglu I. Convolutional capsnet: a novel artificial neural network approach to detect COVID-19 disease from X-ray images using capsule networks. *Chaos Solitons Fractals*. (2020) 140:110122. doi: 10.1016/j.chaos.2020.110122

98. Tsiknakis N, Trivizakis E, Vassalou EE, Papadakis GZ, Spandidos DA, Tsatsakis A, et al. Interpretable artificial intelligence framework for COVID-19 screening on chest X-rays. *Exp Ther Med*. (2020) 20:727–35. doi: 10.3892/etm.2020.8797

99. Tuncer T, Dogan S, Ozyurt F. An automated residual exemplar local binary pattern and iterative ReliefF based COVID-19 detection method using chest X-ray image. *Chemometr Intell Lab Syst*. (2020) 203:104054. doi: 10.1016/j.chemolab.2020.104054

100. Ucar F, Korkmaz D. COVIDiagnosis-Net: deep Bayes-SqueezeNet based diagnosis of the coronavirus disease 2019 (COVID-19) from X-ray images. *Med Hypotheses*. (2020) 140:109761. doi: 10.1016/j.mehy.2020.109761

101. Vaid S, Kalantar R, Bhandari M. Deep learning COVID-19 detection bias: accuracy through artificial intelligence. *Int Orthop*. (2020) 44:1539–42. doi: 10.1007/s00264-020-04609-7

102. Waheed A, Goyal M, Gupta D, Khanna A, Al-Turjman F, Pinheiro PR. CovidGAN: data augmentation using auxiliary classifier GAN for improved Covid-19 detection. *IEEE Access*. (2020) 8:91916–23. doi: 10.1109/ACCESS.2020.2994762

103. Yildirim M, Cinar A. A deep learning based hybrid approach for covid-19 disease detections. *Traitement Signal*. (2020) 37:461–8. doi: 10.18280/ts.370313

104. Yoo SH, Geng H, Chiu TL, Yu SK, Cho DC, Heo J, et al. Deep learning-based decision-tree classifier for COVID-19 diagnosis from chest X-ray imaging. *Front Med*. (2020) 7:427. doi: 10.3389/fmed.2020.00427

105. Ghoshal B, Tucker A. Estimating uncertainty and interpretability in deep learning for coronavirus (COVID-19) detection. *arXiv*. (2020) Preprint arXiv:200310769.

106. Hall LO, Paul R, Goldgof DB, Goldgof GM. Finding covid-19 from chest x-rays using deep learning on a small dataset. *arXiv*. (2020) 40:1–14. doi: 10.36227/techrxiv.12083964

107. Hammoudi K, Benhabiles H, Melkemi M, Dornaika F, Arganda-Carreras I, Collard D, et al. Deep learning on chest X-ray images to detect and evaluate pneumonia cases at the Era of COVID-19. *arXiv*. (2020) Preprint arXiv:200403399.

108. Hemdan EE-D, Shouman MA, Karar ME. Covidx-net: a framework of deep learning classifiers to diagnose covid-19 in x-ray images. *arXiv*. (2020) Preprint arXiv:200311055.

109. Jain G, Mittal D, Thakur D, Mittal MK. A deep learning approach to detect Covid-19 coronavirus with X-Ray images. *Biocybernet Biomed Eng*. (2020). doi: 10.1016/j.bbe.2020.08.008

110. Luz E, Silva PL, Silva R, Moreira G. Towards an efficient deep learning model for covid-19 patterns detection in x-ray images. *arXiv*. (2020) 31:1–10.

111. Ozturk S, Ozkaya U, Barstugan M. Classification of coronavirus images using shrunken features. *medRxiv*. (2020). doi: 10.1101/2020.04.03.20048868

112. Zhang J, Xie Y, Li Y, Shen C, Xia Y. Covid-19 screening on chest x-ray images using deep learning based anomaly detection. *arXiv*. (2020) Preprint arXiv:200312338.

113. Ravishankar H, Sudhakar P, Venkataramani R, Thiruvenkadam S, Annangi P, Babu N, et al. Understanding the mechanisms of deep transfer learning for medical images. In: *Deep Learning and Data Labeling for Medical Applications*: Springer (2016). p. 188–96.

114. Hosny KM, Kassem MA, Foaud MM. Classification of skin lesions using transfer learning and augmentation with Alexnet. *PLoS ONE*. (2019) 14:e0217293. doi: 10.1371/journal.pone. 0217293

115. Khan S, Islam N, Jan Z, Din IU, Rodrigues JJC. A novel deep learning based framework for the detection and classification of breast cancer using transfer learning. *Pattern Recogn Lett*. (2019) 125:1–6. doi: 10.1016/j.patrec.2019. 03.022

116. Singh A, Sengupta S, Lakshminarayanan V. Explainable deep learning models in medical image analysis. *J Imaging*. (2020) 6:52. doi: 10.3390/jimaging6060052

7

Prevalence of Atrial Fibrillation and Associated Mortality Among Hospitalized Patients with COVID-19

Zuwei Li[1†], Wen Shao[2†], Jing Zhang[3], Jianyong Ma[4], Shanshan Huang[2], Peng Yu[2], Wengen Zhu[5*] and Xiao Liu[6,7*]*

[1] Cardiology Department, The Affiliated Hospital of Jiangxi University of Chinese Medicine, Nanchang, China, [2] Endocrine Department, The Second Affiliated Hospital of Nanchang University, Nanchang, China, [3] Anesthesiology Department, The Second Affiliated Hospital of Nanchang University, Nanchang, China, [4] Department of Pharmacology and Systems Physiology, University of Cincinnati College of Medicine, Cincinnati, OH, United States, [5] Department of Cardiology, The First Affiliated Hospital of Sun Yat-sen University, Guangzhou, China, [6] Cardiology Department, The Sun Yat-sen Memorial Hospital of Sun Yat-sen University, Guangzhou, China, [7] Guangdong Province Key Laboratory of Arrhythmia and Electrophysiology, Guangzhou, China

Correspondence:
Peng Yu
yupeng_jxndefy@163.com
Wengen Zhu
zhuwg6@mail.sysu.edu.cn
Xiao Liu
liux587@mail.sysu.edu.cn

[†] These authors share first authorship

Background: Epidemiological studies have shown that atrial fibrillation (AF) is a potential cardiovascular complication of coronavirus disease 2019 (COVID-19). We aimed to perform a systematic review and meta-analysis to clarify the prevalence and clinical impact of AF and new-onset AF in patients with COVID-19.

Methods: PubMed, Embase, the Cochrane Library, and MedRxiv up to February 27, 2021, were searched to identify studies that reported the prevalence and clinical impact of AF and new-onset AF in patients with COVID-19. The study was registered with PROSPERO (CRD42021238423).

Results: Nineteen eligible studies were included with a total of 21,653 hospitalized patients. The pooled prevalence of AF was 11% in patients with COVID-19. Older ($\geq$60 years of age) patients with COVID-19 had a nearly 2.5-fold higher prevalence of AF than younger (<60 years of age) patients with COVID-19 (13 vs. 5%). Europeans had the highest prevalence of AF (15%), followed by Americans (11%), Asians (6%), and Africans (2%). The prevalence of AF in patients with severe COVID-19 was 6-fold higher than in patients with non-severe COVID-19 (19 vs. 3%). Furthermore, AF (OR: 2.98, 95% CI: 1.91 to 4.66) and new-onset AF (OR: 2.32, 95% CI: 1.60 to 3.37) were significantly associated with an increased risk of all-cause mortality among patients with COVID-19.

Conclusion: AF is quite common among hospitalized patients with COVID-19, particularly among older ($\geq$60 years of age) patients with COVID-19 and patients with severe COVID-19. Moreover, AF and new-onset AF were independently associated with an increased risk of all-cause mortality among hospitalized patients with COVID-19.

Keywords: atrial fibrillation, COVID-19, death, prevalence, meta-analysis

INTRODUCTION

Severe acute respiratory syndrome coronavirus 2 (SARS-CoV-2) is the pathogen of coronavirus disease 2019 (COVID-19), which emerged in December 2019 and has since caused a global epidemic. As of November 14, 2020, over 50 million cases of COVID-19 infection have been reported worldwide, resulting in more than 1 million deaths. Previous studies have confirmed that pneumonia is not only an infectious disease affecting the respiratory system, but it also has a significant impact on the cardiovascular system, leading to heart failure, arrhythmias, and myocardial ischemia (1–3). In addition to fever as the primary symptom, there are also initial clinical manifestations of the cardiovascular system among patients with COVID-19, (4, 5) indicating that cardiovascular diseases are potential complications of COVID-19 (6, 7).

Atrial fibrillation (AF) is the most common arrhythmia and can lead to stroke, peripheral embolization, heart failure, and other unfavorable outcomes (8). The prevalence of AF is between approximately 2.3% and 3.4% in the general population (9, 10). However, for patients with pulmonary disease, critical illness, or systemic inflammatory response syndrome, the prevalence and clinical impact of AF are even more substantial (11–13).

More recently, numerous epidemiological studies have shown an increased risk of AF and new-onset AF among patients with COVID-19 but have yielded inconsistent results (14–32). Moreover, accumulating literature has demonstrated that AF or new-onset AF might be significantly associated with the worst outcomes (e.g., mortality) in patients with COVID-19 (21, 25, 29). Subsequently, several meta-analyses have examined the relationship between COVID-19 and AF (33–36). However, these studies focused on arrhythmias or AF and only examined the association between AF and pooled unfavorable outcomes among patients with COVID-19. It is not clear whether AF increases the risk of death among patients with COVID-19. Furthermore, no studies to date have assessed the prevalence and clinical impact of new-onset AF in patients with COVID-19.

To help clinicians understand the potential damage to the cardiovascular system caused by COVID-19 and strengthen the monitoring and preservation of cardiac function, we conducted a systematic review and meta-analysis of observational studies to clarify the prevalence and clinical impact of AF and new-onset AF in patients with COVID-19.

METHODS

Protocol Registration and Search Strategy

This study was registered with PROSPERO (International prospective register of systematic reviews. https://www.crd.york.ac.uk/PROSPERO/ -registration number-CRD 42021238423). We performed this meta-analysis following the Preferred Reporting Items for Systematic Reviews and Meta-Analyses (PRISMA) statement (**Supplemental Table 1**) (37).

Two authors (W. L. and X. L.) independently conducted the database search, selection, data extraction, and statistical analysis. Four databases were searched for all related studies, including PubMed, Embase, the Cochrane Library, and MedRxiv (https://

www.medrxiv.org/), up to February 27, 2021. No language restrictions were applied. The following search terms were used for all databases: ("2019-novel coronavirus" OR "SARS-CoV-2" OR "COVID-19" OR "2019-nCoV" OR "COVID 19" OR "severe acute respiratory syndrome coronavirus 2") AND ("atrial fibrillation" OR "atrial fibrillations" OR "auricular fibrillation" OR "auricular fibrillations"). In addition, the conference abstracts and bibliographies of related literature were scanned to obtain other articles that might meet the requirements.

Selection Criteria and Study Selection

Studies were included if they met the following inclusion criteria: (1) patients in the literature were adults (>18 years of age) who were diagnosed with COVID-19 according to polymerase chain reaction (PCR) tests and had sinus rhythm at admission according to a 12-lead electrocardiogram (ECG); (2) studies reported the prevalence of AF during hospital admission and/or the association between AF and outcomes (e.g., all-cause mortality) in patients with COVID-19; and (3) articles were cohort or nested case–control studies. Accordingly, studies with the following conditions were excluded: (1) reviews, meta-analyses, congress abstracts, practice guidelines, patents, cases, editorials, replies, or comments; and (2) data of the articles remained unavailable after contacting the corresponding authors for further information.

The initial search results were imported into EndNote X8.2 software (Thomson Reuters, New York, NY) for management. Subsequently, duplications were eliminated automatically and manually. First, we examined the citation titles and abstracts. After the preliminary screening, we retrieved full reports that were likely to meet the predefined inclusion criteria. Any inconsistency was resolved through discussion (W. S. and X. L.) until a consensus was reached.

Data Collection and Quality Assessment

Data were extracted based on prespecified inclusion criteria. The following information was abstracted: study characteristics (first author's name, publication year, country, and study design), patient characteristics (sample size, age, sex, and medications), exposure (AF diagnosis and number of episodes during hospitalization), and outcomes (number of events, adjusted OR/RRs and the corresponding 95% CI, and adjustments).

For studies that reported the prevalence of AF, the Joanna Briggs Institute critical appraisal checklist was used to assess the study quality. For studies that reported the association between AF and outcomes in patients with COVID-19, the Newcastle–Ottawa quality scale (NOS) was applied. Case-control studies were appraised on selection, comparability, and exposure, while cohort studies were appraised on selection, comparability, and outcomes. Studies with an NOS of ≥6 stars were considered moderate- to high-quality articles.

Statistical Analysis

RevMan software, version 5.3 (The Cochrane Collaboration 2014, Nordic Cochrane Center Copenhagen, Denmark) and Stata software (Version 14.0, Stata Corp LP, College Station, Texas, USA) were both applied in data analysis. To determine the

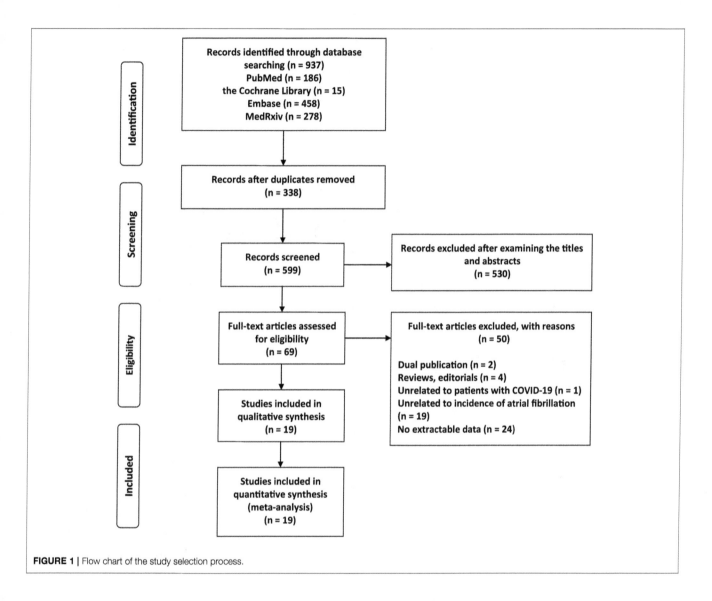

FIGURE 1 | Flow chart of the study selection process.

prevalence of AF in patients with COVID-19, the exact binomial (Clopper–Pearson) method was used to calculate 95% confidence intervals (CIs). Estimates were standardized using the Freeman–Tukey double arcsine transformation. To elucidate the clinical impact of AF in patients with COVID-19, we pooled the crude odds ratios (ORs) for categorical outcomes using the inverse-variance method. The crude ORs were calculated by events and total numbers of patients in the AF groups and control groups. Moreover, we estimated the adjusted effect size by calculating the natural logarithm of the OR (log [OR]) and its standard error (SElog [OR]). The ORs were shown with 95% CIs. We evaluated the degree of heterogeneity among the included studies using the χ^2 statistic (with a P-value of 0.10 considered significant) and the I^2 test (25%, 50%, and 75% represent low, moderate, and high heterogeneity, respectively) (38). We used the random effect model in this study to improve the reliability of our results considering the potential heterogeneity.

Subgroup analyses were performed to research possible modulated factors influencing our primary meta-analysis results,

including age, region, study design, sample size, cases of AF, and severity. We defined patients with severe COVID-19 as those who were admitted to the ICU, while patients who were not admitted to the ICU were considered to have non-severe COVID-19. Additionally, patients with a history of AF were excluded from the analysis of the prevalence of new-onset AF. Publication bias was assessed using funnel plots, Egger's test, and Begg's test. To appraise the robustness and reliability of the primary study outcomes, we also carried out sensitivity analyses by omitting each study in turn. All statistical tests were double-sided, and $P < 0.05$ was considered statistically significant.

RESULTS

Literature Search

The study selection process is shown in **Figure 1**. A total of 937 citations were identified through the initial database search. After a quick screening of the title and abstract, 69 articles remained. We further excluded 50 articles after the full-text review for the

TABLE 1 | Characteristics of included studies in this meta-analysis.

References, country	Sample of size, N	AF diagnosis	Study design	Mean age (years), Male %	History of AF, N	AF cases, N	New-onset AF cases, N	Outcomes reported	Medication (%)	Adjustments
Aajal et al. (20), Morocco	100	ECG	Prospective cohort	55.3, 37	22	2	NR	Prevalence	NR	—
Angeli et al. (23), Italy	50	ECG	Retrospective cohort	64, 72	NR	3	NR	Prevalence	Hydroxychloroquine: 82.0; Macrolides: 56.0; Lopinavir-Ritonavir: 54.0	—
Bhatla et al. (21), USA	700	ECG	Retrospective cohort	50, 45	39	25	NR	Prevalence, Mortality	Hydroxychloroquine: 24.6; Remdesivir: 8.1	None
Chen et al. (39), USA	143	ECG	Retrospective cohort	67, 62.2	19	13	13	Prevalence	NR	—
Colon et al. (14), USA	115	ECG	Retrospective cohort	56, 53.9	6	12	NR	Prevalence	Remdesivir/Placebo Trial: 7.0; Hydroxychloroquine: 6.1; Azithromycin: 43.5	—
Coromilas et al. (32), USA	4,526	ECG	Retrospective cohort	62.8, 57	408	509	NR	Prevalence	Hydroxychloroquine: 57.6; Azithromycin: 49.8; Antiviral: 15.3; IL–6 Inhibitor: 9.6; Anticoagulation: 29.4	—
Iacopino et al. (27), Italy	30	ECG	Prospective cohort	75.2, 66.7	8	10	10	Prevalence	None: 10.0; Antibiotic therapy: 6.7; Hydroxychloroquine+antiviral: 46.7; Hydroxychloroquine+ antiviral+azithromycin: 6.7; Hydroxychloroquine: 30.0; Monoclonal antibodies: 6.7; Low molecular weight heparins: 100.0	—
Kelesoglu et al. (25), Turkey	658	ECG	Retrospective cohort	54, 56.6	NR	33	33	Prevalence Mortality	NR	—
Linschoten et al. (18), Netherlands	3011	ECG	Retrospective cohort	67, 62.8	NR	142	NR	Prevalence	NR	—

(Continued)

TABLE 1 | Continued

References, country	Sample of size, N	AF diagnosis	Study design	Mean age (years), Male %	History of AF, N	AF cases, N	New-onset AF cases, N	Outcomes reported	Medication (%)	Adjustments
Mountantonakis et al. (15), USA	9,564	ECG	Retrospective cohort	64.8, 58.9	687	1,687	1,109	Prevalence Mortality	NR	Matching for age, gender, smoking, race, medical history, lactate, WBC magnesium, procalcitonin, d-dimer, ferritin, CRP, creatinine, bun, AST, lymphocyte count, ALT, ALT phos, serum glucose, potassium, sodium
Oates et al. (31), USA	77	ECG	Retrospective cohort	69, 55	4	5	4	Prevalence	Hydroxychloroquine: 87.0; Azithromycin: 60.0; Remdesivir: 4.0; Tocilizumab: 4.0	–
Peltzer et al. (28), USA	1,053	ECG	Retrospective cohort	62, 62	94	166	101	Prevalence Mortality	Hydroxychloroquine: 70.8; Remdesivir: 4.9; Steroids: 22.9; IL–6 inhibitor: 6.2; Intravenous gamma globulin: 0.9	Age, sex, race, renal disease, hypoxia, heart failure, CAD, hypertension, diabetes, pulmonary disease, renal disease, immunosuppression, smoking status, and cancer
Rav-Acha et al. (16), Israel	390	ECG	Retrospective cohort	57.5, 55.4	21	20	16	Prevalence Mortality	Azithromycin: 24.2; Hydroxychloroquine: 37.9; QT prolonging drug: 17.2	None
Russo et al. (19), Italy	414	ECG	Retrospective cohort	66.9, 61.1	72	71	50	Prevalence Mortality	NR	None
Saleh et al. (22), USA	201	ECG	Prospective cohort	58.5, 57.2	14	17	17	Prevalence	Hydroxychloroquine/Chloroquine: 40.8; (Hydroxychloroquine/Chloroquine) + Azithromycin: 59.2	–
Sanz et al. (26), Spain	160	ECG	Prospective cohort	65.7, 60	30	12	12	Prevalence Mortality	NR	None
Wetterslev et al. (17), Denmark	155	ECG	Retrospective cohort	66, 72.9	NR	52	NR	Prevalence Mortality	NR	–
Yenercag et al. (24), Turkey	140	ECG	Retrospective cohort	51.7, 49.3	NR	13	NR	Prevalence	NR	–
Zylla et al. (29), Germany	166	ECG	Retrospective cohort	64.1, 65.1	NR	11	NR	Prevalence Mortality	Hydroxychloroquine: 44.6; Hydroxychloroquine + azithromycin: 16.3; Anticoagulation therapy: 30.7	None

AF, atrial fibrillation; ECG, electrocardiogram; NR, not reported. WBC, white blood cell; CAD, coronary artery disease; CRP, C-reactive protein; BUN, blood urea nitrogen; AST, Aspartate aminotransferase, ALT, Alanine aminotransferase.

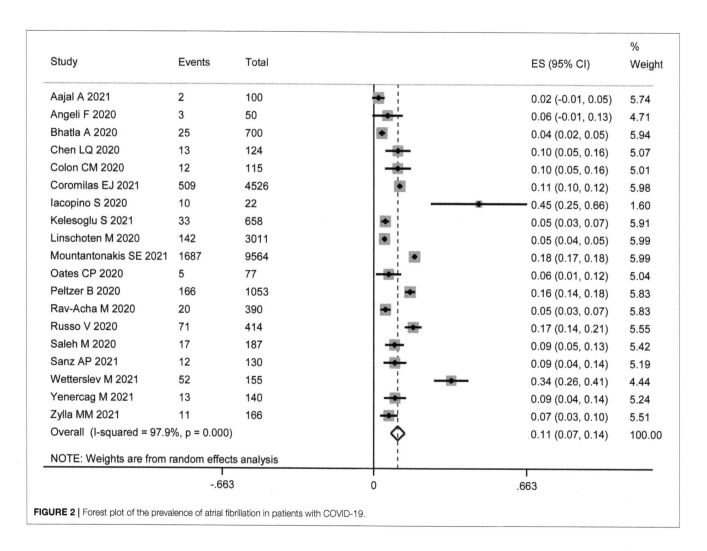

Study	Events	Total	ES (95% CI)	% Weight
Aajal A 2021	2	100	0.02 (-0.01, 0.05)	5.74
Angeli F 2020	3	50	0.06 (-0.01, 0.13)	4.71
Bhatla A 2020	25	700	0.04 (0.02, 0.05)	5.94
Chen LQ 2020	13	124	0.10 (0.05, 0.16)	5.07
Colon CM 2020	12	115	0.10 (0.05, 0.16)	5.01
Coromilas EJ 2021	509	4526	0.11 (0.10, 0.12)	5.98
Iacopino S 2020	10	22	0.45 (0.25, 0.66)	1.60
Kelesoglu S 2021	33	658	0.05 (0.03, 0.07)	5.91
Linschoten M 2020	142	3011	0.05 (0.04, 0.05)	5.99
Mountantonakis SE 2021	1687	9564	0.18 (0.17, 0.18)	5.99
Oates CP 2020	5	77	0.06 (0.01, 0.12)	5.04
Peltzer B 2020	166	1053	0.16 (0.14, 0.18)	5.83
Rav-Acha M 2020	20	390	0.05 (0.03, 0.07)	5.83
Russo V 2020	71	414	0.17 (0.14, 0.21)	5.55
Saleh M 2020	17	187	0.09 (0.05, 0.13)	5.42
Sanz AP 2021	12	130	0.09 (0.04, 0.14)	5.19
Wetterslev M 2021	52	155	0.34 (0.26, 0.41)	4.44
Yenercag M 2021	13	140	0.09 (0.04, 0.14)	5.24
Zylla MM 2021	11	166	0.07 (0.03, 0.10)	5.51
Overall (I-squared = 97.9%, p = 0.000)			0.11 (0.07, 0.14)	100.00

NOTE: Weights are from random effects analysis

-.663   0   .663

FIGURE 2 | Forest plot of the prevalence of atrial fibrillation in patients with COVID-19.

following reasons: (1) dual publication ($n = 2$); (2) editorials or review articles ($n = 4$); (3) unrelated to patients with COVID-19 ($n = 1$); (4) unrelated to the prevalence of AF ($n = 19$); and (5) no extractable data ($n = 24$). As a result, we included 19 eligible studies (14–32).

Study Characteristics and Study Quality

The basic characteristics are shown in **Table 1**. Among the 19 included studies, (14–32) the publishing years ranged from 2020 to 2021. Overall, a total of 21,653 hospitalized patients were included, with 12,700 (58.7%) being men (ranging from 37.0 to 72.9%). The number of individuals ranged from 30 to 9,564, with the mean age of the participants ranging from 50.0 years to 75.2 years. Among the included studies, the diagnosis of AF was based on electrocardiograms. Three reports were from Asia, (16, 24, 25) 1 from Africa, (20) 7 from Europe, (17–19, 23, 26, 27, 29) and 8 from America (14, 15, 21, 22, 28, 30–32). Apart from 4 prospective cohort studies, (20, 22, 26, 27) the remaining 15 articles were designed as retrospective cohort studies (14–19, 21, 23–25, 28–32).

Based on the Joanna Briggs Institute Critical Appraisal Checklist, all 19 studies (14–32) that reported the prevalence

of AF met a minimum of six of the nine criteria, which meant that these articles applied rigorous methodology (**Supplemental Table 2**). In accordance with the NOS, all 8 studies (15, 16, 19, 21, 25, 26, 28, 29) that involved the association between AF and outcomes of patients with COVID-19 were viewed as moderate to high quality, with a score range of 6–8 (**Supplemental Table 3**).

The Prevalence of AF in Patients With COVID-19

Nineteen studies (14–32) with a total of 21,582 participants reported the prevalence of AF in hospitalized patients with COVID-19. The pooled prevalence of AF was 11% (95% CI: 7% to 14%), with high heterogeneity ($I^2 = 97.9\%$) (**Figure 2**).

In the subgroup analysis, older (mean age ≥ 60 years) patients with COVID-19 showed a nearly 2.5-fold higher prevalence of AF than younger (mean age <60 years) patients with COVID-19 (ES: 13 vs. 5%, P for subgroup difference <0.001) (**Figure 3A**). Europeans had the highest prevalence of AF (ES: 15%), followed by Americans (ES: 11%), Asians (ES: 6%), and Africans (ES: 2%) (P for subgroup difference <0.001) (**Figure 3B**). Furthermore, the prevalence of AF in patients with severe COVID-19 was

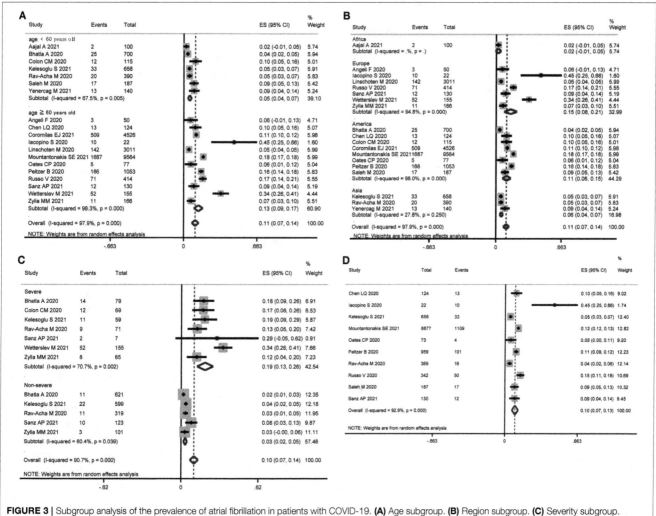

FIGURE 3 | Subgroup analysis of the prevalence of atrial fibrillation in patients with COVID-19. **(A)** Age subgroup. **(B)** Region subgroup. **(C)** Severity subgroup. **(D)** New-onset atrial fibrillation subgroup.

6-fold higher than in patients with nonsevere COVID-19 (ES: 19 vs. 3%, P for subgroup difference <0.001) (**Figure 3C**). Ten articles (15, 16, 19, 22, 25–28, 30, 31) provided data on the prevalence of new-onset AF (ES: 10%, 95% CI: 7% to 13%, I^2 = 92.9%) (**Figure 3D**). There was no significant difference in the study design ($P = 0.92$), sample size ($P = 0.74$), or cases of AF ($P = 0.20$) (**Table 2**).

The Impact of AF on All-Cause Mortality in Patients With COVID-19

Eight articles (15, 16, 19, 21, 25, 26, 28, 29) with a total of 13,075 participants reported the association between AF and all-cause mortality in patients with COVID-19. Ultimately, of the 2,025 patients in the AF group, 1,024 patients died (50.6%). There were 11,050 patients in the control group, with 3,242 deaths (29.3%). As presented in **Figure 4A**, AF was significantly associated with an increased risk of all-cause mortality among patients with COVID-19 (crude OR:

2.98, 95% CI: 1.91 to 4.66, I^2 = 77%). Moreover, the pooled result of the multivariate analysis (15, 28) did not change (adjusted OR: 1.65, 95% CI: 1.16 to 2.35, I^2 = 59%) (**Figure 4B**).

Additionally, 6 publications (15, 16, 19, 25, 26, 28) with a total of 11,335 participants reported the association between new-onset AF and all-cause mortality in patients with COVID-19. There was a strong association between new-onset AF and all-cause mortality among hospitalized patients with COVID-19 (crude OR: 2.32, 95% CI: 1.60 to 3.37, I^2 = 54%) (**Figure 5A**). Consistently, the pooled multivariate analysis (15, 28) showed similar results (adjusted OR: 2.01, 95% CI: 1.12 to 3.62, $P = 0.02$, $I^2 = 82$%) (**Figure 5B**).

As shown in **Supplemental Figure 1**, the funnel plot, Egger's test ($p = 0.19$), and Begg's test ($p = 0.99$) showed no statistically significant potential publication bias, although publication bias was not suggested when the included studies was limited ($N < 10$). Sensitivity analyses performed by omitting each study

TABLE 2 | Subgroup analysis of prevalence of AF in patient with COVID-19.

Items		Number of studies	ES (95%CI)	P	$P^{*}_{h(\%)}$	$P^{\#}$
Result of primary analysis		19	0.105 (0.074–0.136)	<0.001	97.9	–
Mean age	<60 years	7	0.054 (0.037–0.072)	<0.001	67.5	<0.001
	≥60 years	12	0.133 (0.093–0.174)	<0.001	98.3	–
Study design	Retrospective	15	0.106 (0.072–0.140)	<0.001	98.3	0.92
	Prospective	4	0.102 (0.028–0.176)	0.007	88.2	–
Sample size	<300	11	0.110 (0.067–0.154)	<0.001	87.4	0.74
	≥ 300	8	0.100 (0.055–0.145)	<0.001	99.1	–
Cases of AF	<15	9	0.082 (0.049–0.116)	<0.001	73.6	0.20
	≥ 15	10	0.117 (0.076–0.159)	<0.001	98.9	–
Region	Europe	7	0.146 (0.080–0.212)	<0.001	94.8	<0.001
	America	8	0.107 (0.064–0.150)	<0.001	98.0	–
	Asia	3	0.055 (0.039–0.071)	<0.001	27.8	–
	Africa	1	0.020 (−0.007–0.047)	0.153	–	–
Severity of illness	Severe	7	0.191 (0.125–0.257)	<0.001	70.7	<0.001
	Non-severe	5	0.033 (0.018–0.047)	<0.001	60.4	–
Incidence of new-onset AF		10	0.097 (0.067–0.126)	<0.001	92.9	–

*AF, atrial fibrillation. *P for within-group heterogeneity, #P for subgroup difference.*

indicated that our results were stable and reliable, with a range from 2.61 (95% CI: 1.69 to 4.02) to 3.55 (95% CI: 2.14 to 5.91) (**Supplemental Figure 2**).

DISCUSSION

Overall, 19 studies were included in this study with a total of 21,653 hospitalized patients. The pooled prevalence of AF approached 11% in patients with COVID-19. Our results demonstrated that AF is quite common among hospitalized patients with COVID-19, particularly among older patients (≥60 years of age), North American and European patients, and patients with severe COVID-19. Furthermore, AF and new-onset AF were significantly associated with an increased risk of all-cause mortality among hospitalized patients with COVID-19.

Our results seemed to agree with previous studies, (33–36) while there were essential differences between the present meta-analysis and others. Two previous meta-analyses (34, 35) did not specify the type of arrhythmia in COVID-19, which meant that those studies mainly focused on arrhythmias instead of each subtype, such as AF. Our meta-analysis extended these studies and had two important strengths. This is the most comprehensive study to assess the prevalence of AF, as well as new-onset AF, among hospitalized patients with COVID-19, and our results showed that new-onset AF was also independently associated with an increased risk of mortality by excluding data from patients with a prior history of AF. More importantly, our subgroup analyses first revealed regional differences in the prevalence of AF among hospitalized patients with COVID-19 and the correlation between AF and severe COVID-19.

Compared with the prevalence of arrhythmias in hospitalized patients with community-acquired pneumonia (7%, 95% CI: 6 to 9%), (40) this study showed a higher prevalence of AF in hospitalized patients with COVID-19 (11%, 95% CI: 7 to 14%). The exact pathophysiology underlying AF in COVID-19 may be multifactorial and remains elusive. At present, some studies preliminarily speculate that SARS-CoV-2 is similar to SARS-CoV, which may cause a series of cascade reactions leading to pneumonia by combining with angiotensin-converting enzyme-2 (ACE2) in the human respiratory tract and lung tissue (41). The ACE2 receptor is also widely expressed in the cardiovascular system (42). Theoretically, the cardiovascular system is also a potential target organ of SARS-CoV-2 (43). Therefore, ACE2-related signaling pathways may play a key role in myocardial injury, which may affect atrial remodeling and increase susceptibility to AF (44). Moreover, inflammatory factor storms may be the mechanism of disease progression (45). Various inflammatory factors have been proven to be closely related to the development of AF. It has been reported that even mild tension in rat atrial tissue pretreated with IL-6 can lead to the occurrence of AF (46). In addition to the direct damage to myocardial cells caused by virus infection and the systemic inflammatory response syndrome induced by the virus, metabolic abnormalities, (47) hypoxemia, (48–50) respiratory failure, and usage of certain antiviral drugs (51, 52) also play roles in the pathogenesis of AF.

The potential mechanism by which AF contributes to increased mortality in patients with COVID-19 is yet to be determined. Coagulation abnormalities, cardiac injury, and stroke are possible mechanisms. For example, patients with AF had marked elevations in troponin, brain natriuretic peptide, C-reactive protein, and D-dimer, which may be

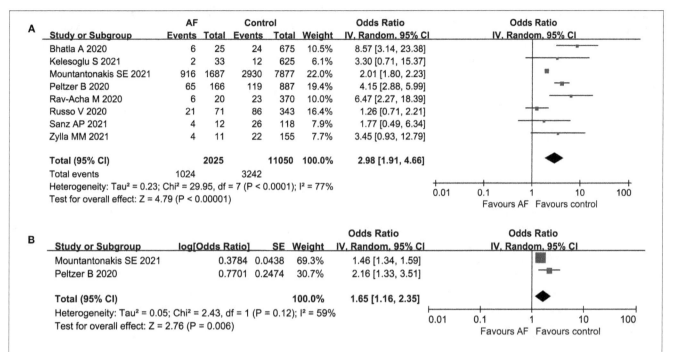

FIGURE 4 | Forest plot of the association between atrial fibrillation and all-cause mortality in patients with COVID-19. **(A)** Crude effect size of the association between atrial fibrillation and all-cause mortality in patients with COVID-19. **(B).** Adjusted effect size of the association between atrial fibrillation and all-cause mortality in patients with COVID-19.

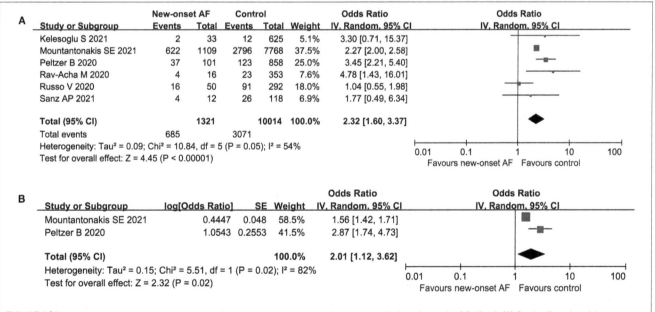

FIGURE 5 | Forest plot of the association between new-onset atrial fibrillation and all-cause mortality in patients with COVID-19. **(A)** Crude effect size of the association between new-onset atrial fibrillation and all-cause mortality in patients with COVID-19. **(B)** Adjusted effect size of the association between new-onset atrial fibrillation and all-cause mortality in patients with COVID-19.

the manifestations of cardiac injury, worsening cardiac function, and inflammatory response (28). Furthermore, hypercoagulability is an important feature in COVID-19, and AF could contribute to poor cardiac output, exacerbate

the hypercoagulable state, and eventually lead to increased mortality (53).

Our prognosis analysis showed that in-hospital mortality was significantly higher among patients with AF than among patients without AF. After adjustment for age, race, body mass index, and comorbidities, AF and new-onset AF were independently associated with a higher risk of all-cause mortality among patients with COVID-19. Moreover, it was notable that a few studies reported that new-onset AF was associated with longer hospital stays, more bleeding events, and more embolic events. These consistent findings indicated that AF and new-onset AF were associated with poor prognosis in patients with COVID-19. Therefore, clinicians should be more attentive to patients with COVID-19 and AF, optimize the clinical management of the disease, and implement more effective treatment regimens. Although no specific therapies have been recommended for patients with COVID-19 with AF to date, anticoagulant therapy may be useful. Systemic anticoagulants were reported to reduce mortality in hospitalized patients with COVID-19 (54). Similarly, low-molecular-weight heparin treatment was associated with lower 28-day mortality in patients with COVID-19 who had symptoms of coagulation disorders (55). In addition, several potential agents have been proposed for the treatment of patients with severe COVID-19, such as the interleukin-6 receptor antagonist tocilizumab (56, 57) and corticosteroids (58). Considering the strong link between inflammation and AF, the effect of these agents on the prevention of AF in patients with severe COVID-19 should be studied further.

Considering the high prevalence of AF among patients with COVID-19 and its poor prognostic implications, clinicians should recognize AF in patients with COVID-19. Careful electrocardiographic monitoring is advisable in patients with COVID-19 to detect AF early. Additionally, screening for AF should be performed in patients with COVID-19 and respective risk factors, particularly in older patients ($\geq$60 years of age), North American and European patients, and patients with severe COVID-19. Moreover, our results highlight the importance of utilizing AF and new-onset AF as clinical markers of in-hospital mortality and poor prognosis in hospitalized patients with COVID-19. Future investigations will need to further explore the association between COVID-19 and AF and to evaluate the safest and most effective strategies for clinical treatment and management of the disease.

Study Limitations

There are several limitations to the present systematic review and meta-analysis that need to be discussed. First, all the included studies were observational studies which cannot prove causality. Most of the studies were retrospective (79%) cohort. Hence, further well-designed, large-scale, prevalence studies are warranted to assessed the prevalence of AF in patient with COVID-19, as well as the potential difference in region, severity and age. Second, a high degree of heterogeneity was observed in our results. Although meta-regression was not performed, the subgroup analysis showed the heterogeneity might derived

from region, age or severity (**Table 2**). Third, many studies did not adjust for clinical confounding factors regarding the outcome of death. However, the positive association between AF and all-cause mortality persisted in the adjusted subgroup, suggesting that our results were relatively stable. Fourth, all the included participants were inpatients, rather than community patients, which may overestimate the prevalence and clinical impact of AF on patients with COVID-19. Fifth, many articles did not report specific drugs for treatment, so we cannot address the effects of these factors on the association between AF and poor prognosis in patients with COVID-19. Sixth, it is well known that AF significantly contributes to the incidence of stroke; however, stroke was not assessed in the present meta-analysis. Nevertheless, studies have shown that stroke is an uncommon complication of COVID-19, and there is no significant association between cerebrovascular disease and fatal outcomes in patients with COVID-19, suggesting that the prognostic damage caused by AF might be independent of stroke (39, 59, 60). Finally, there was only a small number of studies from Asia and Africa. In light of varying population characteristics among different regions, more studies from Asia and Africa are needed to confirm the regional differences in the prevalence of COVID-19.

CONCLUSIONS

AF is quite common among hospitalized patients with COVID-19, particularly among older patients ($\geq$60 years of age), North American and European patients, and patients with severe COVID-19. Moreover, AF and new-onset AF were independently associated with an increased risk of all-cause mortality among hospitalized patients with COVID-19. Our results should be confirmed by further well-designed, prospective studies.

AUTHOR CONTRIBUTIONS

XL, WZ, and PY were responsible for the entire project and revised the draft. ZL and WS performed the study selection, data extraction, statistical analysis, and interpretation of the data. WS and XL drafted the first version of the manuscript. All authors participated in the interpretation of the results and prepared the final version of the manuscript.

REFERENCES

1. Corrales-Medina VF, Musher DM, Shachkina S, Chirinos JA. Acute pneumonia and the cardiovascular system. *Lancet.* (2013) 381:496–505. doi: 10.1016/S0140-6736(12)61266-5

2. Corrales-Medina VF, Musher DM, Wells GA, Chirinos JA, Chen L, Fine MJ. Cardiac complications in patients with community-acquired pneumonia: incidence, timing, risk factors, and association with short-term mortality. *Circulation.* (2012) 125:773–81. doi: 10.1161/CIRCULATIONAHA.111.040766

3. Perry TW, Pugh MJ, Waterer GW, Nakashima B, Orihuela CJ, Copeland LA, et al. Incidence of cardiovascular events after hospital admission for pneumonia. *Am J Med.* (2011) 124:244–51. doi: 10.1016/j.amjmed.2010.11.014

4. Driggin E, Madhavan MV, Bikdeli B, Chuich T, Laracy J, Biondi-Zoccai G, et al. Cardiovascular considerations for patients, health care workers, and health systems during the COVID-19 pandemic. *J Am Coll Cardiol.* (2020) 75:2352–71. doi: 10.1016/j.jacc.2020.03.031

5. Liu K, Fang YY, Deng Y, Liu W, Wang MF, Ma JP, et al. Clinical characteristics of novel coronavirus cases in tertiary hospitals in Hubei Province. *Chin Med J (Engl).* (2020) 133:1025–31. doi: 10.1097/CM9.0000000000000744

6. Guo T, Fan Y, Chen M, Wu X, Zhang L, He T, et al. Cardiovascular implications of fatal outcomes of patients with coronavirus disease 2019 (COVID-19). *JAMA Cardiol.* (2020) 5:811–8. doi: 10.1001/jamacardio.2020.1017

7. Kang Y, Chen T, Mui D, Ferrari V, Jagasia D, Scherrer-Crosbie M, et al. Cardiovascular manifestations and treatment considerations in COVID-19. *Heart.* (2020) 106:1132–41. doi: 10.1136/heartjnl-2020-317056

8. January CT, Wann LS, Calkins H, Chen LY, Cigarroa JE, Cleveland JC Jr, et al. 2019 AHA/ACC/HRS focused update of the 2014 AHA/ACC/HRS guideline for the management of patients with atrial fibrillation: a report of the American college of cardiology/American heart association task force on clinical practice guidelines and the heart rhythm society in collaboration with the society of thoracic surgeons. *Circulation.* (2019) 140:e125–51. doi: 10.1161/CIR.0000000000000665

9. Ball J, Carrington MJ, McMurray JJ, Stewart S. Atrial fibrillation: profile and burden of an evolving epidemic in the 21st century. *Int J Cardiol.* (2013) 167:1807–24. doi: 10.1016/j.ijcard.2012.12.093

10. Lip GYH, Brechin CM, Lane DA. The global burden of atrial fibrillation and stroke: a systematic review of the epidemiology of atrial fibrillation in regions outside North America and Europe. *Chest.* (2012) 142:1489–98. doi: 10.1378/chest.11-2888

11. Chiang CE, Naditch-Brûlé L, Murin J, Goethals M, Inoue H, O'Neill J, et al. Distribution and risk profile of paroxysmal, persistent, and permanent atrial fibrillation in routine clinical practice: insight from the real-life global survey evaluating patients with atrial fibrillation international registry. *Circ Arrhythm Electrophysiol.* (2012) 5:632–9. doi: 10.1161/CIRCEP.112.970749

12. Zoni-Berisso M, Lercari F, Carazza T, Domenicucci S. Epidemiology of atrial fibrillation: European perspective. *Clin Epidemiol.* (2014) 6:213–20. doi: 10.2147/CLEP.S47385

13. McManus DD, Rienstra M, Benjamin EJ. An update on the prognosis of patients with atrial fibrillation. *Circulation.* (2012) 126:e143–6. doi: 10.1161/CIRCULATIONAHA.112.129759

14. Colon CM, Barrios JG, Chiles JW, McElwee SK, Russell DW, Maddox WR, et al. Atrial Arrhythmias in COVID-19 Patients. *JACC Clin Electrophysiol.* (2020) 6:1189–90. doi: 10.1016/j.jacep.2020.05.015

15. Mountantonakis SE, Saleh M, Fishbein J, Gandomi A, Lesser M, Chelico J, et al. Atrial fibrillation is an independent predictor for in-hospital mortality in patients admitted with SARS-CoV-2 infection. *Heart Rhythm.* (2021). doi: 10.1016/j.hrthm.2021.01.018

16. Rav-Acha M, Orlev A, Itzhaki I, Zimmerman SF, Fteiha B, Bohm D, et al. Cardiac arrhythmias among hospitalized Coronavirus 2019 (COVID-19) patients: prevalence, characterization, and clinical algorithm to classify arrhythmic risk. *Int J Clin Pract.* (2020) 75:e13788. doi: 10.22541/au.160071287.74177510

17. Wetterslev M, Jacobsen PK, Hassager C, Jøns C, Risum N, Pehrson S, et al. Cardiac arrhythmias in critically ill patients with coronavirus disease 2019: a retrospective population-based cohort study. *Acta Anaesthesiol Scand.* (2021) 65:770–7. doi: 10.1111/aas.13806

18. Linschoten M, Peters S, van Smeden M, Jewbali LS, Schaap J, Siebelink HM, et al. Cardiac complications in patients hospitalised with COVID-19 *Eur Heart J Acute Cardiovasc Care.* (2020) 9:817–23. doi: 10.1177/2048872620974605

19. Russo V, Di Maio M, Mottola FF, Pagnano G, Attena E, Verde N, et al. Clinical characteristics and prognosis of hospitalized COVID-19 patients with incident sustained tachyarrhythmias: A multicenter observational study. *Eur J Clin Invest.* (2020) 50:e13387. doi: 10.1111/eci.13387

20. Aajal A, El Boussaadani B, Hara L, Benajiba C, Boukouk O, Benali M, et al. The consequences of the lockdown on cardiovascular diseases. *Ann Cardiol Angeiol (Paris).* (2021). doi: 10.1016/S0735-1097(21)04491-0

21. Bhatla A, Mayer MM, Adusumalli S, Hyman MC, Oh E, Tierney A, et al. COVID-19 and cardiac arrhythmias. *Heart Rhythm.* (2020) 17:1439–44. doi: 10.1016/j.hrthm.2020.06.016

22. Saleh M, Gabriels J, Chang D, Soo Kim B, Mansoor A, Mahmood E, et al. Effect of Chloroquine, Hydroxychloroquine, and Azithromycin on the Corrected QT Interval in Patients With SARS-CoV-2 Infection. *Circ Arrhythm Electrophysiol.* (2020) 13:e008662. doi: 10.1161/CIRCEP.120.008662

23. Angeli F, Spanevello A, De Ponti R, Visca D, Marazzato J, Palmiotto G, et al. Electrocardiographic features of patients with COVID-19 pneumonia. *Eur J Intern Med.* (2020) 78:101–6. doi: 10.1016/j.ejim.2020.06.015

24. Yenerçag M, Arslan U, Seker OO, Dereli S, Kaya A, Dogduş M, et al. Evaluation of P-wave dispersion in patients with newly diagnosed coronavirus disease 2019. *J Cardiovasc Med.* (2021) 22:197–203. doi: 10.2459/JCM.0000000000001135

25. Kelesoglu S, Yilmaz Y, Ozkan E, Calapkorur B, Gok M, Dursun ZB, et al. New onset atrial fibrillation and risk faktors in COVID-19. *J Electrocardiol.* (2021) 65:76–81. doi: 10.1016/j.jelectrocard.2020.12.005

26. Pardo Sanz A, Salido Tahoces L, Ortega Pérez R, González Ferrer E, Sánchez Recalde Á, Zamorano Gómez JL. New-onset atrial fibrillation during COVID-19 infection predicts poor prognosis. *Cardiol J.* (2021) 28:34–40. doi: 10.5603/CJ.a2020.0145

27. Iacopino S, Placentino F, Colella J, Pesce F, Pardeo A, Filannino P, et al. New-onset cardiac arrhythmias during COVID-19 hospitalization. *Circ Arrhythm Electrophysiol.* (2020) 13:e009040. doi: 10.1161/CIRCEP.120.009040

28. Peltzer B, Manocha KK, Ying X, Kirzner J, Ip JE, Thomas G, et al. Outcomes and mortality associated with atrial arrhythmias among patients hospitalized with COVID-19. *J Cardiovasc Electrophysiol.* (2020) 31:3077–85. doi: 10.1111/jce.14770

29. Zylla MM, Merle U, Vey JA, Korosoglou G, Hofmann E, Muller M, et al. Predictors and Prognostic Implications of Cardiac Arrhythmias in Patients Hospitalized for COVID-19. *J Clin Med.* (2021) 10:133. doi: 10.3390/jcm10010133

30. Chen LQ, Burdowski J, Marfatia R, Weber J, Gliganic K, Diaz N, et al. Reduced cardiac function is associated with cardiac injury and mortality risk in hospitalized COVID-19 patients. *Clin Cardiol.* (2020) 43:1547–54. doi: 10.1002/clc.23479

31. Oates CP, Turagam MK, Musikantow D, Chu E, Shivamurthy P, Lampert J, et al. Syncope and presyncope in patients with COVID-19. *Pacing Clin Electrophysiol.* (2020) 43:1139–48. doi: 10.1111/pace.14047

32. Coromilas EJ, Kochav S, Goldenthal I, Biviano A, Garan H, Goldbarg S, et al. Worldwide survey of COVID-19 associated arrhythmias. *Circ Arrhythm Electrophysiol.* (2021).

33. Yang H, Liang X, Xu J, Hou H, Wang Y. Meta-analysis of atrial fibrillation in patients With COVID-19. *Am J Cardiol.* (2021) 144:152–6. doi: 10.1016/j.amjcard.2021.01.010

34. Liao SC, Shao SC, Cheng CW, Chen YC, Hung MJ. Incidence rate and clinical impacts of arrhythmia following COVID-19: a systematic review and meta-analysis of 17,435 patients. *Crit Care.* (2020) 24:690. doi: 10.1186/s13054-020-03368-6

35. Pellicori P, Doolub G, Wong CM, Lee KS, Mangion K, Ahmad M, et al. COVID-19 and its cardiovascular effects: a systematic review of prevalence studies. *Cochrane Database Syst Rev.* (2021) 3:Cd013879. doi: 10.1002/14651858.CD013879

36. Mulia EPB, Maghfirah I, Rachmi DA, Jularío R. Atrial arrhythmia and its association with COVID-19 outcome: a pooled analysis. *Diagnosis (Berl).* (2021). doi: 10.1515/dx-2020-0155

37. Moher D, Liberati A, Tetzlaff J, Altman DG. Preferred reporting items for systematic reviews and meta-analyses: the PRISMA statement. *Int J Surg.* (2010) 8:336–41. doi: 10.1016/j.ijsu.2010.02.007

38. Higgins J, Thomas J, Chandler J, Cumpston M, Li T, Page M, et al. Handbook for Systematic Reviews of Interventions version 6.0 (updated August 2019). Available online at: www.training.cochrane.org/handbook. doi: 10.1002/9781119536604

39. Chen J, Bai H, Liu J, Chen G, Liao Q, Yang J, et al. Distinct clinical characteristics and risk factors for mortality in female inpatients with coronavirus disease 2019 (COVID-19): a sex-stratified, large-scale cohort study in Wuhan, China. *Clin Infect Dis.* (2020) 71:3188–95. doi: 10.1093/cid/ciaa920

40. Tralhão A, Póvoa P. Cardiovascular events after community-acquired pneumonia: a global perspective with systematic review and meta-analysis of observational studies. *J Clin Med.* (2020) 9:414. doi: 10.3390/jcm9020414

41. Gralinski LE, Baric RS. Molecular pathology of emerging coronavirus infections. *J Pathol.* (2015) 235:185–95. doi: 10.1002/path.4454

42. Liu X, Long C, Xiong Q, Chen C, Ma J, Su Y, et al. Association of angiotensin converting enzyme inhibitors and angiotensin II receptor blockers with risk of COVID-19, inflammation level, severity, and death in patients with COVID-19: a rapid systematic review and meta-analysis. *Clin Cardiol.* (2020). doi: 10.1002/clc.23421. [Epub ahead of print].

43. Chen L, Li X, Chen M, Feng Y, Xiong C. The ACE2 expression in human heart indicates new potential mechanism of heart injury among patients infected with SARS-CoV-2. *Cardiovasc Res.* (2020) 116:1097–100. doi: 10.1093/cvr/cvaa078

44. Xu X, Chen P, Wang J, Feng J, Zhou H, Li X, et al. Evolution of the novel coronavirus from the ongoing Wuhan outbreak and modeling of its spike protein for risk of human transmission. *Sci China Life Sci.* (2020) 63:457–60. doi: 10.1007/s11427-020-1637-5

45. Huang C, Wang Y, Li X, Ren L, Zhao J, Hu Y, et al. Clinical features of patients infected with 2019 novel coronavirus in Wuhan, China. *Lancet.* (2020) 395:497–506. doi: 10.1016/S0140-6736(20)30183-5

46. Mitrokhin VM, Mladenov MI, Kamkin AG. Effects of interleukin-6 on the bio-electric activity of rat atrial tissue under normal conditions and during gradual stretching. *Immunobiology.* (2015) 220:1107–12. doi: 10.1016/j.imbio.2015.05.003

47. Kwenandar F, Japar KV, Damay V, Hariyanto TI, Tanaka M, Lugito NPH, et al. Coronavirus disease 2019 and cardiovascular system: a narrative review. *Int J Cardiol Heart Vasc.* (2020) 29:100557. doi: 10.1016/j.ijcha.2020.100557

48. Stevenson IH, Roberts-Thomson KC, Kistler PM, Edwards GA, Spence S, Sanders P, et al. Atrial electrophysiology is altered by acute hypercapnia but not hypoxemia: implications for promotion of atrial fibrillation in pulmonary disease and sleep apnea. *Heart Rhythm.* (2010) 7:1263–70. doi: 10.1016/j.hrthm.2010.03.020

49. Linz D, Schotten U, Neuberger HR, Böhm M, Wirth K. Negative tracheal pressure during obstructive respiratory events promotes atrial fibrillation by vagal activation. *Heart Rhythm.* (2011) 8:1436–43. doi: 10.1016/j.hrthm.2011.03.053

50. Linz D, Hohl M, Ukena C, Mahfoud F, Wirth K, Neuberger HR, et al. Obstructive respiratory events and premature atrial contractions after cardioversion. *Eur Respir J.* (2015) 45:1332–40. doi: 10.1183/09031936.00175714

51. Lazzerini PE, Boutjdir M. Capecchi PCOVID-19 L Arrhythmic Risk, and Inflammation: Mind the Gap! *Circulation.* (2020) 142:7–9. doi: 10.1161/CIRCULATIONAHA.120.047293

52. Cvetkovic RS, Goa KL. Lopinavir/ritonavir: a review of its use in the management of HIV infection. *Drugs.* (2003) 63:769–802. doi: 10.2165/00003495-200363080-00004

53. Abou-Ismail MY, Diamond A, Kapoor S, Arafah Y, Nayak L. The hypercoagulable state in COVID-19: Incidence, pathophysiology, and management. *Thromb Res.* (2020) 194:101–15. doi: 10.1016/j.thromres.2020.06.029

54. Bikdeli B, Madhavan MV, Jimenez D, Chuich T, Dreyfus I, Driggin E, et al. COVID-19 and thrombotic or thromboembolic disease: implications for prevention, antithrombotic therapy, and follow-up: JACC state-of-the-art review. *J Am Coll Cardiol.* (2020) 75:2950–73. doi: 10.1016/j.jacc.2020.04.031

55. Tang N, Bai H, Chen X, Gong J, Li D, Sun Z. Anticoagulant treatment is associated with decreased mortality in severe coronavirus disease 2019 patients with coagulopathy. *J Thromb Haemost.* (2020) 18:1094–9. doi: 10.1111/jth.14817

56. Hariyanto TI, Hardyson W, Kurniawan A. Efficacy and safety of tocilizumab for coronavirus disease 2019 (Covid-19) patients: a systematic review and meta-analysis. *Drug Res (Stuttg).* (2021) 71:265–74. doi: 10.1055/a-1336-2371

57. T. Ivan Hariyanto, Kurniawan A. Tocilizumab administration is associated with the reduction in biomarkers of coronavirus disease 2019 infection. *J Med Virol.* (2021) 93:1832–6. doi: 10.1002/jmv.26698

58. Zhao M. Cytokine storm and immunomodulatory therapy in COVID-19: Role of chloroquine and anti-IL-6 monoclonal antibodies. *Int J Antimicrob Agents.* (2020) 55:105982. doi: 10.1016/j.ijantimicag.2020.105982

59. Aggarwal G, G. Lippi, and B. Michael Henry, Cerebrovascular disease is associated with an increased disease severity in patients with Coronavirus Disease 2019 (COVID-19): a pooled analysis of published literature. *Int J Stroke.* (2020) 15:385–9. doi: 10.1177/1747493020921664

60. Siow I, Lee KS, Zhang JJY, Saffari SE, Ng A, Young B. Stroke as a Neurological complication of COVID-19: a systematic review and meta-analysis of incidence, outcomes and predictors. *J Stroke Cerebrovasc Dis.* (2021) 30:105549. doi: 10.1016/j.jstrokecerebrovasdis.2020.105549

8

Promoting a Syndemic Approach for Cardiometabolic Disease Management During COVID-19: The CAPISCO International Expert Panel

Wael Al Mahmeed[1], Khalid Al-Rasadi[2], Yajnavalka Banerjee[3], Antonio Ceriello[4], Francesco Cosentino[5], Massimo Galia[6], Su-Yen Goh[7], Peter Kempler[8], Nader Lessan[9], Nikolaos Papanas[10], Ali A. Rizvi[11,12], Raul D. Santos[13,14], Anca P. Stoian[15], Peter P. Toth[16], Manfredi Rizzo[12,15,17]* and The CArdiometabolic Panel of International experts on Syndemic COvid-19 (CAPISCO)

[1] Cleveland Clinic, Heart and Vascular Institute, Abu Dhabi, United Arab Emirates, [2] Medical Research Center, Sultan Qaboos University, Muscat, Oman, [3] Department of Biochemistry, Mohamed Bin Rashid University, Dubai, United Arab Emirates, [4] IRCCS MultiMedica, Milan, Italy, [5] Unit of Cardiology, Karolinska Institute and Karolinska University Hospital, University of Stockholm, Stockholm, Sweden, [6] Department of Biomedicine, Neurosciences and Advanced Diagnostics (Bind), University of Palermo, Palermo, Italy, [7] Department of Endocrinology, Singapore General Hospital, Singapore, Singapore, [8] Department of Medicine and Oncology, Semmelweis University, Budapest, Hungary, [9] Imperial College London Diabetes Centre, The Research Institute, Abu Dhabi, United Arab Emirates, [10] Second Department of Internal Medicine, Diabetes Center, University Hospital of Alexandroupolis, Democritus University of Thrace, Alexandroupolis, Greece, [11] Department of Medicine, University of Central Florida College of Medicine, Orlando, FL, United States, [12] Division of Endocrinology, Diabetes and Metabolism, University of South Carolina School of Medicine, Columbia, IN, United States, [13] Heart Institute (InCor) University of São Paulo Medical School Hospital, São Paulo, Brazil, [14] Hospital Israelita Albert Einstein, São Paulo, Brazil, [15] Faculty of Medicine, Diabetes, Nutrition and Metabolic Diseases, Carol Davila University, Bucharest, Romania, [16] Cicarrone Center for the Prevention of Cardiovascular Disease, Johns Hopkins University School of Medicine, Baltimore, MD, United States, [17] Department of Health Promotion, Mother and Child Care, Internal Medicine and Medical Specialties (Promise), University of Palermo, Palermo, Italy

*Correspondence:
Manfredi Rizzo
manfredi.rizzo@unipa.it

Efforts in the fight against COVID-19 are achieving success in many parts of the world, although progress remains slow in other regions. We believe that a syndemic approach needs to be adopted to address this pandemic given the strong apparent interplay between COVID-19, its related complications, and the socio-structural environment. We have assembled an international, multidisciplinary group of researchers and clinical practitioners to promote a novel syndemic approach to COVID-19: the CArdiometabolic Panel of International experts on Syndemic COvid-19 (CAPISCO). This geographically diverse group aims to facilitate collaborative-networking and scientific exchanges between researchers and clinicians facing a multitude of challenges on different continents during the pandemic. In the present article we present our "manifesto", with the intent to provide evidence-based guidance to the global medical and scientific community for better management of patients both during and after the current pandemic.

Keywords: diabetes, cardiovascular diseases, complications, COVID-19, pandemic, syndemic

INTRODUCTION

There is a bidirectional pathophysiologic relationship between coronavirus disease 2019 (COVID-19) and cardiometabolic diseases, and individuals at risk of the latter require careful consideration as the global pandemic continues to take its toll. Diabetes, obesity, and cardiovascular disease are associated with an increased risk for severe forms of COVID-19 and resulting death (1–6). At the same time, patients with COVID-19 infection are more prone to the development of new-onset diabetes mellitus (7). Investigators from different areas have emphasized the clinical relevance of the increased incidence of diabetes after severe acute respiratory syndrome coronavirus 2 (SARS-CoV-2) infection (8, 9). Furthermore, COVID-19 is associated with cardiovascular injury attributed to heightened inflammation, endothelial dysfunction and microthrombi formation (10–13). Endothelial dysfunction plays an important role in the pathogenesis of COVID-19, particularly in patients with pre-existing hypertension, diabetes, obesity and cardiovascular diseases (14). The endothelium, and particularly pulmonary endothelium, seems to be a key target organ in COVID-19 patients and its dysfunction has been shown to cause an impaired organ perfusion that can generate acute myocardial injury, renal failure, and a procoagulant state resulting in thromboembolic events (14–16).

It has been shown that SARS-CoV-2 can induce several pro-inflammatory cytokines (17) and that patients with severe COVID-19 develop a "cytokine storm syndrome" (18). Since these first observations it is become clear that the same cytokines that induce aberrant endothelial function may also trigger the acute phase response, which, in combination with local endothelial dysfunction, can lead to clinical consequences (14); indeed, inflammatory cytokines have a major role in both diabetes and cardiovascular diseases (19). Other authors have shown that COVID-19 is associated with myocardial damage such as myocarditis, arrhythmia and reduced left ventricular ejection fraction (20), all of which are associated to increased mortality risk (21). Plasma cardiac biomarkers, such as high sensitivity troponin, creatine kinase and N-terminal pro-B-type natriuretic peptide, are also associated with COVID-19 severity in adults and children (22, 23).

Beyond the direct effect of COVID-19 on the cardiovascular system and metabolic homeostasis, subjects with pre-existing cardiometabolic issues appear to be at a significantly higher risk of complications owing to reduced physical activity, altered eating behaviors, and lack of access to healthcare (24). This encapsulates the so-called "indirect" impact of COVID-19 and indeed a higher incidence of cardiovascular complications and fatalities has been documented secondary to the pandemic, for example in Italy (25). Even in New York City, emergency calls for cardiac arrests rose exponentially in the weeks when COVID-19 infections approached their zenith (26). Beyond deaths attributed directly to COVID-19, a large contribution to the excess mortality reported (27) is attributable to the indirect factors, including the disruption of the proper management of many clinical conditions–including cardiometabolic diseases–by the rapid conversion of entire hospitals or clinical units to deliver COVID-19-specific care (28).

This situation has been exacerbated in some geographical areas by increased unemployment, economic collapse, and widespread poverty (29). Indeed, increasing socio-economic disparities have come to the forefront in many populations during the pandemic, rendering people more vulnerable to economic, nutritional, social, and medical insecurity, particularly during prolonged periods of necessary government-imposed restrictions or lockdowns (30). In addition, the spread of the virus and the related complications and fatalities have been facilitated among subjects with the poorest socio-economic conditions and those living in overcrowded areas (29–31). Socio-economic inequalities are of increasing relevance during the ongoing vaccination campaigns as they contribute to disparities in care across different ethnic populations and geographical areas (32).

IMPORTANCE OF A SYNDEMIC APPROACH

The enormous efforts by many different organizations and individuals involved in the fight against COVID-19 have had some success in many parts of the world. However, this has not been universal and progress has been slow in many other regions. We believe that a syndemic approach needs to be adopted for addressing this pandemic (33) given the strong apparent interplay between COVID-19, its related complications, and the socio-structural environment. The term *syndemic* (from ancient Greek: *syn*, together; *demos*, people) emphasizes the relevance of biological, social, economic, and environmental factors in the health of individuals and populations (29). Physicians have an obligation to understand their patients' social, economic, and environmental situations and to utilize the tools available in existing health systems to improve their access to care. It is also expected that many health systems will continue to be under significant economic pressure, which may contribute to a reduced quality of care for patients with chronic conditions.

Another challenge is represented by the so-called *long-COVID syndrome*, which is a clinical condition present in subjects who have either recovered from COVID-19 but still report lasting effects of the infection or have had the usual symptoms for far longer than would be expected (34). Of increasing current interest are the neurological and neuropsychiatric complications (35), since several studies have reported a broad spectrum of symptoms, from the milder manifestations of memory loss, sleep disorders and impaired concentration to more serious cognitive decline, major depression or persistent delirium (36). Thus, there is an urgent need to better understand the long-term effects of COVID-19 on brain function, behavior and cognition. As a component of a holistic approach to the management of patients with COVID-19, mental health assessment should be included.

CAPISCO: AN INTERNATIONAL, MULTIDISCIPLINARY COLLABORATION

We believe it is crucial to improve interactions between specialists working in different disciplines, since insufficient

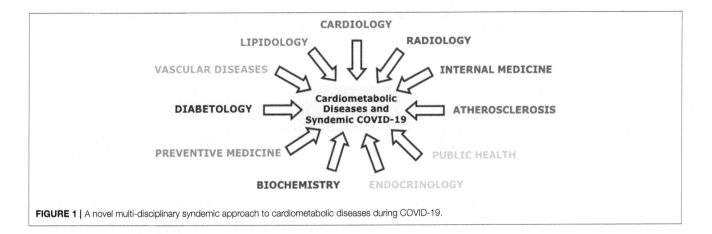

FIGURE 1 | A novel multi-disciplinary syndemic approach to cardiometabolic diseases during COVID-19.

cooperation has contributed to the indirect impact of COVID-19 (37). Furthermore, the pandemic has adversely medical education in many ways, for example owing to shifts to distance-learning modalities and decline in clinical clerkship due to the cancelation of routine patient appointments and surgical procedures and a transition to greater use of telemedicine (38). In response to these challenges we have recently assembled the Cardiometabolic Panel of International Experts on Syndemic COVID-19 (CAPISCO), a group of international researchers and clinical practitioners from many different disciplines including (but not limited to) diabetology, endocrinology, cardiology, lipidology, internal medicine, radiology, preventive medicine, public health and biochemistry–providing a multi-disciplinary representation in a novel approach to COVID-19 (**Figure 1**). We also emphasized geographical diversity when convening the group in order to facilitate collaborative-networking and scientific exchanges between researchers and clinicians facing a multitude of challenges in different continents during the pandemic.

Members of CAPISCO intend to collaboratively investigate:

1. how patients with cardiometabolic diseases and its complications are currently being managed and treated and the extent to which the pandemic impacts proper management, with a view to identifying, categorizing and defining innovative strategies to overcome potential barriers and disparities;

2. why differences in COVID-19 mortality rates have been reported among various countries, beyond the prevalence of the disease *per se*, with the aim to elucidate the social, economic and environmental factors potentially impacting clinical outcomes;

3. whether telemedicine is a reliable and useful tool to deliver high-quality patient care in light of experience gained during the pandemic; across different geographical areas we aim to investigate: what was successfully implemented and how, what was not successfully implemented and why, and what still needs to be improved;

4. how to assess the burden and late consequences of delayed management of cardiometabolic disease and other conditions due to COVID-19.

Ultimately, the overarching aim of CAPISCO is to give evidence-based guidance for the management of patients with cardiometabolic diseases during and after COVID-19 based on a syndemic approach. In terms of methodology, we plan to use a systematic approach, including systematic literature searches, formal quality-grading and analysis of collected studies, resulting in graded levels of recommendations. We also intend to make a roadmap plan of further research avenues once the data from the above indicated tools becomes available; this may also involve cooperation with health authorities and other international organizations.

CONCLUSIONS

In conclusion, we believe it is crucial to view COVID-19 through a syndemic lens to properly tackle the interlinked public health, medical, social and economic challenges that amplify each other in this crisis. The acronym of our expert panel, CAPISCO, is meaningful, since the word *"capisco"* means in Italian, *"I understand"*. CAPISCO contributions will promote a holistic approach for all patients with cardiometabolic diseases based on solid, validated scientific research and clinical expertise. We hope that physicians around the world will be able to use them to help benefit clinical care, follow-up, and monitoring of their patients during and after the COVID-19 pandemic.

AUTHOR CONTRIBUTIONS

This article is the result of three expert panel meetings conducted virtually between May and July 2021. MR and WA, co-chairs of CAPISCO, prepared the first draft of this article, which was first critically discussed and reviewed with AR, AC, and AS, and then extensively reviewed by all the other members. All

authors have equally contributed to the final manuscript and are listed alphabetically.

REFERENCES

1. Ceriello A, Standl E, Catrinoiu D, Itzhak B, Lalic NM, Rahelic D, et al. Issues of cardiovascular risk management in people with diabetes in the COVID-19 era. *Diabetes Care.* (2020) 43:1427–32. doi: 10.2337/dc20-0941

2. Khera A, Baum SJ, Gluckman TJ, Gulati M, Martin SS, Michos ED, et al. Continuity of care and outpatient management for patients with and at high risk for cardiovascular disease during the COVID-19 pandemic: A scientific statement from the American Society for Preventive Cardiology. *Am J Prev Cardiol.* (2020) 1:100009. doi: 10.1016/j.ajpc.2020.100009

3. Schnell O, Cos X, Cosentino F, Forst T, Giorgino F, Heersprink HJL, et al. Report from the CVOT Summit 2020: new cardiovascular and renal outcomes. *Cardiovasc Diabetol.* (2021) 20:75. doi: 10.1186/s12933-021-01254-1

4. Atallah B, El Lababidi R, Jesse W, Noor L, AlMahmeed W. Adapting to the COVID-19 pandemic at a quaternary care hospital in the Middle East Gulf region. *Heart Views.* (2020) 21:133–40.

5. Ceriello A, Stoian AP, Rizzo M. COVID-19 and diabetes management: What should be considered? *Diabetes Res Clin Pract.* (2020) 163:108151. doi: 10.1016/j.diabres.2020.108151

6. Stoian AP, Banerjee Y, Rizvi AA, Rizzo M. Diabetes and the COVID-19 pandemic: How Insights from recent experience might guide future management. *Metab Syndr Relat Disord.* (2020) 18:173–75. doi: 10.1089/met.2020.0037

7. Papachristou S, Stamatiou I, Stoian AP, Papanas N. New-onset diabetes in COVID-19: Time to frame its fearful symmetry. *Diabetes Ther.* (2021) 12:461–4. doi: 10.1007/s13300-020-00988-7

8. Shrestha DB, Budhathoki P, Raut S, Adhikari S, Ghimire P, Thapaliya S, et al. New-onset diabetes in COVID-19 and clinical outcomes: A systematic review and meta-analysis. *World J Virol.* (2021) 10:275–87. doi: 10.5501/wjv.v10.i5.275

9. Mameli C, Scaramuzza A, Macedoni M, Marano G, Frontino G, Luconi E, et al. Type 1 diabetes onset in Lombardy region, Italy, during the COVID-19 pandemic: The double-wave occurrence. *EClinicalMedicine.* (2021) 39:101067. doi: 10.1016/j.eclinm.2021.101067

10. Puntmann VO, Carerj ML, Wieters I, Fahim M, Arendt C, Hoffmann J, et al. Outcomes of cardiovascular magnetic resonance imaging in patients recently recovered from coronavirus disease 2019 (COVID-19). *JAMA Cardiol.* (2020) 5:1265–73. doi: 10.1001/jamacardio.2020.3557

11. Ferrari F, Martins VM, Teixeira M, Santos RD, Stein R. COVID-19 and Thromboinflammation: is there a role for statins? *Clinics (São Paulo).* (2021) 76:e2518. doi: 10.6061/clinics/2021/e2518

12. Libby P, Lüscher T. COVID-19 is, in the end, an endothelial disease. *Eur Heart J.* (2020) 41:3038–44. doi: 10.1093/eurheartj/ehaa623

13. Pellegrini D, Kawakami R, Guagliumi G, Sakamoto A, Kawai K, Gianatti A, et al. Microthrombi as a major cause of cardiac injury in COVID-19: a pathologic study. *Circulation.* (2021) 143:1031–42. doi: 10.1161/CIRCULATIONAHA.120.051828

14. Ionescu M, Stoian AP, Rizzo M, Serban D, Nuzzo D, Mazilu L, et al. The Role of Endothelium in COVID-19. *Int J Mol Sci.* (2021) 22:11920. doi: 10.3390/ijms222111920

15. Kaur S, Tripathi DM, Yadav A. The enigma of endothelium in COVID-19. *Front Physiol.* (2020) 11:989. doi: 10.3389/fphys.2020.00989

16. Sardu C, Gambardella J, Morelli MB, Wang X, Marfella R, Santulli G. Hypertension, thrombosis, kidney failure, and diabetes: Is COVID-19 an endothelial disease? A comprehensive evaluation of clinical and basic evidence. *J Clin Med.* (2020) 9:1417. doi: 10.3390/jcm9051417

17. Conti P, Ronconi G, Caraffa A, Gallenga CE, Ross R, Frydas I. e al. Induction of pro-inflammatory cytokines (IL-1 and IL-6) and lung inflammation by Coronavirus-19 (COVI-19 or SARS-CoV-2): anti-inflammatory strategies. *J Biol Regul Homeost Agents.* (2020) 34:327–31.

18. Mehta P, McAuley DF, Brown M, Sanchez E, Tattersall RS, Manson JJ, et al. Across Speciality Collaboration, UK COVID-19: consider cytokine storm syndromes and immunosuppression. *Lancet.* (2020) 395:1033–4. doi: 10.1016/S0140-6736(20)30628-0

19. Abate N, Sallam HS, Rizzo M, Nikolic D, Obradovic M, Bjelogrlic P, et al. Resistin: an inflammatory cytokine. Role in cardiovascular diseases, diabetes and the metabolic syndrome. *Curr Pharm Des.* (2014) 20:4961–9. doi: 10.2174/1381612819666131206103102

20. Madjid M, Safavi-Naeini P, Solomon SD, Vardeny O. Potential effects of coronaviruses on the cardiovascular system: a review. *JAMA Cardiol.* (2020) 5:831–40. doi: 10.1001/jamacardio.2020.1286

21. Silverio A, Di Maio M, Scudiero F, Russo V, Esposito L, Attena E, et al. Clinical conditions and echocardiographic parameters associated with mortality in COVID-19. *Eur J Clin Invest.* (2021) 51:e13638. doi: 10.1111/eci.13638

22. Zhu Z, Wang M, Lin W, Cai Q, Zhang L, Chen D, et al. Cardiac biomarkers, cardiac injury, and comorbidities associated with severe illness and mortality in coronavirus disease 2019 (COVID-19): A systematic review and meta-analysis. *Immun Inflamm Dis.* (2021) 9:1071–100. doi: 10.1002/iid3.471

23. Zhao Y, Patel J, Huang Y, Yin L, Tang L. Cardiac markers of multisystem inflammatory syndrome in children (MIS-C) in COVID-19 patients: A meta-analysis. *Am J Emerg Med.* (2021) 49:62–70. doi: 10.1016/j.ajem.2021.05.044

24. Bornstein SR, Rubino F, Ludwig B, Rietzsch H, Schwarz PEH, Rodionov RN, et al. Consequences of the COVID-19 pandemic for patients with metabolic diseases. *Nat Metab.* (2021) 3:289–92. doi: 10.1038/s42255-021-00358-y

25. De Rosa S, Spaccarotella C, Basso C, Calabrò MP, Curcio A, Filardi PP, et al. Società Italiana di Cardiologia and the CCU Academy investigators group. Reduction of hospitalizations for myocardial infarction in Italy in the COVID-19 era. *Eur Heart J.* (2020) 41:2083–8. doi: 10.1093/eurheartj/ehaa409

26. Wessler BS, Kent DM, Konstam MA. Fear of coronavirus disease 2019 – an emerging cardiac risk. *JAMA Cardiol.* (2020) 5:981–2. doi: 10.1001/jamacardio.2020.2890

27. Rizzo M, Foresti L, Montano N. Comparison of reported deaths from COVID-19 and increase in total mortality in Italy. *JAMA Intern Med.* (2020) 180:1250–2. doi: 10.1001/jamainternmed.2020.2543

28. Fadaak R, Davies JM, Blaak MJ, Conly J, Haslock J, Kenny A, et al. Rapid conversion of an in-patient hospital unit to accommodate COVID-19: An interdisciplinary human factors, ethnography, and infection prevention and control approach. *PLoS ONE.* (2021) 16:e0245212. doi: 10.1371/journal.pone.0245212

29. Fronteira I, Sidat M, Magalhães JP, de Barros FPC, Delgado AP, Correia T, et al. The SARS-CoV-2 pandemic: A syndemic perspective. *One Health.* (2021) 12:100228. doi: 10.1016/j.onehlt.2021.100228

30. Padmanabhan S. The COVID-19 pan-syndemic – will we ever learn? *Clin Infect Dis.* (2020) 73:e2976–7. doi: 10.1093/cid/ciaa1797

31. Available online at: https://www.nytimes.com/2021/05/04/world/oxygen-shortage-covid.html (accessed September 30th, 2021).

32. Available online at: https://www.kff.org/coronavirus-covid-19/issue-brief/latest-data-on-covid-19-vaccinationsrace-ethnicity/ (accessed September 30th, 2021).

33. Horton R. Offline: COVID-19 is not a pandemic. *Lancet.* (2020) 396:874. doi: 10.1016/S0140-6736(20)32000-6

34. Mahase E. Covid-19: What do we know about "long covid"? *BMJ.* (2020) 370:m2815. doi: 10.1136/bmj.m2815

35. Nuzzo D, Vasto S, Scalisi L, Cottone S, Cambula G, Rizzo M, et al. Post-Acute COVID-19 Neurological Syndrome: A New Medical Challenge. *J Clin Med.* (2021) 10:1947. doi: 10.3390/jcm10091947

36. Pantelis C, Jayaram M, Hannan AJ, Wesselingh R, Nithianantharajah J, Wannan CM, et al. Neurological, neuropsychiatric and neurodevelopmental complications of COVID-19. *Aust N Z J Psychiatry.* (2021) 55:750–62. doi: 10.1177/0004867420961472

37. Ceriello A. Lessons from COVID-19: How human behaviour may influence the science. *Diabetes Res Clin Pract.* (2020) 169:108491. doi: 10.1016/j.diabres.2020.108491

38. Naidoo N, Akhras A, Banerjee Y. Confronting the challenges of anatomy education in a competency-based medical curriculum during normal and unprecedented times (COVID-19 pandemic): pedagogical framework development and implementation. *JMIR Med Educ.* (2020) 6:e21701. doi: 10.2196/21701

9

Lipid Profile Features and their Associations with Disease Severity and Mortality in Patients with COVID-19

Jia Teng Sun [1,2†], Zhongli Chen [3†], Peng Nie [1,2†], Heng Ge [1,2], Long Shen [1,2], Fan Yang [1,2], Xiao Long Qu [1,2], Xiao Ying Ying [1,2], Yong Zhou [1,2], Wei Wang [1,2], Min Zhang [1,2] and Jun Pu [1*]

[1] Division of Cardiology, Renji Hospital, Shanghai Jiao Tong University School of Medicine, Shanghai, China, [2] Division of Pulmonary and Critical Care Medicine, Leishenshan Hospital, Wuhan, China, [3] Institute of Cardiovascular Disease, Ruijin Hospital, Shanghai Jiao Tong University School of Medicine, Shanghai, China

*Correspondence:
Jun Pu
pujun310@hotmail.com

† These authors have contributed equally to this work

Background: Emerging studies have described and analyzed epidemiological, clinical, laboratory, and radiological features of COVID-19 patients. Yet, scarce information is available regarding the association of lipid profile features and disease severity and mortality.

Methods: We conducted a prospective observational cohort study to investigate lipid profile features in patients with COVID-19. From 9 February to 4 April 2020, a total of 99 patients (31 critically ill and 20 severely ill) with confirmed COVID-19 were included in the study. Dynamic alterations in lipid profiles were recorded and tracked. Outcomes were followed up until 4 April 2020.

Results: We found that high-density lipoprotein-cholesterol (HDL-C) and apolipoprotein A-1 (apoA-1) levels were significantly lower in the severe disease group, with mortality cases showing the lowest levels ($p < 0.0001$). Furthermore, HDL-C and apoA-1 levels were independently associated with disease severity (apoA-1: odds ratio (OR): 0.651, 95% confidence interval (CI): 0.456–0.929, $p = 0.018$; HDL-C: OR: 0.643, 95% CI: 0.456–0.906, $p = 0.012$). For predicting disease severity, the areas under the receiver operating characteristic curves (AUCs) of HDL-C and apoA-1 levels at admission were 0.78 (95% CI, 0.70–0.85) and 0.85 (95% CI, 0.76–0.91), respectively. For in-hospital deaths, HDL-C and apoA-1 levels demonstrated similar discrimination ability, with AUCs of 0.75 (95% CI, 0.61–0.88) and 0.74 (95% CI, 0.61–0.88), respectively. Moreover, patients with lower serum concentrations of apoA-1 (<0.95 g/L) or HDL-C (<0.84 mmol/l) had higher mortality rates during hospitalization (log-rank $p < 0.001$). Notably, levels of apoA-1 and HDL-C were inversely proportional to disease severity. The survivors of severe cases showed significant recovery of apoA-1 levels at the end of hospitalization (vs. midterm apoA-1 levels, $p = 0.02$), whereas the mortality cases demonstrated continuously lower apoA-1 levels throughout hospitalization. Correlation analysis revealed that apoA-1 and HDL-C levels were negatively correlated with both admission levels and highest concentrations of C-reactive protein and interleukin-6.

Conclusions: Severely ill COVID-19 patients featured low HDL-C and apoA-1 levels, which were strongly correlated with inflammatory states. Thus, low apoA-1 and HDL-C levels may be promising predictors for severe disease and in-hospital mortality in patients suffering from COVID-19.

Keywords: HDL-C, apoA-1, inflammation, lipid, COVID-19

INTRODUCTION

As Coronavirus Disease 2019 (COVID-19) continues to spread worldwide, millions of people across hundreds of countries have been impacted. Epidemiological data show that although most cases are mild, severely ill patients rapidly progress to acute respiratory disease, multi-organ failure, and septic shock, with a remarkably increased mortality rate. Therefore, early identification of risk factors for COVID-19 severity and progression is of great importance.

Mounting evidence suggests that an impaired immune function and hyper-inflammatory response are characteristics of COVID-19 severity and mortality (1–3). Systemic inflammation and sepsis are prevalent metabolic disorders accompanying severe COVID-19 (4). Furthermore, proteome analysis suggests that patients with severe COVID-19 display dysregulated lipid metabolism (5). Dyslipidemia is associated with damage to the immune, respiratory, and cardiovascular systems, along with high levels of proinflammatory cytokines. Furthermore, dyslipidemia is casually associated with increased risk of thrombotic complications, endothelial dysfunction, and higher platelet activity (6). Thus, lipid dysregulation may contribute to morbidity and mortality from COVID-19 infection. However, the characteristics and dynamic changes in lipid profiles in COVID-19 patients, as well as their predictive value in disease severity and mortality, remain largely unknown.

Here, we performed an observational cohort study to investigate the lipid profile features of patients with COVID-19 and illuminate the associations between lipid features and disease severity/mortality.

MATERIALS AND METHODS
Study Population

This observational cohort study prospectively included 99 COVID-19-confirmed inpatients treated from 9 February to 4 April 2020 in Leishenshan Hospital, an urgently constructed hospital designated for COVID-19 patients located in Wuhan, China. All patients were diagnosed with COVID-19 according to interim guidance provided by the World Health Organization (WHO) (7). COVID-19 severity was classified according to the Guidelines on the Diagnosis and Treatment of COVID-19 released by the National Health Commission of China (version 7). Criteria for severe cases included any of the following: (1) respiratory rate $\geq$ 30 per min; (2) blood oxygen saturation (SPO$_2$) $\leq$ 93% at rest; (3) partial pressure of arterial oxygen to fraction of inspired oxygen ratio <300; (4) more than 50% of lung infiltrates within 24–48 h; or (5) patients needing mechanical

respiratory support or presenting with septic shock or multi-organ dysfunction or failure. All patients had a definite outcome (discharged, continued treatment, deceased) before data analysis.

Data Collection

Time from symptom onset to hospitalization and length of hospital stay were recorded. All epidemiological, clinical, laboratory, and outcome data were collected with standardized data collection forms from the electronic medical records system at Leishenshan Hospital. Personal history, including comorbidities, was confirmed with patients or family members. For information not available from the electronic medical records, researchers also communicated directly with patients or their families to obtain additional epidemiological and symptom data. Lipid profiles, including total cholesterol (TC), triglycerides (TG), low-density lipoprotein-cholesterol (LDL-C), high-density lipoprotein-cholesterol (HDL-C), apolipoprotein A-1 (apoA-1), and apolipoprotein B (apoB), were first determined within 24 h of admission. A subset of patients had multiple lipid and cytokine metrics (i.e., collected more than once); therefore, these data were included for longitudinal analysis. Dynamic alterations in the above indicators were recorded. The Sequential Organ Failure Assessment (SOFA) score (https://www.mdcalc.com/sequential-organ-failure-assessmment-sofa-score) were calculated for each participant on admission. Two researchers independently reviewed the forms to double-check the data collected.

Outcome Definition

Outcomes were followed up until 4 April 2020. The primary outcome in the study was defined as in-hospital death.

Statistics Analysis

No preliminary sample size calculation was evaluated, considering the observational nature of our study about this emerging infectious disease. Continuous variables were expressed as medians with interquartile ranges (IQR) and compared using unpaired Student's t-test or Mann-Whitney U test. Categorical data were expressed as absolute values and percentages and were compared using chi-square or Fisher's exact tests. Univariate and multivariable analyses were conducted to examine the associations between lipids and disease severity. To assess the discrimination ability of each lipid marker for outcome, receiver operating characteristic (ROC) curves were calculated, and the optimal cutoff values were determined by maximizing the Youden index. Spearman tests were used to analyze the correlations between lipids and inflammatory factors. Survival differences among groups with different lipid concentrations were compared by Kaplan-Meier analysis using the log-rank test. Significance levels were set based on two-sided α < 0.05. Data analyses were performed in statistical packages R (The R Foundation; http://www.r-project.org; version 3.6.1) and SPSS 22.0. Diagrams were plotted by GraphPad Prism 8.0 (GraphPad Software, USA).

RESULTS
Baseline Characteristics
A total of 99 laboratory-confirmed COVID-19 patients were prospectively enrolled in this study. As shown in **Table 1**, the median time from symptom onset to admission was comparable between mild and severe cases [20.00 (IQR: 14.00–26.00) days vs. 19.00 (IQR, 10.25–30.00) days, $p = 0.841$] as well as between severe-surviving and severe-non-surviving groups [20.00 (IQR: 10.50–30.00) days vs. 17.00 (IQR, 10.00–30.00) days, $p = 0.663$]. Compared with mild cases, severely ill patients were older (severe: median 70.5 years: IQR, 61.3–81.8 vs. mild: 52 years: IQR, 42.0–62.0) and more likely to have comorbidities (severe: 84% vs. mild: 59.2%) and higher SOFA scores (severe: median, 5, IQR, 2–7 vs. mild: median, 0, IQR, 0–1). No sex differences were found between the mild and severe groups. Fourteen patients received mechanical ventilation in the severe group, whereas no mechanical ventilation was used in the mild cases. A total of 15 severe group patients died in hospital. Mechanical ventilation was more frequently applied among non-survivors. Severe-non-surviving cases presented significantly higher SOFA scores (median, 8.00, IQR, 7.50–10.00) than severe-surviving cases (median, 3.00, IQR, 1.25–5.00). Statin and antiviral treatment were similar among the groups. However, corticosteroid and antibiotic use differed significantly between severe and mild patients. Of note, more deceased patients received corticosteroid therapy compared with severe-surviving patients. The time from symptom onset to admission was comparable between the mild and severe groups [20 IQR (14–26) days vs. 19 IQR (10.25–30) days, $p = 0.841$] as well as between the severe-surviving and severe-non-surviving groups [20 IQR (10.5–30) days vs. 17 IQR (10–30) days, $p = 0.663$]. Mild patients experienced a longer hospitalization stay compared to severe patients [20 IQR (15–25) days vs. 15 IQR (9–20.5) days, $p = 0.012$]. Length of hospitalization was similar between the severe-surviving and severe-non-surviving groups [15 IQR (9–22.5) days vs. 15 IQR (10–18.5) days, $p = 0.706$].

Laboratory Parameters and Lipid Variation on Admission
For major laboratory characteristics, mild and severe COVID-19 cases demonstrated significant deviation in terms of blood cell proportions, coagulation functions, cardiac and renal functions, inflammatory indicators, and lipid profiles. Hierarchical clustering was performed to visualize the differences in laboratory parameters between mild and severe COVID-19 patients. The resulting heatmap illustrated different enrichment in blood indicators between mild and severe cases (**Figure 1, Supplementary Figure 1**). Notably, inflammatory cytokines, which are organ injury-associated indicators, were found at higher concentrations in the severe cases, whereas certain blood indicators, including lymphocytes, erythrocytes, hemoglobin, and albumin, were higher in the mild group.

In terms of lipid profiles, we detected lower concentrations of HDL-C, apoA-1, LDL-C, and TC in the severe group compared with the mild group (**Figures 2A–D**). The TG level was significantly increased in the severe-non-surviving cases compared with the severe-surviving cases (**Figure 2E**), while HDL-C, apoA-1, LDL-C, TC and apoB concentrations were comparable between these two groups (**Figures 2A–D,F**).

Lipid Profiles and Risk of Severe Condition
Based on the distinct lipid profile features between the severe and mild cases, we performed univariate and multivariate logistic regression analyses to explore the associations between lipid concentrations and disease severity. According to univariate analysis, TC, HDL-C, and apoA-1 levels were associated with severe disease as both continuous and categorical variables (divided by tertiles), whereas LDL-C and TG did not reach statistical significance. Remarkably, based on multivariate analysis, we found that apoA-1 (OR: 0.651 95% CI: 0.456–0.929, $p = 0.018$) and HDL-C (OR: 0.643 95% CI: 0.456–0.906, $p = 0.012$) were still independently associated with severity after adjusting for well-recognized risk factors: i.e., age and albumin, D-dimer, C-reactive protein (CRP), and interleukin-6 (IL-6) levels (**Table 2**). Moreover, patients with the highest tertile of HDL-C and apoA-1 displayed the lowest risk for severe COVID-19. Even after considering comorbidities and SOFA scores for further adjustment, apoA-1 and HDL-C levels remained independently associated with severe status of the disease (**Supplementary Table 1**). The ROC curves confirmed the significant predictive value of HDL-C and apoA-1 for the presence of severe cases. As shown in **Table 3**, apoA-1 ≤ 1.16 g/L predicted severity with a specificity of 0.86, sensitivity of 0.66, and area under ROC curve (AUC) of 0.85 (95% CI: 0.76–0.91; $p < 0.001$). An optimal serum HDL-C cut-off of 1.00 mmol/L provided diagnostic specificity and sensitivity of 75.5 and 68.2%, respectively, for severe cases. TC also displayed prognostic capability, but LDL-C, apoB, and TG showed weak discrimination of the severe condition.

Association of Lipid Biomarkers With COVID-19 Mortality
We further detected the predictive performance of lipid profiles for in-hospital death. Notably, ROC analysis revealed that HDL-C and apoA-1 remained valuable for predicting in-hospital death. At a threshold of 0.95 g/L, the AUC of the ROC curve of apoA-1 for death was 0.74 (95% CI 0.61–0.88, $p = 0.002$). With a cut-off of 0.84 mmol/L, the AUC of HDL-C for death was 0.75 (95% CI: 0.61–0.88, $p = 0.002$) (**Table 4**). Moreover, the Kaplan-Meier survival curves and log-rank tests demonstrated that patients with lower apoA-1 or HDL-C levels had a higher rate of in-hospital mortality (divided according to the best threshold) (**Figure 3**).

Dynamic Alterations in Lipid Profiles and Associations With Inflammatory Indicators
Figure 4 shows the changes in inflammatory factors and lipid profiles in the mild, severe-surviving, and severe-non-surviving

TABLE 1 | Clinical characteristics and laboratory assessments in COVID-19 patients.

	Mild (n = 49)	Severe(n = 50)	p-value	Severe (n = 50)		p-value
				Severe-surviving (n = 35)	Severe-non-surviving (n = 15)	
Age, years	52.00 (42.00–62.00)	70.50 (61.25–80.75)	<0.001	69.00 (61.50–80.50)	73.00 (63.50–78.50)	0.695
Male, n%	26 (53.06%)	34 (68.00%)	0.128	26 (74.29%)	8 (53.33%)	0.191
SOFA score	0 (0–1)	5.0 (2.0–7.0)	<0.001	3.00 (1.25–5.00)	8.00 (7.50–10.00)	<0.001
Mechanical ventilation, n%	0 (0.00%)	15 (30.00%)	<0.001	5 (14.29%)	10 (66.67%)	<0.001
Symptom to admission duration, days	20.00 (14.00–26.00)	19.00 (10.25–30.00)	0.841	20.00 (10.50–30.00)	17.00 (10.00–30.00)	0.663
Length of hospitalization, days	20.00 (15.00–25.00)	15.00 (9.00–20.50)	0.012	15.00 (9.00–22.50)	15.00 (10.00–18.50)	0.706
Symptom						
- Fever, n%	38 (77.55%)	28 (56.0%)	0.023	20 (57.14%)	8 (53.33%)	0.804
- Diarrhea, n%	9 (18.37%)	6 (12.0%)	0.377	6 (17.14%)	0 (0.00%)	0.160
- Fatigue, n%	13 (26.53%)	19 (38.0%)	0.222	16 (45.71%)	3 (20.00%)	0.117
- Cough, n%	29 (59.18%)	26 (52.0%)	0.472	19 (54.29%)	7 (46.67%)	0.760
- Chest pain, n%	19 (38.78%)	23 (46.0%)	0.467	18 (51.43%)	5 (33.33%)	0.355
- Dyspnea, n%	13 (26.53%)	24 (48.0%)	0.027	21 (60.00%)	3 (20.00%)	0.014
Comorbidities, n%	29 (59.18%)	42 (84.0%)	0.006	27 (77.14%)	15 (100.00%)	0.086
- Diabetes, n%	7 (14.29%)	24 (48.00%)	<0.001	16 (45.71%)	7 (46.67%)	1.000
- Hypertension, n%	18 (36.73%)	28 (56.00%)	0.085	19 (54.29%)	9 (60.00%)	0.765
- Pulmonary disease, n%	5 (10.20%)	6 (12.00%)	0.563	4 (11.43%)	2 (13.33%)	0.849
- Heart failure, n%	3 (6.12%)	14 (26.00%)	0.007	11 (31.43%)	3 (20.00%)	0.507
- CKD, n%	0 (0.00%)	16 (32.00%)	<0.001	11 (31.43%)	5 (33.33%)	1.000
- CAD, n%	1 (2.04%)	13 (26.00%)	<0.001	10 (28.57%)	3 (20.00%)	0.728
- Tumor, n%	3 (6.12%)	4 (8.00%)	0.716	2 (5.71%)	2 (13.33%)	0.574
- Autoimmune disease, n%	0 (0.00%)	2 (4.00%)	0.157	1 (2.86%)	1 (6.67%)	0.514
- Dyslipidemia, n%	4 (8.16%)	8 (16.00%)	0.147	4 (11.43%)	4 (26.67%)	0.178
Laboratory findings						
- Leukocytes × 10^9/L	5.68 (4.67–7.02)	7.42 (5.27–10.41)	<0.001	7.33 (5.68–9.68)	9.69 (5.00–14.82)	0.403
- Neutrophil × 10^9/L	3.04 (2.61–3.94)	6.01 (3.96–8.91)	<0.001	5.64 (3.96–7.28)	8.00 (4.26–11.82)	0.182
- Lymphocyte × 10^9/L	1.66 (1.04–2.26)	0.83 (0.67–1.24)	<0.001	0.90 (0.71–1.33)	0.70 (0.28–0.89)	0.020
- Platelets × 10^9/L	199.00 (171.00–256.00)	199.00 (133.75–274.50)	0.378	216.00 (174.00–281.00)	117.00 (80.50–152.50)	0.003
- Erythrocytes × 10^{12}/L	4.13 (3.87–4.51)	3.35 (2.83–3.80)	<0.001	3.31 (2.88–3.77)	3.39 (2.55–3.74)	0.594
- Hemoglobin, g/L	128.00 (119.00–137.00)	103.00 (84.00–117.50)	<0.001	105.0–3.74 (84.50–120.00)	101.00 (84.00–112.00)	0.775
- CRP, mg/L	0.81 (0.52–2.61)	33.91 (9.14–82.47)	<0.001	22.66 (6.26–63.94)	69.53 (30.16–114.89)	0.014
- Procalcitonin, ng/mL	0.03 (0.02–0.04)	0.32 (0.09–1.04)	<0.001	0.16 (0.09–0.52)	0.87 (0.44–1.53)	0.017
- ESR, mm/H	12.00 (7.00–23.00)	43.00 (21.25–60.75)	<0.001	42.00 (21.50–59.50)	44.00 (17.00–67.50)	0.916
- SAA, mg/L	5.00 (5.00–5.30)	54.78 (13.61–214.33)	<0.001	35.44 (9.61–244.24)	102 (32.4–270.46)	0.016
- PT, s	11.40 (10.90–11.70)	12.10 (11.43–13.55)	<0.001	12.10 (11.35–13.60)	12.10 (11.55–14.40)	0.491
- INR	0.98 (0.93–1.01)	1.05 (0.98–1.18)	<0.001	1.05 (0.97–1.19)	1.05 (0.99–1.27)	0.484
- Fibrinogen, g/L	2.66 (2.40–2.95)	4.04 (3.21–5.60)	<0.001	3.99 (3.24–5.72)	4.75 (3.25–5.60)	0.832
- D-Dimer, mg/L	0.29 (0.15–0.59)	2.94 (1.64–4.09)	<0.001	2.31 (1.45–3.74)	4.03 (2.57–6.42)	0.088
- BNP, pg/mL	7.00 (6.00–13.87)	117.66 (28.15–342.00)	<0.001	119.79 (26.27–593.00)	115.22 (33.84–189.34)	0.695
- Hs-cTnl, ng/ml	0.01 (0.01–0.01)	0.03 (0.01–0.06)	<0.001	0.02 (0.01–0.06)	0.03 (0.03–0.06)	0.078
- ALT, μ/L	28.00 (19.00–42.00)	21.00 (12.50–29.50)	0.059	21.00 (13.00–27.00)	24.00 (16.50–36.50)	0.532
- AST, μ/L	20.00 (17.00–26.00)	24.00 (18.00–32.75)	0.053	22.00 (18.00–31.00)	28.00 (18.50–44.00)	0.385
- Albumin, g/L	38.10 (36.10–41.30)	30.50 (28.40–35.68)	<0.001	30.50 (28.80–34.55)	29.40 (25.10–34.90)	0.346
- TBIL, μmol/L	9.24 (7.40–12.70)	9.40 (6.55–14.10)	0.607	8.40 (6.35–11.65)	14.10 (7.25–18.10)	0.159
- Glucose, mmol/L	4.69 (4.38–5.03)	5.97 (4.88–8.20)	<0.001	5.73 (4.89–7.48)	6.69 (4.62–12.05)	0.498

(Continued)

TABLE 1 | Continued

	Mild (n = 49)	Severe(n = 50)	p-value	Severe (n = 50) Severe-surviving (n = 35)	Severe-non-surviving (n = 15)	p-value
- BUN, mmol/L	4.70 (4.00–5.30)	8.70 (5.32–15.60)	<0.001	7.20 (4.60–11.05)	14.40 (8.80–37.40)	0.026
- Creatinine, μmol/L	60.20 (50.70–70.40)	82.20 (56.73–154.83)	<0.001	75.00 (56.25–108.45)	98.20 (68.20–235.20)	0.295
- Total cholesterol, mmol/L	4.52 (3.63–4.9)	3.51 (2.90–4.48)	<0.001	3.59 (2.98–4.48)	3.18 (2.58–4.25)	0.553
- Triglycerides, mmol/L	1.21 (0.81–1.80)	0.96 (0.70–1.62)	0.114	0.90 (0.70–1.38)	1.00 (0.82–2.71)	0.010
- LDL-C, mmol/L	2.57 (2.04–2.96)	2.16 (1.58–2.68)	0.016	2.19 (1.64–2.83)	1.76 (1.49–2.64)	0.494
- HDL-C, mmol/L	1.18 (1.00–1.42)	0.94 (0.74–1.12)	<0.001	0.97 (0.76–1.08)	0.77 (0.61–0.99)	0.112
- apoA-1, g/L	1.42 (1.22–1.64)	1.01 (0.79–1.23)	<0.001	1.03 (0.80–1.25)	0.84 (0.64–1.19)	0.277
- apoB, g/L	0.93 (0.79–1.08)	0.80 (0.69–1.14)	0.205	0.86 (0.73–1.14)	0.70 (0.66–1.07)	0.277
- IL.6, pg/mL	1.29 (0.75–3.37)	38.45 (12.59–80.07)	<0.001	23.84 (10.55–41.88)	124.90 (58.45–241.45)	<0.001
- IL.1β, pg/mL	3.00 (2.00–3.29)	3.75 (3.00–5.00)	0.009	3.00 (3.00–4.07)	5.00 (3.67–6.32)	0.023
- IL.8, pg/mL	6.00 (3.80–8.60)	16.70 (13.00–27.80)	<0.001	16.00 (11.50–22.00)	28.40 (19.50–49.00)	0.005
- IL.10, pg/mL	3.00 (2.00–3.56)	4.01 (3.00–8.97)	<0.001	4.00 (3.00–7.55)	8.20 (3.43–15.00)	0.146
- IL2R, U/mL	0.31 (0.22–0.43)	0.81 (0.57–1.65)	<0.001	0.72 (0.58–1.42)	1.56 (0.60–2.94)	0.147
- TNF α, pg/mL	6.50 (5.50–7.16)	10.61 (7.75–14.73)	<0.001	10.70 (7.45–14.38)	11.50 (8.50–19.45)	0.427
Treatment, n%						
Antibiotic therapy	17 (34.70%)	50 (100%)	<0.001	35 (100%)	15 (100%)	–
Antiviral therapy	47 (95.92%)	48 (96.00%)	0.984	34 (97.14%)	14 (93.33%)	0.529
Use of corticosteroids	0 (0%)	19 (38.00%)	<0.001	10 (28.57%)	9 (60.00%)	0.036
Statin	8 (16.32%)	15 (30.00%)	0.107	11 (31.42%)	4 (26.67%)	0.736

Categorical data are expressed as absolute values and percentages and were compared using chi-square or Fisher exact tests. Continuous variables were expressed as medians with interquartile ranges (IQR) and compared by unpaired Student's t-test or Mann-Whitney U test. AST, aspartate aminotransferase; ALT,alanine aminotransferase; BUN, blood urea nitrogen; BNP, brain natriuretic peptide; Hs-cTnI, hypersensitive troponin I;CRP, C-reactive protein; CKD, chronic kidney disease; CAD, coronary artery disease; ESR, erythrocyte sedimentation rate; SAA, serum amyloid A; IL, interleukin; IL2R, interleukin2 receptor; LDL-C, low-densitylipoprotein-cholesterol; HDL-C, high-density lipoprotein-cholesterol; apoA-1, apolipoproteinA-1; apoB, apolipoproteinB; INR,international standard ratio; PT, prothrombin time; TNF α, tumor necrosis factorα; TBIL, total bilirubin; SOFA, Sequential Organ Failure Assessment.

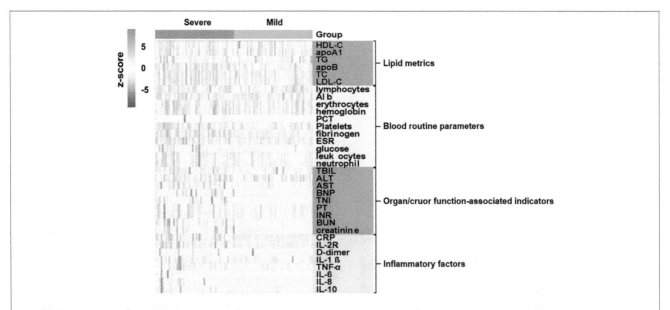

FIGURE 1 | Admission characteristics of laboratory parameters between mild and severe COVID-19 patients. Hierarchical clustering was applied based on laboratory parameters. Heatmap indicates enriched concentration of laboratory indicators in mild and severe cases. Levels of laboratory metrics were scaled by calculating z-scores (subtracting mean, then dividing by standard deviation of each row). Laboratory metrics were categorized into four major groups, i.e., lipid metrics, routine blood parameters, organ/cruor function-associated indicators, and inflammatory factors, with color bars on right side of plot indicating each analyte category. Y-axis represents laboratory values after z-scoring by row; x-axis represents individual cases. Annotations show severe cases in pink and mild cases in cyan.

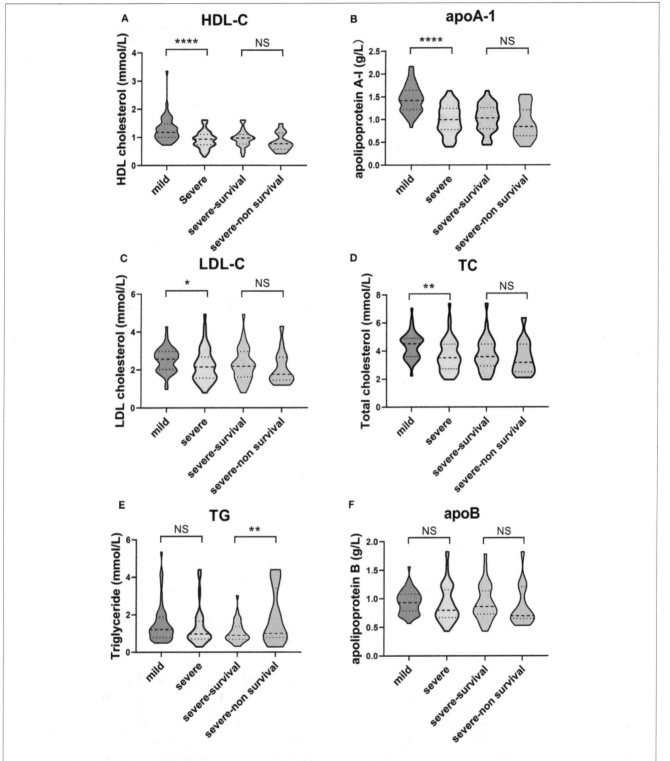

FIGURE 2 | Violin plots of lipid features of mild vs. severe and severe survivors vs. severe non-survivors. Plots demonstrate lipid concentration within each group. Horizontal dotted lines represent first and third quartiles; horizontal dashed lines within plot indicate median of lipid levels. Dunnett's test was applied to assess significance of differences with mild cases serving as the control. (****$p < 0.0001$, **$p < 0.01$, *$p < 0.05$).

TABLE 2 | Logistic regression analysis for severity in COVID-19 patients.

	Univariate OR (95% CI)	p-value	Adjusted OR* (95% CI)	p-value
apoA-1 (10⁻¹g/L)	0.617 (0.507, 0.751)	<0.001	0.651 (0.456, 0.929)	0.018
apoA-1 group				
Q1 (4–10.4)	Ref		Ref	
Q2 (10.5–13.8)	0.126 (0.036, 0.443)	0.001	0.538 (0.059, 4.882)	0.581
Q3 (14.0–21.7)	0.036 (0.009, 0.136)	<0.001	0.066 (0.005, 0.823)	0.034
apoA-1 group trend		<0.001		0.023
HDL-C (10⁻¹mmol/L)	0.709 (0.602, 0.835)	<0.001	0.643 (0.456, 0.906)	0.012
HDL-C group				
Q1 (3.1–9.1)	Ref		Ref	
Q2 (9.3–11.78)	0.400 (0.139, 1.147)	0.090	0.264 (0.028, 2.469)	0.242
Q3 (11.8–33.5)	0.103 (0.033, 0.316)	<0.001	0.065 (0.005, 0.778) 0.03093	0.031
HDL-C group trend		<0.001		0.029
Total cholesterol (mmol/L)	0.505 (0.328, 0.776)	0.002	0.866 (0.425, 1.766)	0.693
TC group				
Q1 (1.97–3.44)	Ref		Ref	
Q2 (3.49–4.54)	0.301 (0.106, 0.860)	0.025	0.497 (0.079, 3.146)	0.458
Q3 (4.56–7.38)	0.120 (0.040, 0.362)	<0.001	0.338 (0.048, 2.360)	0.274
TC group trend		<0.001		0.281
Triglycerides (mmol/L)	0.808 (0.538, 1.214)	0.304	0.808 (0.269, 2.423)	0.703
TG group				
Q1 (0.29–0.82)	Ref		Ref	
Q2 (0.84–1.43)	0.778 (0.295, 2.051)	0.611	1.212 (0.242, 6.079)	0.815
Q3 (1.44–5.35)	0.648 (0.244, 1.724)	0.385	1.006 (0.119, 8.472)	0.996
TG group trend		0.402		0.993
LDL-C (mmol/L)	0.588 (0.343, 1.007)	0.053	1.281 (0.508, 3.230)	0.599
LDL-C group				
Q1 (0.79–1.96)	Ref		Ref	
Q2 (2.01–2.68)	0.471 (0.174, 1.273)	0.137	1.614 (0.208, 12.524)	0.647
Q3 (2.70–4.93)	0.286 (0.104, 0.787)	0.015	1.709 (0.241, 12.144)	0.592
LDL-C group trend		0.01545		0.62094
apoB (g/L)	0.638 (0.147, 2.766)	0.548	3.908 (0.279, 54.710)	0.311
apoB group				
Q1 (0.43–0.76)	Ref		Ref	
Q2 (0.77–1.02)	0.300 (0.108, 0.830)	0.02	1.022 (0.147, 7.105)	0.982
Q3 (1.03–1.82)	0.444 (0.165, 1.194)	0.108	1.706 (0.270, 10.797)	0.57
apoB group trend		0.145		0.512

*Logistic regression was used to determine association between lipid profile with severity of COVID-19. *Adjusted for age and albumin, D-dimer, CRP, and IL-6 levels. LDL-C, low-densitylipoprotein-cholesterol; HDL-C, high-density lipoprotein-cholesterol; apoA-1, apolipoproteinA-1; apoB, apolipoprotein B; TG, triglycerides; TC, total cholesterol.*

groups from hospital admission, mid-term hospitalization, and end of hospitalization. As illustrated in **Figures 4A,B**, throughout hospitalization, CRP and IL-6 levels were significantly and continuously high in the severe-surviving and mortality cases but showed low levels among mild cases. Notably, compared with that in the severe-surviving group, both CRP and IL-6 levels in mortality cases were significantly higher at the end of hospitalization ($p < 0.05$).

On admission, regardless of severity or outcome, most patients presented comparable TG and LDL-C levels (**Figures 4C,D**). By the end of hospitalization, however, TG levels displayed a slight upward trend in the mortality cases

and were significantly higher than that in the severe survivors ($p = 0.013$); in addition, LDL-C levels were significantly lower in severe survivors and non-survivors compared to that in the mild cases (both $p < 0.01$). Levels of apoA-1 and HDL-C were inversely proportional to disease severity, with mortality cases showing continuously lower levels across hospitalization (**Figures 4E,F**). Of note, after a slight downward trend in mid-term apoA-1 levels, severe survivors showed a significant recovery in apoA-1 levels at the end of hospitalization (vs. mid-term apoA-1 levels, $p = 0.02$). By the end of hospitalization, the lowest apoA-1 levels were found in severe cases with a fatal outcome ($p < 0.01$). For TC and apoB, no significant differences

TABLE 3 | Diagnostic values of lipid profiles in assessment of COVID-19 severity.

	AUC (95% CI)	Best threshold	Specificity	Sensitivity	p-value
apoA-1	0.85 (0.76–0.91)	1.16	0.86	0.66	<0.001
HDL-C	0.78 (0.69–0.85)	1.00	0.76	0.68	<0.001
TC	0.71 (0.61–0.81)	3.24	0.94	0.42	<0.001
apoB	0.58 (0.46–0.68)	0.78	0.78	0.46	0.192
LDL-C	0.62 (0.52–0.76)	1.78	0.92	0.40	0.016
TG	0.59 (0.46–0.70)	1.13	0.61	0.62	0.126
apoA-1 + HDL-C	0.85 (0.77–0.92)	–	0.86	0.66	<0.001

AUC, area under the curve; LDL-C, low-density lipoprotein-cholesterol; HDL-C, high-density lipoprotein-cholesterol; apoA-1, apolipoprotein A-1; apoB, apolipoprotein B; TG, triglycerides; TC, total cholesterol.

TABLE 4 | Diagnostic values of lipid profiles in assessment of COVID-19 mortality.

	AUC (95% CI)	Best threshold	Specificity	Sensitivity	p-value
apoA-1	0.74 (0.61–0.88)	0.95	0.83	0.67	0.002
HDL-C	0.75 (0.61–0.88)	0.84	0.81	0.73	0.002
apoB	0.62 (0.43–0.79)	0.71	0.85	0.53	0.093
LDL-C	0.64 (0.46–0.80)	1.83	0.80	0.60	0.054
TG	0.44 (0.27–0.61)	1.01	0.58	0.53	0.444
TC	0.66 (0.51–0.80)	3.18	0.83	0.53	0.040
apoA-1 + HDL-C	0.77 (0.63–0.90)	–	0.83	0.67	0.002

AUC, area under the curve; LDL-C, low-density lipoprotein-cholesterol; HDL-C, high-density lipoprotein-cholesterol; apoA-1, apolipoprotein A-1; apoB, apolipoprotein B; TG, triglycerides; TC, total cholesterol.

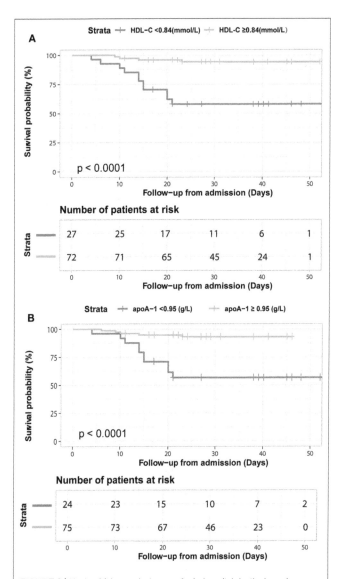

FIGURE 3 | Kaplan-Meier survival curves for in-hospital deaths based on dichotomized HDL-C and apoA-1 concentrations. COVID-19 patients with apoA-1 **(A)** and HDL-C **(B)** levels above and below the optimal cutoff value (calculated by ROC analysis) showed obvious disparity in survival time ($p <$ 0.0001).

were observed among the three groups across the three time points (**Figures 4G,H**).

Correlation analysis was performed to detect potential factors related to lipid characteristics. As shown in **Figure 5A**, admission lipid profiles, especially apoA-1 and HDL-C, were negatively correlated with inflammatory factors, such as CRP and IL-6. Admission apoA-1 and HDL-C levels were inversely correlated with peak CRP and IL-6 concentrations during the clinical course of the disease (**Figure 5B**).

DISCUSSION

Our study highlighted an important association between lipid profiles and fatal clinical outcomes in COVID patients. The main findings are as follows: (1) COVID-19 patients in severe disease were characterized by decreased apoA-1 and HDL-C levels; (2) low apoA-1 and HDL-C levels on admission were able to predict COVID-19 severity and mortality during hospitalization; and (3) apoA-1 and HDL-C levels were strongly correlated with inflammatory indicators, and deviated markedly from the normal reference range in severe cases throughout the course of the disease.

Previous studies have shown that infection and sepsis are accompanied by a metabolic change in the lipid profile, featuring hypertriglyceridemia and reduced HDL-C levels in serum (4, 8).

Lipid metabolism dysregulation has also been confirmed in septic patients secondary to both community and hospital-acquired pneumonia (9, 10). In the context of COVID-19, excessive cytokine activation in response to SARS-CoV-2 infection appears to contribute to multiple organ dysfunction. As a result, sepsis and septic shock are frequently observed complications in severe COVID-19 patients (11, 12). Therefore, it is not surprising that serum apoA-1 and HDL-C levels were lower in severely ill patients, especially non-survivors, compared to mild cases.

Both apoA-1 ($r = -0.55; p < 0.001$) and HDL-C ($r = -0.45;$ $p < 0.001$) levels were negatively related to SOFA scores, a common diagnostic tool for identifying sepsis severity (13). Based on multivariate analyses, decreased apoA-1 and HDL-C levels

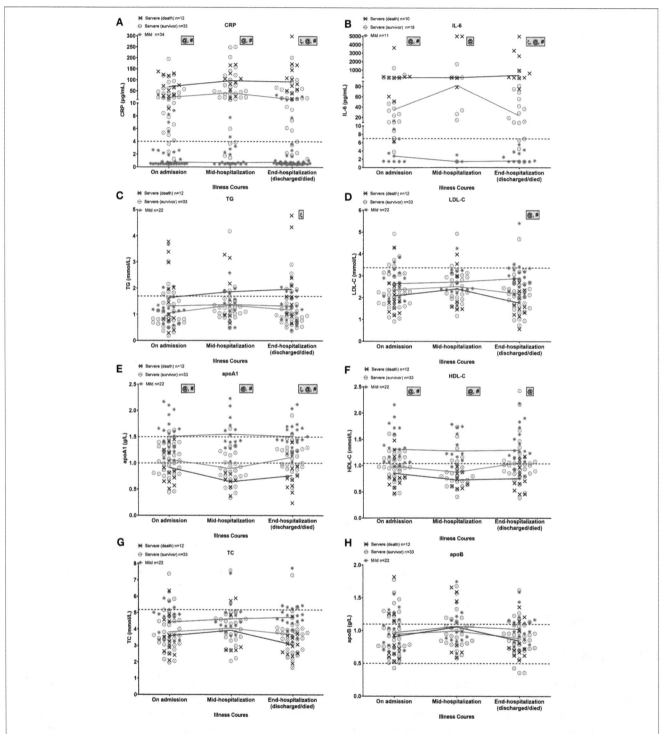

FIGURE 4 | Dynamic alterations in lipid and major laboratory markers from admission in COVID-19 patients. Temporal changes in CRP **(A)**, IL-6 **(B)**, TG **(C)**, LDL-C **(D)**, apoA-1 **(E)**, HDL-C **(F)**, TC **(G)**, and apoB **(H)** in a subset of COVID-19 patients with ≥2 longitudinal data across three time periods, including on admission, mid-hospitalization, and end of hospitalization. Horizontal dashed lines indicate normal reference range of factors. Mean values of normally distributed parameters (lipid metrics) and median values of non-normally distributed factors (CRP and IL-6) in each group at three time periods are linked by lines. Significant differences among three groups at each time point were compared using one-way ANOVA with Tukey's multiple comparisons test or Kruskal-Wallis test as appropriate. Statistical significance ($p < 0.05$) is indicated by ξ between severe (death) and severe (survivor) cases, @ between severe (death) and mild cases, and # between severe (survivor) and mild cases. IL-6, interleukin-6; CRP, C-reactive protein; TG, triglycerides; TC, total cholesterol; LDL-C, low-density lipoprotein-cholesterol; HDL-C, high-density lipoprotein-cholesterol, apoA-1, apolipoprotein A-1; apoB, apolipoprotein B.

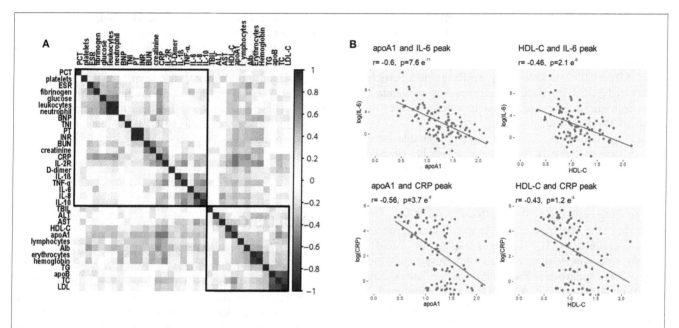

FIGURE 5 | Correlations among lipid profiles and laboratory parameters. **(A)** Heatmap values represent pairwise Spearman rank correlation coefficients. Blue indicates positive correlation, red indicates negative correlation. **(B)** Spearman correlation coefficient analysis shows that initial HDL-C and apoA-1 levels were significantly inversely correlated with peak values of CRP and IL-6 during disease course.

were independently associated with COVID-19 severity after adjusting for established indicators of severity, such as age, low albumin, and increased D-dimer, CRP, and IL-6 levels (14, 15). These covariates were included in the multivariate analysis due to their close association with sepsis development reported in previous studies (16, 17). In addition, ROC analysis illustrated that decreased apoA-1 and HDL-C levels were strong predictors of COVID-19 severity. In line with our findings, Groin et al. found that low serum HDL-C concentration on admission is a risk factor for the development of severe sepsis (18).

Our results also highlighted the predictive value of decreased HDL/apoA-1 levels on admission to in-hospital death in COVID-19 patients. Almost half of our research population developed into severe cases, with a relatively high mortality rate of 15.1%. This may be because Leishenshan Hospital was a designated hospital for treating complicated patients transferred from other local hospitals. Our study, for the first time, illustrated that in-hospital death increased significantly in patients with low serum apoA-1 (<0.95 g/L) or HDL-C (<0.84 mmol/L). In addition, ROC analysis verified the predictive value of HDL-C and apoA-1 levels for in-hospital death among COVID-19 patients. This is in agreement with previous study, which found that low apoA-1 concentration is independently associated with the 30-day mortality rate in septic patients (19). Interestingly, here, the temporal recording of lipid profiles showed that the initial decrease in apoA-1/HDL-C levels in survivors began to recover at the end of hospitalization. A similar tendency in HDL-C change has also been observed in patients recovering from sepsis (20). Here, however, apoA-1 rapidly deteriorated in non-survivors throughout the clinical course of the disease.

The underlying mechanisms of HDL-C reduction in severe COVID-19 patients and its association with increased mortality are not fully understood. HDL-C and its major structural protein (apoA-1) directly exert anti-inflammatory effects by neutralizing lipopolysaccharides (LPS), thus playing an important role in host resistance to bacterial, viral, and parasitic infection (21). The protective role of apoA-1 is also evidenced in acute lung injury and acute respiratory distress syndrome. Specifically, apoA-1-deficient mice exhibit enhanced recruitment of neutrophils and monocytes to airspace under LPS inhalation (22). However, both HDL-C and its beneficial effects can be disturbed by inflammation (23, 24). For example, pro-inflammatory cytokines like IL-6 and CRP directly inhibit apolipoprotein synthesis enzyme activity, resulting in reduced apoA-1 and HDL-C production (25). In our study, IL-6 and CRP concentrations were significantly higher in the severe group, and were negatively correlated with lipid indicators apoA-1 and HDL-C. We also found that serum amyloid A (SAA), an acute phase protein, was markedly increased in severe patients. SAA-enriched HDL is reported to clear more rapidly from circulation than normal HDL (26). Hence, the inflammatory-induced humoral innate response to scavenge lipoprotein from circulation may be another potential mechanism leading to low-HDL-C levels. As a result, a vicious cycle occurs in severely ill COVID-19 patients, with a deficiency in HDL-C resulting in cytokine overproduction and a further depletion of HDL-C.

In our study, TC and LDL-C levels in severe patients tended to follow a pattern similar to that of HDL-C. Low TC and LDL-C levels are considered as markers of malnutrition, as nutrition provides the basic substrate for cholesterol synthesis

(27). Furthermore, early enteral nutrition is reported to accelerate the recovery of TC levels (20). Consistently, the nutrition states of patients deteriorated in our study, as reflected by continuously decreased levels of albumin in the severe group. Like HDL-C, inflammatory mediators also participate in impaired LDL-C synthesis. Thus, hypocholesterolemia may reflect both malnutrition and an overactive inflammatory status in severe COVID-19 patients.

Although admission TG levels were comparable between mild and severe cases, TG levels were remarkably elevated in non-survivors. Serum TG frequently increases under a septic environment due to reduced TG hydrolysis. Inflammatory cytokines also contribute to inhibit LPL activity, overproduction of free fatty acid, and TG synthesis (26). Besides, after comparing the survival rates between four groups of patients stratified by TG and apoA-1 levels, we found that patients with lower apoA-1 levels and elevated TG levels displayed the unfavorable prognosis with the lowest survival rate (**Supplementary Figure 2**). Thus, we considered that elevated TG levels, together with persistently low lipoprotein cholesterol concentrations, might be a marker of uncontrolled inflammation and increased risk of death in COVID-19 patients. And further assessment in larger cohorts are required for validation.

STUDY LIMITATIONS

There are several limitations in our study. First, given the small sample size, to avoid overfitting, we only calculated the Kaplan-Meier survival curve to evaluate the prognostic values of apoA-1 and HDL-C but did not conduct multivariate cox regression to assess the independent prognostic values of these lipid metrics. Thus, further larger cohorts are warranted to verify our conclusions. Second, some patients were already in poor condition when transferred from

the local hospital to Leishenshan Hospital, resulting in a higher rate of severe cases in our study. Further studies on outpatients and other mobile hospitals are required to provide a more complete picture of the relationship between lipid profiles and disease progression. Third, our study only focused on lipid concentrations rather than their quality. Therefore, whether lipid particle composition and functional alteration can affect COVID-19 outcomes deserves further investigation.

CONCLUSIONS

Lipid metabolism disorders, characterized by low HDL-C and apoA-1 levels, were found in severely ill COVID-19 patients. The altered HDL-C and apoA-1 levels were negatively correlated with inflammatory indicators. Low apoA-1 and HDL-C levels on admission exhibited predictive value in discriminating disease severity and mortality during hospitalization. Our study examined COVID-19 in regard to lipid metabolism, and thus provides new insights into the disease.

AUTHOR CONTRIBUTIONS

JS and JP: conceived and designed the experiments. ZC, PN, HG, LS, FY, XQ, WW, MZ, XY, and YZ: collected and analyzed the data. JS, ZC, and JP: wrote the manuscript. All authors contributed to the article and approved the submitted version.

REFERENCES

1. Verity R, Okell LC, Dorigatti I, Winskill P, Whittaker C, Imai N, et al. Estimates of the severity of coronavirus disease 2019: a model-based analysis. *Lancet Infect Dis.* (2020) 20:669–77. doi: 10.1016/S1473-3099(20)30243-7
2. Huang C, Wang Y, Li X, Ren L, Zhao J, Hu Y, et al. Clinical features of patients infected with 2019 novel coronavirus in Wuhan, China. *Lancet.* (2020) 395:497–506. doi: 10.1016/S0140-6736(20)30183-5
3. Li X, Xu S, Yu M, Wang K, Tao Y, Zhou Y, et al. Risk factors for severity and mortality in adult COVID-19 inpatients in Wuhan. *J Allergy Clin Immunol.* (2020) 146:110–18. doi: 10.1016/j.jaci.2020.04.006
4. Golucci A, Marson FAL, Ribeiro AF, Nogueira RJN. Lipid profile associated with the systemic inflammatory response syndrome and sepsis in critically ill patients. *Nutrition.* (2018) 55–6:7–14. doi: 10.1016/j.nut.2018.04.007
5. Shen B, Yi X, Sun Y, Bi X, Du J, Zhang C, et al. Proteomic and metabolomic characterization of COVID-19 patient sera. *Cell* (2020) 182:59–72.e15. doi: 10.1016/j.cell.2020.05.032
6. Sorokin AV, Karathanasis SK, Yang ZH, Freeman L, Kotani K, Remaley AT. Covid-19-associated dyslipidemia: implications for mechanism

of impaired resolution and novel therapeutic approaches. *Faseb J.* (2020). doi: 10.1096/fj.202001451. [Epub ahead of print].
7. World Health Organization. *Clinical Management of Severe Acute Respiratory Infection When Novel Coronavirus (2019-nCoV) Infection is Suspected: Interim Guidance.* World Health Organization (2020). Available online at: https://apps.who.int/iris/handle/10665/330893
8. Tanaka S, Diallo D, Delbosc S, Genève C, Zappella N, Yong-Sang J, et al. High-density lipoprotein (HDL) particle size and concentration changes in septic shock patients. *Ann Intensive Care.* (2019) 9:68. doi: 10.1186/s13613-019-0541-8
9. Sharma NK, Ferreira BL, Tashima AK, Brunialti MKC, Torquato RJS, Bafi A, et al. Lipid metabolism impairment in patients with sepsis secondary to hospital acquired pneumonia, a proteomic analysis. *Clin Proteomics.* (2019) 16:29. doi: 10.1186/s12014-019-9252-2
10. Sharma NK, Tashima AK, Brunialti MKC, Ferreira ER, Torquato RJS, Mortara RA, et al. Proteomic study revealed cellular assembly and lipid metabolism dysregulation in sepsis secondary to community-acquired pneumonia. *Sci Rep.* (2017) 7:15606. doi: 10.1038/s41598-017-15755-1
11. Alhazzani W, Møller MH, Arabi YM, Loeb M, Gong MN, Fan E, et al. Surviving sepsis campaign: guidelines on the management of critically Ill

adults with coronavirus disease 2019 (COVID-19). *Crit Care Med.* (2020) 48:e440–69. doi: 10.1097/CCM.0000000000004363

12. Li H, Liu L, Zhang D, Xu J, Dai H, Tang N, et al. SARS-CoV-2 and viral sepsis: observations and hypotheses. *Lancet.* (2020) 395:1517–20. doi: 10.1016/S0140-6736(20)30920-X

13. Singer M, Deutschman CS, Seymour CW, Shankar-Hari M, Annane D, Bauer M, et al. The third international consensus definitions for sepsis and septic shock (sepsis-3). *JAMA.* (2016) 315:801–10. doi: 10.1001/jama.2016.0287

14. Feng Y, Ling Y, Bai T, Xie Y, Huang J, Li J, et al. COVID-19 with different severity: a multi-center study of clinical features. *Am J Respir Crit Care Med.* (2020) 201:1380–88. doi: 10.1164/rccm.202002-0445OC

15. Chen T, Wu D, Chen H, Yan W, Yang D, Chen G, et al. Clinical characteristics of 113 deceased patients with coronavirus disease 2019: retrospective study. *BMJ.* (2020) 368:m1295. doi: 10.1136/bmj.m1091

16. Rodelo JR, De la Rosa G, Valencia ML, Ospina S, Arango CM, Gómez CI, et al. D-dimer is a significant prognostic factor in patients with suspected infection and sepsis. *Am J Emerg Med.* (2012) 30:1991–9. doi: 10.1016/j.ajem.2012.04.033

17. Pierrakos C, Vincent JL. Sepsis biomarkers: a review. *Crit Care.* (2010) 14:R15. doi: 10.1186/cc8872

18. Grion CM, Cardoso LT, Perazolo TF, Garcia AS, Barbosa DS, Morimoto HK, et al. Lipoproteins and CETP levels as risk factors for severe sepsis in hospitalized patients. *Eur J Clin Invest.* (2010) 40:330–8. doi: 10.1111/j.1365-2362.2010.02269.x

19. Chien JY, Jerng JS, Yu CJ, Yang PC. Low serum level of high-density lipoprotein cholesterol is a poor prognostic factor for severe sepsis. *Crit Care Med.* (2005) 33:1688–93. doi: 10.1097/01.CCM.0000171183.79525.6B

20. Marik PE. Dyslipidemia in the critically ill. *Crit Care Clin.* (2006) 22:151–9, viii. doi: 10.1016/j.ccc.2005.08.008

21. Tanaka S, Couret D, Tran-Dinh A, Duranteau J, Montravers P, Schwendeman A, et al. High-density lipoproteins during sepsis: from bench to bedside. *Crit Care.* (2020) 24:134. doi: 10.1186/s13054-020-02860-3

22. Gordon EM, Figueroa DM, Barochia AV, Yao X, Levine SJ. High-density lipoproteins and apolipoprotein a-i. Potential new players in the prevention and treatment of lung disease. *Front Pharmacol.* (2016) 7:323. doi: 10.3389/fphar.2016.00323

23. Jahangiri A, de Beer MC, Noffsinger V, Tannock LR, Ramaiah C, Webb NR, et al. HDL remodeling during the acute phase response. *Arterioscler Thromb Vasc Biol.* (2009) 29:261–7. doi: 10.1161/ATVBAHA.108.178681

24. Sun JT, Liu Y, Lu L, Liu HJ, Shen WF, Yang K, et al. Diabetes-invoked high-density lipoprotein and its association with coronary artery disease in patients with type 2 diabetes mellitus. *Am J Cardiol.* (2016) 118:1674–9. doi: 10.1016/j.amjcard.2016.08.044

25. Pirillo A, Catapano AL, Norata GD. HDL in infectious diseases and sepsis. *Handb Exp Pharmacol.* (2015) 224:483–508. doi: 10.1007/978-3-319-09665-0_15

26. Wendel M, Paul R, Heller AR. Lipoproteins in inflammation and sepsis. II. Clinical aspects. *Intensive Care Med.* (2007) 33:25–35. doi: 10.1007/s00134-006-0433-x

27. Chiarla C, Giovannini I, Giuliante F, Zadak Z, Vellone M, Ardito F, et al. Severe hypocholesterolemia in surgical patients, sepsis, and critical illness. *J Crit Care.* (2010) 25:361 e7–12. doi: 10.1016/j.jcrc.2009.08.006

10

Telemedicine in Heart Failure During COVID-19: A Step into the Future

Gregorio Tersalvi [1,2*], Dario Winterton [3], Giacomo Maria Cioffi [1,4], Simone Ghidini [5], Marco Roberto [1], Luigi Biasco [6,7], Giovanni Pedrazzini [1,7], Jeroen Dauw [8,9], Pietro Ameri [10,11] and Marco Vicenzi [5,12]

[1] Division of Cardiology, Fondazione Cardiocentro Ticino, Lugano, Switzerland, [2] Department of Internal Medicine, Hirslanden Klinik St. Anna, Lucerne, Switzerland, [3] Department of Anesthesia and Intensive Care Medicine, ASST Monza, Monza, Italy, [4] Department of Cardiology, Kantonsspital Luzern, Lucerne, Switzerland, [5] Dyspnea Lab, Department of Clinical Sciences and Community Health, University of Milan, Milan, Italy, [6] Division of Cardiology, Azienda Sanitaria Locale Torino 4, Ospedale di Cirié, Cirié, Italy, [7] Department of Biomedical Sciences, University of Italian Switzerland, Lugano, Switzerland, [8] Department of Cardiology, Ziekenhuis Oost-Limburg, Genk, Belgium, [9] Doctoral School for Medicine and Life Sciences, Hasselt University, Diepenbeek, Belgium, [10] Cardiovascular Diseases Unit, IRCCS Ospedale Policlinico San Martino, Genoa, Italy, [11] Department of Internal Medicine, University of Genoa, Genoa, Italy, [12] Cardiovascular Disease Unit, Fondazione IRCCS Ca' Granda Ospedale Maggiore Policlinico, Milan, Italy

*Correspondence:
Gregorio Tersalvi
tersalvi@gmail.com

During the Coronavirus Disease 2019 worldwide pandemic, patients with heart failure are a high-risk group with potential higher mortality if infected. Although lockdown represents a solution to prevent viral spreading, it endangers regular follow-up visits and precludes direct medical assessment in order to detect heart failure progression and optimize treatment. Furthermore, lifestyle changes during quarantine may trigger heart failure decompensations. During the pandemic, a paradoxical reduction of heart failure hospitalization rates was observed, supposedly caused by patient reluctance to visit emergency departments and hospitals. This may result in an increased patient mortality and/or in more complicated heart failure admissions in the future. In this scenario, different telemedicine strategies can be implemented to ensure continuity of care to patients with heart failure. Patients at home can be monitored through dedicated apps, telephone calls, or devices. Virtual visits and forward triage screen the patients with signs or symptoms of decompensated heart failure. In-hospital care may benefit from remote communication platforms. After discharge, patients may undergo remote follow-up or telerehabilitation to prevent early readmissions. This review provides a comprehensive appraisal of the many possible applications of telemedicine for patients with heart failure during Coronavirus disease 2019 and elucidates practical limitations and challenges regarding specific telemedicine modalities.

Keywords: COVID-19, coronavirus, telemedicine, heart failure, remote monitoring, virtual visits, forward triage, telerehabilitation

INTRODUCTION

The Coronavirus Disease 2019 (COVID-19) pandemic has caused considerable morbidity and mortality worldwide. Epidemiological data from China indicate that patients with concomitant cardiovascular disease are more likely to develop life-threatening complications from severe acute respiratory syndrome coronavirus 2 (SARS-CoV-2) infection (1–7). The risk of complications may be even higher in patients with heart failure (HF) because they are older and have more comorbidities, but also due to the specific characteristics of this syndrome (8). Lockdown of social activities has allowed limiting the spreading of SARS-CoV-2, but it has also decreased medical contacts. For HF patients, this might have led to late recognition and treatment of episodes of decompensation and missed opportunities for optimization of medical and nonmedical therapy. In addition, lifestyle changes adopted during lockdown, such as dietary changes, increased alcohol consumption and decreased physical activity, may trigger HF decompensations (9, 10).

Telemedicine represents a useful tool to prevent negative direct and indirect consequences of SARS-CoV-2, and the present situation might be the right moment to implement a structured telemedicine program in clinical practice. Its main benefits include guiding the treatment of patients in primary care to minimize the risk of disease transmission during referral, continuing to provide optimal treatment to the patients with cardiovascular disease who are isolated at home or are discharged from the hospital to prevent clinical deterioration, monitoring early signs of new onset or worsening HF, and reducing unnecessary visits to the hospital to decrease the incidence of cluster infections (11).

In this review, we provide an overview of the many possible applications of telemedicine, its limitations and challenges, in patients with HF during COVID-19.

IMPACT OF COVID-19 ON THE MANAGEMENT OF HEART FAILURE

Already in the first months of the COVID-19 pandemic, the impact of cardiovascular comorbidities on disease course became clear in observational studies, indicating that patients with previous cardiovascular disease had higher COVID-19 disease severity and mortality (2, 6, 7). In addition, myocardial injury in COVID-19 has been broadly described (6, 7, 12, 13), which might further impair myocardial function and worsen prognosis in patients with known HF.

Patients with chronic HF represent a vulnerable group during a pandemic of infectious respiratory disease. Previous studies have shown that they are at increased risk for adverse consequences of seasonal influenza (14) and other causes of pneumonia (15). Furthermore, acute infections may trigger HF exacerbations (16).

The social and environmental effects of lockdown must also be mentioned. A significant decline in hospitalization rates for acute HF during the COVID-19 pandemic, compared to before the pandemic and each of the preceding 3 years, was described, which might be the consequence of fear for infection leading to reluctance to seek medical attention when needed (17). Notably, hospitalized patients had more severe symptoms on admission, possibly suggesting that patients have waited longer before presenting to the hospital or less severe cases did not come to the hospital at all. Further, lifestyle changes during lockdown, such as dietary changes, increased alcohol consumption and decreased physical activity, may trigger HF decompensations (9, 10).

Although lockdown represents a solution to prevent viral spreading, it may complicate regular follow-up visits, therefore encumbering optimization of medical therapy and limiting detection of development of complications or disease progression that may require a change in management.

For these reasons, the great challenge of patients with HF during COVID-19 is keeping them safe from infection risk, but equally continuing with strict monitoring in order to prevent hospitalizations. As a result, health systems have largely transitioned to noncontact care delivery methods for ambulatory care (9). In this setting, various strategies of telemedicine and remote monitoring were developed rapidly and implemented more widely in HF patients (**Table 1**, **Figure 1**).

TELEMEDICINE STRATEGIES DURING COVID-19

Home Monitoring

Several strategies can be applied to perform home monitoring of HF patients. Two small studies performed in Boston and New York City showed initial encouraging results of implantable hemodynamic monitoring in COVID-19 (18, 19). However, device and hemodynamic monitoring can only be performed in those patients, which had implanted a device or hemodynamic sensor before the lockdown, which are a minority of the HF population.

A new home monitoring system should be easy to install, be intuitive to users, and provide robust communication (20). Hence, structured telephone support (STS), defined as monitoring, self-care management, or both, delivered using telephone calls (21), may represent the most simple and affordable system for HF centers starting with telemedicine during COVID-19.

A recent study on 103 patients in an Italian tertiary referral center investigated whether a telemedicine service expressly set up during the COVID-19 outbreak changed HF outcomes compared with the same period of 2019 without telemedicine (22). Around 60% of patients accessed telemedicine services at least once, and half of contacts led to a clinical decision (e.g., adjustment of diuretic doses, change of blood pressure drugs, rate controls, and anticoagulant management). In this study, the telemedicine service reduced the composite of HF hospitalization and death compared to patients in the 2019 cohort, which is nevertheless to be interpreted cautiously in light of the previously mentioned reduction of HF hospitalizations during lockdown. In fact, new-established STS interventions are expected to give significant advantages only in the long term, since they could be influenced by a learning-to-care curve due to staff training (23). However, the main goal of telemonitoring during COVID-19 is not to provide superior care than standard, but to offer patients with HF a "health maintenance strategy" which provides an individualized target for each HF patient and adjusts treatment to maintain the monitored parameters as close as possible to ideal (20).

Besides HF patients in general, HF patients who suffer SARS-CoV-2 infection and are treated at home

TABLE 1 | Strengths and weaknesses of different telemedicine strategies for patients with heart failure during COVID-19.

Strategies	Definition	Objectives	Challenges
Home monitoring	Remote monitoring of vital parameters and transmission (via devices, telephone, apps) to a care center for interpretation and management	Individualized targets Therapy optimization Patients' empowerment Avoiding social disparities	Device delivery and patients' education Staff training Initial investment
Virtual visits	Remote visits with audiovisual telecommunication system or through an online portal	Assessment of symptoms Therapy optimization Maintain connection between patient and physician Seeing new HF patients	Adequate assessment of volume status or congestion Availability of stable internet connection and devices
Forward triage	Sorting of patients before presentation in the ED	Early assignation to the right path Protect patients from high-risk exposure	Logistic reorganization of ED triage models Software implementation
In-hospital telemedicine	Implementation of telemedicine in the in-hospital setting	Limiting unnecessary exposure to affected patients Favor communication and reduce social isolation	Staff training Hardware costs
Telerehabilitation	Delivery of rehabilitation services remotely	Allow cardiac rehabilitation during lockdown	Initial assessment Patients' compliance and motivation Costs and reimbursement

ED, emergency department.

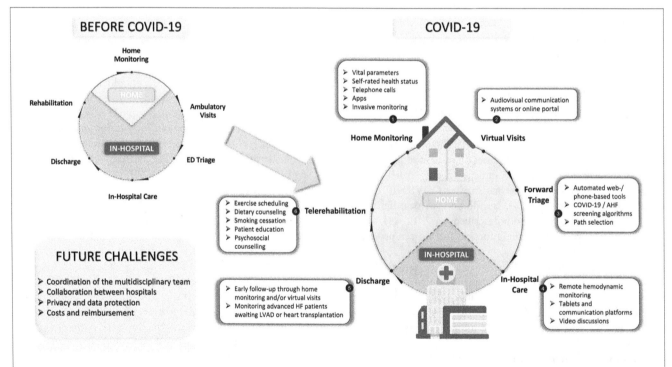

FIGURE 1 | Telemedicine in patients with heart failure before and during COVID-19. AHF, acute heart failure; COVID-19, coronavirus disease 2019; ED, emergency department; LVAD, left ventricular assist device. Modified from https://github.com/emojione/emojione/tree/2.2.7 and https://github.com/twitter/twemoji/. Licensed under a CC BY-SA License (https://creativecommons.org/licenses/by-sa/4.0).

could even more benefit from STS as they are at high risk for complications (8). Remote monitoring can also encourage patients to maintain home isolation and assist in correct timing of stopping the isolation precautions (24).

Virtual Visits

Virtual visits (VV) include remote visits, in which an audiovisual telecommunication system is used, and e-visits, which are communications between patients and providers through an online portal (9).

A recent statement from the Heart Failure Society of America provides information regarding platforms, workflows, and care models for VV in HF patients (25). Some institutions have already balanced the deferred or canceled face-to-face HF visits with rapid adoption of VV while employing several novel virtual health technologies with overall positive results (26). Specifically, the potential benefits of VV for HF patients are providing access to care and medical advice which would be otherwise difficult to obtain and reducing in-person exposure to SARS-CoV-2. Involvement of caregivers who may be present at home, but not in the outpatient clinic because of restrictions to hospital access, is an additional advantage of VV during the pandemic (25).

Hypothetically, this might represent also a smart working possibility for healthcare personnel, a class of workers for which this possibility is not usually considered or available.

VV may be best utilized for medication titration and optimization in stable patients with chronic HF. While substantial patient information can be gained from such visits, certain challenges remain, such as the adequate assessment of volume status or congestion (27). Thus, in-person visits should be reserved for recently hospitalized patients, patients approaching or with advanced HF, who are new post implantation of a left ventricular assist device (LVAD) or heart transplant, and those with new-onset HF (9).

Forward Triage

Respiratory symptoms, as well as functional decline and fatigue, may be early signs of both COVID-19 and of decompensated HF. Hence, stratification of patients before arriving in the emergency department (ED), the so-called *forward triage*, represents another potential strategy for health care surge control.

Before COVID-19, many EDs modified their triage model by allowing a remote provider to perform intake (28). In an emergency situation, web-conferencing software with a direct line from a triage room to a clinician can be rapidly implemented (29). An automated web- or phone-based tool could guide HF patients with concerning symptoms to determine the need for self-isolation, symptom monitoring, urgent VV, or presenting to the ED (30). Through a structured telemedicine program, detailed medical and exposure histories might be easily obtained. Screening algorithms can be integrated and local epidemiological information can be used to standardize screening and practice patterns across providers (29). The ultimate goal is to guide patients to the right diagnostic–therapeutic pathway while protecting them from unnecessary risk and exposure.

Patients with suspected COVID-19 are isolated immediately upon arrival to emergency departments. In several centers in the USA, telemedicine carts (i.e., systems that integrate displays, cameras, microphones, speakers, and network access) were already successfully deployed into COVID-19 isolation rooms. This initiative increased provider/patient communication and attention to staff safety, improved palliative care and patient support services, lowered consumption of personal protective equipment, increased patient comfort, and reduced the psychological toll of isolation (31).

In-Hospital Telemedicine

Certain principles of virtual medicine might be considered when approaching an HF patient seeking acute cardiac care during COVID-19. In this setting, telemedicine measures must aim at limiting unnecessary exposure to affected patients, utilizing remote hemodynamic monitoring and ICU flowcharts to evaluate patient progress and adjust medications (32). These data can be implemented with clinical assessments performed by a single bedside operator to generate operable conditions for safe, remote decision-making, using tools such as electronic stethoscopes and mobile ultrasound probes (32). Initial results of basic thoracic ultrasound programs in ICU are encouraging with rapid adoption of point-of-care ultrasound and commensurate reduction in formal imaging studies (26).

Importantly, COVID-19 has presented healthcare professionals with new and unusual barriers to effective communication between physician, patient, and family. As hospital visits are now frequently prohibited to patients' relatives, novel telecommunication and video options might be considered for patients to speak with loved ones, review treatment choices, and even discuss objectives of care (32). For this purpose, several hospitals introduced use of tablets and video calls with the ultimate goal to favor communication and reduce social isolation of hospitalized patients (33).

Telerehabilitation

Cardiovascular rehabilitation (CR) represents a cornerstone in the treatment of patients with HF. The term *telerehabilitation* has been used in much of the literature to date and is defined as the delivery of rehabilitation services via information and communication technologies (34). Before COVID-19, it has been shown to be a viable and effective alternative for individuals who are unable to access in-person healthcare services for the management of many conditions. During COVID-19, the reallocation of medical resources as well as the lockdown caused the cessation of all nonurgent medical services, including CR. Therefore, centers had to switch to alternative ways to deliver the core components of CR remotely.

A technology-driven CR model has been proposed, with the assistance of any form of technology (e.g., smartphones, mobile apps, internet, e-mail, webcams, and use of wearable sensors) (35). A recent survey about the implementation of cardiac telerehabilitation services during the COVID-19 pandemic in Belgium (36) showed that half of the answering centers switched to telerehabilitation during the pandemic, mainly for patients that were already undergoing CR. The most frequently used medium to deliver the CR components were online videos (71%) followed by website information (64%) and emails (64%). As the authors of this survey suggested, the remote delivery of CR can also play an important role after the reopening of the rehabilitation centers because of a reduced capacity due to social distancing measures (36). For this purpose, a recent call for action paper of the European Association of Preventive Cardiology provides a practical guide for the setup of a comprehensive cardiac telerehabilitation intervention during the COVID-19 pandemic, which could also be relevant to any cardiovascular disease patient not able to visit CR centers regularly after the COVID-19 pandemic ceases (37).

Advanced Heart Failure

The evaluation of patients with advanced HF awaiting LVAD placement or heart transplantation may be interrupted during the pandemic, as traditional social work, nutrition, pharmacy referrals, and diagnostic procedures are delayed. Telemedicine offers a platform for these multidisciplinary assessments to occur serially or simultaneously without delay (10). Furthermore, heart transplant recipients on stable immunosuppression at low risk for allograft rejection and hemodynamically optimized LVAD patients may be managed remotely without exposing them to further unnecessary risks (9). A telemonitoring algorithm for patients with LVAD has been recently proposed (38), and it is potentially adaptable to every LVAD center, regardless of the number of LVAD patients or previous experiences.

Clinical Trials

Since the first wave of the pandemic, clinical trials unrelated to COVID-19 have been paused in most institutions. Telemedicine might avoid the loss of data during lockdown, which can jeopardize the entire research validity. In clinical trials, measurements and data collection are traditionally performed during patient visits. As stated by a recent document of the Heart Failure Association (39), endpoints like symptom status, quality of life questionnaires, or even vital signs could be assessed using home-based testing, with alternative methods such as telephone contacts, app-based self-assessments, or video links.

DISCUSSION

Practical Considerations and Limitations of Telemedicine

Although telemedicine provides numerous advantages in many fields, it currently still carries practical limitations and pitfalls, which must be taken into consideration.

First, the hardware required for telemonitoring (i.e., smartphones, tablets, as well as blood pressure machines, scales, etc.) and exercise equipment for telerehabilitation (i.e., treadmill, stationary bike, etc.) may represent a significant financial burden, so either patients must be able to afford this or their health insurance/national health service must provide or reimburse the equipment. Moreover, patients who are unable to utilize the required devices or participate in a telemedicine session unaided either because of old age, poor hearing, cognitive dysfunction, language barriers, or limited education which may require the assistance of a family member or caregiver, who may not be available (40, 41). Finally, the use of telemedicine may be technically limited by poor phone and internet connectivity in rural areas (42, 43).

Telephone support is the most readily applicable and can be performed competently by trained nurses. However, home monitoring creates a large amount of data which must be screened and interpreted by trained staff (44), a process that could be time-consuming. In addition, it requires a dedicated physician to act on critical laboratory abnormalities, all of which can be

challenging for physicians managing their practices and possibly receiving limited reimbursement.

The care of a patient with HF requires a multidisciplinary collaboration among physicians, pharmacologists, nurses, physical therapists, nutritionists, and medical social workers. Hence, technology should be conjugated also to ensure communication between the team (e.g., virtual multidisciplinary meetings using video calling in times of social restrictions) (37). In addition, patients with HF often have several comorbidities and may be looked after by more than one hospital, thus requiring intensive collaboration between different specialists and clinics. Authors analyzing the impact of the first COVID-19 wave on patients with chronic diseases described a poor interconnection between telemedicine services operating at higher levels (i.e., secondary or tertiary care facilities) and those deployed in primary care clinics or community pharmacies, preventing to obtain the maximum benefit from these digital solutions (45). Future developments should encourage the collaboration between different professional figures, departments, hospitals, and care institutions.

Due to the fact that telemedicine involves the transmission of patients' confidential information, whether those data are processed and transferred via telephone calls, videoconference, mobile apps, or other platforms, their monitoring requires safe encrypted storage systems which only allow for authorized access to data and protect patient privacy. The interfaces used must be compliant with local regulations both regarding data protection (i.e., GDPR) and encryption (i.e., HIPAA requirements) (46, 47). Physicians implementing telemedicine in clinical practice during COVID-19 suggest using device management software for telehealth devices to create security settings and enforce encryption for devices given to patients (48).

The inclusion of new patients in a telerehabilitation program will be challenging during lockdown, especially with respect to the initial assessment (i.e., baseline stress test) and initial interview, a hurdle that may be overcome by a structured technology-based program with predefined remote assessment methods and audio-visual communication systems (35). However, not all patients could be comfortable with this mode of action, and the problem of financing and delivering technologies to the single patients still persists. An effective approach to reorganize CR could be to start a rehabilitation path in person and subsequently integrate this with a patient-tailored remote telerehabilitation program in order to optimize performance and extend patients' education.

Finally, telemedicine services are not yet included in the essential levels of care in many countries (9, 29, 45). During COVID-19, some efforts were already made by agencies like the US Food and Drug Administration, which is facilitating the use of remote monitoring devices, and Centers for Medicare and Medicaid Services, which is paying for telehealth services at the same rate they would have been paid, if provided in person (27). However, these costs were covered only due to the emergency situation. In order to continue after the pandemic, the shift to telemedicine should be done in parallel with developments in policymaking (27).

Future Perspectives

Evidence coming from observational studies on telemedicine during COVID-19 is of great importance. Centers having a dedicated HF unit should collect information regarding their own telemedicine approach, with the aim of defining strengths and weaknesses of each program and its impact on HF patients' care. This enormous amount of data provided during the pandemic should then be evaluated to be wisely implemented in daily clinical practice also after the crisis.

By evaluating results of telemedicine programs during COVID-19, one should keep in mind that in the particular setting of a pandemic, a system that is cost-efficient, user-friendly, and person-centered does not need to show that it improves outcome, but only that it is not inferior to traditional ways of delivering care and thus allows a safe maintenance of the *status quo* (20).

Although this pandemic has accelerated implementation of technology in the clinical setting, telemedicine should not be considered a cure-all for clinical scenarios. At its core, it remains a synergistic extension of the care team (49) and cannot entirely reproduce the bond-forming element of the traditional doctor–patient relationship based on direct face-to-face interactions (50).

CONCLUSIONS

COVID-19 represents a serious threat for the HF population due to both higher risk of severe disease and death and reduced availability of outpatient care. Telemedicine in all its different forms and possibilities can be adopted to ensure continued healthcare delivery to patients with HF. Thus, we are witnessing its rapid, large-scale implementation during the pandemic. However, there are still several limitations and issues that should be solved in order to continue providing high-quality telemedicine services in patients with HF also after COVID-19.

AUTHOR CONTRIBUTIONS

GT and DW drafted the manuscript. GMC, SG, MR, LB, GP, JD, PA, and MV critically reviewed the manuscript. All authors have participated in the work and have reviewed and agreed with the content of the article. None of the article contents are under consideration for publication in any other journal or have been published in any journal.

REFERENCES

1. Wang D, Hu B, Hu C, Zhu F, Liu X, Zhang J, et al. Clinical characteristics of 138 hospitalized patients with 2019 novel coronavirus-infected pneumonia in Wuhan, China. *JAMA*. (2020) 323:1061. doi: 10.1001/jama.2020.1585
2. Huang C, Wang Y, Li X, Ren L, Zhao J, Hu Y, et al. Clinical features of patients infected with 2019 novel coronavirus in Wuhan, China. *Lancet*. (2020) 395:497–506. doi: 10.1016/S0140-6736(20)30183-5
3. Chen N, Zhou M, Dong X, Qu J, Gong F, Han Y, et al. Epidemiological and clinical characteristics of 99 cases of 2019 novel coronavirus pneumonia in Wuhan, China: a descriptive study. *Lancet*. (2020) 395:507–13. doi: 10.1016/S0140-6736(20)30211-7
4. Guan W, Ni Z, Hu Y, Liang W-h, Qu C-q, He J-x, et al. Clinical characteristics of coronavirus disease 2019 in China. *N Engl J Med*. (2020) 382:1708–20. doi: 10.1056/NEJMoa2002032
5. Zhou F, Yu T, Du R, Fan G, Liu Y, Liu Z, et al. Clinical course and risk factors for mortality of adult inpatients with COVID-19 in Wuhan, China: a retrospective cohort study. *Lancet*. (2020) 395:1054–62. doi: 10.1016/S0140-6736(20)30566-3
6. Shi S, Qin M, Shen B, Cai Y, Liu T, Yang F, et al. Association of cardiac injury with mortality in hospitalized patients with COVID-19 in Wuhan, China. *JAMA Cardiol*. (2020) 5:802–10. doi: 10.1001/jamacardio.2020.0950
7. Guo T, Fan Y, Chen M, Wu X, Zhang L, He T, et al. Cardiovascular implications of fatal outcomes of patients with coronavirus disease 2019 (COVID-19). *JAMA Cardiol*. (2020) 5:811–18. doi: 10.1001/jamacardio.2020.1017
8. Zhang Y, Stewart Coats AJ, Zheng Z, Adamo M, Ambrosio G, Anker SD, et al. Management of heart failure patients with COVID-19. A Joint Position Paper of the Chinese Heart Failure Association & National Heart Failure Committee and the Heart Failure Association of the European Society of Cardiology. *Eur J Heart Fail*. (2020) 22:941–56. doi: 10.1002/ejhf.1915
9. DeFilippis EM, Reza N, Donald E, Givertz MM, Lindenfeld J, Jessup M. Considerations for heart failure care during the coronavirus disease 2019 (COVID-19) pandemic. *JACC Heart Fail*. (2020) 8:681–91. doi: 10.1016/j.jchf.2020.05.006
10. Reza N, DeFilippis EM, Jessup M. Secondary impact of the COVID-19 pandemic on patients with heart failure. *Circ Heart Fail*. (2020) 13:e007219. doi: 10.1161/CIRCHEARTFAILURE.120.007219
11. Han Y, Zeng H, Jiang H, Yang Y, Yuan Z, Cheng X, et al. CSC expert consensus on principles of clinical management of patients with severe emergent cardiovascular diseases during the COVID-19 epidemic. *Circulation*. (2020) 141:e810–e816. doi: 10.1161/CIRCULATIONAHA.120.047011
12. Tersalvi G, Vicenzi M, Calabretta D, Biasco L, Pedrazzini G, Winterton D. Elevated troponin in patients with coronavirus disease 2019: possible mechanisms. *J Card Fail*. (2020) 26:470–5. doi: 10.1016/j.cardfail.2020.04.009
13. Tersalvi G, Veronese G, Winterton D. Emerging evidence of myocardial injury in COVID-19: a path through the smoke. *Theranostics*. (2020) 10:9888–9. doi: 10.7150/thno.50788
14. Alon D, Stein GY, Korenfeld R, Fuchs S. Predictors and outcomes of infection-related hospital admissions of heart failure patients. *PLoS One*. (2013) 8:e72476. doi: 10.1371/journal.pone.0072476
15. Sandoval C, Walter SD, Krueger P, Smieja M, Smith A, Yusuf S, et al. Risk of hospitalization during influenza season among a cohort of patients with congestive heart failure. *Epidemiol Infect*. (2007) 135:574–82. doi: 10.1017/S095026880600714X
16. Kytömaa S, Hegde S, Claggett B, Udell JA, Rosamond W, Temte J, et al. Association of influenza-like illness activity with hospitalizations for heart failure: the atherosclerosis risk in communities study. *JAMA Cardiol*. (2019) 4:363. doi: 10.1001/jamacardio.2019.0549
17. Bromage DI, Cannatà A, Rind IA, Gregorio C, Piper S, Shah AM, et al. The impact of COVID-19 on heart failure hospitalization and management: report from a Heart Failure Unit in London during the peak of the pandemic. *Eur J Heart Fail*. (2020) 22:978–84. doi: 10.1002/ejhf.1925
18. Almufleh A, Ahluwalia M, Givertz MM, Weintraub J, Young M, Cooper I, et al. Short-term outcomes in ambulatory heart failure during the COVID-19

pandemic: insights from pulmonary artery pressure monitoring. *J Card Fail.* (2020) 26:633–4. doi: 10.1016/j.cardfail.2020.05.021

19. Oliveros E, Mahmood K, Mitter S, Pinney SP, Lala A. Letter to the Editor: pulmonary artery pressure monitoring during the COVID-19 pandemic in New York city. *J Card Fail.* (2020) 26:900–1. doi: 10.1016/j.cardfail.2020.08.003

20. Cleland JGF, Clark RA, Pellicori P, Inglis SC. Caring for people with heart failure and many other medical problems through and beyond the COVID-19 pandemic: the advantages of universal access to home telemonitoring. *Eur J Heart Fail.* (2020) 22:995–8. doi: 10.1002/ejhf.1864

21. Bui AL, Fonarow GC. Home monitoring for heart failure management. *J Am Coll Cardiol.* (2012) 59:97–104. doi: 10.1016/j.jacc.2011.09.044

22. Salzano A, D'Assante R, Stagnaro FM, Valente V, Crisci G, Giardino F, et al. Heart failure management during COVID-19 outbreak in Italy. Telemedicine experience from a heart failure university tertiary referral centre. *Eur J Heart Fail.* (2020) 22:1048–50. doi: 10.1002/ejhf.1911

23. Tersalvi G, Vicenzi M, Kirsch K, Gunold H, Thiele H, Lombardi F, et al. Structured telephone support programs in chronic heart failure may be affected by a learning curve. *J Cardiovasc Med.* (2020) 21:231–7. doi: 10.2459/JCM.0000000000000934

24. Razonable RR, Pennington KM, Meehan AM, Wilson JW, Froemming AT, Bennett CE, et al. A collaborative multidisciplinary approach to the management of coronavirus disease 2019 in the hospital setting. *Mayo Clin Proc.* (2020) 95:1467–81. doi: 10.1016/j.mayocp.2020.05.010

25. Gorodeski EZ, Goyal P, Cox ZL, Thibodeau JT, Reay RE, Rasmusson K, et al. Virtual visits for care of patients with heart failure in the era of COVID-19: a statement from the heart failure society of America. *J Card Fail.* (2020) 26:448–56. doi: 10.1016/j.cardfail.2020.04.008

26. Almufleh A, Givertz MM. Virtual health during a pandemic: redesigning care to protect our most vulnerable patients. *Circ Heart Fail.* (2020) 13:e007317. doi: 10.1161/CIRCHEARTFAILURE.120.007317

27. Abraham WT, Fiuzat M, Psotka MA, O'Connor CM. Heart failure collaboratory statement on heart failure remote monitoring in the landscape of COVID-19 and social distancing. *JACC Heart Fail.* (2020) 8:423–5. doi: 10.1016/j.jchf.2020.03.005

28. Joshi AU, Randolph FT, Chang AM, Slovis BH, Rising KL, Sabonjian M, et al. Impact of emergency department tele-intake on left without being seen and throughput metrics. *Acad Emerg Med.* (2020) 27:139–47. doi: 10.1111/acem.13890

29. Hollander JE, Carr BG. Virtually perfect? Telemedicine for Covid-19. *N Engl J Med.* (2020) 382:1679–81. doi: 10.1056/NEJMp2003539

30. Alwashmi MF. The use of digital health in the detection and management of COVID-19. *Int J Environ Res Public Health.* (2020) 17:2906. doi: 10.3390/ijerph17082906

31. Bains J, Greenwald PW, Mulcare MR, Leyden D, Kim J, Shemesh AJ, et al. Utilizing telemedicine in a novel approach to COVID-19 management and patient experience in the emergency department. *Telemed J E Health.* (2020). doi: 10.1089/tmj.2020.0162. [Epub ahead of print].

32. Katz JN, Sinha SS, Alviar CL, Dudzinski DM, Gage A, Brusca SB, et al. Disruptive modifications to cardiac critical care delivery during the Covid-19 pandemic: an international perspective. *J Am Coll Cardiol.* (2020) 76:72–84. doi: 10.1016/j.jacc.2020.04.029

33. Goulabchand R, Boclé H, Vignet R, Sotto A, Loubet P. Digital tablets to improve quality of life of COVID-19 older inpatients during lockdown. *Eur Geriatr Med.* (2020) 11:705–6. doi: 10.1007/s41999-020-00344-9

34. Brennan D, Tindall L, Theodoros D, Brown J, Campbell M, Christiana D, et al. A blueprint for telerehabilitation guidelines. *Int J Telerehab.* (2010) 2:31–4. doi: 10.5195/IJT.2010.6063

35. Babu AS, Arena R, Ozemek C, Lavie CJ. COVID-19: a time for alternate models in cardiac rehabilitation to take centre stage. *Can J Cardiol.* (2020) 36:792–4. doi: 10.1016/j.cjca.2020.04.023

36. Scherrenberg M, Frederix I, De Sutter J, Dendale P. Use of cardiac telerehabilitation during COVID-19 pandemic in Belgium. *Acta Cardiol.* (2020) :1-4. doi: 10.1080/00015385.2020.1786625

37. Scherrenberg M, Wilhelm M, Hansen D, Völler H, Cornelissen V, Frederix I, et al. The future is now: a call for action for cardiac telerehabilitation in the COVID-19 pandemic from the secondary prevention and rehabilitation section of the European Association of Preventive Cardiology. *Eur J Prev Cardiol.* (2020). doi: 10.1177/2047487320939671. [Epub ahead of print].

38. Mariani S, Hanke JS, Dogan G, Schmitto JD. Out of hospital management of LVAD patients during COVID-19 outbreak. *Artif Organs.* (2020) 44:873–6. doi: 10.1111/aor.13744

39. Anker SD, Butler J, Khan MS, Abraham WT, Bauersachs J, Bocchi E, et al. Conducting clinical trials in heart failure during (and after) the COVID-19 pandemic: an Expert Consensus Position Paper from the Heart Failure Association (HFA) of the European Society of Cardiology (ESC). *Eur Heart J.* (2020) 41:2109–17. doi: 10.1093/eurheartj/ehaa461

40. Orlando JF, Beard M, Kumar S. Systematic review of patient and caregivers' satisfaction with telehealth videoconferencing as a mode of service delivery in managing patients' health. *PLoS One.* (2019) 14:e0221848. doi: 10.1371/journal.pone.0221848

41. Scott Kruse C, Karem P, Shifflett K, Vegi L, Ravi K, Brooks M. Evaluating barriers to adopting telemedicine worldwide: a systematic review. *J Telemed Telecare.* (2018) 24:4–12. doi: 10.1177/1357633X16674087

42. Hirko KA, Kerver JM, Ford S, Szafranski C, Beckett J, Kitchen C, et al. Telehealth in response to the Covid-19 Pandemic: implications for rural health disparities. *J Am Med Inform Assoc.* (2020) 27:1816–8. doi: 10.1093/jamia/ocaa156

43. Zachrison KS, Boggs KM, Hayden EM, Espinola JA, Camargo CA. Understanding barriers to telemedicine implementation in rural emergency departments. *Ann Emerg Med.* (2020) 75:392–9. doi: 10.1016/j.annemergmed.2019.06.026

44. Angermann CE, Störk S, Gelbrich G, Faller H, Jahns R, Frantz S, et al. Mode of action and effects of standardized collaborative disease management on mortality and morbidity in patients with systolic heart failure: the interdisciplinary network for heart failure (INH) study. *Circ Heart Fail.* (2012) 5:25–35. doi: 10.1161/CIRCHEARTFAILURE.111.962969

45. Omboni S. Telemedicine during the COVID-19 in Italy: a missed opportunity? *Telemed J E Health.* (2020) 26:973–5. doi: 10.1089/tmj.2020.0106

46. HealthITSecurity. *Healthcare Data Encryption not 'Required,' but Very Necessary.* HealthITSecurity (2017). Available online at: https://healthitsecurity.com/news/healthcare-data-encryption-not-required-but-very-necessary (accessed September 17, 2020).

47. HIPAA Encryption Requirements. HIPAA Journal. Available online at: https://www.hipaajournal.com/hipaa-encryption-requirements/ (accessed September 17, 2020).

48. Heslin SM, Nappi M, Kelly G, Crawford J, Morley EJ, Lingam V, et al. Rapid creation of an emergency department telehealth program during the COVID-19 pandemic. *J Telemed Telecare.* (2020). doi: 10.1177/1357633X2095 2632. [Epub ahead of print].

49. Czartoski T. *Commentary: Telehealth Holds Promise, but Human Touch Still Needed.* Articles, Abstracts, and Reports. 1278 (2019). Available online at: https://digitalcommons.psjhealth.org/publications/1278

50. Romanick-Schmiedl S, Raghu G. Telemedicine - maintaining quality during times of transition. *Nat Rev Dis Primer.* (2020) 6:45. doi: 10.1038/s41572-020-0199-4

11

Outcomes of Patients with ST-Segment Elevation Myocardial Infarction Admitted During COVID-19 Pandemic Lockdown in Germany

Manuel Rattka [1]*, Lina Stuhler [1], Claudia Winsauer [1], Jens Dreyhaupt [2], Kevin Thiessen [1], Michael Baumhardt [1], Sinisa Markovic [1], Wolfgang Rottbauer [1] and Armin Imhof [1]*

[1] Clinic for Internal Medicine II, University Hospital Ulm - Medical Center, Ulm, Germany, [2] Institute of Epidemiology and Medical Biometry, Ulm University, Ulm, Germany

*Correspondence:
Manuel Rattka
manuel.rattka@uniklinik-ulm.de
orcid.org/0000-0002-3269-3871
Armin Imhof
armin.imhof@uniklinik-ulm.de
orcid.org/0000-0001-7452-303X

Objective: Since the outbreak of the COVID-19 pandemic, healthcare professionals reported declining numbers of patients admitted with ST-segment myocardial infarction (STEMI) associated with increased in-hospital morbidity and mortality. However, the effect of lockdown on outcomes of STEMI patients admitted during the COVID-19 crisis has not been prospectively evaluated.

Methods: A prospective, observational study on STEMI patients admitted to our tertiary care center during the COVID-19 pandemic was conducted. Outcomes of patients admitted during lockdown were compared to those patients admitted before and after pandemic-related lockdown.

Results: A total of 147 patients were enrolled in our study, including 57 patients in the pre-lockdown group (November 1, 2019 to March 20, 2020), 16 patients in the lockdown group (March 21 to April 19, 2020), and 74 patients in the post-lockdown group (April 20 to September 30, 2020). Patients admitted during lockdown had significantly longer time to first medical contact, longer door-to-needle-time, higher serum troponin T levels, worse left ventricular end-diastolic pressure, and higher need for circulatory support. After a median follow-up of 142 days, survival was significantly worse in STEMI patients of the lockdown group (log-rank: $p = 0.0035$).

Conclusions: This is the first prospective study on outcomes of STEMI patients admitted during public lockdown amid the COVID-19 pandemic. Our results suggest that lockdown might deteriorate outcomes of STEMI patients. Public health strategies to constrain spread of COVID-19, such as lockdown, have to be accompanied by distinct public instructions to ensure timely medical care in acute diseases such as STEMI.

Keywords: COVID-19, STEMI, myocardial infarction, lockdown, outcome, epidemiology, Germany

INTRODUCTION

Soon after the severe acute respiratory syndrome coronavirus 2 (SARS-CoV-2) spread globally, physicians warned about potential side effects of the COVID-19 pandemic compromising medical care (1, 2). It has been suggested that the pandemic keeps patients from seeking and receiving needed medical attention despite suffering from physical symptoms. Social containment measures (i.e., lockdown and stay-at-home orders), stress, and fear of COVID-19 may influence an individual's health behavior (3–5). Patients with ST-segment elevation myocardial infarction (STEMI) are an especially vulnerable population, as total ischemic time severely influences their outcome (6). There have been several reports on diminishing numbers of STEMI admissions during the outbreak in both epicenters and non-epicenters of the COVID-19 pandemic. This has been associated with significantly prolonged times from symptom onset to first medical contact (FMC) and increased in-hospital morbidity and mortality (7–11). However, the reasons underlying this phenomenon have rarely been assessed. The influence of factors such as lockdown, stress, and fear of COVID-19 on the patient's long-term outcome, has not yet been evaluated.

METHODS

Study Design and Study Population

In this prospective, observational cohort study, we aimed for inclusion of all patients with STEMI admitted between March 21, 2020 and September 30, 2020. STEMI patients admitted between November 1, 2019 and March 20, 2020 were enrolled retrospectively.

Patients had to be ≥18 years old and give written informed consent to be eligible for inclusion. Diagnosis of STEMI was made according to contemporary guidelines and all STEMI patients underwent cardiac catheterization and subsequent percutaneous coronary intervention (PCI) immediately after admission as indicated by current recommendations (6). During the COVID-19 pandemic, all patients were treated with personal protection gear in the case of an unknown COVID-19 status. The study complies with the Declaration of Helsinki and was approved by the local ethics committee (number of application and positive vote 250/20). This study adheres to the STROBE statement (12).

Data Collection

Demographic, clinical, laboratory, interventional, and in-hospital outcome data were extracted from our patient management system by two medical practitioners (CW and LS) and adjudicated by a third one (MR) in case of any kind of difference. Left ventricular systolic function at admissions was measured by cardiac ventriculography during cardiac catheterization and categorized as normal, mildly impaired, moderately impaired, or severely impaired, according to the expertise of the attending physician. Left ventricular systolic function at follow-up was assessed by automated echocardiographic quantification (outpatient visit: EPIQ 7, Koninklijke Philips N.V., Eindhoven,

Netherlands; home visit: Butterfly IQ, Butterfly Network. Inc., Guilford, CT, USA).

Clinical Follow-Up

Patients were scheduled for outpatient clinic visits (clinical assessment, 12-lead ECG, and echocardiography) after 1 month, 3 months and, then, at least every 3 months after discharge. If, for any reason, an outpatient clinic visit could not be realized, a home visit was offered to the patient.

Laboratory Measurements

Blood samples were drawn at the time of hospital admission or at the outpatient clinic visits for measurements of high sensitivity cardiac troponin T (hsTnT), NT-pro BNP, and creatinine (ElectroChemiLumineszenz ImmunoAssay "ECLIA" Roche, Cobas 8000, Modul e801 and e601) as part of the clinical routine. In addition, every patient was tested for SARS- CoV-2 by throat swab test at admissions (Sigma-Virocult® with 2 ml Virocult® medium, Check Diagnostics GmbH, Germany) and analyzed by RT-PCR at the local Institute for Virology.

Assessment of the Effect of Lockdown on STEMI Patients

Measures of social restriction in Germany came into effect on March 21, 2020 and public reopening was partly initiated on April 20, 2020. Consequently, patients admitted between November 1, 2019 and March 20, 2020 were classified as the "pre-lockdown" (pre-COVID-19) group, patients admitted between March 21 and April 19, 2020 were assigned to the "lockdown" group, and patients admitted between April 20 and September 30, 2020 to the "post-lockdown" group. Comparisons were made on patient characteristics, clinical data, and outcomes of patients of the lockdown group and the combined pre-/post-lockdown group. Outcomes were heart failure symptoms as measured by NYHA class, serum levels of cardiac biomarkers, left ventricular ejection fraction, and survival. Additionally, baseline characteristics, laboratory parameters, in-hospital clinical characteristics and time to FMC were assessed and compared between the groups.

Assessment of the Effect of Stress and Fear of COVID-19 on STEMI Patients Admitted During the COVID-19 Pandemic

To assess the level of stress and fear of COVID-19 at baseline in STEMI patients admitted during the pandemic, we utilized well-established questionnaires. The COVID Stress Scales (CSS) were used to assess COVID-19 related distress and the Fear of COVID-19 Scale (FCV-19S) was implemented to measure COVID-19 related fear (13, 14).

Statistical Analysis

Continuous variables were described as mean ± standard deviation or median together with interquartile range (IQR), as appropriate. Categorical variables were described as absolute and relative frequencies, respectively. Group comparison (lockdown vs. pre-/post-lockdown combined) of continuous variables was performed by two-sample t-test or Wilcoxon rank sum test

TABLE 1 | Patient characteristics at baseline.

	Total n = 147	Lockdown n = 16	Pre-/Post-Lockdown n = 131	p-value
Age	64 ± 13	69 ± 12	64 ± 14	0.1519*
Sex (male)	112 (76)	12 (75)	100 (76)	1.0000§
Arterial hypertension	89 (61)	11 (69)	78 (60)	0.4768§§
Diabetes	39 (27)	3 (19)	36 (27)	0.5608§
Family history	35 (24)	3 (19)	32 (24)	0.7627§
Smoking	71 (48)	8 (50)	63 (48)	0.8853§§
Obesity	21 (14)	2 (13)	19 (15)	1.0000§
TIA/stroke	8 (5)	2 (13)	6 (5)	0.2109§
OSAS	7 (5)	1 (6)	6 (5)	0.5616§
COPD	2 (3)	1 (6)	4 (3)	0.4427§
CKD	35 (24)	5 (31)	30 (23)	0.5345§
FCV-19S questionnaire (score)	14 (9, 17)	12 (9, 17)	14 (9, 17)	0.8976**
CSS questionnaire (score)	38 (25, 70)	31 (13, 50]	39 (27, 71)	0.2018**

TIA, transient ischemic attack; OSAS, obstructive sleep apnea syndrome; COPD, chronic obstructive pulmonary disease; CKD, chronic kidney disease; FCV-19S, Fear of COVID-19 Scale; CSS, COVID-19 Stress Scales.
*two-sample t-test.
**Wilcoxon rank sum test.
§Fisher's exact test.
§§ chi² test.

as appropriate. Group comparison (pre-lockdown vs. lockdown vs. post-lockdown) of continuous variables was performed by one-way ANOVA or Kruskal-Wallis test as appropriate. The chi² test or Fisher's exact test was used for group comparison of categorical variables. The Fisher's exact test was used if >20% of cells of the table contain expected values of <5, as appropriate. Otherwise the chi-squared test was used. The Kaplan-Meier estimator was used to assess the time to event and groups were compared using the log-rank test. Logistic regression analysis was done to investigate potential predictors on delayed presentation. Association of outcomes and total sums of both CSS and FCV-19S were assessed by scatter plots and either point-biserial correlation coefficient (in the case of dichotomous variables) or Spearman rank correlation coefficient (in the case of continuous variables).

Statistical analysis was performed by SAS version 9.4 under Windows. A two-sided p-value of <0.05 was considered statistically significant. Due to the explorative nature of this study, all results from statistical tests have to be interpreted as hypothesis generating. An adjustment for multiple testing was not done.

RESULTS

Patient Characteristics

From March 21, 2020, when measures of social restrictions were implemented for the first time during the COVID-19 pandemic in Germany, until the end of our inclusion period on September 31, 2020, 90 patients with STEMI had been

admitted to our tertiary care center. Amongst those, 16 patients had been admitted during the lockdown period (March 21, 2020 to April 19, 2020; "lockdown group") and 74 patients in the post-lockdown period (April 20, 2020 to September 30, 2020; "post-lockdown group"). Furthermore, characteristics of 57 STEMI patients admitted before the COVID-19 pandemic ("pre-lockdown group") were assessed. For main analyses, the "pre-lockdown group" and the "post-lockdown group" were combined ("pre-/post-lockdown group"). In total, the mean age was 64 ± 13 years with 76% (112 out of 147 patients) being male. There were no significant differences in baseline characteristics between groups. No patients tested positive for SARS-CoV-2 virus during hospitalization. No patient was lost to follow-up. Detailed baseline characteristics are shown in **Table 1** and **Supplementary Table 1**.

Clinical Characteristics at Admission

To assess the effect of lockdown on STEMI patients admitted to hospital during the COVID-19 outbreak, clinical characteristics were assessed and compared to patients admitted before the outbreak and those admitted after measures of social restrictions had been lifted. Remarkably, a significantly higher rate of patients in the lockdown period reported that they intentionally did not go to the hospital or inform the emergency medical services immediately after the onset of symptoms (pre-/post-lockdown: 39 out of 120 patients (33%), lockdown: 11 out of 13 patients (85%); p = 0.0004). Likewise, 46% of patients in the lockdown group acknowledged that the time from symptom onset to FMC was longer than 24 h compared to 11% of patients in the pre-/post-lockdown group. Overall, time to FMC (in hours) was significantly prolonged in the lockdown group [pre-/post-lockdown: 2.0 (0.3, 16.0), lockdown: 11.0 (2.0, 144.0); p = 0.0193]. Additionally, door-to-needle time (in minutes) was significantly prolonged in patients admitted during lockdown [pre-/post-lockdown: 46 (28, 74); lockdown: 83 (59, 117); p = 0.0277]. Interestingly, patients in the lockdown group were more symptomatic at admission, as measured by NYHA class. However, there was no significant difference for measurements of vital signs at admission. Evaluation of laboratory parameters at admissions revealed that patients admitted due to STEMI during lockdown had significantly higher serum troponin T levels compared to those admitted before and after the pandemic lockdown [pre-/post-lockdown: 244 (53, 1124) ng/L, lockdown: 746 (292, 3899) ng/L; p = 0.0105]. Additionally, measures for NT-pro BNP and creatinine showed no significant difference. However, mean left ventricular end diastolic pressure (LVEDP) was significantly higher in the lockdown group compared to the pre-/post-lockdown group [pre-/post-lockdown: 24 (17, 29) mmHg, lockdown: 34 (27, 36) mmHg; p = 0.0116]. Lastly, STEMI patients admitted during lockdown had significantly higher need for circulatory support than those admitted before after the lockdown period [pre-/post lockdown: 18 out of 122 patients (15%), lockdown: nine out of 16 patients (56%), p = 0.0005]. Clinical characteristics at admission are summarized in **Table 2** and **Supplementary Table 2**.

TABLE 2 | Clinical characteristics at baseline.

	Total	Lockdown	Pre-/Post-Lockdown	p-value
	n = 147	n = 16	n = 131	
NYHA class				
I	34 (27)	1 (8)	33 (29)	**0.0087**[§]
II	25 (20)	0 (0)	25 (22)	
III	10 (8)	3 (23)	7 (6)	
IV	57 (45)	9 (69)	48 (42)	
Delayed presentation				
Yes	50 (38)	11 (85)	39 (33)	**0.0004**[§]
No	83 (62)	2 (15)	81 (68)	
Time to FMC				
Immediately	60 (45)	2 (15)	58 (49)	**0.0032**[§]
≤ 3 h	27 (20)	2 (15)	25 (21)	
≤ 12 h	14 (11)	3 (23)	11 (9)	
≤ 24 h	12 (9)	0 (0)	12 (10)	
> 24 h	19 (14)	6 (46)	13 (11)	
Time to FMC (hours)	2.0 (0.3, 24.0)	11.0 (2.0, 144.0)	2.0 (0.3, 16.0)	**0.0193**[**]
Systolic bp (mmHg)	117 ± 28	116 ± 29	117 ± 29	0.9009[*]
Diastolic bp (mmHg)	67 ± 20	76 ± 19	65 ± 19	0.0579[*]
Troponin T (ng/L)	318 (63, 1,301)	746 (292, 3,899)	244 (53, 1,124)	**0.0105**[**]
NT-pro BNP (pg/ml)	354 (91, 1,879)	1,120 (237, 6,459)	331 (83, 1,712)	0.0717[**]
Creatinine (µmol/L)	84 (71, 110)	86 (74, 115)	84 (71, 109)	0.6503[**]
Laevocardiography				
Normal	4 (3)	0 (0)	4 (3)	0.2620[§]
Mildly reduced	31 (23)	4 (27)	27 (22)	
Moderately reduced	55 (40)	3 (20)	52 (43)	
Severely reduced	46 (34)	8 (53)	38 (31)	
LVEDP (mmHg)	26 (17, 32)	34 (27, 36)	24 (17, 29)	**0.0116**[**]
Door-to-needle-time (min)	54 (28, 80)	83 (59, 117)	46 (28, 74)	**0.0277**[**]
Culprit lesion				
LAD	67 (49)	11 (79)	56 (46)	0.0815[§]
LCX	19 (14)	1 (7)	18 (15)	
RCA	51 (37)	2 (14)	49 (40)	
Circulatory support				
Yes	27 (20)	9 (56)	18 (15)	**0.0005**[§]
No	111 (80)	7 (44)	104 (85)	
Time at hospital (days)	4 (3, 6)	5 (2, 6)	4 (3, 6)	0.9445[**]

FMC, first medical contact; BNP, brain natriuretic peptide; bp, blood pressure; LVED, left ventricular end diastolic pressure; LAD, left anterior descending; LCX, left circumflex artery; RCA, right coronary artery.
[*]two-sample t-test.
[**]Wilcoxon rank sum test.
[§]Fisher's exact test.
[§§]chi² test.
Boldface denotes significance of p-values.

Clinical Outcomes

Patients included in our analysis had a median follow-up time of 142 days. Intriguingly, a comparison of survival time of patients of the lockdown group and patients of the pre-/post-lockdown group showed that STEMI patients admitted during lockdown had a significantly lower survival (confirmed deaths; pre-/post-lockdown: 21 out of 131 patients; lockdown: 7 out of 16 patients; log-rank test: $p = 0.0035$; **Figure 1**). This was associated with a higher rate of patients in the lockdown group (30%) reporting the presence of heart failure symptoms at rest compared to the pre-/post-lockdown period (11%). However, the overall difference in NYHA-class between both groups was only a non-significant result ($p = 0.1367$; **Table 3**). Analysis of laboratory measures at follow-up showed no significant difference. Clinical outcomes are shown in **Table 3** and **Supplementary Table 3**.

Effect of Stress of COVID-19 and Fear of COVID-19 on Outcomes

Since the association of fear of COVID-19 and outcomes of STEMI patients has not been comprehensively evaluated so far, we assessed the level of stress and fear of COVID-19 by two well-established questionnaires (FCV-19S and CSS). Patients in the lockdown period had a median FCV-19S Score of 12 (9, 17) and CSS score of 31 (13, 50), compared to a FCV-19S score of 14 (9, 17) ($p = 0.8976$), and CSS Score of 39 (27, 71) ($p = 0.2018$) in the pre-/post-lockdown group (**Table 1**). Association analysis of total test scores with baseline and follow-up parameters showed a significant relationship between the total CCS score and left ventricular contractile function as assessed by laevocardiography. However, no association between the total FCS-19V score and laevocardiography at admission could be demonstrated. There was no relationship between anxiety of COVID-19 and other parameters (**Supplementary Table 4**).

Predictors of Intentionally Delayed Presentation

To identify predictors of delayed presentation, we performed both univariate as well as multiple logistic regression analysis of the parameters that potentially keep STEMI patients from seeking timely medical care amid the COVID-19 pandemic. After multiple analysis, only "admission during lockdown" remained significantly associated with intentionally delayed presentation (**Table 4**).

DISCUSSION

To the best of our knowledge, this is the first study prospectively evaluating the outcome of STEMI patients admitted during the COVID-19 pandemic caused lockdown, which also analyzes the effects of stress and fear of COVID-19 on patient outcomes. We found that patients with STEMI admitted during the lockdown period to our tertiary center showed lower survival compared to both those admitted before the COVID-19 pandemic and after measures of social restriction have been partly lifted. This was associated with a longer time from symptom onset to FMC and

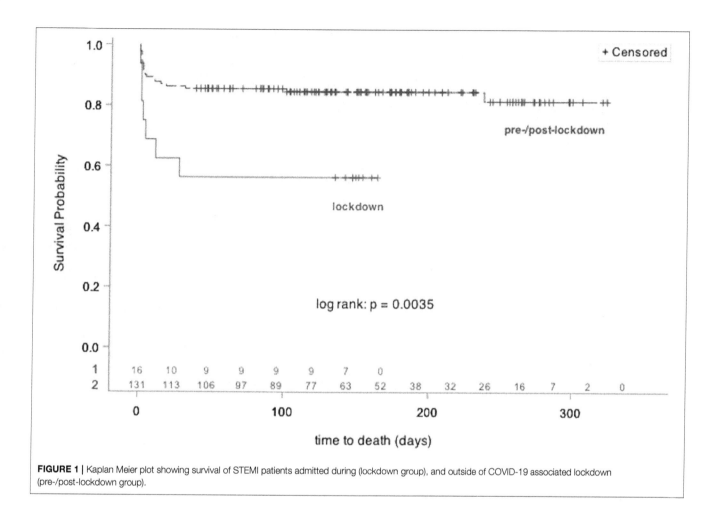

FIGURE 1 | Kaplan Meier plot showing survival of STEMI patients admitted during (lockdown group), and outside of COVID-19 associated lockdown (pre-/post-lockdown group).

a prolonged door-to-needle time. Additionally, patients in the lockdown group had significantly higher serum troponin T levels, a worse left ventricular end-diastolic pressure, and a higher need of circulatory support at admission.

Effect of Fear of COVID-19 and Stress of COVID-19 on STEMI Patients

Observations since the beginning of the COVID-19 crisis have suggested that various factors, such as altruistic behavior, information by the media, and especially fear of contagion with SARS-CoV-2 in hospital, contributed to reduced admissions of patients with acute myocardial infarction and prolonged times from symptom onset to FMC (4, 15). It has been reported, that patients who avoided an emergency room visit timely because they feared getting infected with SARS-CoV-2 in hospital, suffered catastrophic complications such as ventricular septal defect, which has become rare due to steadily improving medical care (16). As fear displays one characteristic of infectious disease and is associated with its transmission rate, morbidity, and mortality, Ahorsu et al. developed and validated a 7-item scale (Fear of COVID-19 Scale, FCV-19S) assessing the level of fear of SARS-CoV-2 (14). As there is currently no systematic study on the effect of fear on patients with myocardial infarction, we

employed the FCV-19S to estimate if the extent of fear of COVID-19 is associated with worsened outcomes in STEMI patients. To do so, we conducted association analysis of the scores of the FCV-19S, and relevant clinical patient characteristics. Our results indicate that overall fear of COVID-19 is not related to adverse outcomes in STEMI patients. To substantiate this finding, we applied the COVID Stress Scales, a 36-item scale developed by Taylor et al. to better understand and assess COVID-19-related stress and anxiety (13). Besides a single relationship between the total CSS score and left ventricular systolic contractility as assessed by laevocardiography, we could not demonstrate an association between the totaled item scores and outcomes of STEMI patients. Therefore, fear of COVID-19 was not associated with lockdown, higher measures of cardiac biomarkers, outcomes at follow-up, and prolonged times from symptom onset to FMC. Since our study population represents a region which has been rather spared from overwhelming infection rates in the early phase of the pandemic, these results might deviate if STEMI patients in epicenters of the pandemic are interviewed.

Effect of Lockdown on STEMI Patients

Soon after SARS-CoV-2 surfaced around the world, several countermeasures were initiated to contain further spread as

TABLE 3 | Patient characteristics at follow up.

	Total	Lockdown	Pre-/Post-Lockdown	p-value
	n = 147	n = 16	n = 131	
NYHA class				
I	46 (45)	5 (50)	41 (44)	0.1367§
II	35 (34)	1 (10)	34 (37)	
III	9 (9)	1 (10)	8 (9)	
IV	13 (13)	3 (30)	10 (11)	
LVEF	53 (45, 60)	47 (35, 63)	53 (45, 60)	0.4327**
Troponin T (ng/L)	19 (10, 39)	26 (19, 81)	17 (10, 33)	0.1300**
NT-pro BNP (pg/ml)	483 (187, 1,092)	1,014 (187, 3,559)	483 (195, 964)	0.4976**
Creatinine (µmol/L)	81 (74, 93)	83 (74, 131)	80 (74, 93)	0.5377**

NYHA, New York Heart Association; LVEF, left ventricular ejection fraction; BNP, brain natriuretic peptide.
**Wilcoxon rank sum test.
§Fisher's exact test.

TABLE 4 | Identification of predictors of intentionally delayed presentation.

	Multiple analysis		
Variables	**Odds Ratio (OR)**	**95% CI of OR**	**p-value**
Age	0.965	0.924–1.008	0.1133
Sex (female)	2.187	0.567–8.437	0.2558
Admission during lockdown	16.393	1.692–166.67	**0.0159**
FCV-19S questionnaire (score)	1.083	0.939–1.249	0.2760
CSS questionnaire (score)	0.986	0.952–1.021	0.4280

FCV-19S, Fear of COVID-19 Scale; CSS, COVID-19 Stress Scales. Boldface denotes significance of p-values.

much as possible. Drastic measures of social distancing and public lockdown were implemented, among other policies. In Germany, public facilities were closed, sporting events were canceled, and the physical contact of more than two persons outside of families was prohibited (9). Depending on the region, even curfews were enforced to minimize the inter-personal contact. For patients suffering from acute myocardial infarction, it has been suggested that measures of public lockdown might interfere with timely and adequate medical care (1, 2, 4, 10). It has been observed that the implementation of regional lockdown was associated with a significant decline in admission numbers of STEMI patients compared to times before the pandemic (10, 17). Furthermore, a concomitant increase of patient-related as well as system-related delay times, as measured by the time from symptom onset to FMC and door-to-balloon time, has been registered (18). However, it is difficult to distinguish if these findings were related specifically to the lockdown or to the COVID-19 crisis as a whole. To date, there are only a few retrospective cohort and register studies available with data on STEMI patients admitted during and after regional lockdown (19, 20). While these studies confirm the decrease

in incidence during lockdown period, there is a lack of information regarding delay times, mortality and survival (19, 20). To compensate for this issue, we prospectively assessed and compared survival of STEMI patients admitted during the COVID-19 pandemic and outside of lockdown. Intriguingly, we found that the lockdown group had a significantly lower survival. This might be attributed to our finding that during lockdown, patients were admitted in worse condition. This is substantiated by (1) worse symptoms as measured by NYHA-class, (2) significantly increased serum troponin T levels, (3) a significantly higher LVEDP, and (4) significantly higher need for circulatory support in the lockdown-group. This could be related to a significantly prolonged time from symptom onset to FMC during lockdown, which is known to be associated with larger infarct size and infarct transmurality (21). Additionally, we observed that the door-to-needle time was significantly prolonged in the lockdown-group, too. Evidently, this is related to the indispensable adaptation of emergency processes, such as employment of personal protective gear, to mitigate the risk of getting infected with SARS-CoV-2 (22). Nevertheless, it remains possible that the increase in system-related delay time, as measured by door-to-needle time, contributed to the worse outcome of STEMI patients admitted during lockdown. Assessment of other outcomes did not show differences, which might be related to the higher number of deceased patients in the lockdown group, who, therefore, did not receive a follow-up visit.

Moreover, by multiple logistic regression analysis, we show that amongst several aforementioned factors that potentially keep STEMI patients from seeking timely medical attention despite experiencing ischemic symptoms, that lockdown (not stress or fear of COVID-19) was significantly associated with an intentionally delayed presentation. These findings substantiate our hypothesis that measures of social distancing such as lockdown adversely affect the health behavior and outcomes of STEMI patients.

As a consequence, public lockdown appears to considerably deteriorate the prognosis of patients suffering from myocardial ischemia. In the presence of the currently rising incidence of SARS-CoV-2 virus infections worldwide and imminent recurrence of lockdown measures, public health policy has to carefully decide on the extent of social policies to avoid potential excess morbidity and mortality. Implementation of lockdown measures have to be accompanied by distinct public instructions on how to act in health emergencies such as STEMI and others.

Limitations

As this is a prospective, observational explorative study on the outcomes of STEMI patients admitted during and outside of social lockdown related to the COVID-19 pandemic, it inherently has limitations. Since this is a study from a single center, only a limited number of patients could be included. Due to the explorative character of this study, our results have to be interpreted as hypothesis generating. Studies reporting the outcomes a larger number of participants, which might be achievable by a multi-center design or a prolonged time to select cases, are of the essence to verify our results and to further investigate the drivers of increased mortality (e.g., by pathway analysis). Nonetheless, these results are the first prospective data on the outcomes of STEMI patients admitted during, before and after lockdown, which reveal a significant decrease in survival during lockdown. For further analysis, the raw data underlying our analyses are available upon publication.

CONCLUSION

This is the first prospective study comparing the outcomes of STEMI patients admitted during lockdown, to outcomes of patients admitted before and after public lockdown in a non-COVID-19 epicenter. Our results suggest that enforced lockdown is associated with reduced survival of STEMI patients, which supposedly is related to prolonged patients delay times. Patient related factors such as the fear of getting infected in the hospital or stress factors related to COVID-19 seem to have less impact on outcomes among these patients. Public health care strategies to constrain SARS-CoV-2 or other pandemics at present and

in future including public lockdown measures have to assure timely medical treatment beyond COVID-19. Implementation of lockdown measures should be accompanied by distinct public instructions on how to act in acute life-threatening diseases such as STEMI and others.

AUTHOR CONTRIBUTIONS

MR and AI had the idea for and designed the study and had full access to all data and take responsibility for the integrity of the data and the accuracy of the data analysis. MR, CW, and LS collected the data. JD performed the statistical analysis. MR and KT mainly wrote the manuscript with support from AI, CW, LS, SM, and MB. MR, AI, and WR were mainly responsible for the interpretation of the data. AI and WR supervised the project. All authors contributed to the article and approved the submitted version.

REFERENCES

1. Rosenbaum L. The untold toll — the pandemic's effects on patients without Covid-19. *N Engl J Med.* (2020) 382:2368–71. doi: 10.1056/NEJMms2009984

2. Kittleson MM. The invisible hand — medical care during the pandemic. *N Engl J Med.* (2020) 382:1586–7. doi: 10.1056/NEJMp2006607

3. Dubey S, Biswas P, Ghosh R, Chatterjee S, Dubey MJ, Chatterjee S, et al. Psychosocial impact of COVID-19. *Diabetes Metab Syndr Clin Res Rev.* (2020) 14:779–88. doi: 10.1016/j.dsx.2020.05.035

4. Pessoa-Amorim G, Camm CF, Gajendragadkar P, De Maria GL, Arsac C, Laroche C, et al. Admission of patients with STEMI since the outbreak of the COVID-19 pandemic: a survey by the European society of cardiology. *Eur Hear J Qual Care Clin Outcomes.* (2020) 6:210–6. doi: 10.1093/ehjqcco/qcaa046

5. Ahmed T, Lodhi SH, Kapadia S, Shah G V. Community and healthcare system-related factors feeding the phenomenon of evading medical attention for time-dependent emergencies during COVID-19 crisis. *BMJ Case Rep.* (2020) 13:e237817. doi: 10.1136/bcr-2020-237817

6. Ibanez B, James S, Agewall S, Antunes MJ, Bucciarelli-Ducci C, Bueno H, et al. 2017 ESC guidelines for the management of acute myocardial infarction in patients presenting with ST-segment elevation. *Eur Heart J.* (2018) 39:119–77. doi: 10.1093/eurheartj/ehx393

7. Xiang D, Xiang X, Zhang W, Yi S, Zhang J, Gu X, et al. Management and outcomes of patients with STEMI during the COVID-19 pandemic in China. *J Am Coll Cardiol.* (2020) 76:1318–24. doi: 10.1016/j.jacc.2020.06.039

8. De Rosa S, Spaccarotella C, Basso C, Calabrò MP, Curcio A, Filardi PP, et al. Reduction of hospitalizations for myocardial infarction in Italy in the COVID-19 era. *Eur Heart J.* (2020) 41:2083–8. doi: 10.1093/eurheartj/ehaa409

9. Rattka M, Baumhardt M, Dreyhaupt J, Rothenbacher D, Thiessen K, Markovic S, et al. 31 days of COVID-19-cardiac events during restriction of public life-a comparative study. *Clin Res Cardiol.* (2020) 109:1476–82. doi: 10.2139/ssrn.3594561

10. Claeys MJ, Argacha J-F, Collart P, Carlier M, Van Caenegem O, Sinnaeve PR, et al. Impact of COVID-19-related public containment measures on the ST elevation myocardial infarction epidemic in Belgium: a nationwide, serial, cross-sectional study. *Acta Cardiol.* (2020). doi: 10.1080/00015385.2020.1796035. [Epub ahead of print].

11. Gramegna M, Baldetti L, Beneduce A, Pannone L, Falasconi G, Calvo F, et al. ST-segment–elevation myocardial infarction during COVID-19 pandemic. *Circ Cardiovasc Interv.* (2020) 13:e009413. doi: 10.1161/CIRCINTERVENTIONS.120.009413

12. Von Elm E, Altman DG, Egger M, Pocock SJ, Gøtzsche PC, Vandenbroucke JP. STROBE initiative. The strengthening the reporting of observational studies in epidemiology (STROBE) statement: guidelines for reporting observational studies. *Lancet.* (2007) 370:1453–7. doi: 10.1016/S0140-6736(07)61602-X

13. Taylor S, Landry CA, Paluszek MM, Fergus TA, McKay D, Asmundson GJG. Development and initial validation of the COVID stress scales. *J Anxiety Disord.* (2020) 72:102232. doi: 10.1016/j.janxdis.2020.102232

14. Ahorsu DK, Lin C-Y, Imani V, Saffari M, Griffiths MD, Pakpour AH. The fear of COVID-19 scale: development and initial validation. *Int J Ment Health Addict.* (2020). doi: 10.1007/s11469-020-00270-8. [Epub ahead of print].

15. Hammad TA, Parikh M, Tashtish N, Lowry CM, Gorbey D, Forouzandeh F, et al. Impact of COVID-19 pandemic on ST-elevation myocardial infarction in a non-COVID-19 epicenter. *Catheter Card Interv.* (2021) 97:208–14. doi: 10.1002/ccd.28997

16. Masroor S. Collateral damage of COVID-19 pandemic: delayed medical care. *J Card Surg.* (2020) 35:1345–7. doi: 10.1111/jocs.14638

17. Rebollal-Leal F, Aldama-López G, Flores-Ríos X, Piñón-Esteban P, Salgado-Fernández J, Calviño-Santos R, et al. Impact of COVID-19 outbreak and public lockdown on ST-segment elevation myocardial infarction care in Spain. *Cardiol J.* (2020) 27:425–6. doi: 10.5603/CJ.a2020.0098

18. Kwok CS, Gale CP, Kinnaird T, Curzen N, Ludman P, Kontopantelis E, et al. Impact of COVID-19 on percutaneous coronary intervention for ST-elevation myocardial infarction. *Heart.* (2020) 106:1805–11. doi: 10.1136/heartjnl-2020-317650

19. Oikonomou E, Aznaouridis K, Barbetseas J, Charalambous G, Gastouniotis I, Fotopoulos V, et al. Hospital attendance and admission trends for cardiac diseases during the COVID-19 outbreak and lockdown in Greece. *Public Health.* (2020) 187:115–9. doi: 10.1016/j.puhe.2020.08.007

20. Wu J, Mamas M, Rashid M, Weston C, Hains J, Luescher T, et al. Patient response, treatments and mortality for acute myocardial infarction during the COVID-19 pandemic. *Eur Hear J Qual Care Clin Outcomes.* (2020) 53:1689–99. doi: 10.1093/ehjqcco/qcaa062

21. Thiele H, Kappl MJ, Linke A, Erbs S, Boudriot E, Lembcke A, et al. Influence of time-to-treatment, TIMI-flow grades, and ST-segment resolution on infarct size and infarct transmurality as assessed by delayed enhancement magnetic resonance imaging. *Eur Heart J.* (2006) 28:1433–9. doi: 10.1093/eurheartj/ehm173

22. Han Y. A treatment strategy for acute myocardial infarction and personal protection for medical staff during the COVID-19 epidemic: the Chinese experience. *Eur Heart J.* (2020) 41:2148–9. doi: 10.1093/eurheartj/ehaa358

12

Myocardial Work Efficiency, a Novel Measure of Myocardial Dysfunction, is Reduced in COVID-19 Patients and Associated with In-Hospital Mortality

Anum S. Minhas[1†], Nisha A. Gilotra[1†], Erin Goerlich[1], Thomas Metkus[1], Brian T. Garibaldi[2], Garima Sharma[1], Nicole Bavaro[1], Susan Phillip[1], Erin D. Michos[1] and Allison G. Hays[1*]

[1] Division of Cardiology, Department of Medicine, Johns Hopkins University School of Medicine, Baltimore, MD, United States, [2] Division of Pulmonary and Critical Care Medicine, Department of Medicine, Johns Hopkins University School of Medicine, Baltimore, MD, United States

*Correspondence:
Allison G. Hays
ahays2@jhmi.edu

[†] These authors have contributed equally to this work

Background: Although troponin elevation is common in COVID-19, the extent of myocardial dysfunction and its contributors to dysfunction are less well-characterized. We aimed to determine the prevalence of subclinical myocardial dysfunction and its association with mortality using speckle tracking echocardiography (STE), specifically global longitudinal strain (GLS) and myocardial work efficiency (MWE). We also tested the hypothesis that reduced myocardial function was associated with increased systemic inflammation in COVID-19.

Methods and Results: We conducted a retrospective study of hospitalized COVID-19 patients undergoing echocardiography ($n = 136$), of whom 83 and 75 had GLS (abnormal $>-16\%$) and MWE (abnormal $<95\%$) assessed, respectively. We performed adjusted logistic regression to examine associations of GLS and MWE with in-hospital mortality. Patients were mean 62 ± 14 years old (58% men). While 81% had normal left ventricular ejection fraction (LVEF), prevalence of myocardial dysfunction was high by STE; [39/83 (47%) had abnormal GLS; 59/75 (79%) had abnormal MWE]. Higher MWE was associated with lower in-hospital mortality in unadjusted [OR 0.92 (95% CI 0.85–0.99); $p = 0.048$] and adjusted models [aOR 0.87 (95% CI 0.78–0.97); $p = 0.009$]. In addition, increased systemic inflammation measured by interleukin-6 level was associated with reduced MWE.

Conclusions: Subclinical myocardial dysfunction is common in COVID-19 patients with clinical echocardiograms, even in those with normal LVEF. Reduced MWE is associated with higher interleukin-6 levels and increased in-hospital mortality. Non-invasive STE represents a readily available method to rapidly evaluate myocardial dysfunction in COVID-19 patients and can play an important role in risk stratification.

Keywords: echo, strain, COVID-19, non-invasive, ultrasoud diagnosis

INTRODUCTION

COVID-19, the disease caused by the novel coronavirus SARS-CoV2, carries high acute cardiovascular morbidity and mortality (1, 2). The mechanisms for cardiac injury are not fully understood, with hypotheses ranging from systemic inflammation due to cytokine release syndrome, angiotensin converting enzyme-2 mediated direct viral myocardial toxicity, autoimmune myocarditis, and sympathetic stress response (1, 3). Over 25% of hospitalized COVID-19 patients have acute cardiac injury as detected by elevated cardiac troponin, associated with greater in-hospital mortality (1, 3, 4). However, troponin alone has limited specificity and sensitivity in myocarditis and can also rise in acute respiratory distress syndrome (ARDS), another recognized complication of COVID-19 (5–7). Additionally, although multiple inflammatory pathways, such as interleukin-6 (IL-6), are implicated in myocardial injury in COVID-19, their effect on indices of cardiac function is unknown and a better understanding of the degree and determinants of myocardial function may improve risk stratification and lead to new therapeutic approaches (8–10).

Studies examining the degree of myocardial dysfunction in COVID-19 are limited, and assessment with cardiac imaging has been challenging due to exposure concerns to echocardiography staff. Thus, it is likely that the true prevalence of cardiac dysfunction is underreported (11). Speckle tracking echocardiography (STE) can rapidly quantify myocardial dysfunction (e.g., using global longitudinal strain [GLS]) with increased sensitivity compared with standard echocardiographic measures (12–14). More recently, a novel technique to measure LV function based on STE, global myocardial work (MW), was developed (15, 16). The advantage of MW [assessed by myocardial work index (MWI) and myocardial work efficiency (MWE)], is that it provides a more load independent measure of LV function by accounting for afterload; MW is also highly reproducible and adds incremental value to GLS in predicting adverse events (17).

Given the high mortality and severity of complications with COVID-19, we conducted a clinical cardiac imaging study in hospitalized COVID-19 patients with echocardiograms performed with the following aims: (1) to determine the prevalence and extent of myocardial dysfunction using STE (GLS and MWE), (2) to examine the association of myocardial dysfunction with in-hospital mortality, and (3) to investigate clinical and inflammatory biomarker risk factors associated with worsened subclinical myocardial dysfunction.

Abbreviations: COVID-19, SARS-CoV2; ARDS, acute respiratory distress syndrome; GLS, global longitudinal strain; MW, myocardial work; MWI, myocardial work index; MWE, myocardial work efficiency; LV, left ventricular; RV, right ventricular; EF, ejection fraction; LVEDD, left ventricular end diastolic diameter; RVEDD, right ventricular end diastolic diameter; TAPSE, tricuspid annular plane systolic excursion; TR, tricuspid regurgitation; STE, speckle tracking echocardiography; ASE, American Society of Echocardiography; BMI, body mass index; CRP, C-reactive protein; IL-6, interleukin 6; Pro-BNP, N-terminal pro-hormone B-type natriuretic peptide.

METHODS

Study Design

This retrospective, single-center cohort study included 136 consecutive patients with confirmed COVID-19 who were hospitalized at Johns Hopkins Hospital and underwent clinically indicated transthoracic echocardiogram between March 25, 2020 and May 19, 2020, with follow-up completed by June 22, 2020. All echocardiograms were ordered by the patient's clinical care team. The study was approved by the Johns Hopkins Institutional Review Board and informed consent was waived per IRB guidelines.

Clinical Data

Patient characteristics, including demographics, medical history, clinical presentation, laboratory testing, and clinical outcomes were extracted from the electronic medical record. Initial values after admission for the following serum biomarkers were collected: cardiac troponin I, IL-6, C-reactive protein (CRP), ferritin, fibrinogen, and d-dimer. In- hospital all-cause mortality during index hospitalization was ascertained from electronic medical records through the end of follow-up. Two separate investigators independently reviewed the data.

Transthoracic Echocardiography
Conventional 2D Echocardiographic Analysis

Bedside transthoracic echocardiographic (TTE) examinations were performed by experienced sonographers using Vivid™ E95 ultrasound system (GE Vingmed Ultrasound; Horten, Norway). Both standard 2D and Doppler echocardiography were acquired. Measurements including LV, right ventricular (RV) parameters and diastology were performed by a dedicated research sonographer based on the American Society of Echocardiography (ASE) guidelines (18, 19). To limit exposure to patients and staff, measurements that were not essential, including STE analyses, were performed offline, removed from the patient's room, and limited studies were performed according to COVID-19 specific imaging guidelines (20).

Speckle Tracking Echocardiography Analysis

STE analyses were conducted according to ASE recommendations in a subset of TTEs that were (1) deemed to be of fair quality or greater for subendocardial image visualization by two independent readers and (2) in a patient free of atrial or ventricular arrhythmias at the time of exam ($n = 83$) (18). Two-dimensional images from the apical four-chamber, two-chamber, and long-axis views were acquired with frame rates between 50 and 80 frames/s to enable GLS. GLS was quantified using semiautomated analysis software (EchoPAC version 202; GE Vingmed Ultrasound). The automated algorithm traces and tracks the LV myocardium, with manual adjustments made when appropriate, and the software calculates GLS from the weighted average of the peak systolic longitudinal strain of all segments using the 17 segment model. GLS is quantified as a negative number with cutoff as −18%, and more negative as normal for this system, but based on prior literature supporting use of a cutoff of −16% as the threshold for normal, analyses were conducted with > −16% as the cutoff for normal (21–25). Tracking quality was assessed by the operator and over-ridden in segments with two or fewer rejected regions where the operator deemed tracking quality to be acceptable. Images were analyzed by two independent observers blinded to clinical data on a dedicated offline research workstation. Intraobserver and interobserver variability of STE measures, specifically MWE, were assessed by intra- class correlation coefficient (individual ICC of 0.994 and average ICC of 0.997 for intraobserver and 0.992 and 0.995 for interobserver, respectively), and Bland-Altman analysis (all differences in measurements within ±1 SD). The time between intraobserver measurements was 1 day.

Myocardial Work

Myocardial work (MW) was determined from non-invasive LV pressure-strain analysis, which has previously been described and validated (26, 27). MW is calculated as the area of the pressure-strain loop, similar in concept to deriving LV stroke work using pressure volume loops invasively. In this technique, pressures are assessed using brachial systolic pressure and valvular event timing and strain measured with STE (15, 16). MW indices were calculated with the same software as above to evaluate LV performance by incorporating afterload determination using blood pressure; this provides a more load-independent measure compared with GLS (27). Blood pressure was measured by sphygmomanometry at the time of the

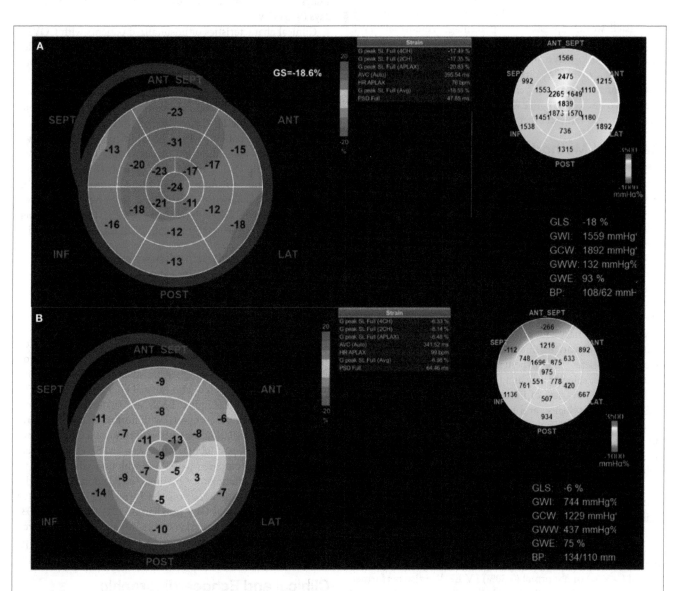

FIGURE 1 | Global longitudinal strain and myocardial work efficiency measurement in patients with COVID-19. Global longitudinal strain and myocardial work index bull's eye mapping for two patients with COVID-19. **(A)** representative patient with relatively normal strain and myocardial work; **(B)** representative patient with severely reduced global longitudinal strain (apical predominant), myocardial work index, and work efficiency. ANT, anterior; ANT SEPT, anterospetal; APLAX, apical long axis; AVC, aortic valve closure; CH, chamber; GS, global strain; HR, heart rate; INF, inferior; LAT, lateral; POST, posterior; PSD, peak systolic dispersion; SEPT, septal; SL, strain length.

echocardiogram immediately before acquiring images for STE. The MW software then constructs a non-invasive LV pressure curve adjusted according to the duration of isovolumic and ejection phases defined by the timing of aortic and mitral valve opening and closing events (28). Global MW was quantified by calculating the rate of regional shortening by differentiation of the strain tracing and multiplying by instantaneous LV pressure (estimated) integrated over time. During LV ejection time, segments were analyzed for wasted work and constructive work, with global values determined as the averages of all segmental values (see example **Figure 1**). The following parameters were acquired using EchoPAC software: Global MW index (MWI, mmHg%) defined as the area within the global LV pressure-strain loop and global MW efficiency (MWE, %), defined as constructive MW divided by the sum of constructed work and wasted work, expressed as a percentage. Abnormal MWE was defined as <95%, consistent with other studies (16). For myocardial work, MWE was chosen as the primary variable of interest as it provides a comprehensive assessment of the ratio between constructive work performed by the LV and the sum of both wasted and constructive work, and has previously shown to have prognostic value in other populations (29–31).

Statistical Methods

Descriptive statistical analyses were performed for clinical and echocardiographic parameters. Continuous variables are presented as mean ± standard deviation (normally distributed variables) or median (IQR) (non-normally distributed variables). Differences between groups were compared using parametric two-sample Student's t-test or non-parametric Mann–Whitney U-test. Categorical variables are presented as number (%) and groups compared using Chi-squared test. For relevant analyses, normal LVEF was defined as >50%.

We then performed unadjusted and adjusted logistic regression to estimate the odds of mortality with either GLS or MWE as the primary independent variable of interest, analyzed continuously. Covariates included were clinical characteristics (age, sex, diabetes, and hypertension) and echocardiographic measurements, selected one at a time for addition to the model as the primary covariate of interest (LVEF, GLS, MWE, TAPSE, RVSP, TR peak velocity, and E/E'). Clinical covariates selected for inclusion in the adjusted models were chosen based on prior literature suggesting possible confounding, and included age, sex, history of hypertension, and diabetes (32–36). Model 1 included the echocardiographic covariate of interest, adjusted for age and sex. Model 2 included the echocardiographic covariate of interest, adjusted for age, sex, diabetes, and hypertension. All variables for logistic regression were analyzed as continuous variables.

To further understand the incremental value of STE analysis over standard echocardiographic LVEF assessment for mortality prediction, we performed subgroup analyses in patients with normal (>50%) or abnormal (<50%) LV EF. We also performed subgroup analyses in patients with the presence or absence of acute respiratory distress syndrome (ARDS). A $p \leq 0.05$ was considered significant.

Last, for a subset of the cohort, linear regression was then performed to evaluate inflammatory markers (divided into

tertiles given non-normal distribution) as predictors of MWE. Values within each tertile are included in the supplement. These markers included IL6, troponin, ferritin, C-reactive protein (CRP), d-dimer, and fibrinogen. Missing data were considered to occur at random, and patients with missing inflammatory data were not included in this analysis.

RESULTS

Clinical Characteristics of Patients Undergoing Echocardiogram

Median time of symptom duration prior to admission was 6 days (3–8 days). Median time to echocardiogram after admission was 4 days (2–8 days) and median overall time of admission was 16.5 days (9–31 days).

Clinical characteristics of hospitalized patients with COVID-19 who had echocardiogram performed are shown in **Table 1** ($n = 136$). The mean age was 62 years, 79 (58%) were men and 63 (47%) African American. Approximately 63% of patients required mechanical ventilation, 57% were diagnosed with ARDS and 53% had shock (septic, distributive, cardiogenic or otherwise) (**Table 1**).

The cohort of patients with echocardiograms performed was comparable to the subset of patients with GLS and MWE measured (**Table 1**). The majority of patients (81%) undergoing echocardiogram had normal LV systolic function by LVEF measurement. Follow-up (discharged as alive or deceased) was complete for 131/136 patients, while 5/136 (3.7%) were administratively censored (still admitted at the time of analysis).

Clinical and Echocardiographic Characteristics for Patients With Global Longitudinal Strain Assessed

Among the patients with GLS performed ($n = 83$), 44 patients had normal GLS and 39 (47%) had abnormal GLS (**Table 1**). There were no significant differences in age, sex, race, or history of hypertension or CAD between patients with and without abnormal GLS. There was higher prevalence of diabetes mellitus in the abnormal compared with normal GLS group (51 vs. 27%, $p = 0.025$). Body mass index (BMI) was significantly higher in patients with abnormal compared with normal GLS (median 31.4 vs. 27.8 kg/m², $p = 0.017$). Patients with abnormal GLS had lower LVEF (55 vs. 62%, $p < 0.001$), and lower TAPSE (1.7 vs. 2.0 cm, $p = 0.005$) when compared with those with normal GLS.

Among the inflammatory markers, interleukin-6 was higher among patients with abnormal GLS [median 164 (69–815)] compared with normal GLS [median 86 (32–167)], $p = 0.034$. All other inflammatory markers were not significantly different (**Table 1**). The value ranges of each inflammatory marker per tertile are presented in **Supplementary Table 1**.

Clinical and Echocardiographic Characteristics for Patients With Myocardial Work Efficiency Assessed

Among the subgroup of patients with myocardial work imaging performed ($N = 75$), abnormal MWE (defined as <95%) was

TABLE 1 | Comparison of clinical characteristics and echocardiographic parameters in the cohort of hospitalized patients with COVID-19 and subgroups with normal vs. abnormal global longitudinal strain (GLS) and myocardial work efficiency (MWE).

Variables	Overall cohort $N = 136$	Normal GLS $N = 44$	Abnormal GLS $N = 39$	p-value	Normal MWE $N = 16$	Abnormal MWE $N = 59$	p-value
Age, years	62.4 ± 13.9	61.9 ± 13.4	63.4 ± 14.4	0.614	55.2 ± 16.5	64.3 ± 13.1	**0.023**
Male	79 (58%)	27 (61%)	22 (56%)	0.647	13 (81%)	32 (53%)	**0.039**
Race				0.347			0.082
White	34 (25%)	10 (23%)	5 (13%)		3 (19%)	12 (21%)	
African American	63 (47%)	20 (45%)	23 (61%)		5 (31%)	33 (57%)	
Other	37 (27%)	14 (32%)	10 (26%)		8 (50%)	13 (22%)	
Body mass index, kg/m^2	30.0 (26.4–35.8)	27.8 (25.6–31.3)	31.4 (26.5–38.4)	**0.017**	27.7 (25.7–31.8)	28.7 (25.7–34.5)	0.544
Comorbidities							
Hypertension	97 (72%)	29 (66%)	30 (77%)	0.269	7 (44%)	46 (78%)	**0.008**
Diabetes mellitus	55 (41%)	12 (27%)	20 (51%)	**0.025**	1 (6%)	29 (49%)	**0.002**
Coronary artery disease	20 (15%)	4 (9%)	8 (21%)	0.140	0 (0%)	10 (17%)	0.077
Heart failure	20 (15%)	2 (5%)	12 (31%)	**0.001**	0 (0%)	12 (20%)	**0.049**
Clinical presentation							
Heart rate, beats per min	99 ± 20	97 ± 17	103 ± 21	0.151	95 ± 18	100 ± 20	0.392
Systolic blood pressure, mmHg	129 ± 25	129 ± 24	134 ± 24	0.368	126 ± 27	132 ± 23	0.343
Diastolic blood pressure, mmHg	71 ± 16	71 ± 16	74 ± 15	0.389	74 ± 16	71 ± 16	0.546
Laboratory measurements							
White blood cell count, K/cu mm	6.7 (5.0–9.3)	6.4 (4.6–8.7)	6.0 (4.8–8.3)	0.773	6.4 (4.8–9.0)	6.4 (4.8–9.1)	0.946
Absolute lymphocyte count, K/cu mm	0.6 (0.1–1.1)	0.6 (0.1–1.0)	0.5 (0.0–1.3)	0.794	0.7 (0.0–1.2)	0.7 (0.03–1.2)	0.992
D-dimer, mg/L	2.0 (0.8–5.3)	2.0 (0.8–4.6)	2.2 (0.9–7.3)	0.433	2.0 (0.4–4.7)	2.2 (0.9–4.5)	0.213
Interleukin-6, pg/ml	130 (51–409)	86 (32–167)	164 (69–815)	**0.034**	114 (47–422)	125 (45–406)	0.695
CRP, mg/dl	15.3 (4.9–34.7)	11.7 (3.3–20.5)	13.7 (5.1–37.7)	0.410	4.9 (2.3–15.3)	15 (6.6–34.3)	**0.009**
Ferritin, ng/ml	735 (395–1,424)	737 (427–1,130)	800 (402–2,898)	0.525	830 (289–1,677)	719 (412–1,125)	0.897
Fibrinogen, mg/dl	596 (445–703)	737 (427–1,130)	800 (402–2,898)	0.695	568 (463–729)	597 (457–722)	0.694
Pro-BNP, pg/ml	422 (157–1,956)	242 (99–589)	564 (164–3,992)	**0.044**	176 (70–385)	392 (164–2,611)	**0.032**
Troponin I, ng/ml	0.03 (0.03–0.05)	0.03 (0.03–0.03)	0.03 (0.03–0.08)	0.454	0.03 (0.03–0.03)	0.03 (0.03–0.05)	0.305
Clinical events							
Shock	72 (53%)	17 (39%)	23 (59%)	0.064	4 (25%)	30 (51%)	0.065
Mechanical ventilation	86 (63%)	22 (50%)	26 (67%)	0.125	5 (31%)	38 (64%)	**0.017**
ARDS	78 (57%)	19 (43%)	25 (64%)	0.057	5 (31%)	32 (54%)	0.103
DVT or PE	31 (23%)	8 (18%)	8 (21%)	0.788	3 (19%)	12 (20%)	0.888
Death	25 (19%)	7 (16%)	8 (21%)	0.620	2 (12%)	9 (16%)	0.764
Echocardiographic parameters							
LA volume, ml	44 (35–71)	41 (29–45)	48 (39–95)	**0.046**	39.5 (28–42)	47 (39–55)	0.222
LVEDD, cm	4.2 (3.7–4.8)	4.1 (3.8–4.6)	4.3 (3.4–4.9)	0.378	4.4 (3.8–4.9)	4.1 (3.5–4.7)	0.276
LVEF, %	62 (52–62)	62 (57–64)	55 (40–62)	<0.001	62 (62–64)	57 (50–62)	**0.011**
Normal LVEF (>50%)	109 (81%)	43 (64%)	24 (36%)	<0.001	16 (100%)	45 (74%)	**0.031**
RVEDD, cm	3.6 ± 0.7	3.4 ± 0.6	3.6 ± 0.7	0.224	3.4 ± 0.7	3.6 ± 0.6	0.225
Normal RV function	63 (81%)	22 (85%)	18 (72%)	0.274	12 (92%)	24 (73%)	0.147
TAPSE, cm	1.8 ± 0.4	2.0 ± 0.4	1.7 ± 0.4	**0.005**	2.1 ± 0.3	1.8 ± 0.4	**0.003**
RVSP, mmHg	37 (30–50)	37 (29–48)	34 (32–53)	0.742	31 (30–33)	37 (29–49)	0.288
Mean PAP, mmHg	34 ± 12	35 ± 9	34 ± 11	0.754	27 ± 12	35 ± 9	0.087
Peak TR gradient, mmHg	31 (25–42)	32 (25–42)	31 (25–40)	0.899	29 (25–38)	31 (24–43)	0.832
PCWP, mmHg	14 (10–18)	13 (9–17)	12 (9–16)	0.820	12 (10–16)	15 (12–21)	0.422
E/E'	10 (8–13)	10 (7–12)	9 (7–13)	0.665	9 (7–11)	9 (7–13)	0.561
GLS, %	−16.1 ± 4.3	−19.2 ± 2.4	−12.6 ± 3.0	<0.001	−19.7 ± 3.1	−15.5 ± 4.1	<0.001
MWI, mmHg%	1,412 ± 425	1,579 ± 362	1,227 ± 417	<0.001	1,723 ± 399	1,331 ± 396	<0.001
MWE, %	92 (87–94)	94 (91–95)	89 (82–92)	<0.001	96 (95–96)	91 (86–93)	<0.001

Categorical variables are presented as number (%) and continuous variables are presented as mean ± standard deviation or median (interquartile range).
CRP, C-reactive protein; Pro-BNP, N-terminal pro-hormone B-type natriuretic peptide; ARDS, acute respiratory distress syndrome; DVT, deep venous thrombosis; PE, pulmonary embolism; LA, left atrium; LVEDD, left ventricular end diastolic diameter; LVEF, left ventricular ejection fraction; GLS, global longitudinal strain; RVEDD, right ventricular end diastolic diameter; TAPSE, tricuspid annular plane systolic excursion; RVSP, right ventricular systolic pressure; PAP, pulmonary artery pressure; TR, tricuspid regurgitation; GLS, global longitudinal strain; MWI, myocardial work index; MWE, myocardial work efficiency.
The bold values represent significant p-values, with significant defined as <0.05.

present in the majority (59/75, 79%). There were no significant differences in demographics or clinical presentation between patients with normal vs. abnormal MWE (**Table 1**). A history of hypertension was more common among patients with abnormal MWE compared with normal MWE (78 vs. 44%, $p = 0.008$), as was a prior history of diabetes (29 vs. 1%, $p = 0.002$). Patients with abnormal MWE compared with those with normal MWE had lower LVEF (57 vs. 62%, $p = 0.011$), and lower TAPSE (1.8 vs. 2.1 cm, $p = 0.003$).

Among patients with normal LVEF ($n = 67$), a high percentage had evidence of subclinical myocardial dysfunction using STE: 36% had abnormal GLS (GLS>−16%) and 74% had abnormal MWE (MWE <95%) (**Figure 2**).

Association of Clinical Characteristics and Speckle Tracking Echocardiography Measurements With Mortality

During hospital admission, 25 (19%) of patients experienced in-hospital death. No clinical characteristics were independently associated with mortality in univariate analysis. MWE was the only echocardiographic parameter independently associated with mortality [unadjusted OR 0.92 (95% CI 0.85–0.999), $p = 0.048$]. In adjusted Models 1–2, MWE remained associated with mortality, with the strongest association in Model 2 [OR 0.87 (95% CI 0.78–0.97), $p = 0.009$] (**Table 2**), suggesting that a 1% increase in MWE was associated with 13% lower odds of death.

Additional subgroup analyses performed to confirm the relationship of MWE and mortality showed similar findings. Among patients with normal LVEF, higher MWE was again independently inversely associated with death [unadjusted OR 0.89 (95% CI 0.78–1.00), $p = 0.050$]. MWE was also associated with in-hospital death after adjusting for age and sex [aOR 0.85 (95% CI 0.74–0.99), $p = 0.038$]. GLS was not associated with death in adjusted or unadjusted analysis. No echocardiographic parameter (LVEF, GLS, or MWE) was associated with mortality in subgroup analyses of patients with and without ARDS (**Supplementary Table 2**).

As MWE was the only echocardiographic parameter associated with mortality, we then evaluated systemic inflammatory markers as predictors of abnormal MWE in a subset of patients with available inflammatory marker data. We observed that MWE was 2.04% lower per higher tertile of IL-6 level ($p = 0.021$), indicating that greater degree of inflammation reflected by IL-6 levels were associated with worse myocardial function as measured using MWE. All other inflammatory markers tested were associated with no difference in MWE (**Figure 3**).

DISCUSSION

We report that subclinical cardiac dysfunction measured by GLS and MWE on STE is common in hospitalized COVID-19 patients with clinically indicated echocardiograms performed. To our knowledge, this is one of the first reports characterizing novel echocardiographic indices of myocardial dysfunction (GLS and the newer imaging parameter MWE)

in hospitalized patients with COVID-19. We report several unique findings in our population: (1) Subclinical myocardial dysfunction is prevalent among COVID-19 patients even in the setting of normal LVEF, especially in those with traditional cardiovascular risk factors, (2) lower, more abnormal MWE, which is a sensitive measure of load independent myocardial dysfunction, is associated with greater in-hospital mortality, and (3) higher level of the inflammatory marker, IL-6, is predictive of lower MWE. Importantly, the finding of the association of MWE with mortality held true even after analyzing patients with normal LVEF, suggesting the prognostic benefit of MWE over LVEF and supporting use of MWE in addition to LVEF for hospitalized patients with COVID-19.

Speckle Tracking Echocardiography for the Detection of Subclinical Myocardial Dysfunction in COVID-19 Patients

Both GLS and MWE are sensitive measures of LV function and cardiac injury, and the current study is among the first to characterize these indices in the setting of acute COVID-19 (37, 38). Compared with LVEF, GLS improves risk stratification, enhances disease classification, and may guide the treatment approach in asymptomatic patients with subclinical LV dysfunction (14, 38). Both GLS and MWE measurements are validated, reproducible, and do not require additional imaging beyond standard TTE, reducing potential additional provider exposure during image acquisition. Prior studies have consistently demonstrated reduced GLS despite a preserved LVEF among patients at increased risk for cardiac injury and dysfunction (39). MWE is a newer load-independent measure that permits both global and regional ventricular mechanics to be analyzed through the relationship between myocardial contractility and LV pressure (15). A previous study showed that non-invasive indices of myocardial work are more sensitive than GLS for the detection of significant CAD in patients with normal regional wall motion and preserved LVEF (17). The present study supports these prior findings, as abnormal MWE was even more prevalent than abnormal GLS (79 vs. 46% of patients). Additionally, patients with abnormal STE indices were more likely to have cardiovascular risk factors than those with normal indices, even among those with normal LVEF.

Myocardial Work Efficiency and Mortality

While recent data has suggested high incidence of acute cardiac injury by troponin levels in COVID-19, investigations into the extent and implications of myocardial dysfunction on adverse outcomes such as death are limited (1, 7, 13, 40–42). In the present study, in a cohort with comparable in-hospital mortality to prior studies in COVID-19, we demonstrate the ability of MWE to predict mortality while GLS and LVEF did not. Prior studies suggest that the amount of myocardial work is related to uptake of fluro-deoxy-glucose at myocardial positron emission tomography scan, suggesting a relationship between myocardial work efficiency and metabolism (27). It is possible that impaired

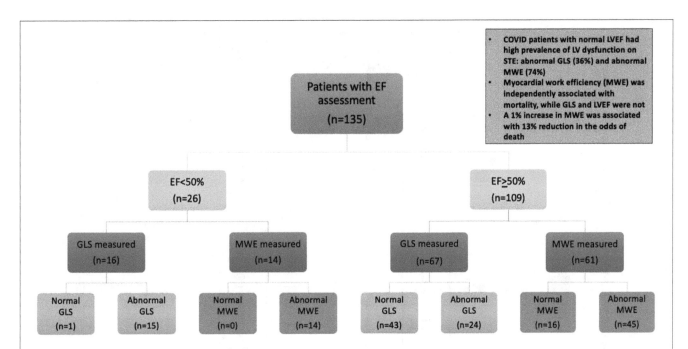

FIGURE 2 | Echocardiogram evaluation and main findings in hospitalized patients with COVID-19. Flow diagram of the study shows number of patients undergoing echocardiogram, including with speckle tracking technique for strain measures. GLS, global longitudinal strain; LVEF, left ventricular ejection fraction; MWE, myocardial work efficiency. Abnormal GLS is defined as ≤16% (the absolute value of −16%). Additional abbreviations in **Figure 1**.

TABLE 2 | Association of each echocardiographic parameter with mortality in hospitalized patients with COVID-19.

	Unadjusted	Model 1 (age and sex) odds ratio (95% CI)	Model 2 (age, sex, diabetes, hypertension) odds ratio (95% CI)
LVEF	1.00 (0.96–1.03) P = 0.248	1.00 (0.96–1.04) P = 0.934	1.00 (0.96–1.04) P = 0.918
GLS	1.07 (0.94–1.22) P = 0.287	1.08 (0.94–1.23) P = 0.287	1.15 (0.98–1.35) P = 0.089
MWE	0.92 (0.85–0.999) **P = 0.048**	0.90 (0.81–0.98) **P = 0.021**	0.87 (0.78–0.97) **P = 0.009**
TAPSE	0.43 (0.11–1.71) P = 0.230	0.41 (0.10–1.74) P = 0.228	0.30 (0.06–1.45) P = 0.135
RVSP	1.04 (1.00–1.09) P = 0.051	1.04 (1.00–1.09) P = 0.073	1.04 (1.0–1.09) P = 0.081
TR peak velocity	1.03 (0.99–1.07) P = 0.182	1.03 (0.98–1.07) P = 0.219	1.03 (0.98–1.07) P = 0.235
E/E'	0.97 (0.91–1.05) P = 0.459	0.96 (0.87–1.06) P = 0.392	0.97 (0.90–1.05) P = 0.498

The bold values represent significant p-values, with significant defined as <0.05.

MWE may be related to derangements in myocardial metabolism that can occur in the setting of increased systemic inflammation.

Based on these findings, it is possible that STE measures of subclinical LV dysfunction may provide incremental value to standard echo measures in patients with COVID-19. Given the acuity of presentation and cardiovascular complications of COVID-19, a better understanding of the extent of myocardial injury and dysfunction early in the disease course may help triage at risk patients and implement early interventions aimed at reducing mortality.

Systemic Inflammation and Cardiac Dysfunction

Although recent studies have aimed to describe pathophysiologic processes leading to RV strain and dilation in acute COVID-19 (43, 44), LV dysfunction and particularly subclinical dysfunction on STE, have not been as well-investigated. Studies suggest that increased systemic inflammation and impaired immune function may play a role (6, 7). Potential causes of myocardial dysfunction include myocarditis, ischemic injury (caused by microvascular dysfunction or epicardial CAD), stress cardiomyopathy or

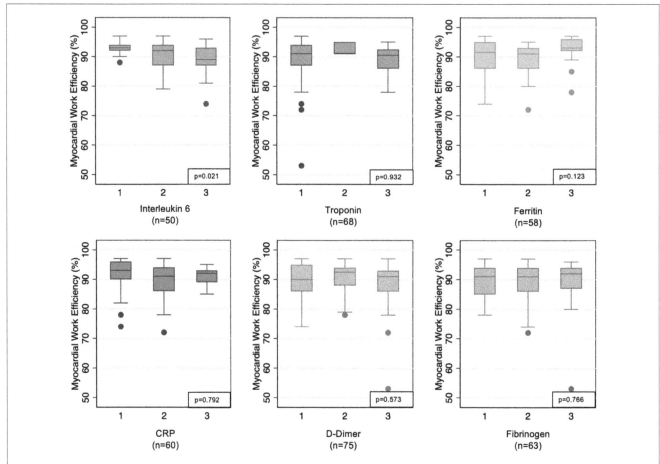

FIGURE 3 | Association of myocardial work efficiency with inflammatory markers. Inflammatory markers are analyzed by tertile of each marker given non-normal distribution.

cytokine release syndrome (45). Autopsy studies of severe COVID-19 disease suggest there can also be direct viral-induced injury of multiple organs, including the heart (46). However, the relative contribution and determinants of myocardial dysfunction have not been well-characterized, partially due to limited ability to obtain widespread cardiac testing in these patients. Given these limitations, the true prevalence of cardiac dysfunction has likely been underreported thus far, and is mainly limited to case reports (6, 7).

In our study, patients underwent echocardiography at a median 4 days after hospital admission and 6 days of symptom onset, suggesting that impaired GLS and MWE occur early in COVID-19 during the systemic inflammatory response, and cannot entirely be explained by a more chronic myocardial process such as fibrosis. In addition, COVID-19 patients with LV dysfunction on STE had more obesity, which is a pro-inflammatory state that initiates oxidative stress and adversely affects immune function, leading to cardiac injury (40, 47, 48). Finally, although inflammatory pathways have been implicated in myocardial injury related to COVID-19, their effect on important indices of cardiac function has not been well-characterized. In the present study, we show that subclinical myocardial dysfunction is related to the degree of systemic inflammation measured by IL-6. IL-6 has previously been shown to act as a key cytokine

in producing downstream effects resulting in organ damage, including reduced myocardial contractility (49–51).

Additionally, IL-6 levels in the setting of COVID-19 have been reported to be elevated in several studies and have been shown to correlate with mortality (52–54). Our study, along with these prior studies, supports a potential role of IL-6 and heightened inflammation in mediating myocardial dysfunction, thereby increasing risk of death. Of note, we did not find a similar relationship with troponin and myocardial dysfunction, likely related to the primarily normal-range troponin values for the majority of patients.

By characterizing subclinical myocardial dysfunction using STE, the present study provides incremental knowledge, linking increased systemic inflammation (by IL-6 levels) to the pathophysiology of myocardial injury and dysfunction in COVID-19.

Limitations

The main limitation of this study is the relatively small sample size and retrospective cohort study design. Larger prospective studies are needed to further explore these novel echocardiographic parameters (GLS and MWE) with regard to cardiovascular mortality and other clinically meaningful outcomes in COVID-19 disease. Also, not all hospitalized

COVID-19 patients underwent echocardiogram and STE, which could result in selection bias and inability to detect true prevalence of abnormal GLS or MWE among COVID-19 patients. Lastly, a minority of patients with GLS and MWE performed did not have all inflammatory markers tested clinically, thus limiting the analyses.

CONCLUSIONS

In summary, sensitive indices of LV dysfunction, GLS and MWE, measured with STE are abnormal in a substantial portion of hospitalized COVID-19 patients who underwent echocardiograms, even in those with normal LVEF. Impaired MWE is independently associated with in-hospital mortality in COVID-19 patients. Higher IL-6 levels are associated with reduced MWE, providing a possible pathophysiologic link between increased inflammation and adverse outcomes in COVID-19. Based on these findings, it is possible that STE

measures of subclinical LV dysfunction may provide incremental value to standard echocardiographic measures in patients with COVID-19. Given the acuity of presentation and cardiovascular complications of COVID-19, a better understanding of the extent of myocardial injury and dysfunction early in the disease course may help triage at risk patients and implement early interventions aimed at reducing mortality. Further longitudinal studies are needed to investigate persistence of impaired cardiac function in the setting of COVID-19.

AUTHOR CONTRIBUTIONS

AM, NG, EG, and AH drafted the manuscript. BG, TM, GS, SP, and NB edited the manuscript. AM, NG, EG, and NB collected the data. AM analyzed the data and performed statistical analysis. All authors contributed to the article and approved the submitted version.

REFERENCES

1. Guo T, Fan Y, Chen M, Wu X, Zhang L, He T, et al. Cardiovascular implications of fatal outcomes of patients with coronavirus disease 2019 (COVID-19). *JAMA Cardiol.* (2020) 5:811–8. doi: 10.1001/jamacardio.2020.1017

2. Shi S, Qin M, Shen B, Cai Y, Liu T, Yang F, et al. Association of cardiac injury with mortality in hospitalized patients with COVID-19 in Wuhan, China. *JAMA Cardiol.* (2020) 5:802–10. doi: 10.1001/jamacardio.2020.0950

3. Hoffmann M, Kleine-Weber H, Schroeder S, Krüger N, Herrler T, Erichsen S, et al. SARS-CoV-2 cell entry depends on ACE2 and TMPRSS2 and is blocked by a clinically proven protease inhibitor. *Cell.* (2020) 181:271–80.e8. doi: 10.1016/j.cell.2020.02.052

4. Richardson S, Hirsch JS, Narasimhan M, Crawford JM, McGinn T, Davidson KW, et al. Presenting characteristics, comorbidities, and outcomes among 5700 patients hospitalized with COVID-19 in the New York City area. *JAMA.* (2020) 323:2052–9. doi: 10.1001/jama.2020.6775

5. Gilotra NA, Minkove N, Bennett MK, Tedford RJ, Steenbergen C, Judge DP, et al. Lack of relationship between serum cardiac troponin I level and giant cell myocarditis diagnosis and outcomes. *J Cardiac Fail.* (2016) 22:583–5. doi: 10.1016/j.cardfail.2015.12.022

6. Hu H, Ma F, Wei X, Fang Y. Coronavirus fulminant myocarditis treated with glucocorticoid and human immunoglobulin. *Eur Heart J.* (2020) 4:260. doi: 10.1093/eurheartj/ehaa190

7. Inciardi RM, Lupi L, Zaccone G, Italia L, Raffo M, Tomasoni D, et al. Cardiac involvement in a patient with coronavirus disease 2019 (COVID-19). *JAMA Cardiol.* (2020) 5:819–24. doi: 10.1001/jamacardio.2020.1096

8. Zeng F, Huang Y, Guo Y, Yin M, Chen X, Xiao L, et al. Association of inflammatory markers with the severity of COVID-19: A meta-analysis. *Int J Infect Dis.* (2020) 96:467–74. doi: 10.1016/j.ijid.2020.05.055

9. Rali AS, Ranka S, Shah Z, Sauer AJ. Mechanisms of myocardial injury in coronavirus disease 2019. *Card Fail Rev.* (2020) 6:e15. doi: 10.15420/cfr.2020.10

10. Chen C, Zhou Y, Wang DW. SARS-CoV-2: a potential novel etiology of fulminant myocarditis. *Herz.* (2020) 45:230–2. doi: 10.1007/s00059-020-04909-z

11. Cooper LT, Baughman KL, Feldman AM, Frustaci A, Jessup M, Kuhl U, et al. The role of endomyocardial biopsy in the management of cardiovascular disease. *J Am Coll Cardiol.* (2007) 50:1914–31. doi: 10.1016/j.jacc.2007.09.008

12. Kostakou PM, Kostopoulos VS, Tryfou ES, Giannaris VD, Rodis IE, Olympios CD, et al. Subclinical left ventricular dysfunction and correlation with regional strain analysis in myocarditis with normal ejection fraction. A new diagnostic criterion. *Int J Cardiol.* (2018) 259:116–21. doi: 10.1016/j.ijcard.2018.01.058

13. Han J, Mou Y, Yan D, Zhang Y-T, Jiang T-A, Zhang Y-Y, et al. Transient cardiac injury during H7N9 infection. *Eur J Clin Invest.* (2015) 45:117–25. doi: 10.1111/eci.12386

14. Awadalla M, Mahmood SS, Groarke JD, Hassan MZO, Nohria A, Rokicki A, et al. Global longitudinal strain and cardiac events in patients with immune checkpoint inhibitor-related myocarditis. *J Am College Cardiol.* (2020) 75:467–78. doi: 10.1016/j.jacc.2019.11.049

15. Sörensen J, Harms HJ, Aalen JM, Baron T, Smiseth OA, Flachskampf FA. Myocardial efficiency. *JACC: Cardiovasc Imag.* (2019) 13:1564–76. doi: 10.1016/j.jcmg.2019.08.030

16. Chan J, Edwards NFA, Khandheria BK, Shiino K, Sabapathy S, Anderson B, et al. A new approach to assess myocardial work by non-invasive left ventricular pressure–strain relations in hypertension and dilated cardiomyopathy. *Eur Heart J Cardiovasc Imaging.* (2019) 20:31–9. doi: 10.1093/ehjci/jey131

17. Edwards NFA, Scalia GM, Shiino K, Sabapathy S, Anderson B, Chamberlain R, et al. Global myocardial work is superior to global longitudinal strain to predict significant coronary artery disease in patients with normal left ventricular function and wall motion. *J Am Soc Echocardiogr.* (2019) 32:947–57. doi: 10.1016/j.echo.2019.02.014

18. Lang RM, Badano LP, Mor-Avi V, Afilalo J, Armstrong A, Ernande L, et al. Recommendations for cardiac chamber quantification by echocardiography in adults: an update from the American society of echocardiography and the European association of cardiovascular imaging. *J Am Soc Echocardiogr.* (2015) 28:1–39.e14. doi: 10.1016/j.echo.2014.10.003

19. Nagueh SF, Smiseth OA, Appleton CP, Byrd BF, Dokainish H, Edvardsen T, et al. Recommendations for the evaluation of left ventricular diastolic function by echocardiography: an update from the American society of echocardiography and the European association of cardiovascular imaging. *J Am Soc Echocardiograp.* (2016) 29:277–314. doi: 10.1016/j.echo.2016.01.011

20. Kirkpatrick JN, Mitchell C, Taub C, Kort S, Hung J, Swaminathan M. ASE statement on protection of patients and echocardiography service providers during the 2019 novel coronavirus outbreak. *J Am College Cardiol.* (2020) 75:3078–84. doi: 10.1016/j.jacc.2020.04.002

21. Farsalinos KE, Daraban AM, Ünlü S, Thomas JD, Badano LP, Voigt J-U. Head-to-head comparison of global longitudinal strain measurements among

nine different vendors. *J Am Soc Echocardiograp.* (2015) 28:1171–81.e2. doi: 10.1016/j.echo.2015.06.011

22. Haji K, Marwick TH. Clinical utility of echocardiographic strain and strain rate measurements. *Curr Cardiol Rep.* (2021) 23:18. doi: 10.1007/s11886-021-01444-z

23. D'Elia N, Caselli S, Kosmala W, Lancellotti P, Morris D, Muraru D, et al. Normal global longitudinal strain. *JACC: Cardiovasc Imaging.* (2020) 13:167–9. doi: 10.1016/j.jcmg.2019.07.020

24. Pieske B, Tschöpe C, de Boer RA, Fraser AG, Anker SD, Donal E, et al. How to diagnose heart failure with preserved ejection fraction: the HFA–PEFF diagnostic algorithm: a consensus recommendation from the heart failure association (HFA) of the European Society of Cardiology (ESC). *Eur Heart J.* (2019) 40:3297–317. doi: 10.1093/eurheartj/ehz641

25. Potter E, Marwick TH. Assessment of left ventricular function by echocardiography. *JACC: Cardiovascu Imaging.* (2018) 11:260–74. doi: 10.1016/j.jcmg.2017.11.017

26. Russell K, Eriksen M, Aaberge L, Wilhelmsen N, Skulstad H, Gjesdal O, et al. Assessment of wasted myocardial work: a novel method to quantify energy loss due to uncoordinated left ventricular contractions. *Am J Physiol Heart Circul Physiol.* (2013) 305:H996–1003. doi: 10.1152/ajpheart.001 91.2013

27. Russell K, Eriksen M, Aaberge L, Wilhelmsen N, Skulstad H, Remme EW, et al. A novel clinical method for quantification of regional left ventricular pressure-strain loop area: a non-invasive index of myocardial work. *Eur Heart J.* (2012) 33:724–33. doi: 10.1093/eurheartj/ehs016

28. Hubert A, Le Rolle V, Leclercq C, Galli E, Samset E, Casset C, et al. Estimation of myocardial work from pressure-strain loops analysis: an experimental evaluation. *Eur Heart J Cardiovasc Imaging.* (2018) 19:1372–9. doi: 10.1093/ehjci/jey024

29. Manganaro R, Marchetta S, Dulgheru R, Ilardi F, Sugimoto T, Robinet S, et al. Echocardiographic reference ranges for normal non-invasive myocardial work indices: results from the EACVI NORRE study. *Eur Heart J Cardiovasc Imaging.* (2019) 20:582–90. doi: 10.1093/ehjci/jey188

30. El Mahdiui M, van der Bijl P, Abou R, Ajmone Marsan N, Delgado V, Bax JJ. Global left ventricular myocardial work efficiency in healthy individuals and patients with cardiovascular disease. *J Am Soc Echocardiograp.* (2019) 32:1120–7. doi: 10.1016/j.echo.2019.05.002

31. Bouali Y, Donal E, Gallard A, Laurin C, Hubert A, Bidaut A, et al. Prognostic usefulness of myocardial work in patients with heart failure and reduced ejection fraction treated by sacubitril/valsartan. *Am J Cardiol.* (2020) 125:1856–62. doi: 10.1016/j.amjcard.2020.03.031

32. Abou R, Leung M, Khidir MJH, Wolterbeek R, Schalij MJ, Ajmone Marsan N, et al. Influence of aging on level and layer-specific left ventricular longitudinal strain in subjects without structural heart disease. *Am J Cardiol.* (2017) 120:2065–72. doi: 10.1016/j.amjcard.2017.08.027

33. Liu J-H, Chen Y, Yuen M, Zhen Z, Chan CW-S, Lam KS-L, et al. Incremental prognostic value of global longitudinal strain in patients with type 2 diabetes mellitus. *Cardiovasc Diabetol.* (2016) 15:22. doi: 10.1186/s12933-016-0333-5

34. Wierzbowska-Drabik K, Trzos E, Kurpesa M, Rechciński T, Miśkowiec D, Cieślik-Guerra U, et al. Diabetes as an independent predictor of left ventricular longitudinal strain reduction at rest and during dobutamine stress test in patients with significant coronary artery disease. *Eur Heart J Cardiovasc Imaging.* (2018) 19:1276–86. doi: 10.1093/ehjci/jex315

35. Vrettos A, Dawson D, Grigoratos C, Nihoyannopoulos P. Correlation between global longitudinal peak systolic strain and coronary artery disease severity as assessed by the angiographically derived SYNTAX score. *Echo Res Pract.* (2016) 3:29–34. doi: 10.1530/ERP-16-0005

36. Liou K, Negishi K, Ho S, Russell EA, Cranney G, Ooi S-Y. Detection of obstructive coronary artery disease using peak systolic global longitudinal strain derived by two-dimensional speckle-tracking: a systematic review and meta-analysis. *J Am Soc Echocardiograp.* (2016) 29:724–35.e4. doi: 10.1016/j.echo.2016.03.002

37. Smiseth OA, Torp H, Opdahl A, Haugaa KH, Urheim S. Myocardial strain imaging: how useful is it in clinical decision making? *Eur Heart J.* (2016) 37:1196–207. doi: 10.1093/eurheartj/ehv529

38. Thavendiranathan P, Poulin F, Lim K-D, Plana JC, Woo A, Marwick TH. Use of myocardial strain imaging by echocardiography for the early detection of cardiotoxicity in patients during and after cancer chemotherapy. *J Am College Cardiol.* (2014) 63:2751–68. doi: 10.1016/j.jacc.2014.01.073

39. Stokke TM, Hasselberg NE, Smedsrud MK, Sarvari SI, Haugaa KH, Smiseth OA, et al. Geometry as a confounder when assessing ventricular systolic function. *J Am College Cardiol.* (2017) 70:942–54. doi: 10.1016/j.jacc.2017.06.046

40. Honce R, Schultz-Cherry S. Impact of obesity on influenza A virus pathogenesis, immune response, and evolution. *Front Immunol.* (2019) 10:1071. doi: 10.3389/fimmu.2019.01071

41. Estabragh ZR, Mamas MA. The cardiovascular manifestations of influenza: A systematic review. *Int J Cardiol.* (2013) 167:2397–403. doi: 10.1016/j.ijcard.2013.01.274

42. Cummings MJ, Baldwin MR, Abrams D, Jacobson SD, Meyer BJ, Balough EM, et al. Epidemiology, clinical course, and outcomes of critically ill adults with COVID-19 in New York City: a prospective cohort study. *Lancet.* (2020) 395:1763–70. doi: 10.1016/S0140-6736(20)31189-2

43. Li Y, Li H, Zhu S, Xie Y, Wang B, He L, et al. Prognostic value of right ventricular longitudinal strain in patients with COVID-19. *JACC: Cardiovasc Imaging.* (2020) 13:2287–99. doi: 10.1016/j.jcmg.2020.04.014

44. Argulian E, Sud K, Vogel B, Bohra C, Garg VP, Talebi S, et al. Right ventricular dilation in hospitalized patients with COVID-19 infection. *JACC: Cardiovasc Imaging.* (2020) 13:2459–61. doi: 10.1016/j.jcmg.2020.05.010

45. Atri D, Siddiqi HK, Lang J, Nauffal V, Morrow DA, Bohula EA. COVID-19 for the cardiologist: a current review of the virology, clinical epidemiology, cardiac and other clinical manifestations and potential therapeutic strategies. *JACC: Basic Transl Sci.* (2020) 5:518–36. doi: 10.1016/j.jacbts.2020.04.002

46. Buja LM, Wolf DA, Zhao B, Akkanti B, McDonald M, Lelenwa L, et al. The emerging spectrum of cardiopulmonary pathology of the coronavirus disease 2019 (COVID-19): report of 3 autopsies from Houston, Texas, and review of autopsy findings from other United States cities. *Cardiovasc Pathol.* (2020) 48:107233. doi: 10.1016/j.carpath.2020.107233

47. The GBD 2015 Obesity Collaborators. Health effects of overweight and obesity in 195 countries over 25 years. *N Engl J Med.* (2017) 377:13–27. doi: 10.1056/NEJMoa1614362

48. Kass DA, Duggal P, Cingolani O. Obesity could shift severe COVID-19 disease to younger ages. *Lancet.* (2020) 395:1544–5. doi: 10.1016/S0140-6736(20)31024-2

49. Pathan N, Hemingway CA, Alizadeh AA, Stephens AC, Boldrick JC, Oragui EE, et al. Role of interleukin 6 in myocardial dysfunction of meningococcal septic shock. *Lancet.* (2004) 363:203–9. doi: 10.1016/S0140-6736(03)15326-3

50. Johnson DE, O'Keefe RA, Grandis JR. Targeting the IL-6/JAK/STAT3 signalling axis in cancer. *Nat Rev Clin Oncol.* (2018) 15:234–8. doi: 10.1038/nrclinonc.2018.8

51. Liu B, Li M, Zhou Z, Guan X, Xiang Y. Can we use interleukin-6 (IL-6) blockade for coronavirus disease 2019 (COVID-19)-induced cytokine release syndrome (CRS)? *J Autoimmun.* (2020) 111:102452. doi: 10.1016/j.jaut.2020.102452

52. Huang C, Wang Y, Li X, Ren L, Zhao J, Hu Y, et al. Clinical features of patients infected with 2019 novel coronavirus in Wuhan, China. *Lancet.* (2020) 395:497–506. doi: 10.1016/S0140-6736(20) 30183-5

53. Chen N, Zhou M, Dong X, Qu J, Gong F, Han Y, et al. Epidemiological and clinical characteristics of 99 cases of 2019 novel coronavirus pneumonia in Wuhan, China: a descriptive study. *Lancet.* (2020) 395:507–13. doi: 10.1016/S0140-6736(20)30211-7

54. Gao Y, Li T, Han M, Li X, Wu D, Xu Y, et al. Diagnostic utility of clinical laboratory data determinations for patients with the severe COVID-19. *J Med Virol.* (2020) 92:791–6. doi: 10.1002/jmv.25770

13

Impact of COVID-19 Pandemic on Mechanical Reperfusion in ST-Segment-Elevation Myocardial Infarction Undergoing Primary Percutaneous Coronary Intervention: A Multicenter Retrospective Study from a Non-Epicenter Region

Qi Mao[1], Jianhua Zhao[1], Youmei Li[1], Li Xie[1], Han Xiao[1], Ke Wang[1], Youzhu Qiu[1], Jianfei Chen[2], Qiang Xu[3], Zhonglin Xu[4], Yang Yu[5], Ying Zhang[6], Qiang Li[7], Xiaohua Pang[8], Zhenggong Li[9], Boli Ran[10], Zhihui Zhang[11], Zhifeng Li[12], Chunyu Zeng[13], Shifei Tong[14], Jun Jin[1], Lan Huang[1]* and Xiaohui Zhao[1]*

[1] Department of Cardiology, Institute of Cardiovascular Research, Xinqiao Hospital, Army Medical University, Chongqing, China, [2] Department of Cardiology, People's Hospital of Banan District, Chongqing, China, [3] Department of Cardiology, The Fifth People's Hospital, Chongqing, China, [4] Department of Cardiology, The Ninth People's Hospital, Chongqing, China, [5] Department of Cardiology, People's Hospital of Dianjiang District, Chongqing, China, [6] Department of Cardiology, Emergency Medical Center, Chongqing, China, [7] Department of Cardiovascular Medicine, People's Hospital of Nanchuan District, Chongqing, China, [8] Department of Cardiovascular Medicine, The Three Gorges Central Hospital, Chongqing, China, [9] Department of Cardiac Intervention Therapy, Zhongshan Hospital District, Chongqing General Hospital, University of Chinese Academy of Sciences, Chongqing, China, [10] Department of Cardiology, The Third Hospital District, Chongqing General Hospital, University of Chinese Academy of Sciences, Chongqing, China, [11] Department of Cardiology, Southwest Hospital, Army Medical University, Chongqing, China, [12] Department of Cardiology, Yongchuan Hospital, Chongqing Medical University, Chongqing, China, [13] Department of Cardiology, Daping Hospital, Army Medical University, Chongqing, China, [14] Department of Cardiology, The Third Affiliated Hospital of Chongqing Medical University, Chongqing, China

Correspondence:
Lan Huang
huanglan260@126.com
Xiaohui Zhao
doctorzhaoxiaohui@yahoo.com

Objective: The COVID-19 pandemic placed heavy burdens on emergency care and posed severe challenges to ST-segment-elevation myocardial infarction (STEMI) treatment. This study aimed to investigate the impact of COVID-19 pandemic on mechanical reperfusion characteristics in STEMI undergoing primary percutaneous coronary intervention (PPCI) in a non-epicenter region.

Methods: STEMI cases undergoing PPCI from January 23 to March 29 between 2019 and 2020 were retrospectively compared. PPCI parameters mainly included total ischemic time (TIT), the period from symptom onset to first medical contact (S-to-FMC), the period from FMC to wire (FMC-to-W) and the period from door to wire (D-to-W). Furthermore, the association of COVID-19 pandemic with delayed PPCI risk was further analyzed.

Results: A total of 14 PPCI centers were included, with 100 and 220 STEMI cases undergoing PPCI in 2020 and 2019, respectively. As compared to 2019, significant prolongations occurred in reperfusion procedures ($P < 0.001$) including TIT (420 vs. 264 min), S-to-FMC (5 vs. 3 h), FMC-to-W (113 vs. 95 min) and D-to-W (83 vs. 65 min).

Consistently, delayed reperfusion surged including TIT $\geq$ 12 h (22.0 vs.3.6%), FMC-to-W $\geq$ 120 min (34.0 vs. 6.8%) and D-to-W $\geq$ 90 min (19.0 vs. 4.1%). During the pandemic, the patients with FMC-to-W $\geq$ 120 min had longer durations in FMC to ECG completed (6 vs. 5 min, $P = 0.007$), FMC to DAPT (24 vs. 21 min, $P = 0.001$), catheter arrival to wire (54 vs. 43 min, $P < 0.001$) and D-to-W (91 vs. 78 min, $P < 0.001$). The pandemic was significantly associated with high risk of delayed PPCI (OR = 7.040, 95% CI 3.610–13.729, $P < 0.001$).

Conclusions: Even in a non-epicenter region, the risk of delayed STEMI reperfusion significantly increased due to cumulative impact of multiple procedures prolongation.

Keywords: COVID-19, ST-segment-elevation myocardial infarction, primary percutaneous coronary intervention, mechanical reperfusion, non-epicenter region

INTRODUCTION

ST-segment-elevation myocardial infarction (STEMI) is a major cardiovascular emergency requiring early diagnosis and timely reperfusion (1). Mechanical reperfusion is mainly based on rapid and standardized emergency procedures for chest pain (2). Since the outbreak in December 2019, over 110 million coronavirus-2019 disease (COVID-19) infected cases have been diagnosed and 2.4 million confirmed deaths (3). The continuing pandemic placed heavy burdens on emergency care and posed severe challenges to STEMI treatment (4).

On the one hand, protective measures against COVID-19 cause delays in primary percutaneous coronary intervention (PPCI) and prolonged ischemia time thus may lead to poor prognosis. On the other hand, emergency process without protection greatly increases the risk of virus spread, especially serious infection in hospital (5, 6). Therefore, how to balance prevention and treatment is a great ordeal for medical institutions. Considering the pandemic may last for a long time, as a core issue in health governance, it will profoundly affect the public health system and chest pain practice. In previous studies, decline of admitted STEMI was reported both in Europe, US etc, and increased delays in PPCI were also observed in COVID-19 epicenters (7–9). However, in non-epicenters, few studies on detailed mechanical reperfusion characteristics were reported.

METHODS
Study Population
This multicenter retrospective study included 14 PPCI centers, which were certified by the China Chest Pain Center (CCPC) with standardized catheterization lab. In light of changes in epidemic and adjustments in public health response, the COVID-19 pandemic was defined as the period from January 23 (the

day on which Wuhan City entered into a state of full-scale wartime through the lockdown, and then other regions including Chongqing City also upgraded their public health response to prevent the spread of the epidemic) to March 29 in 2020 (the day on which Chongqing City downgraded local public health response due to the absolute clearance of COVID-19 cases). Also, similar patients at the same period last year were included to reduce the biases of seasonal variation and festive events on the incidence. The patients with confirmed or suspected COVID-19 were excluded. Our study protocol complied with the Declaration of Helsinki and was approved by Xinqiao Hospital Ethics Committee, Army Medical University.

Treatment Procedure During the Pandemic
Although Chongqing City was a non-epicenter during the pandemic, local public health response was still upgraded on January 23 to minimize the spread of virus. Except for the lockdown, social restrictive measures were implemented to reduce external input and local transmission. For medical institutions, all admitted patients were screened for SARS-COV-2 according to Clinical Guideline of COVID-19 Diagnosis and Treatment (7 th edition) (10). In brief, the patients with confirmed or suspected COVID-19 would be transferred to the designated hospitals as soon as possible; the patients without exclusion of COVID-19 temporarily would be first transferred to the special clinics for isolation and treatment, if further tests were positive, they would be immediately transferred to the designated hospitals; while non-COVID-19 patients underwent conventional treatment procedures (11). Reperfusion therapy was determined based on benefit/risk assessment and consensus recommendation (12). Compared to the epicenters, PPCI remained the preferred option for local reperfusion therapy rather than thrombolysis-first. The flowchart of emergency procedure was shown in **Figure 1**.

Definition and Data Collection
Acute myocardial infarction refers to the fourth universal definition, when troponin value exceeds the 99 th percentile upper reference limit and combines at least one of following characteristics: (1) symptoms of myocardial ischemia; (2) new changes in ischemic electrocardiogram or emerging pathological

Abbreviations: COVID-19, coronavirus-2019 disease; STEMI, ST-segment-elevation myocardial infarction; PPCI, primary percutaneous coronary intervention; SBP, systolic blood pressure; DBP, diastolic blood pressure; Scr, serum creatinine; EMS, emergency medical service; CCPC, China Chest Pain Center; FMC, first medical contact; S-to-FMC, symptom onset to FMC; DAPT, dual antiplalet therapy; D-to-W, door to wire; FMC-to-W, FMC to wire; TIT, total ischemic time.

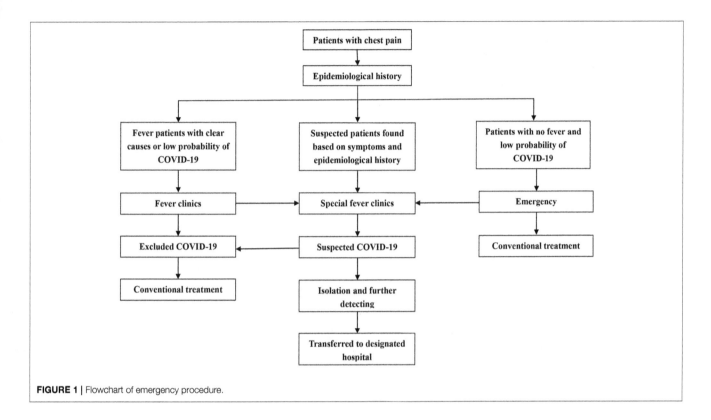

FIGURE 1 | Flowchart of emergency procedure.

Q waves; (3) imaging evidence of new loss of viable myocardium or new regional wall motion abnormality (13). Global Registry of Acute Coronary Events (GRACE) risk score is applied to stratification and prediction of risk in patients with ACS and is calculated based on the clinical data, electrocardiogram (ECG), and laboratory parameters at admission (14).

Arrival patterns included walk-in, in-hospital onset, emergency medical services (EMS) and inter-facility transports; walk-in and in-hospital onset were defined as non-transferred pattern, while EMS and inter-facility transports were regarded as transferred pattern. PPCI parameters mainly included the period from symptom onset to first medical contact (S-to-FMC), the period from FMC to wire through culprit (FMC-to-W), and the period from door to wire through culprit (D-to-W) (15). Total ischemic time (TIT) was composed of S-to-FMC and FMC-to-W. D-to-W $\geq$ 90 min, FMC-to-W $\geq$ 120 min and TIT $\geq$ 12 h were deemed as pivotal timelines for delayed mechanical reperfusion (16). Clinical data and mechanical reperfusion characteristics were obtained from medical records.

Statistical Analysis

Continuous variables are presented as mean ± SD for symmetric distributions and median (interquartile range, IQR) for skewed distributions. Categorical variables are expressed as frequency (percentage). In comparisons between groups, the t-test was performed for symmetric distributed variables, and nonparametric Mann-Whitney U test was applied for skewed distributed variables. Differences in categorical variables were compared by the Chi-squared test or Fisher exact

test. Taking the dichotomous delay PPCI indicators as the dependent variables, we conducted logistic regression analysis to explore the association of COVID-19 pandemic with delayed mechanical reperfusion, and sub-group analysis was utilized to further assess this correlation. Two-tailed P-values < 0.05 were considered statistically significant. All statistical analyses were performed using SPSS software version 24.0 (SPSS, Inc, Chicago, Illinois).

RESULTS
Composition and Grouping

STEMI collaboration network from 14 PPCI centers implemented a unified procedure in accordance with CCPC specification in chest pain emergency (17). During the pandemic from 23 th January 2020 to 29 th March 2020 in China, a total of 145 consecutive patients admitted to chest pain emergency were diagnosed with STEMI, and 100 patients (69.0%) met the inclusion criteria after exclusion of non-mechanical reperfusion cases among these cases. During the same period in 2019, a total of 278 consecutive STEMI patients arrived in chest pain emergency after symptom onset, and 220 cases (79.1%) were included after screening (**Figure 2**).

Comparison of Study Population Before and During the Pandemic

Overall, we identified 320 non-COVID-19 patients with STEMI undergoing PPCI as the study population (**Table 1**). As compared to 2019, the cases of STEMI (decreased by 47.8%) and PPCI (decreased by 54.5%) had a significant reduction. In terms of

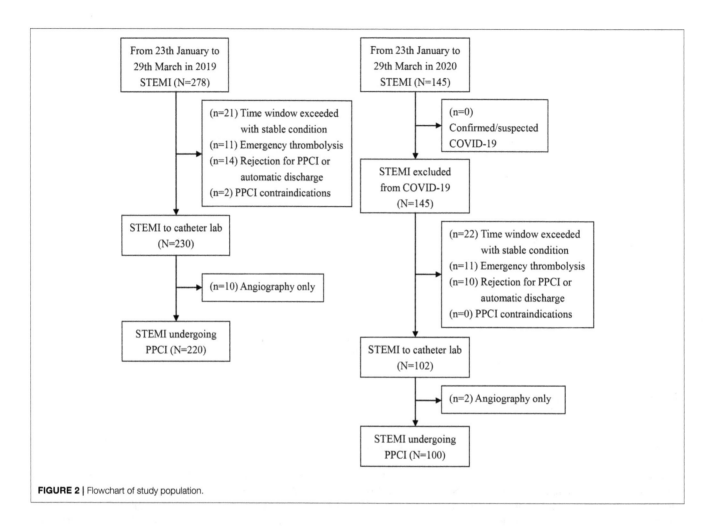

FIGURE 2 | Flowchart of study population.

clinical characteristics, there were no differences in age, gender, heart rate, Killip class, serum creatinine and GRACE scores between the two groups ($P > 0.05$). Although arrival during non-offices hours did not differ significantly between the two groups ($P > 0.05$), more non-transferred patients with less inter-facility transports (24.0 vs. 41.4%) and more walk-in (61.0 vs. 48.6%) appeared during the pandemic ($P < 0.05$). In terms of mechanical reperfusion characteristics, significant prolongations occurred in PPCI parameters ($P < 0.001$) including TIT (420 vs. 264 min), S-to-FMC (5 vs. 3 h), FMC-to-W (113 vs. 95 min) and D-to-W (83 vs. 65 min). Further analysis revealed that median time of TIT increased by 156 min during the pandemic; COVID-19 outbreak delayed the median time of FMC-to-W for 18 min. Consistently, delayed reperfusion surged including TIT $\geq$ 12 h (22.0 vs.3.6%), FMC-to-W $\geq$ 120 min (34.0 vs. 6.8%) and D-to-W $\geq$ 90 min (19.0 vs. 4.1%) significantly ($P < 0.001$). Of note, the ratio of S-to-FMC to TIT increased significantly during the pandemic (72.8 vs. 63.7%, $P < 0.001$).

PPCI Parameters Between Different Groups During the Pandemic

No differences occurred in PPCI parameters between office periods and non-office periods during the pandemic ($P > 0.05$)

(Table 2). Compared to the transferred patients, the periods of FMC to ECG completed and FMC to DAPT were decreased by 2 and 3 min, respectively, in non-transferred patients ($P = 0.002$); whereas the periods of telephone to catheter activated (15 vs. 9 min, $P < 0.001$) and catheter arrival to wire (47 vs. 44 min, $P < 0.042$) significantly extended for non-transferred patients; non-transferred pattern increased the proportion of patients with TIT $\geq$ 12 h ($P = 0.045$) (Table 3).

In Table 4, the patients with FMC-to-W $\geq$ 120 min had longer durations in FMC to ECG completed (6 vs. 5 min, $P = 0.007$), FMC to DAPT (24 vs. 21 min, $P = 0.001$), catheter arrival to wire (54 vs. 43 min, $P < 0.001$) and D-to-W (91 vs. 78 min, $P < 0.001$) than the patients with FMC-to-W < 120 min; while S-to-FMC and TIT showed no differences between the two groups ($P > 0.05$).

Association of the Pandemic With the Risk of Delayed PPCI

Logistic regression analysis was used to explore the association between the pandemic and delayed PPCI. The binary delayed PPCI indicators and COVID-19 pandemic status were included as dependent and independent variables in the model, respectively. The results indicated the pandemic was

TABLE 1 | Characteristics of study population before and during COVID-19 pandemic.

Characteristics	From 23rd January to 29th March in 2019 (N = 220)	From 23 rd January to 29th March in 2020 (N = 100)	P-value
Male, n (%)	177 (80.5)	77 (77.0)	0.479
Age (years)	63 (54–73)	64 (55–75)	0.768
Heart rate (min)	78 (70–89)	75 (65–88)	0.082
SBP (mmHg)	122 (110–142)	125 (110–150)	0.790
DBP (mmHg)	77 (68–88)	78 (68–92)	0.667
Killip class			
Killip class I, n (%)	138 (62.7)	62 (62.0)	
Killip class II, n (%)	57 (25.9)	22 (22.0)	
Killip class III, n (%)	9 (4.1)	2 (2.0)	
Killip class IV, n (%)	15 (6.8)	15 (15.0)	
Killip class ≥ II, n (%)	82 (37.3)	39 (39.0)	0.768
Scr (μmol/L)	74.0 (61.9–90.4)	71.3 (60.3–91.4)	0.624
GRACE scores in hospital	143 (121–163)	139 (119–166)	0.804
Arrival During non-office hours, n (%)	99 (45.0)	51 (51.0)	0.319
Pattern of patients arrival			
Walk-in	107 (48.6)	61 (61.0)	
In-hospital onset	2 (0.9)	1 (1.0)	
EMS	20 (9.1)	14 (14.0)	
Inter-facility transports	91 (41.4)	24 (24.0)	
Non-transferred patients, n (%)	109 (49.5)	62 (62.0)	0.038
S-to-FMC (hours)	3.0 (2.0–4.5)	5.0 (3.0–10.0)	<0.001
FMC to ECG completed (min)	3 (2–6)	5 (3–7)	<0.001
Door to Troponin completed (min)	12 (11–15)	13 (12–14)	0.475
FMC to DAPT (min)	19 (17–22)	22 (19–25)	<0.001
Telephone to catheter activated (min)	9 (6–12)	13 (9–17)	<0.001
Catheter arrival to wire (min)	36 (31–42)	45 (41–53)	<0.001
D-to-W (min)	65 (57–76)	83 (75–89)	<0.001
D-to-W ≥ 90 min, n (%)	9 (4.1)	19 (19.0)	<0.001
FMC-to-W (min)	95 (87–108)	113 (106–124)	<0.001
FMC-to-W ≥120 min, n (%)	15 (6.8)	34 (34.0)	<0.001
TIT (min)	264 (204–367)	420 (295–688)	<0.001
TIT ≥ 12 h, n (%)	8 (3.6)	22 (22.0)	<0.001
S-to-FMC/TIT ratio (%)	63.7 (50.4–74.5)	72.8 (62.6–83.8)	<0.001
FMC-to-W/TIT ratio (%)	36.3 (25.5–49.6)	27.2 (16.2–37.4)	

Data are expressed as median (interquartile range) or number (percentage) as appropriate.

TABLE 2 | Comparison of PPCI parameters between different arrival periods during COVID-19 pandemic.

Parameters	During office hours (N = 49)	During non-office hours (N = 51)	P-value
Killip class≥II, n (%)	18 (36.7)	21 (41.2)	0.649
GRACE scores in hospital	137 (120–161)	147 (118–172)	0.546
Non-transferred patients, n (%)	32 (65.3)	30 (58.8)	0.504
S-to-FMC (hours)	6.0 (3.0–11.0)	4.0 (3.0–9.0)	0.076
FMC to ECG completed (min)	5 (3–7)	6 (4–7)	0.113
Door to Troponin completed (min)	13 (11–14)	13 (12–15)	0.186
FMC to DAPT (min)	22 (19–25)	22 (19–27)	0.836
Telephone to catheter activated (min)	14 (10–17)	13 (9–18)	0.751
Catheter arrival to wire (min)	45 (41–53)	46 (42–54)	0.394
D-to-W (min)	82 (75–89)	83 (75–87)	0.753
D-to-W ≥ 90 min, n (%)	10 (20.4)	9 (17.6)	0.725
FMC-to-W (min)	113 (106–121)	114 (107–127)	0.574
FMC-to-W ≥ 120 min, n (%)	14 (28.6)	20 (39.2)	0.261
TIT (min)	462 (315–750)	374 (289–639)	0.116
TIT ≥ 12 h, n (%)	14 (28.6)	8 (15.7)	0.120
S-to-FMC/TIT ratio (%)	77.3 (64.3–84.0)	67.3 (58.4–82.9)	0.073
FMC-to-W/TIT ratio (%)	22.7 (16.0–35.7)	32.7 (17.1–41.6)	

Data are expressed as median (interquartile range) or number (percentage) as appropriate.

association (**Table 5**). Meanwhile, constituent ratios of TIT and PPCI were shown in **Figure 3**.

DISCUSSION

In this study, we found that risk of delayed STEMI reperfusion significantly increased due to cumulative impact of multiple procedures in a non-epicenter region.

Evidence from Europe indicated that compared with the same period in 2019, PPCI cases decreased by 19.3%, and the median time of TIT and D-to-W were delayed by 9 and 2 min, respectively (18). The data from North America showed an estimated 38% reduction in U.S. cardiac catheterization activation after the outbreak (19). Consistently, the analysis from China's epicenter (Hubei Province) also revealed a 62.3% decline in STEMI cases during the pandemic, while the proportion of non-transferred patients characterized by walk-in increased significantly (8). In a non-epicenter, our results also revealed that a significant reduction occurred in cases of admitted STEMI and PPCI during the pandemic. Common reasons had been formulated to explain the reduction in cases including fear of infection, social distancing, and medical care avoidance. However, the decline in cases could not be simply ascribed to

significantly associated with high risk of delayed TIT (OR = 7.474, 95% CI 3.195–17.484, P < 0.001), delayed FMC-to-W (OR = 7.040, 95% CI 3.610–13.729, P < 0.001) and delayed D-to-W (OR = 5.499, 95% CI 2.390–12.655, P < 0.001). Sub-group analysis stratified by clinical characteristics further examined this

TABLE 3 | Comparison of PPCI parameters between different transferred methods during COVID-19 pandemic.

Parameters	Non-transferred Patients (*N* = 62)	Transferred Patients (*N* = 38)	*P*-value
Killip class≥II, *n* (%)	21 (33.9)	18 (47.4)	0.179
GRACE scores in hospital	134 (115–160)	143 (133–177)	0.053
Arrival during non-office hours, *n* (%)	30 (48.4)	21 (55.3)	0.504
S-to-FMC (hours)	5.5 (3.0–11.0)	5.0 (3.0–9.0)	0.322
FMC to ECG completed (min)	5 (3–6)	7 (4–10)	0.002
Door to Troponin completed (min)	13 (11–14)	14 (12–15)	0.377
FMC to DAPT (min)	21 (18–24)	24 (20–30)	0.002
Telephone to catheter activated (min)	15 (12–18)	9 (6–14)	<0.001
Catheter arrival to wire (min)	47 (42–54)	44 (36–50)	0.042
D-to-W (min)	83 (77–89)	83 (74–88)	0.511
D-to-W ≥ 90 min, *n* (%)	12 (19.4)	7 (18.4)	0.908
FMC-to-W (min)	113 (106–122)	115 (107–126)	0.649
FMC-to-W ≥ 120 min, *n* (%)	17 (27.4)	17 (44.7)	0.076
TIT (min)	443 (294–774)	400 (303–641)	0.347
TIT ≥ 12 h, *n* (%)	18 (29.0)	4 (10.5)	0.045
S-to-FMC/TIT ratio (%)	76.0 (63.1–84.5)	68.1 (62.2–82.6)	0.248
FMC-to-W/TIT ratio (%)	24.0 (15.5–36.9)	31.9 (17.4–37.8)	

Data are expressed as median (interquartile range) or number (percentage) as appropriate.

TABLE 4 | Comparison of parameters between timely PPCI and delayed PPCI during COVID-19 pandemic.

Parameters	FMC-to-W <120 min (*N* = 66)	FMC-to-W ≥ 120 min (*N* = 34)	*P*-value
Killip class ≥ II, *n* (%)	26 (39.4)	13 (38.2)	0.910
GRACE scores in hospital	137 (115–162)	142 (123–177)	0.142
Arrival during non-office hours, *n* (%)	31 (47.0)	20 (58.8)	0.261
Non-transferred patients, *n* (%)	45 (68.2)	17 (50.0)	0.076
S-to-FMC (hours)	6.0 (3.0–9.0)	4.0 (3.0–10.0)	0.818
FMC to ECG completed (min)	5 (3–6)	6 (4–9)	0.007
Door to Troponin completed (min)	13 (11–14)	14 (12–15)	0.181
FMC to DAPT (min)	21 (18–23)	24 (20–29)	0.001
Telephone to catheter activated (min)	12 (9–16)	14 (11–20)	0.050
Catheter arrival to wire (min)	43 (40–48)	54 (47–57)	<0.001
D-to-W (min)	78 (69–83)	91 (85–106)	<0.001
D-to-W ≥ 90 min, *n* (%)	0	19 (55.9)	<0.001
FMC-to-W (min)	108 (101–113)	128 (124–138)	<0.001
TIT (min)	462 (289–654)	396 (320–724)	0.702
TIT ≥ 12 h, *n* (%)	12 (18.2)	10 (29.4)	0.199
S-to-FMC/TIT ratio (%)	77.1 (63.3–84.1)	66.3 (58.3–83.0)	0.137
FMC-to-W/TIT ratio (%)	22.9 (15.9–36.7)	33.7 (17.0–41.7)	

Data are expressed as median (interquartile range) or number (percentage) as appropriate.

individual behaviors, and we should also pay attention to the comprehensive impact of the pandemic on chest pain procedure. STEMI rescue includes pre-hospital and in-hospital segments. Both S-to-FMC and D-to-W were apparently prolonged, which led to cumulative delays in reperfusion procedure.

Mechanical reperfusion for STEMI is a competition with time. The 1-year mortality of STEMI increases by 15% with every 1 h extension in time to reperfusion (20). Quality control of PPCI based on standardized procedure can help shorten TIT, reduce infarction sizes and mortality (21). Although COVID-19 has been shown to directly cause myocardial injury and induce thrombosis, heart failure, arrhythmia and even cardiac arrest; for non-COVID-19 patients, delayed PPCI affected by the pandemic might be the determinant for the poor prognosis in STEMI (22). In previous studies, Tam et al. (23) showed longer median time in all components of PPCI parameters compared with historical data from prior year in Hong Kong, yet limited by very small sample size (7 cases) and non-contemporaneous data comparison. Siudak et al. (24) reported that time from FMC to inflation significantly increased compared with analogous time period last year in Poland, but the impact of the virus infection on delayed PPCI had not been ruled out. An observational study from Canada revealed that significant delay appeared in

reperfusion procedure and predominantly ascribed to patient-level and transfer-level during the pandemic (25). Of note, our study found that delays in mechanical reperfusion should be attributed to the cumulative effect of multiple processes. In addition to pre-hospital level, in-hospital delays should also not be ignored. In a non-hot spot region from America, Hammad et al. found that although no difference occurred in total D-to-B between pre-COVID-19 and post-COVID-19, a higher proportion of patients in the post-COVID-19 period presented with >12-h delay compared with the pre-COVID-19 period, and those patients with >12-h delay also had a longer average D-to-B time (26). Similarly, we also observed the adverse effect of COVID-19 pandemic on reperfusion procedure in another non-epicenter region. However, our results revealed the apparent prolongations in S-to-FMC and FMC-to-W after the outbreak through detailed parameter analysis. We speculated that this might be associated with stricter social restrictions and upgraded public health response after the first wave pandemic in China. In epicenter region (Hubei Province) from China, although differences of median time in S-to-FMC and FMC-to-W seemed to be not significant, delays in timelines was still apparent due to the highly fluctuated time and limited sample size (8). Compared with our study, reperfusion strategy of this epicenter had been adjusted to meet the needs of high-intensity epidemic control. A

TABLE 5 | Logistic analyses for the association of COVID-19 pandemic with delayed PPCI.

	Delayed PPCI								
	TIT ≥ 12 h			FMC-to-W ≥ 120 min			D-to-W ≥ 90 min		
	OR	95% CI	*P*-value	OR	95% CI	*P*-value	OR	95% CI	*P*-value
Overall	7.474	(3.195–17.484)	<0.001	7.040	(3.610–13.729)	<0.001	5.499	(2.390–12.655)	<0.001
Age									
≥65 years	4.694	(1.733–12.717)	0.002	7.759	(3.090–19.479)	<0.001	6.803	(2.039–22.694)	0.002
<65 years	25.929	(3.189–210.805)	0.002	6.216	(2.333–16.563)	<0.001	4.353	(1.350–14.037)	0.014
Gender									
Male	7.475	(2.798–19.973)	<0.001	8.514	(3.849–18.832)	<0.001	5.541	(2.258–13.598)	<0.001
Female	7.235	(1.325–39.497)	0.022	4.053	(1.142–14.392)	0.030	6.300	(0.616–64.426)	0.121
Killip class									
Killip class ≥ II	5.850	(1.675–20.435)	0.006	6.333	(2.183–18.370)	0.001	2.868	(0.725–11.343)	0.133
Killip class < II	9.073	(2.821–29.179)	<0.001	7.525	(3.192–17.741)	<0.001	7.923	(2.707–23.190)	<0.001
GRACE score									
GRACE > 140	5.294	(1.930–14.524)	0.001	8.053	(3.277–19.793)	<0.001	6.568	(1.909–22.594)	0.003
GRACE ≤ 140	24.318	(3.022–195.704)	0.003	6.538	(2.367–18.062)	<0.001	4.682	(1.512–14.494)	0.007
Office hours or not									
Non–office hours	18.233	(2.211–150.318)	0.007	5.742	(2.425–13.598)	<0.001	3.321	(1.111–9.932)	0.032
Office hours	6.514	(2.437–17.412)	<0.001	9.280	(3.124–27.569)	<0.001	10.085	(2.641–38.518)	0.001
Transferred or not									
Transferred	6.412	(1.125–36.548)	0.036	9.175	(3.603–23.359)	<0.001	8.129	(1.984–33.304)	0.004
Non-transferred	7.023	(2.612–18.882)	<0.001	6.485	(2.399–17.530)	<0.001	4.120	(1.461–11.617)	0.007

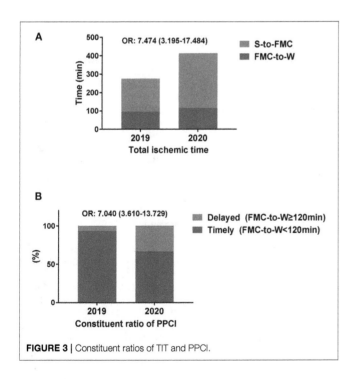

FIGURE 3 | Constituent ratios of TIT and PPCI.

large number of patients from epicenter received thrombolytic therapy at the first time, given that thrombolysis could be considered as the recommended reperfusion option during the pandemic (12).

Compared to other regions, we discovered that delays in mechanical reperfusion were still rather serious in non-COVID-19 STEMI patients from a non-epicenter implying severe condition might be not the only driving factor for admission. Medical responses affected by the pandemic might be also important for seeking assistance at symptom onset. Interestingly, an observational study from Italy found that although myocardial infarction hospitalizations significantly decreased, FMC-balloon time remained unchanged after the outbreak (27). The result might be firstly attributed to the excellent reorganization for local hospital activities. Secondly, compared with our study, Italian patients were younger and had fewer cardiovascular risk factors, and were more likely to seek medical assistance timely due to striking symptoms and maintain high medical compliance in rescue procedure. FITT-STEMI study from Germany showed high-standard treatment and management for STEMI, reperfusion parameters were almost unaffected during the pandemic (16). This achievement was due to quick public response, very high proportion of EMS transport, high-level routine procedure and pre-existing care network. Based on our findings, we noticed that the pandemic might magnify the shortcomings of the pre-existing treatment pathway, thus still caused a significant delay even in a non-epicenter region. This also meant that only a high-level treatment pathway maintained for a long time could effectively deal with medical burden caused by the pandemic. In the present study, we further provided new evidence for cumulative delays in reperfusion procedure; S-to-FMC was the determinant for prolonged TIT, while slow activation in hospital was pivotal to delayed PPCI. Furthermore, our findings showed the significant correlation between the pandemic and high risk of delayed PPCI. In our opinion, longer FMC-to-W might be interpreted by institutional delays due to protective protocols for screening patients, preparing for equipment and activating personnel in catheter lab. Meanwhile, emergency care overload and staff fatigue should also be taken into consideration certainly. Hence, we proposed the insight as optimizing mechanical reperfusion by controlling cumulative delays.

LIMITATIONS

Our study had several limitations. First, this study was subject to the biases inherent to its retrospective design. Second, clinical characteristics and PPCI parameters were evaluated by trained investigators in each center, without central reconfirmation, potentially resulting biases and errors. Third, our study had a small sample size and no follow-up data for *post-hoc* analysis.

CONCLUSION

The COVID-19 pandemic significantly increased the risk of delayed STEMI reperfusion in a non-epicenter region, probably due to cumulative impact of multiple procedures prolongation.

AUTHOR CONTRIBUTIONS

XZ was responsible for the design. QM, JZ, JC, QX, ZX, YY, YZ, QL, XP, ZheL, BR, ZZ, ZhiL, CZ, and ST contributed to collect and clean the data. QM, JZ, YL, LX, HX, KW, and YQ performed the data analysis. QM wrote the draft of this manuscript. JJ, LH, and XZ contributed to the writing and revision of the paper. All authors contributed to the article and approved the submitted version.

ACKNOWLEDGMENTS

We are grateful for all the participants and investigators for their support.

REFERENCES

1. Ibanez B, James S, Agewall S, Antunes MJ, Bucciarelli-Ducci C, Bueno H, et al. 2017 ESC Guidelines for the management of acute myocardial infarction in patients presenting with ST-segment elevation. *Eur Heart J.* (2018) 39:119–77. doi: 10.1093/eurheartj/ehx393
2. Danchin N, Popovic B, Puymirat E, Goldstein P, Belle L, Cayla G, et al. Five-year outcomes following timely primary percutaneous intervention, late primary percutaneous intervention, or a pharmaco-invasive strategy in ST-segment elevation myocardial infarction: the FAST-MI programme. *Eur Heart J.* (2020) 41:858–66. doi: 10.1093/eurheartj/ehz665
3. World Health Organization. *Coronavirus Disease 2019 Situation Report.* Available online at: https://www.who.int/emergencies/diseases/novel-coronavirus-2019/situation-reports/ (accessed February 24, 2021).
4. Boukhris M, Hillani A, Moroni F, Annabi MS, Addad F, Ribeiro MH, et al. Cardiovascular implications of the COVID-19 pandemic: a global perspective. *Can J Cardiol.* (2020) 36:1068–80. doi: 10.1016/j.cjca.2020.05.018
5. Jacobs AK, Ali M, Best PJ, Bieniarz M, Cohen MG, French WJ, et al. Temporary emergency guidance to STEMI systems of care during the COVID-19 pandemic. *Circulation.* (2020) 142:199–202. doi: 10.1161/CIRCULATIONAHA.120.048180
6. Roffi M, Guagliumi G, Ibanez B. The obstacle course of reperfusion for ST-segment-elevation myocardial infarction in the COVID-19 pandemic. *Circulation.* (2020) 141:1951–3. doi: 10.1161/CIRCULATIONAHA.120.047523
7. Rodríguez-Leor O, Cid-Álvarez B, Pérez De Prado A, Rossello X, Ojeda S, Serrador A, et al. Impact of COVID-19 on ST-segment elevation myocardial infarction care. The Spanish experience. *Rev Esp Cardiol.* (2020) 73:994–1002. doi: 10.1016/j.recesp.2020.07.033
8. Xiang D, Xiang X, Zhang W, Yi S, Zhang J, Gu X, et al. Management and outcomes of patients with STEMI during the COVID-19 pandemic in China. *J Am Coll Cardiol.* (2020) 76:1318–24. doi: 10.1016/j.jacc.2020.06.039
9. Garcia S, Albaghdadi MS, Meraj PM, Schmidt C, Garberich R, Jaffer FA, et al. Reduction in ST-segment elevation cardiac catheterization laboratory activations in the United States during COVID-19 pandemic. *J Am Coll Cardiol.* (2020) 75:2871–2. doi: 10.1016/j.jacc.2020.04.011
10. NHCotPsRo, China. *Chinese Clinical Guideline for COVID-19 Diagnosis and Treatment.* 7th ed. National Health Committee (2020). Available online at: http://www.nhc.gov.cn/yzygj/s7653p/202003/46c9294a7dfe4cef80dc7f5912eb1989.shtml (accessed March 4, 2020).
11. Xiang D, Huo Y, Ge J. Expert consensus on operating procedures at chest pain centers in China during the coronavirus infectious disease-19 epidemic. *Cardiol Plus.* (2020) 5:21–32. doi: 10.4103/cp.cp_5_20
12. Han Y, Zeng H, Jiang H, Yang Y, Yuan Z, Cheng X, et al. CSC expert consensus on principles of clinical management of patients with severe emergent cardiovascular diseases during the COVID-19 epidemic. *Circulation.* (2020) 141:e810–6. doi: 10.1161/CIRCULATIONAHA.120.047011
13. Thygesen K, Alpert JS, Jaffe AS, Chaitman BR, Bax JJ, Morrow DA, et al. Fourth universal definition of myocardial infarction (2018). *Circulation.* (2018) 138:e618–51. doi: 10.1161/CIR.0000000000000617
14. Fox KA, Dabbous OH, Goldberg RJ, Pieper KS, Eagle KA, Van de Werf F, et al. Prediction of risk of death and myocardial infarction in the six months after presentation with acute coronary syndrome: prospective multinational observational study (GRACE). *BMJ.* (2006) 333:1091. doi: 10.1136/bmj.38985.646481.55
15. Mahmud E, Dauerman HL, Welt FGP, Messenger JC, Rao SV, Grines C, et al. Management of acute myocardial infarction during the COVID-19 pandemic: a position statement from the society for cardiovascular angiography and interventions (SCAI), the American college of cardiology (ACC), and the American college of emergency physicians (ACEP). *J Am Coll Cardiol.* (2020) 76:1375–84. doi: 10.1016/j.jacc.2020.04.039
16. Scholz KH, Lengenfelder B, Thilo C, Jeron A, Stefanow S, Janssens U, et al. Impact of COVID-19 outbreak on regional STEMI care in Germany. *Clin Res Cardiol.* (2020) 109:1511–21. doi: 10.1007/s00392-020-01703-z
17. Zhang Y, Yu B, Han Y, Wang J, Yang L, Wan Z, et al. Protocol of the China ST-segment elevation myocardial infarction (STEMI) care project (CSCAP): a 10-year project to improve quality of care by building up a regional STEMI care network. *BMJ Open.* (2019) 9:e26362. doi: 10.1136/bmjopen-2018-026362
18. De Luca G, Verdoia M, Cercek M, Jensen LO, Vavlukis M, Calmac L, et al. Impact of COVID-19 pandemic on mechanical reperfusion for patients with STEMI. *J Am Coll Cardiol.* (2020) 76:2321–30. doi: 10.1016/j.jacc.2020.09.546
19. Welt F, Shah PB, Aronow HD, Bortnick AE, Henry TD, Sherwood MW, et al. Catheterization laboratory considerations during the coronavirus (COVID-

19) pandemic: from the ACC's interventional council and SCAI. *J Am Coll Cardiol.* (2020) 75:2372–5. doi: 10.1016/j.jacc.2020.03.021

20. Hannan EL, Zhong Y, Jacobs AK, Holmes DR, Walford G, Venditti FJ, et al. Effect of onset-to-door time and door-to-balloon time on mortality in patients undergoing percutaneous coronary interventions for ST-segment elevation myocardial infarction. *Am J Cardiol.* (2010) 106:143–7. doi: 10.1016/j.amjcard.2010.02.029

21. Vogel B, Claessen BE, Arnold SV, Chan D, Cohen DJ, Giannitsis E, et al. ST-segment elevation myocardial infarction. *Nat Rev Dis Primers.* (2019) 5:39. doi: 10.1038/s41572-019-0090-3

22. Zheng YY, Ma YT, Zhang JY, Xie X. COVID-19 and the cardiovascular system. *Nat Rev Cardiol.* (2020) 17:259–60. doi: 10.1038/s41569-020-0360-5

23. Tam CF, Cheung K, Lam S, Wong A, Yung A, Sze M, et al. Impact of coronavirus disease 2019 (COVID-19) outbreak on ST-segment-elevation myocardial infarction care in Hong Kong, China. *Circ Cardiovasc Qual Outcomes.* (2020) 13:e6631. doi: 10.1161/CIRCOUTCOMES.120.006631

24. Siudak Z, Grygier M, Wojakowski W, Malinowski KP, Witkowski A, Gasior M, et al. Clinical and procedural characteristics of COVID-19 patients treated with percutaneous coronary interventions. *Catheter Cardiovasc Interv.* (2020) 96:E568–75. doi: 10.1002/ccd.29134

25. Clifford C R, Le May M, Chow A, Boudreau R, Fu A, Barry Q, et al. Delays in ST-elevation myocardial infarction care during the COVID-19 lockdown: an observational study. *CJC Open.* (2020) 3:565–73. doi: 10.1016/j.cjco.2020.12.009

26. Hammad T A, Parikh M, Tashtish N, Lowry CM, Gorbey D, Forouzandeh F, et al. Impact of COVID-19 pandemic on ST-elevation myocardial infarction in a non-COVID-19 epicenter. *Catheter Cardiovasc Interv.* (2021) 97:208–14. doi: 10.1002/ccd.28997

27. Campo G, Fortuna D, Berti E, De Palma R, Pasquale GD, Galvani M, et al. In- and out-of-hospital mortality for myocardial infarction during the first wave of the COVID-19 pandemic in Emilia-Romagna, Italy: a population-based observational study. *Lancet Reg Health Eur.* (2021) 3:100055. doi: 10.1016/j.lanepe.2021.100055

14

Myocarditis Associated with COVID-19 mRNA Vaccination Following Myocarditis Associated with *Campylobacter Jejuni*

Nobuko Kojima[1], Hayato Tada[1]*, Hirofumi Okada[1], Shohei Yoshida[1], Kenji Sakata[1], Soichiro Usui[1], Hiroko Ikeda[2], Masaki Okajima[3], Masa-aki Kawashiri[1] and Masayuki Takamura[1]

[1] Department of Cardiovascular Medicine, Kanazawa University Graduate School of Medical Sciences, Kanazawa, Japan,
[2] Diagnostic Pathology, Kanazawa University Hospital, Kanazawa, Japan, [3] Department of Emergency Medicine, Kanazawa University Hospital, Kanazawa, Japan

*Correspondence:
Hayato Tada
ht240z@sa3.so-net.ne.jp

We herein present our experience with a case involving a 17-year-old Japanese boy suffering from acute myocarditis after his second coronavirus disease-2019 (COVID-19) messenger RNA (mRNA) vaccine shot. The patients had a history of myocarditis associated with *Campylobacter jejuni* 3 years prior. This has been the first-ever documented case of myocarditis associated with COVID-19 mRNA vaccination in a patient with a history of myocarditis. We present a series of images and blood biomarkers for different types of myocarditis that developed in this single patient.

Keywords: cardiomyopathy, left ventricle, chest pain, myocarditis, COVID-19

LEARNING OBJECTIVE

History of myocarditis may be a risk factor for COVID-19 mRNA vaccine-associated myocarditis. Thus, vigilance is required for patients with such a history when considering indications for COVID-19 mRNA vaccination, especially among young boys.

INTRODUCTION

Myocarditis, the main cause of which is viral infections such as coronavirus disease 2019 (COVID-19), is a rare condition, wherein signs of inflammation can be observed in the myocardium (1, 2). Studies have shown that other conditions such as nonviral infections, autoimmune syndromes, and vaccines can also cause myocarditis (1). Soon after the introduction of COVID-19 mRNA vaccination, many case reports exhibiting acute myocarditis associated with the vaccination had emerged (3–5). Accumulated data appear to suggest that the occurrence of myocarditis is more frequent among young adult and adolescent males (6–8). However, it remains unclear whether other risk factors, particularly a history of myocarditis, are present for this condition. Given the current global situation caused by the COVID-19 pandemic, additional data regarding this issue, especially among younger individuals, need to be accumulated. We herein present the first-ever documented case of acute myocarditis associated with COVID-19 mRNA vaccination in a patient who had a history of myocarditis.

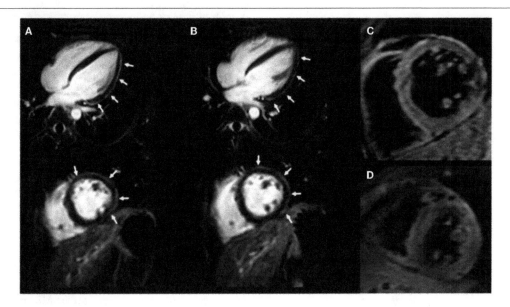

FIGURE 1 | Cardiac MRI imaging. Diffuse late gadolinium enhancement at the epicardium was observed in both images. **(A)** Images obtained 3 years ago when he suffered from his previous myocarditis (top: long-axis view, bottom: short-axis view). **(B)** Images obtained during the current myocarditis episode associated with coronavirus disease-2019 (COVID-19) messenger RNA (mRNA) vaccination (top: long-axis view, bottom: short-axis view). T2-weighted MR images. **(C)** Image obtained 3 years ago when he suffered from his previous myocarditis episode. **(D)** Image obtained during the current myocarditis episode associated with COVID-19 mRNA vaccination.

CASE DESCRIPTION

History of Presentation

A 17-year-old Japanese boy, with chest pain occurring 2 days after his second COVID-19 mRNA vaccination (BNT 162b2, manufactured by Pfizer and BioNTech), was presented to a previous hospital. Electrocardiography showed ST elevation in V2 to V5 leads (**Supplemental Material**). Moreover, his serum cardiac enzymes, including cardiac troponin T (1.605 ng/ml, normal range ≤0.014 ng/ml) and creatinine kinase (CK, 462 IU/L, normal range 62–287 IU/L) were elevated. He was then referred to Kanazawa University Hospital for further investigation and treatment of his chest symptom.

Medical History

The patient had a history of myocarditis (causative bacteria was *Campylobacter*) when he was 13 years old, which was treated with intravenous immunoglobulin (IVIG). His initial symptoms included fever, chest pain, and diarrhea. His maximum CK was 1,682 IU/L. Cardiac MRI revealed diffuse late gadolinium enhancement at the epicardium (**Figure 1A**). A cardiac biopsy was not performed. After the introduction of IVIG, his symptoms improved, for which he was discharged from the hospital without any apparent cardiac dysfunction assessed by echocardiography and myocardial scintigraphy. Enalapril 5 mg/day was introduced and was discontinued 1 year after this episode. He received regular follow-up at our institute, during which, his serum cardiac enzymes were assessed, and electrocardiography and

Abbreviations: CK, creatinine kinase; IVIG, intravenous immunoglobulin; MRI, magnetic resonance imaging; LVEF, left ventricular ejection fraction.

echocardiography were performed. No signs of recurrence had been observed until his last visit 6 days before his second COVID-19 mRNA vaccination. Echocardiography revealed a normal left ventricular ejection fraction (LVEF = 75%), without other dilatations in any chambers, and his cardiac troponin T level was within the normal range (0.006 ng/ml) in his last visit (6 days before his second COVID-19 mRNA vaccination).

Differential Diagnosis

Acute coronary syndrome and acute systolic heart failure of any cause were considered as differential diagnoses.

Diagnostic Assessment

Upon admission to our hospital, the patient had blood pressure, heart rate, and body temperature of 135/65 mmHg, 97 bpm, and 37.3°C, respectively. Chest radiography showed no signs of cardiomegaly or pulmonary congestion. Blood tests revealed an elevation in white blood cells (9,560/μl) and C-reactive protein (4.44 mg/dl, normal range ≤0.3 mg/dl), together with elevations in cardiac enzymes, including CK (818 IU/L, normal range 62–287 IU/L), CK-MB (59 IU/L, normal range 2–21 IU/L), and cardiac troponin T (1.41 ng/ml, normal range ≤0.014 ng/ml). The N-terminal pro-brain natriuretic peptide (NT-pro BNP) level was also elevated (221.2 pg/ml, normal range ≤ 125 pg/ml). Electrocardiography revealed ST elevations in V2–V5 leads, whereas echocardiography revealed systolic dysfunction (LVEF = 55%) associated with left ventricular dilatation (LVDd, 55 mm) without any pericardial effusion. Coronary CT showed no signs of coronary atherosclerosis. A myocardial specimen obtained from the septum of the right

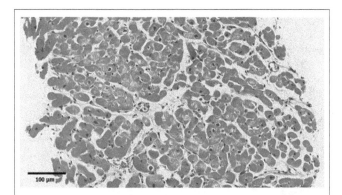

FIGURE 2 | Pathological specimens. Hematoxylin and eosin staining (original magnification ×200). The black bar indicates 100 μm. No apparent signs of inflammation were observed.

ventricle showed no apparent signs of myocardial destruction or inflammation (**Figure 2**). Hemodynamic evaluation by Swan–Ganz catheterization revealed a pulmonary artery pressure of 27/11 (19) mmHg, pulmonary capillary wedge pressure of 13 mmHg, and cardiac output of 6.62 L/min. Cardiac MRI revealed diffuse late gadolinium enhancement at the epicardium (**Figure 1B**) that was similar but somewhat different from the images observed 3 years prior when he suffered from his previous myocarditis (**Figure 1A**). A T2-weighted MRI revealed diffuse high-intensity areas, suggesting edematous changes in the left ventricle during his previous bout of myocarditis, as well as during the current myocarditis (**Figures 1C,D**). Enzyme-linked immunosorbent assays of sera were all negative for potential causes of viral myocarditis (Coxsackie, echo, influenza A and B, cytomegalovirus, and Epstein-Barr virus (EBV)]. Negative T waves were observed in V3 to V6 leads following electrocardiography on day 5 (**Supplemental Material**). All the aforementioned results, except for pathological findings from the myocardial specimen, were consistent with a diagnosis of COVID-19 mRNA vaccination-related myocarditis. We ruled out acute coronary syndrome given the absence of cardiac asynergy and cardiac MRI findings. We also ruled out acute systolic heart failure of any cause based on the hemodynamic evaluation findings by Swan–Ganz catheterization.

Management

The patient was started on IVIG treatment (5 g/day × 3 days), colchicine (0.5 g/day × 14 days), and aspirin (300 mg/day × 14 days) (**Figure 3**). The Japanese guideline (9) utilized by our institute has no clear first-choice therapy for this situation. Among several potential medical therapies, we opted to use IVIG to avoid complications when using immunosuppressive agents. The CK, CK–MB, cardiac troponin T, and NT-proBNP levels gradually returned to normal, and follow-up echocardiography showed normal cardiac function (LVEF = 68%). After being hospitalized for a total of 23 days, the patient was discharged without any symptoms.

DISCUSSION

Currently, myocarditis is being recognized as one of the complications of COVID-19 mRNA vaccination (1–3). Albeit rare, the prognosis of this condition seems to be quite good. Nonetheless, more information on risk factors for this unfavorable phenomenon needs to be collected (6–8). So far, epidemiological studies have suggested that this condition is more frequently observed among young adult and adolescent males (6–8). However, it is unclear whether a history of other types of myocarditis can be considered a risk factor. In this report, we present the first-ever documented case of myocarditis associated with COVID-19 mRNA vaccination in a patient who had a history of myocarditis (**Supplemental Material**). Based on a series of investigations, including cardiac enzymes, electrocardiogram, echocardiography, and cardiac MRI, we found similarities between COVID-19 mRNA vaccination-related myocarditis and myocarditis associated with *Campylobacter jejuni*. We observed unique yet similar patterns on cardiac MRI wherein diffuse late gadolinium enhancement was located mainly at the epicardium during both the current COVID-19 mRNA vaccination-related myocarditis and the previous myocarditis episode associated with *Campylobacter jejuni*. Cardiac MRI has been considered a useful modality for diagnosing acute myocarditis (10, 11) given its great potential for not only diagnosis but also understanding of the pathophysiological mechanism of COVID-19 mRNA vaccination-related myocarditis (12–14). There are several limitations to be considered. First, we obtained three specimens at the time of endomyocardial biopsy. Although the patient had no apparent signs of myocardial destruction or inflammation from the endomyocardial biopsy, a diagnosis of myocarditis was established because of his elevated cardiac troponin T, elevated creatinine kinase, reduced EF, changes in the electrocardiogram, and MRI findings. Second, we could not determine the causal association between the history of myocarditis and the current vaccination-associated myocarditis. Third, we did not compare the cardiac MR images between the previous and current myocarditis episodes. Thus, the diffuse late gadolinium enhancement at the epicardium observed during the current myocarditis episode may not have represented acute myocarditis. However, we observed edematous changes in the myocardium using T2-weighted MR images. In addition, the area of late gadolinium enhancement at the epicardium observed in the current myocarditis episode was somewhat different from that of the previous one. These facts support the notion that late gadolinium enhancement at the epicardium observed in the current episode represents acute myocarditis. Lastly, we were unable to perform the suggested immunohistochemical testing on our biopsy specimens to investigate whether there were any autoantibodies against the myocardium. The second episode might, indeed, be associated with post-infectious autoimmune syndrome; however, this situation has been described as a chronic condition rather than an acute one with complications in multiple organs (1). Of note is that the mechanism of myocarditis induced by mRNA vaccination remains unclear. In most cases without a history of previous myocarditis,

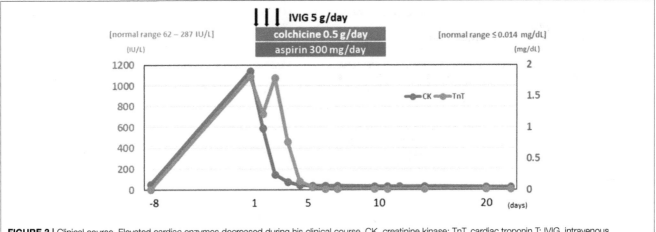

FIGURE 3 | Clinical course. Elevated cardiac enzymes decreased during his clinical course. CK, creatinine kinase; TnT, cardiac troponin T; IVIG, intravenous immunoglobulin.

molecular mimicry between the spike protein of virus and self-antigens, trigger of pre-existing dysregulated immune pathways in certain individuals, immune response to mRNA, activation of immunologic pathways, and dysregulated cytokine expression have been proposed (8). However, in this case with a history of myocarditis, there may be something more in addition to these common mechanisms, although observations from a single case cannot produce any concrete evidence.

In conclusion, special attention may be needed when introducing COVID-19 mRNA vaccination to individuals who have a history of myocarditis. Cardiac MRI can be useful for diagnosing COVID-19 mRNA vaccination-related myocarditis.

PATIENT PERSPECTIVE

We suggest that this episode would not have any serious impact on his cardiac function. However, we will advise the patient

to avoid the booster COVID-19 mRNA vaccine because of this episode.

AUTHOR CONTRIBUTIONS

NK, HT, HO, SY, KS, SU, HI, MO, M-aK, and MT contributed to the patient's care and contributed to the preparation of the manuscript. All authors approved the final version of the manuscript.

ACKNOWLEDGMENTS

We thank Ms. Kazuko Honda and Sachio Yamamoto for their technical assistance.

REFERENCES

1. Heymans S, Eriksson U, Lehtonen J, Cooper LT Jr. The quest for new approaches in myocarditis and inflammatory cardiomyopathy. *J Am Coll Cardiol.* (2016) 68:2348–64. doi: 10.1016/j.jacc.2016.09.937
2. Siripanthong B, Nazarian S, Muser D, Deo R, Santangeli P, Khanji MY, et al. Recognizing COVID-19-related myocarditis: the possible pathophysiology and proposed guideline for diagnosis and management. *Heart Rhythm.* (2020) 17:1463–71. doi: 10.1016/j.hrthm.2020.05.001
3. Abu Mouch S, Roguin A, Hellou E, Ishai A, Shoshan U, Mahamid L, et al. Myocarditis following COVID-19 mRNA vaccination. *Vaccine.* (2021) 39:3790–3. doi: 10.1016/j.vaccine.2021.05.087
4. Mansour J, Short RG, Bhalla S, Woodard PK, Verma A, Robinson X, et al. Acute myocarditis after a second dose of the mRNA COVID-19 vaccine: a report of two cases. *Clin Imaging.* (2021) 78:247–9. doi: 10.1016/j.clinimag.2021.06.019

5. Dickey JB, Albert E, Badr M, Laraja KM, Sena LM, Gerson DS, et al. A series of patients with myocarditis following SARS-CoV-2 vaccination with mRNA-1279 and BNT162b2. *JACC Cardiovasc Imaging.* (2021) 14:1862–3. doi: 10.1016/j.jcmg.2021.06.003
6. Barda N, Dagan N, Ben-Shlomo Y, Kepten E, Waxman J, Ohana R, et al. Safety of the BNT162b2 mRNA Covid-19 vaccine in a nationwide setting. *N Engl J Med.* (2021) 385:1078–90. doi: 10.1056/NEJMoa2110475
7. Dionne A, Sperotto F, Chamberlain S, Baker AL, Powell AJ, Prakash A, et al. Association of myocarditis with BNT162b2 messenger RNA COVID-19 vaccine in a case series of children. *JAMA Cardiol.* (2021) 6:1446–50. doi: 10.1001/jamacardio.2021.3471
8. Bozkurt B, Kamat I, Hotez PJ. Myocarditis with COVID-19 mRNA vaccines. *Circulation.* (2021) 144:471–84. doi: 10.1161/CIRCULATIONAHA.121.056135
9. JCS Joint Working Group. Guidelines for diagnosis and treatment of myocarditis (JCS 2009): digest version. *Circ J.* (2011) 75:734–43. doi: 10.1253/circj.CJ-88-0008
10. Liguori C, Farina D, Vaccher F, Ferrandino G, Bellini D, Carbone I. Myocarditis: imaging up to date. *Radiol Med.* (2020) 125:1124–34. doi: 10.1007/s11547-020-01279-8

11. Ammirati E, Veronese G, Bottiroli M, Wang DW, Cipriani M, Garascia A, et al. Update on acute myocarditis. *Trends Cardiovasc Med.* (2021) 31:370–9. doi: 10.1016/j.tcm.2020.05.008

12. Isaak A, Feisst A, Luetkens JA. Myocarditis following COVID-19 vaccination. *Radiology.* (2021) 301:E378–9. doi: 10.1148/radiol.2021211766

13. Maurus S, Weckbach LT, Marschner C, Kunz WG, Ricke J, Kazmierczak PM, et al. Differences in cardiac magnetic resonance imaging markers between patients with COVID-19-associated myocardial injury and patients with clinically suspected myocarditis. *J Thorac Imaging.* (2021) 36:279–85. doi: 10.1097/RTI.0000000000000599

14. Tanacli R, Doeblin P, Götze C, Zieschang V, Faragli A, Stehning C, et al. COVID-19 vs. classical myocarditis associated myocardial injury evaluated by cardiac magnetic resonance and endomyocardial biopsy. *Front Cardiovasc Med.* (2021) 8:737257. doi: 10.3389/fcvm.2021.737257

15

Innovation in Precision Cardio-Oncology During the Coronavirus Pandemic and into a Post-Pandemic World

Sherry-Ann Brown[1]*, June-Wha Rhee[2], Avirup Guha[3] and Vijay U. Rao[4]

[1] Cardio-Oncology Program, Division of Cardiovascular Medicine, Medical College of Wisconsin, Milwaukee, WI, United States, [2] Stanford Cardiovascular Institute, Stanford University, Stanford, CA, United States, [3] Harrington Heart and Vascular Institute, Case Western Reserve University, Cleveland, OH, United States, [4] Franciscan Health, Indianapolis, Indiana Heart Physicians, Indianapolis, IN, United States

*Correspondence:
Sherry-Ann Brown
shbrown@mcw.edu

Keywords: innovation, precision, cardio-oncology, artificial intelligence, machine learning, big data, digital health, telemedicine

INTRODUCTION

Almost 2 million new cancer diagnoses will be made and more than 600,000 cancer deaths will occur in 2020, the equivalent of 5,000 new cases and 1,600 deaths daily (1). Juxtaposed with these staggering numbers is the prevalence of ~17 million cancer survivors in the United States, with a projected estimate of 26 million in 2040 (2); advances in cancer treatments have significantly improved survival across cancers. With growing numbers of survivors comes a growing number of individuals at risk for or living with higher rates of cardiovascular disease than in the general population. In fact, cardiovascular disease is a leading cause of death in cancer survivors, second only to cancer recurrence or the development of new primary cancers (3). Consequently, Cardio-Oncology has emerged as a new field of medicine to specifically address cardiovascular care of cancer patients and survivors, with a particular focus on prevention.

Reminiscent of cardiovascular toxicities from cancer therapies, the recent coronavirus disease of 2019 (COVID-19) pandemic is a clear example of how cardiotoxicities can arise unexpectedly and how adaptable clinicians need to be to deal with a constant flow of new cardiotoxic agents and their complications. The severe acute respiratory syndrome coronavirus 2 (SARS-CoV-2) has arisen as an emergent cardiotoxic agent, underlying COVID-19. By July 2020, more than 18 million confirmed cases and 600,000 deaths had been reported globally (4). In positive cases, direct and indirect cardiovascular (CV) injury has been noted as a prominent feature (5, 6), mediated by hypoxia, inflammation, demand ischemia, microvascular dysfunction, or thrombosis (7–10). Around the world, our patients have been physically and socially distancing themselves from others and avoiding physical entrance of health care facilities, in order to limit exposure in COVID-19. Correspondingly, health care institutions have restricted non-emergent in-person visits, to curb the rates of morbidity and mortality from COVID-19. Individuals with known CV disease or risk factors have been at greater risk of morbidity and mortality in COVID-19 (11–16), as is similar in Cardio-Oncology (17). Therefore, there is an urgent need for various avenues of innovation to predict cardiovascular risk and customize preventive, diagnostic, and management care plans in the setting of cancer therapies, especially during the pandemic and beyond. Here, we briefly describe forms of innovation implemented during the pandemic, as well as innovative tools being explored for utility beyond the pandemic (**Figure 1**).

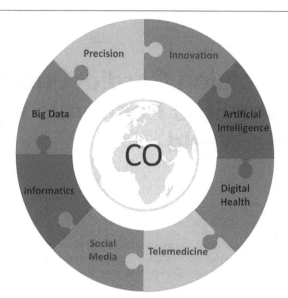

Precision

Personalize care based on therapies, genotypes, 'omics', clinical variables, biomarkers, and environmental exposures

Big Data

Collect and harmonize abundant health data from EHRs, payer records, imaging, digital technologies, and research

Informatics

Integrate, synthesize, and mine clinical and biomedical data to provide epidemiologic insights and inform research

Social Media

Share knowledge, research, advocacy, and support in a global community involving patients, families and health care workers

Innovation

Customize and innovate preventive, diagnostic, and management care plans in the setting of therapies

Artificial Intelligence

Employ artificial intelligence algorithms for survivorship tracking, risk stratification, diagnostics, and therapeutic discoveries

Digital Health

Augment health care through mobile health, information technology, wearables, and virtual platforms

Telemedicine

Improve access to care, enhance preventive services, and reduce health care costs through virtual visit platforms

FIGURE 1 | Various forms of Innovation advance Precision Medicine in Cardio-Oncology or COVID-19, with the use of Informatics to integrate Big Data from Artificial Intelligence, Digital Health, Telemedicine, and Social Media. CO denotes either Cardio-Oncology or COVID-19 or both.

INNOVATION DURING THE PANDEMIC

Digital Health

Digital health technologies include mobile health (mHealth), wearable devices, health information technologies, wireless technologies, virtual platforms and applications, telehealth, telemedicine, artificial intelligence, machine learning, and personalized medicine, with a common goal of improving health care outcomes and efficiency (18). With more and more personalized health and lifestyle information available through digital technologies, care providers are better able to monitor patients' conditions in real time or by retrieving remote data recently stored by patients' local devices, identify treatment side effects, and personalize prevention and intervention strategies. Digital technologies can also empower and engage patients to proactively monitor their health while preventing unnecessary hospital visits, which is especially critical in times of a pandemic such as COVID-19 (19). With the implementation of shelter-in-place and subsequent rapid adaptation of virtual visits during this COVID-19 outbreak, the ability to remotely monitor patients' clinical conditions through digital technologies has become more important than ever.

Remote monitoring can enhance our care of cancer patients and survivors. For example, a wearable cardiac rhythm monitoring device such as an Apple watch can detect abnormal heart rates or rhythms (20). As atrial fibrillation is a common side effect of various cancer therapies, including multiple classes of novel tyrosine kinase inhibitors, the ability to detect this rhythm abnormality early and accurately through a wearable cardiac rhythm monitoring device would have an important impact in the ongoing care, as well as future treatment decisions, for cancer patients (21). Abnormal rhythm strips detected from these devices can now be shared and reviewed by the

care team, which can potentially alter the treatment course and prevent undesirable toxicities. Another example is virtual cardiac rehabilitation and monitoring (22). Cancer therapies such as doxorubicin can cause myocardial injury and cardiac dysfunction, requiring close monitoring and preferably a tailored rehabilitation program as patients work to recover (23). Virtual rehab programs enable remote collection and evaluation of health data such as activity levels, blood pressures, heart rate/rhythms, and weight, which can be reviewed and acted upon when necessary by health care providers, allowing cancer patients and survivors to safely and efficiently recover from their cardiac complications. This has been of particular importance during COVID-19 pandemic, as many have avoided or limited outdoor physical activities. Guided virtual indoor rehabilitation would allow cancer patients and survivors to continue physical conditioning and rehabilitation and thereby remain physically active during the pandemic.

Digital technologies can provide the unique ability to quickly scale to larger populations with less time, money, and resources, and thereby facilitate near real-time data insights that allow for point-of-service execution (24). These technologies will be critical in caring for cancer patients and survivors, as their numbers continue to increase, with more cancer therapies and related cardiotoxicity profiles dynamically changing daily.

Telemedicine

Telemedicine or telehealth is the delivery of healthcare at a distance utilizing various technology platforms. Health care systems have recently devoted increased resources to implementation of telemedicine or telehealth services during the pandemic, building upon prior goals of improving access to specialty care, enhancing preventive services, reducing health care costs, and improving patient and provider safety and satisfaction (25, 26). Numerous platforms have been actualized (27), including those embedded within electronic health records (e.g., In-Touch through EPIC) or third-party vendors such as *Doxy.me* or Zoom. Many of the software solutions are cloud-based, accessible (requiring only a desktop, tablet, or smartphone), and free, and have prioritized being HIPAA (Health Insurance Portability and Accountability Act)-compliant. However, security concerns have arisen with some vendors, leading to more careful attention to cybersecurity to enable telemedicine. Indeed, to facilitate wide-spread adoption of telemedicine, great emphasis on protection of patient information through cybersecurity technology will be key, in tandem with the persistence of government-supported regulations and initiatives.

Adoption of these platforms has been expedited during the pandemic to dramatically reduce in-person clinical visits and conform to social distancing (28). The US federal government has taken steps to support rapid and widespread utilization of telemedicine by allowing cross-state accreditation, developing new telemedicine billing codes, and temporarily reducing strict privacy restrictions while still protecting patients and providers (29). As a result, practices across the country converted to virtual clinics in a matter of weeks. This conversion has been especially important for our cardio-oncology patients, who are particularly vulnerable, given their high cardiovascular disease burden and immunocompromised states placing them at high risk for COVID-19 (30). Cardio-oncology, which relies heavily on the patient history and our understanding of cancer therapy regimens, is ideally suited to make the transition to telemedicine.

A recent report described the virtual adaptation of a Cardio-Oncology clinic (31). Suggestions for ensuring a successful patient-centered telemedicine visit include making eye contact with the patient, thanking the patient for inviting the provider into their home, and intentionally offering an excellent "webside" manner. It may become commonplace for initial cardio-oncology consultations to occur via a virtual platform, with follow-up visits (e.g., for reports on home blood pressures) occurring via telephone or secure messaging. Telemedicine could optimize cardio-oncologic care with (i) three-way video or teleconferences enabling the patient/oncologist/cardio-oncologist to collaboratively initiate treatment plans and monitoring algorithms similar to virtual multidisciplinary tumor boards, (ii) follow-up visits to monitor for hypertension and review cardiac function on surveillance imaging in patients on active cancer therapy, and (iii) access points to specialized cardio-oncologist expertise for oncologists in the community (32). While COVID-19 has exposed many limitations in our healthcare system, the expansion and integration of telemedicine in clinical practice will undoubtedly continue to play a larger role than ever before (33), and we are well-poised in cardio-oncology to help lead the way and benefit from this widespread adoption. The Association of American Medical Colleges has submitted a letter to the Centers for Medicare and Medicaid Services to appeal for the permanence of the widescale telemonitoring

provisions made during the pandemic[1]. Bipartisan senators and other groups have also submitted similar letters in their respective spheres. With support from the senate and other governmental bodies, telemedicine will likely prevail after the pandemic.

Social Media

Social media provides an incredible opportunity for healthcare workers and patients and their families to share and exchange knowledge, research, and advocacy, and support in a global community. Spreading education and awareness on social media can propagate messages for prevention and disseminate discoveries and innovation (34–36). Online resources provide timely and timeless sources of information that can have tremendous impact for patients and health professionals if curated appropriately and accurately.

Social distancing during the COVID-19 pandemic has led to enhanced experiences of social networking online, as both patients and healthcare workers reached out to strengthen community and further buttress knowledge, for example, on Facebook (Facebook, Inc.; www.facebook.com) and Twitter (Twitter, Inc.; www.twitter.com) (37–42). Community and sharing of information were developed by patients among each other, healthcare workers among each other, and with cross-pollination between the two sets of communities as healthcare workers themselves became patients in the pandemic.

Social media integrated with the rise of telemedicine or telehealth, with creation of the hashtag #TelemedNow on Twitter (43), with associated twitter chats and threads. Individuals from various public and private healthcare sectors joined in the real-time discussions to share stories, successes, and challenges from implementing telemedicine or telehealth in response to COVID-19.

At no point did the impact of social media wane during the COVID-19 pandemic. In fact, social media became even more important for innovation, information, and prevention. Preventive Cardio-Oncology, Precision Cardio-Oncology, and other Cardio-Oncology tweets would spread across Twitter before the pandemic. These messages continued throughout the time of COVID-19, as preventive and innovative cardio-oncologic care of our patients remained of paramount value. Several pandemic-related Cardio-Oncology papers have been rapidly published, including one on the role of telehealth (31). Within a few hours, this paper was being disseminated on social media, to be assessed and validated or rebutted by healthcare workers and patients alike. Cardio-Oncology can learn much from the time of COVID-19. Rapid and persistent propagation of information can place relevant details in the palms of cancer patients and survivors and their healthcare providers in real-time. Such innovation should help protect the hearts and wellness of our patients and clinicians.

---

[1]https://www.aamc.org/system/files/2020-05/ocomm-hca-aamclettterto
CMS5132020.pdf

INNOVATION BEYOND THE PANDEMIC

Artificial Intelligence

Much of digital health is driven by artificial intelligence. Remote monitoring, wearables, mobile health (mHealth), voice apps, voice analysis, and drones all depend on the simulation of human intelligence. All of these components can be useful in both the COVID-19 pandemic and the practice of Cardio-Oncology. Many of these technologies are also being explored for various scenarios in cardiology (44–51), and have great clinical utility for cardio-oncology and COVID-19. Remote monitoring from wearable biosensors and mHealth is being investigated to improve outcomes in heart rhythm and heart failure and other cardiovascular conditions (44, 46–50), and may have utility for COVID-19 (19, 52–58) and Cardio-Oncology (59–61). Voice apps and voice analysis have shown promise in cardiology for heart failure, ischemic heart disease, pulmonary hypertension, and other forms of cardiovascular disease (45, 62–64), as well as cardio-oncology (65), and have been considered for COVID-19. Drones built on artificial intelligence are being used to deliver healthcare equipment, medicines, personal protective equipment, and food, especially to remote areas with high rates of illness with COVID-19, and are also being dispatched to dense urban locations to urge pedestrians to maintain social distancing (66–68). Similar drones could be used to transport healthcare equipment, medicines, and supplies to cancer patients and survivors with limited mobilities and care support. Particularly in rural America, where advanced cancer and heart care services are limited (69), drones may facilitate delivery of point-of-care equipment and specialty medicines recommended by cardio-oncologists following remote assessment of cancer patients and survivors through virtual care.

Artificial intelligence algorithms could also be used to track cancer survivors and detect any early signs of cardiovascular risk features, saving lives of those who fought and overcame cancer years before. Other relevant AI applications currently being explored include (1) *in silico* screening to develop novel or repurposed therapeutics, (2) patient tracking by location or geography, (3) online voice apps on smartphones, tablets, and smart speakers to promote drug compliance as well as screen for new symptoms or disseminate educational information, and (4) big data predictive analytics to enhance prediction of disease incidence, severity, spread, and recovery (42, 70–80). There is a myriad of lessons to be learned from incredible technological progress being made during these epic times. The algorithms created or adapted for the era of COVID-19 should remain available for use and wide application in medicine, and especially in cardio-oncology, far beyond the pandemic.

Artificial intelligence has also been integrated with social media and interaction during the pandemic (42, 81). Twitter chatter has been monitored to assess individuals' self-reports of COVID-19 symptoms, testing experience, and recovery from illness (81). Gaps in care for symptomatic individuals have been revealed, due to limited testing capacity, and this has likely compromised accurate case counts of COVID-19 positivity at the city, state, and national, and global level. Interactive chatbots have utilized artificial intelligence to spread COVID-19 awareness and education and provide information and patient guidance (42). Analysis of social media chatter could help identify cancer patients and survivors with symptoms suggestive of cardiovascular toxicity and connect them with healthcare resources in cardio-oncology. Monitoring of social media channels could also help recruit patients into cohort studies and build national and international networks to optimize connectivity and care of cancer survivors.

Precision

Recent advances in multi-omics technologies may help us to collect in-depth large-scale data to better understand disease mechanisms, identify populations at risk, and discover preventive or therapeutic interventions (82). For example, the current state of the sequencing technologies renders whole genome sequencing to be performed in an accelerated and cost-effective (<$1,000) fashion (83). The consequent exponentially increasing genetic knowledge combined with deep cardiovascular phenotyping of cancer patients may allow us to identify genetic variants predicting either increased susceptibility or tolerance for specific drug-induced cardiotoxicity and thereby to risk stratify patients based on their genetic backgrounds (84). The same type of genomic data may also be applied and utilized to identify those at risk for COVID-19 complications. For example, a genome wide association study was recently completed on two case–control panels (835 patients and 1,255 control participants from Italy, and 775 patients and 950 control participants from Spain). The study identified COVID-19 susceptibility genetic loci (3p21.31 gene cluster) which could help risk stratify patients (85).

Additionally, novel biomarker discoveries may be possible through transcriptomics, metabolomics, or proteomics of patients' biological samples (e.g., serum), to complement current imaging-based screening strategies for early detection of cardiotoxicities (86) in cancer and in COVID-19. This is particularly relevant in the era of the COVID-19 pandemic, as we work to avoid clinical encounters or diagnostic studies such as echocardiography that would require in-person interactions (87). More refined biomarkers discovered through multi-omics investigations may allow physicians to closely and accurately monitor cardiotoxicities while minimizing in-person evaluations.

Finally, deeper understanding of ethnic disparities and socioeconomic factors may be achieved through population data-based epigenomics, environmentomics, or populomics, which in turn allows clinicians to assess patients holistically and tailor treatment strategies accordingly (88). Taken together, with accumulating comprehensive omics data, physicians may be able to deliver patients' individualized care based on their cancer therapies, genotypes, phenotypes, biomarker profiles, lifestyle, and surrounding environment, enabling precision cardio-oncology.

Big Data and Informatics

All aforementioned technologies have the potential to create an ever-increasing volume of data on our patients in the COVID-19 and post-pandemic world. Biomedical and clinical informatics

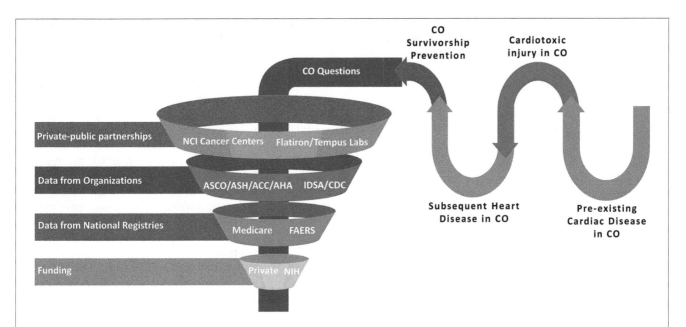

FIGURE 2 | Realms of Big Data such as national medical societies, data science companies (which specialize in patient electronic medical record data management), pharmaceutical industry partners, national databases, and multiple institutions can intersect with CO patient and survivor needs to optimize clinical care and research. This approach can be used to investigate cardiovascular toxic disease or therapy, heart disease predating or as a consequence of CO, survivorship and prevention initiatives, and other relevant themes. Regulatory processes will be needed to ensure preservation of privacy, fairness, inclusiveness, transparency, accountability, and appropriate oversight (79), to ensure the safety of our patients and their protected information. ACC, American College of Cardiology; AHA, American Heart Association; ASCO, American Society of Clinical Oncology; ASH, American Society of Hematology; CDC, Centers for Disease Control and Prevention; CO, either Cardio-Oncology or COVID-19 or both; FAERS, Food and Drug Administration Adverse Event Reporting System; IDSA, Infectious Diseased Society of America; NIH, National Institute of Health. CO denotes either Cardio-Oncology or COVID-19 or both.

can be useful for combining or mining the data and integrating data sources with the electronic health records. In addition, due to social distancing and reduced in-person work hours, traditional pathways of clinical research have been put on hold or disrupted completely. Big data generated from various government and non-government sources can supplement and help restart some of these endeavors amenable to informatics.

Claims-based information from Medicare registries, as well as Surveillance, Epidemiology, and End Results (SEER) databases, in addition to Truven and Healthcare Cost and Utilization Project (HCUP) datasets, can also reveal epidemiological insights regarding incidence, prevalence, trends, costs, and "codable" outcomes (89–91). The International Classification of Disease (ICD) version 10 and Healthcare Common Procedure Coding System (HCPCS) codes that have been created for COVID-19 will be helpful for capturing large-scale data on signs, symptoms, exposure, testing, diagnosis and treatment of this condition (92, 93). These codes may be used across the globe, including in countries which have nationalized healthcare system repositories like Sweden (94), Denmark (95), and the United Kingdom (96). These repositories can also overcome challenges faced when mining anti-cancer therapy information, since drug coverage in the US is heterogenous among insurance companies, resulting in more variability of administration of particular neoplastic drugs.

Several barriers to meaningful collection and use of big data are being quickly overcome during the pandemic, with rapid data-sharing. Challenges with physical recruitment of study participants for prospective studies have halted some pre-existing clinical trials or cohort studies. However, new trials and paradigms have emerged during the pandemic particularly in cancer patients, to facilitate digital clinical trials and cohort studies based on remote monitoring and virtual care (97, 98). Such paradigms enable novel methodology and also allow for continuation of biomedical inquiry in the midst of COVID-19. These tools will not be limited to the pandemic and will likely enrich our conduct of prospective studies in Cardio-Oncology.

Structured multi-pronged approaches should continue to be developed (**Figure 2**), similar to a vision for integrative and collaborative cardio-oncology practice and research laid out in the 2019 Global Cardio-Oncology summit meeting (99). Collective research and clinical practice targets in precision cardio-oncology could be divided among institutions and societies like the American College of Cardiology or American Heart Association, in partnership with large cancer centers. Industry partners should continue to sponsor clinical trials of anti-cancer therapies. Large oncological organizations such as the American Society of Clinical Oncology or the American Society of Hematology should also participate, and privately owned data science companies [e.g., Flatiron Health Inc. and Tempus Labs Inc. (100)] should create databases which are granular to the study of cardio-oncology epidemiology, multi-omics, and biomarkers to inform basic, translational and clinical research to further these aims. These companies work in the field of data management of patient electronic medical record data into analyzable back ends with heavy focus in the field of oncology. However, in light of the recent major retractions of COVID-19 articles that used a large dataset from a private enterprise, a detailed public reporting of data source architecture, data dictionary, and signed attestation by all authors should be mandated while collaborating with private enterprises.

CONCLUSION

The COVID-19 pandemic has dramatically transformed health care and delivery, accelerating and actualizing a wide spectrum of technology solutions. Over the course of just a few weeks, outpatient practices across the country have been converted to virtual clinics to conform to social distancing. Digital technologies have also been rapidly incorporated into clinical care to further complement virtual care. Social media has played more important roles than ever in sharing and disseminating important health care information particularly relevant to cardiovascular complications of COVID-19. Healthcare and biomedical data, as well as precision health, have been assimilated through innovative ways to advance the care of our patients. These advances, along with the lessons learned through our experiences with COVID-19 will undoubtedly reshape our long-term care of patients and survivors in cardio-oncology.

Clinical implementation of these forms of innovation was heralded with the incorporation of "remote patient monitoring" or telemonitoring in the 2016 European Society of Cardiology guidelines for management of heart failure (101). The ACC and AHA have now followed suit and expanded indications for telehealth, remote monitoring, wearables, and other tools in digital medicine throughout the specialty of Cardiology during and after the pandemic (57). New guidelines and recommendations in subsequent years should also encourage the integration of remote monitoring, telemedicine, precision medicine, informatics, and other forms of digital health in electronic health records in Cardio-Oncology, among other medical and surgical specialties. Social media and artificial intelligence should also coalesce with these tools for synergistic monitoring, assessment, and health education. Such integration will help propel optimal care of patients and survivors further along the innovation spectrum in the Digital Post-Pandemic Era.

AUTHOR CONTRIBUTIONS

S-AB conceptualized the manuscript. S-AB, J-WR, AG, and VR drafted, edited, and approved the manuscript for publication. All authors contributed to the article and approved the submitted version.

REFERENCES

1. Siegel RL, Miller KD, Jemal A. Cancer statistics, 2020. *CA Cancer J Clin.* (2020) 70:7–30. doi: 10.3322/caac.21590
2. National Cancer Institute Office of Cancer Survivorship. *Statistics: National Cancer Institute.* (2019). Available online at: https://cancercontrol.cancer.gov/ocs/statistics/index.html (accessed June 30, 2020).
3. Mehta LS, Watson KE, Barac A, Beckie TM, Bittner V, Cruz-Flores S, et al. Cardiovascular disease and breast cancer: where these entities intersect: a scientific statement from the American heart association. *Circulation.* (2018) 137:e30–66. doi: 10.1161/CIR.0000000000000556
4. WHO. *WHO Coronavirus Disease (COVID-19) Dashboard 2020.* Available online at: https://covid19.who.int/ (accessed June 30, 2020).
5. Cheng P, Zhu H, Witteles RM, Wu JC, Quertermous T, Wu SM, et al. Cardiovascular risks in patients with COVID-19: potential mechanisms and areas of uncertainty. *Curr Cardiol Rep.* (2020) 22:34. doi: 10.1007/s11886-020-01293-2
6. Oudit GY, Kassiri Z, Jiang C, Liu PP, Poutanen SM, Penninger JM, et al. SARS-coronavirus modulation of myocardial ACE2 expression and inflammation in patients with SARS. *Eur J Clin Invest.* (2009) 39:618–25. doi: 10.1111/j.1365-2362.2009.02153.x
7. Musher DM, Abers MS, Corrales-Medina VF. Acute infection and myocardial infarction. *N Engl J Med.* (2019) 380:171–6. doi: 10.1056/NEJMc1901647
8. Inciardi RM, Lupi L, Zaccone G, Italia L, Raffo M, Tomasoni D, et al. Cardiac involvement in a patient with coronavirus disease 2019 (COVID-19). *JAMA Cardiol.* (2020) 5:1–6. doi: 10.1001/jamacardio.2020.1096
9. Libby P, Loscalzo J, Ridker PM, Farkouh ME, Hsue PY, Fuster V, et al. Inflammation, immunity, and infection in Atherothrombosis: JACC review topic of the week. *J Am Coll Cardiol.* (2018) 72:2071–81. doi: 10.1016/j.jacc.2018.08.1043
10. Lax SF, Skok K, Zechner P, Kessler HH, Kaufmann N, Koelblinger C, et al. Pulmonary arterial thrombosis in COVID-19 with fatal outcome: results from a prospective, single-center, clinicopathologic case series. *Ann Intern Med.* (2020) 14:M20–2566. doi: 10.7326/M20-2566

11. Ganatra S, Hammond SP, Nohria A. The novel coronavirus disease (COVID-19) threat for patients with cardiovascular disease and cancer. *JACC CardioOncol.* (2020) 2:350–5. doi: 10.1016/j.jaccao.2020.03.001
12. Wu Z, McGoogan JM. Characteristics of and important lessons from the coronavirus disease 2019 (COVID-19) outbreak in China: summary of a Report of 72314 cases from the Chinese center for disease control and prevention. *JAMA.* (2020) 323:1239–42. doi: 10.1001/jama.2020.2648
13. Ky B, Mann DL. COVID-19 clinical trials: a primer for the cardiovascular and cardio-oncology communities. *JACC CardioOncol.* (2020) 2:254–69. doi: 10.1016/j.jaccao.2020.04.002
14. Patel AB, Verma A. COVID-19 and angiotensin-converting enzyme inhibitors and angiotensin receptor blockers: what is the evidence? *JAMA.* (2020) 323:1769–70. doi: 10.1001/jama.2020.4812
15. Asokan I, Rabadia SV, Yang EH. The COVID-19 pandemic and its impact on the cardio-oncology population. *Curr Oncol Rep.* (2020) 22:60. doi: 10.1007/s11912-020-00945-4
16. Lee LYW, Cazier JB, Starkey T, Turnbull CD, Kerr R, Middleton G, et al. COVID-19 mortality in patients with cancer on chemotherapy or other anticancer treatments: a prospective cohort study. *Lancet.* (2020) 395:1919–26. doi: 10.1016/S0140-6736(20)31173-9
17. Armenian SH, Lacchetti C, Barac A, Carver J, Constine LS, Denduluri N, et al. Prevention and monitoring of cardiac dysfunction in survivors of adult cancers: American society of clinical oncology clinical practice guideline. *J Clin Oncol.* (2017) 35:893–911. doi: 10.1200/JCO.2016.70.5400
18. Sharma A, Harrington RA, McClellan MB, Turakhia MP, Eapen ZJ, Steinhubl S, et al. Using digital health technology to better generate evidence and deliver evidence-based care. *J Am Coll Cardiol.* (2018) 71:2680–90. doi: 10.1016/j.jacc.2018.03.523
19. Keesara S, Jonas A, Schulman K. Covid-19 and health care's digital revolution. *N Engl J Med.* (2020) 382:e82. doi: 10.1056/NEJMp2005835
20. Perez MV, Mahaffey KW, Hedlin H, Rumsfeld JS, Garcia A, Ferris T, et al. Large-scale assessment of a smartwatch to identify atrial fibrillation. *N Engl J Med.* (2019) 381:1909–17. doi: 10.1056/NEJMoa1901183
21. Buza V, Rajagopalan B, Curtis AB. Cancer treatment-induced arrhythmias: focus on chemotherapy and targeted therapies. *Circ Arrhythm Electrophysiol.* (2017) 10:e005443. doi: 10.1161/CIRCEP.117.005443

22. Hwang R, Morris NR, Mandrusiak A, Bruning J, Peters R, Korczyk D, et al. Cost-utility analysis of home-based telerehabilitation compared with centre-based rehabilitation in patients with heart failure. *Heart Lung Circ.* (2019) 28:1795–803. doi: 10.1016/j.hlc.2018.11.010

23. Gilchrist SC, Barac A, Ades PA, Alfano CM, Franklin BA, Jones LW, et al. Cardio-oncology rehabilitation to manage cardiovascular outcomes in cancer patients and survivors: a scientific statement from the American heart association. *Circulation.* (2019) 139:e997–1012. doi: 10.1161/CIR.0000000000000679

24. Marceglia S, D'Antrassi P, Prenassi M, Rossi L, Barbieri S. Point of care research: integrating patient-generated data into electronic health records for clinical trials. *AMIA Annu Symp Proc.* (2017) 2017:1262–71.

25. Schwamm LH, Chumbler N, Brown E, Fonarow GC, Berube D, Nystrom K, et al. Recommendations for the implementation of telehealth in cardiovascular and stroke care: a policy statement from the American heart association. *Circulation.* (2017) 135:e24–44. doi: 10.1161/CIR.0000000000000475

26. Mann DM, Chen J, Chunara R, Testa PA, Nov O. COVID-19 transforms health care through telemedicine: evidence from the field. *J Am Med Inform Assoc.* (2020) 27:1132–5. doi: 10.1093/jamia/ocaa072

27. Hollander JE, Carr BG. Virtually perfect? Telemedicine for Covid-19. *N Engl J Med.* (2020) 382:1679–81. doi: 10.1056/NEJMp2003539

28. Gorodeski EZ, Goyal P, Cox ZL, Thibodeau JT, Reay RE, Rasmusson K, et al. Virtual visits for care of patients with heart failure in the Era of COVID-19: a statement from the heart failure society of America. *J Card Fail.* (2020) 26:448–56. doi: 10.1016/j.cardfail.2020.04.008

29. Centers for Medicare and Medicaid Services. *COVID-19 Emergency Declaration Blanket Waivers for Health Care Providers.* (2020). Available online at: https://www.cms.gov/files/document/summary-covid-19-emergency-declaration-waivers.pdf (accessed June 30, 2020).

30. Al-Shamsi HO, Alhazzani W, Alhuraiji A, Coomes EA, Chemaly RF, Almuhanna M, et al. A practical approach to the management of cancer patients during the novel coronavirus disease 2019 (COVID-19) pandemic: an international collaborative group. *Oncologist.* (2020) 25:e936–45. doi: 10.1634/theoncologist.2020-0213

31. Parikh A, Kumar AA, Jahangir E. Cardio-oncology care in the time of COVID-19 and the role of telehealth. *JACC Cardio Oncol.* (2020) 2:356–8. doi: 10.1016/j.jaccao.2020.04.003

32. Dharmarajan H, Anderson JL, Kim S, Sridharan S, Duvvuri U, Ferris RL, et al. Transition to a virtual multidisciplinary tumor board during the COVID-19 pandemic: University of Pittsburgh experience. *Head Neck.* (2020) 42:1310–6. doi: 10.1002/hed.26195

33. Wosik J, Fudim M, Cameron B, Gellad ZF, Cho A, Phinney D, et al. Telehealth transformation: COVID-19 and the rise of virtual care. *J Am Med Inform Assoc.* (2020) 27:957–62. doi: 10.1093/jamia/ocaa067

34. Basch CH, Hillyer GC, Meleo-Erwin ZC, Jaime C, Mohlman J, Basch CE. Preventive behaviors conveyed on youtube to mitigate transmission of COVID-19: cross-sectional study. *JMIR Public Health Surveill.* (2020) 6:e18807. doi: 10.2196/18807

35. Basch CE, Basch CH, Hillyer GC, Jaime C. The role of youtube and the entertainment industry in saving lives by educating and mobilizing the public to adopt behaviors for community mitigation of COVID-19: successive sampling design study. *JMIR Public Health Surveill.* (2020) 6:e19145. doi: 10.2196/19145

36. Sun K, Chen J, Viboud C. Early epidemiological analysis of the coronavirus disease 2019 outbreak based on crowdsourced data: a population-level observational study. *Lancet Digit Health.* (2020) 2:e201–8. doi: 10.1016/S2589-7500(20)30026-1

37. Limaye RJ, Sauer M, Ali J, Bernstein J, Wahl B, Barnhill A, et al. Building trust while influencing online COVID-19 content in the social media world. *Lancet Digit Health.* (2020) 2:e277–8. doi: 10.1016/S2589-7500(20)30084-4

38. Wahbeh A, Nasralah T, Al-Ramahi M, El-Gayar O. Mining physicians' opinions on social media to obtain insights into COVID-19: mixed methods analysis. *JMIR Public Health Surveill.* (2020) 6:e19276. doi: 10.2196/19276

39. Sesagiri Raamkumar A, Tan SG, Wee HL. Measuring the outreach efforts of public health authorities and the public response on facebook during the COVID-19 pandemic in early 2020: cross-country comparison. *J Med Internet Res.* (2020) 22:e19334. doi: 10.2196/preprints.19334

40. Lwin MO, Lu J, Sheldenkar A, Schulz PJ, Shin W, Gupta R, et al. Global sentiments surrounding the COVID-19 pandemic on twitter: analysis of twitter trends. *JMIR Public Health Surveill.* (2020) 6:e19447. doi: 10.2196/19447

41. Chen E, Lerman K, Ferrara E. Tracking social media discourse about the COVID-19 pandemic: development of a public coronavirus twitter data set. *JMIR Public Health Surveill.* (2020) 6:e19273. doi: 10.2196/19273

42. Ting DSW, Carin L, Dzau V, Wong TY. Digital technology and COVID-19. *Nat Med.* (2020) 26:459–61. doi: 10.1038/s41591-020-0824-5

43. Symplur. *#TelemedNow - Healthcare Social Media Analytics and Transcripts.* (2020). Available online at: https://www.symplur.com/healthcare-hashtags/telemednow/ (accessed June 30, 2020).

44. Sana F, Isselbacher EM, Singh JP, Heist EK, Pathik B, Armoundas AA. Wearable devices for ambulatory cardiac monitoring: JACC state-of-the-art review. *J Am Coll Cardiol.* (2020) 75:1582–92. doi: 10.1016/j.jacc.2020.01.046

45. Jadczyk T, Kiwic O, Khandwalla RM, Grabowski K, Rudawski S, Magaczewski P, et al. Feasibility of a voice-enabled automated platform for medical data collection: cardioCube. *Int J Med Inform.* (2019) 129:388–93. doi: 10.1016/j.ijmedinf.2019.07.001

46. Shufelt C, Dzubur E, Joung S, Fuller G, Mouapi KN, van Den Broek I, et al. A protocol integrating remote patient monitoring patient reported outcomes and cardiovascular biomarkers. *NPJ Digit Med.* (2019) 2:84. doi: 10.1038/s41746-019-0145-6

47. Treskes RW, van der Velde ET, Barendse R, Bruining N. Mobile health in cardiology: a review of currently available medical apps and equipment for remote monitoring. *Expert Rev Med Devices.* (2016) 13:823–30. doi: 10.1080/17434440.2016.1218277

48. Ong MK, Romano PS, Edgington S, Aronow HU, Auerbach AD, Black JT, et al. Effectiveness of remote patient monitoring after discharge of hospitalized patients with heart failure: the better effectiveness after transition – heart failure (BEAT-HF) randomized clinical trial. *JAMA Intern Med.* (2016) 176:310–8. doi: 10.1001/jamainternmed.2015.7712

49. Zakeri R, Morgan JM, Phillips P, Kitt S, Ng GA, McComb JM, et al. Impact of remote monitoring on clinical outcomes for patients with heart failure and atrial fibrillation: results from the REM-HF trial. *Eur J Heart Fail.* (2020) 22:543–53. doi: 10.1002/ejhf.1709

50. Sohn A, Speier W, Lan E, Aoki K, Fonarow G, Ong M, et al. Assessment of heart failure patients' interest in mobile health apps for self-care: survey study. *JMIR Cardio.* (2019) 3:e14332. doi: 10.2196/14332

51. Gensini GF, Alderighi C, Rasoini R, Mazzanti M, Casolo G. Value of telemonitoring and telemedicine in heart failure management. *Card Fail Rev.* (2017) 3:116–21. doi: 10.15420/cfr.2017:6:2

52. Greiwe J, Nyenhuis SM. Wearable technology and how this can be implemented into clinical practice. *Curr Allergy Asthma Rep.* (2020) 20:36. doi: 10.1007/s11882-020-00927-3

53. Zamberg I, Manzano S, Posfay-Barbe K, Windisch O, Agoritsas T, Schiffer E. a mobile health platform to disseminate validated institutional measurements during the COVID-19 outbreak: utilization-focused evaluation study. *JMIR Public Health Surveill.* (2020) 6:e18668. doi: 10.2196/18668

54. Timmers T, Janssen L, Stohr J, Murk JL, Berrevoets M. Using mHealth to support COVID-19 education, self-assessment, and symptom monitoring: an observational study in The Netherlands. *JMIR Mhealth Uhealth.* (2020) 8:e19822. doi: 10.2196/preprints.19822

55. Abeler J, Bäcker M, Buermeyer U, Zillessen H. COVID-19 contact tracing and data protection can go together. *JMIR Mhealth Uhealth.* (2020) 8:e19359. doi: 10.2196/19359

56. Annis T, Pleasants S, Hultman G, Lindemann E, Thompson JA, Billecke S, et al. Rapid implementation of a COVID-19 remote patient monitoring program. *J Am Med Inform Assoc.* (2020) 2020:ocaa097. doi: 10.1093/jamia/ocaa097

57. Varma N, Marrouche NF, Aguinaga L, Albert CM, Arbelo E, Choi JI, et al. HRS/EHRA/APHRS/LAHRS/ACC/AHA worldwide practice update for telehealth and arrhythmia monitoring during and after a pandemic. *J Am Coll Cardiol.* (2020). doi: 10.1002/joa3.12389. [Epub ahead of print].

58. Schinköthe T, Gabri MR, Mitterer M, Gouveia P, Heinemann V, Harbeck N, et al. A web- and app-based connected care solution for COVID-19 in- and

outpatient care: qualitative study and application development. *JMIR Public Health Surveill.* (2020) 6:e19033. doi: 10.2196/19033

59. Kim Y, Seo J, An SY, Sinn DH, Hwang JH. Efficacy and safety of an mhealth app and wearable device in physical performance for patients with hepatocellular carcinoma: development and usability study. *JMIR Mhealth Uhealth.* (2020) 8:e14435. doi: 10.2196/14435

60. Lynch BM, Nguyen NH, Moore MM, Reeves MM, Rosenberg DE, Boyle T, et al. A randomized controlled trial of a wearable technology-based intervention for increasing moderate to vigorous physical activity and reducing sedentary behavior in breast cancer survivors: the ACTIVATE trial. *Cancer.* (2019) 125:2846–55. doi: 10.1002/cncr.32143

61. Wright AA, Raman N, Staples P, Schonholz S, Cronin A, Carlson K, et al. The HOPE pilot study: harnessing patient-reported outcomes and biometric data to enhance cancer care. *JCO Clin Cancer Inform.* (2018) 2:1–12. doi: 10.1200/CCI.17.00149

62. Sara JDS, Maor E, Borlaug B, Lewis BR, Orbelo D, Lerman LO, et al. Non-invasive vocal biomarker is associated with pulmonary hypertension. *PLoS ONE.* (2020) 15:e0231441. doi: 10.1371/journal.pone.0231441

63. Maor E, Perry D, Mevorach D, Taiblum N, Luz Y, Mazin I, et al. Vocal biomarker is associated with hospitalization and mortality among heart failure patients. *J Am Heart Assoc.* (2020) 9:e013359. doi: 10.1161/JAHA.119.013359

64. Maor E, Sara JD, Orbelo DM, Lerman LO, Levanon Y, Lerman A. Voice signal characteristics are independently associated with coronary artery disease. *Mayo Clin Proc.* (2018) 93:840–7. doi: 10.1016/j.mayocp.2017.12.025

65. Hassoon A, Schrack J, Naiman D, Lansey D, Baig Y, Stearns V, et al. Increasing physical activity amongst overweight and obese cancer survivors using an alexa-based intelligent agent for patient coaching: protocol for the physical activity by technology help (PATH) trial. *JMIR Res Protoc.* (2018) 7:e27. doi: 10.2196/resprot.9096

66. Forum WE. *How Drones are Used for Life-Saving Healthcare 2020.* Available online at: https://www.weforum.org/agenda/2020/04/medicines-from-the-sky-how-a-drone-may-save-your-life/ (accessed June 30, 2020).

67. Transportation NCDo. *NCDOT Helping in Effort to Use Drones in COVID-19 Relief Efforts.* (2020). Available online at: https://www.ncdot.gov/news/press-releases/Pages/2020/2020-04-22-ncdot-drones-covid-19.aspx (accessed June 30, 2020).

68. Ye Q, Zhou J, Wu H. Using information technology to manage the COVID-19 pandemic: development of a technical framework based on practical experience in China. *JMIR Med Inform.* (2020) 8:e19515. doi: 10.2196/19515

69. Harrington RA, Califf RM, Balamurugan A, Brown N, Benjamin RM, Braund WE, et al. Call to action: rural health: a presidential advisory from the American heart association and american stroke association. *Circulation.* (2020) 141:e615–44. doi: 10.1161/CIR.0000000000000753

70. British Broadcasting Corporation. *Coronavirus: Covid-19 Detecting Apps Face Teething Problems 2020.* Available online at: https://www.bbc.com/news/technology-52215290 (accessed June 30, 2020).

71. National Public Radio. *Use of Smart Speakers in the US Increases During Quarantine.* Available online at: https://www.npr.org/about-npr/848319916/use-of-smart-speakers-in-the-u-s-increases-during-quarantine (accessed June 30, 2020).

72. Insilico Medicine. *In silico Medicine To Support The Drug Discovery Efforts Against Coronavirus 2019-nCoV.* (2020). Available online at: https://insilico.com/ncov-sprint (accessed June 30, 2020).

73. McCall B. COVID-19 and artificial intelligence: protecting health-care workers and curbing the spread. *Lancet Digit Health.* (2020) 2:e166–7. doi: 10.1016/S2589-7500(20)30054-6

74. Knight W. *How AI Is Tracking the Coronavirus Outbreak 2020.* Available online at: https://www.wired.com/story/how-ai-tracking-coronavirus-outbreak/ (accessed June 30, 2020).

75. Li L, Qin L, Xu Z, Yin Y, Wang X, Kong B, et al. Artificial intelligence distinguishes COVID-19 from community acquired pneumonia on chest CT. *Radiology.* (2020) 19:200905. doi: 10.1148/radiol.2020200905

76. Neri E, Miele V, Coppola F, Grassi R. Use of CT and artificial intelligence in suspected or COVID-19 positive patients: statement of the Italian Society of Medical and Interventional Radiology. *Radiol Med.* (2020) 2020:1–4. doi: 10.1007/s11547-020-01197-9

77. Rao ASRS, Vazquez JA. Identification of COVID-19 can be quicker through artificial intelligence framework using a mobile phone-based survey in the populations when cities/towns are under quarantine. *Infect Control Hosp Epidemiol.* (2020) 2020:1–5. doi: 10.1017/ice.2020.61

78. Alimadadi A, Aryal S, Manandhar I, Munroe PB, Joe B, Cheng X. Artificial intelligence and machine learning to fight COVID-19. *Physiol Genomics.* (2020) 52:200–2. doi: 10.1152/physiolgenomics.00029.2020

79. Ienca M, Vayena E. On the responsible use of digital data to tackle the COVID-19 pandemic. *Nat Med.* (2020) 26:463–4. doi: 10.1038/s41591-020-0832-5

80. Mei X, Lee HC, Diao KY, Huang M, Lin B, Liu C, et al. Artificial intelligence-enabled rapid diagnosis of patients with COVID-19. *Nat Med.* (2020). doi: 10.1038/s41591-020-0931-3. [Epub ahead of print].

81. Mackey T, Purushothaman V, Li J, Shah N, Nali M, Bardier C, et al. Machine learning to detect self-reporting of symptoms, testing access, and recovery associated with COVID-19 on Twitter: retrospective big data infoveillance study. *JMIR Public Health Surveill.* (2020) 6:e19509. doi: 10.2196/19509

82. Hasin Y, Seldin M, Lusis A. Multi-omics approaches to disease. *Genome Biol.* (2017) 18:83. doi: 10.1186/s13059-017-1215-1

83. Suwinski P, Ong C, Ling MHT, Poh YM, Khan AM, Ong HS. Advancing personalized medicine through the application of whole exome sequencing and big data analytics. *Front Genet.* (2019) 10:49. doi: 10.3389/fgene.2019.00049

84. Roden DM, McLeod HL, Relling MV, Williams MS, Mensah GA, Peterson JF, et al. Pharmacogenomics. *Lancet.* (2019) 394:521–32. doi: 10.1016/S0140-6736(19)31276-0

85. Ellinghaus D, Degenhardt F, Bujanda L, Buti M, Albillos A, Invernizzi P, et al. Genomewide association study of severe covid-19 with respiratory failure. *N Engl J Med.* (2020). doi: 10.1056/NEJMoa2020283. [Epub ahead of print].

86. Vohra A, Asnani A. Biomarker discovery in cardio-oncology. *Curr Cardiol Rep.* (2018) 20:52. doi: 10.1007/s11886-018-1002-y

87. Saleh M, Gabriels J, Chang D, Kim BS, Mansoor A, Mahmood E, et al. The effect of chloroquine, hydroxychloroquine and azithromycin on the corrected QT interval in patients with SARS-CoV-2 infection. *Circ Arrhythm Electrophysiol.* (2020) 13:e008662. doi: 10.1161/CIRCEP.120.008662

88. Saban KL, Mathews HL, deVon HA, Janusek LW. Epigenetics and social context: implications for disparity in cardiovascular disease. *Aging Dis.* (2014) 5:346–55. doi: 10.14336/AD.2014.0500346

89. National Cancer Institute. *Surveillance, Epidemiology, and End Results.* Available online at: https://seer.cancer.gov/ (accessed June 30, 2020).

90. International Business Machines. *Truven Health Analytics.* Available online at: https://www.ibm.com/watson-health/about/truven-health-analytics (accessed June 30, 2020).

91. Agency for Healthcare Research and Quality. *Healthcare Cost and Utilization Project.* Available online at: https://www.ahrq.gov/data/hcup/index.html (accessed June 30, 2020).

92. CDC. *ICD-10-CM Official Coding and Reporting Guidelines: CDC.* (2020). Available online at: https://www.cdc.gov/nchs/data/icd/COVID-19-guidelines-final.pdf (accessed March 31, 2020).

93. CMS. *Coverage and Payment Related to COVID-19 Medicare: CMS.* (2020). Available online at: https://www.cms.gov/files/document/03052020-medicare-covid-19-fact-sheet.pdf (accessed March 23, 2020).

94. Swedish registers › *Cancer.* (2020). Available online at: https://www.lupop.lu.se/lupop-for-researchers/registers/cancer (accessed March 3, 2020).

95. Schmidt M, Schmidt SAJ, Sandegaard JL, Ehrenstein V, Pedersen L, Sørensen HT. The Danish National patient registry: a review of content, data quality, and research potential. *Clin Epidemiol.* (2015) 7:449–90. doi: 10.2147/CLEP.S91125

96. Welch CA, Sweeting MJ, Lambert PC, Rutherford MJ, Jack RH, West D, et al. Impact on survival of modelling increased surgical resection rates in patients with non-small-cell lung cancer and cardiovascular comorbidities: a VICORI study. *Br J Cancer.* (2020). doi: 10.1038/s41416-020-0869-8. [Epub ahead of print].

97. Waterhouse DM, Harvey RD, Hurley P, Levit LA, Kim ES, Klepin HD, et al. Early impact of COVID-19 on the conduct of oncology clinical trials and long-term opportunities for transformation: findings from an American society of clinical oncology survey. *JCO Oncol Pract.* (2020) 16:417–21. doi: 10.1200/OP.20.00275

98. Goldsack JC, Izmailova ES, Menetski JP, Hoffmann SC, Groenen PMA, Wagner JA. Remote digital monitoring in clinical trials in the time of COVID-19. *Nat Rev Drug Discov.* (2020) 19:378–9. doi: 10.1038/d41573-020-00094-0

99. Lenihan DJ, Fradley MG, Dent S, Brezden-Masley C, Carver J, Filho RK, et al. Proceedings from the global cardio-oncology summit. *JACC CardioOncol.* (2019) 1:256. doi: 10.1016/j.jaccao.2019.11.007

100. *Real-World Data For The Precision Medicine Era.* Available online at: https://www.tempus.com/data-solutions/

101. Ponikowski P, Voors AA, Anker SD, Bueno H, Cleland JGF, Coats AJS, et al. 2016 ESC guidelines for the diagnosis treatment of acute chronic heart failure: the task force for the diagnosis treatment of acute chronic heart failure of the European Society of Cardiology (ESC)Developed with the special contribution of the Heart Failure Association (HFA) of the ESC. *Eur Heart J.* (2016) 37:2129–200. doi: 10.1093/eurheartj/ehx158

16

COVID-19 and Acute Coronary Syndromes: Current Data and Future Implications

Matteo Cameli[1], Maria Concetta Pastore[1,2]*, Giulia Elena Mandoli[1], Flavio D'Ascenzi[1], Marta Focardi[1], Giulia Biagioni[1], Paolo Cameli[3], Giuseppe Patti[2], Federico Franchi[4], Sergio Mondillo[1] and Serafina Valente[1]

[1] Department of Medical Biotechnologies, Division of Cardiology, University of Siena, Siena, Italy, [2] University of Eastern Piedmont, Maggiore della Carità Hospital, Novara, Italy, [3] Department of Clinical Medical and Neurosciences, Respiratory Disease and Lung Transplantation Section, Le Scotte Hospital, University of Siena, Siena, Italy, [4] Department of Medical Biotechnologies, Anesthesia and Intensive Care, University of Siena, Siena, Italy

*Correspondence:
Maria Concetta Pastore
pastore2411@gmail.com

Coronavirus disease-2019 (COVID-19) pandemic is a global healthcare burden, characterized by high mortality and morbidity rates all over the world. During the outbreak period, the topic of acute coronary syndromes (ACS) has raised several clinical issues, due to the risks of COVID-19 induced myocardial injury and to the uncertainties about the management of these cardiologic emergency conditions, which should be organized optimizing the diagnostic and therapeutic resources and ensuring the maximum protection to healthcare personnel and hospital environment. COVID-19 status should be assessed as soon as possible. Moreover, considerably lower rates of hospitalization for ACS have been reported all over the world, due to patients' hesitations to refer to hospital and to missed diagnosis. As a result, short- and long-term complications of myocardial infarction are expected in the near future; therefore, great efforts of healthcare providers will be required to limit the effects of this issue. In the present review we discuss the impact of COVID-19 pandemic on ACS diagnosis and management, with possible incoming consequences, providing an overview of the available evidence and suggesting future changes in social and clinical approach to ACS.

Keywords: SARS-CoV2, myocardial injury, NSTEMI, STEMI, acute coronary syndromes, COVID-19

INTRODUCTION

Background

Coronavirus-2019 (COVID-19) outbreak is currently the most discussed public health issue, caused by the highly infectious severe acute respiratory syndrome coronavirus 2 (SARS-CoV-2). COVID-19 was declared a pandemic by the World Health Organization in early March 2020 and it was characterized by an exponential rise in contagions worldwide, with continuously increasing number of victims (1). The typical clinical spectrum of COVID-19 includes fever, cough, myalgia, dyspnea (2), with frequent progression to pneumonia, which in one third of the cases eventually leads to acute respiratory distress syndrome (ARDS), of which another third warrant critical care (3). Therefore, prevention and treatment of COVID-19 are currently the primary focus of clinical and scientific debates. However, acute coronary syndromes (ACS) management during this emergency period is gaining growing interest, yielding many scientific researches as well as national and international societies consensus documents, stimulated by four major concerns:

- an increase in short-term risk of myocardial injury and infarction has been reported, particularly for patients with underlying CAD and/or pro-inflammatory cardiovascular risk factors (such as diabetes mellitus, hypertension, and obesity);
- differential diagnosis between non-COVID ACS and COVID-19 induced acute myocardial injury (COVID-AMI), and within COVID-AMI, among myocardial infarction (MI), acute viral myocarditis, stress cardiomyopathy, is currently challenging, due also to the restricted availability of diagnostic tools;
- a sensible reduction of the rates of ACS has been recorded all over the world (4), probably not only as a consequence of lower patients' referral to the emergency department (ED), but also of misdiagnosis;
- lack of preparation and standardized protocols to balance between timely management of ACS and protection of healthcare personnel and hospital environment has provoked delays in the treatment of high-risk ACS; this fact, in conjunction with the previous point, has led to an increased incidence of short-term MI complications and estimated higher long-term MI complications, which will probably require changes in public health resources and system.

Aims

In the present review we sought to address these four important issues, discussing the earliest evidence and recommendations present in literature, and providing hints and previsions for the future, in order to prepare clinicians and solve their uncertainties on the matter of ACS during and after COVID-19 pandemic.

ACUTE MYOCARDIAL INJURY TRIGGERED BY COVID-19

The development of myocardial injury is not uncommon among patients with COVID-19 and correlates with disease severity. In fact, a meta-analysis involving 1,527 COVID-19 patients revealed that at least 8% of the patients had acute myocardial injury and that the risk of myocardial injury is 13-fold higher in patients with severe clinical presentation (5).

COVID-AMI has been defined as the elevation of high-sensitivity cardiac troponin (hs-cTn) above the 99th percentile of its upper limit of normal or evidence of new electrocardiographic (ECG) or echocardiographic abnormalities (6). In fact, the presence of increased levels of hs-cTn was found to be an independent predictor of disease severity and mortality rate in COVID-19 (7) even after adjustment for baseline characteristics and medical comorbidities, also showing an association with the need for intensive care unit (ICU) admittance (RR 13.48, 95%CI 3.60 to 50.47, $p = 0.0001$) (5).

DIFFERENTIAL DIAGNOSIS

There are different potential etiologies of COVID-AMI: ACS due to plaque rupture or thrombosis (type I MI) or to supply-demand mismatch (type II MI), myocardial injury due to disseminated intravascular coagulation (DIC), and non-ischemic injury (myocarditis, stress-induced cardiomyopathy, cytokine release syndrome, acute pulmonary embolism). Each one is the result of a direct or indirect effect of severe viral infection, as explained in **Table 1**. It is essential to recognize ACS and ACS-mimicker in order to provide an adequate treatment and avoid additional risks (e.g., fibrinolysis in case of myocarditis or stress-cardiomyopathy would expose patients to bleeding risk and eventual invasive coronary angiography (ICA) for unresolved ST-elevation rather than being beneficial) (6).

Differential Diagnosis: First Contact With Patients

The distinction between primary ACS and COVID-AMI for outpatients referring to ED would be crucial for the subsequent patient management, not only for treatment but also for the safety measures to employ (i.e., isolation, use of adequate personal protective equipment [PPE]). In accordance to the European Association of Percutaneous Cardiovascular Interventions (EAPCI) recommendations (27), for patients with suspected ACS, the likelihood of COVID-19 status should be assessed through accurate clinical interview, investigating the presence of typical symptoms (e.g., fever, cough, dyspnea, cold) or contacts with COVID-19 infected, together with the execution of nasal and/or oropharyngeal swab for SARS-CoV2 Nucleic Acid test as soon as the patient arrives in the ED, if possible. Fast-track pathways for the exclusion of COVID status would expedite the management of these patients. Until the result of the swab is ready, each patient should be considered as COVID infected; this is also valid for STEMI patients who are transferred to the catheterization laboratory (Cath-lab) before having the results. Healthcare workers and patients must always wear at least droplets PPE (i.e., surgical mask, gloves, cup, goggles, and single-use gown for clinicians, surgical mask and gloves for patient). Moreover,

- in case of patients with asymptomatic/negative anamnesis and negative SARS-CoV2 Nucleic Acid test the common ACS-pathway should be followed;
- in case of patients with symptomatic/positive anamnesis and negative SARS-CoV2 Nucleic Acid test, the swab should be repeated;
- in case of positive SARS-CoV2 Nucleic Acid test, patients are considered as COVID infected, healthcare professionals must wear total-protection PPE (i.e., cup, facial protection, waterproof single-use gown and gloves) and filtering face piece class 3 (FFP3) or N95 mask.

Based on our clinical experience, we suggest that it could be reasonable, while awaiting swab results, prioritize timely treatment in high-risk patients, considering them as COVID-19 infected in order to provide timely treatment and perform ICA, whenever indicated, using airborne PPE (coverall or disposable gown, gloves, headcover, eye shield, FFP3/N99 respirators masks, and shoe covers); then, after revascularization, assess COVID-19 status in order to organize hospitalization in a dedicated ward or isolation in coronary care unit, and subsequent healthcare workers' use of different types of PPE.

TABLE 1 | Different etiologies and hypothesized mechanism of COVID-induced myocardial injury.

Type of myocardial injury	Possible mechanism	Clinical consequences	Available evidence
Type 1 myocardial infarction	*Systemic inflammatory response syndrome*: ↑risk of plaque rupture and thrombus formation **Cytokine storm** due to imbalanced TH1/TH2 response ⇒**DIC** [*71.4% non-survivors vs. 0.6% survivors* (8)]: MOF	STEMI or NSTEMI (9) **Thrombosis** of coronary epi- and subepicardial arteries ⇒focal myocardial necrosis and dysfunction (10)	Bangalore et al. (11) Xhuan et al. (12) Tang et al. (8) Sugiura et al. (10)
Type 2 myocardial infarction	**Myocardial oxygen imbalance** (↑demand for sepsis state, not satisfiable for COVID-19 induced hypoxaemia and vasoconstriction)	Severe myocardial ischaemia, ++ in patients with underlying CAD	Li et al. (5) Shi et al. (13) Guo et al. (14)
Venous thromboembolism	Hypercoagulable status + active inflammation + propensity for DIC + prolonged immobilization + oxidative stress + endothelial dysfunction + increased platelet reactivity + mechanical ventilation + liver dysfunction + central venous catheters + nutritional deficit	↑D-dimer *(>1µg/mL on admission ⇒↑ in-hospital death)*, FDP, fibrinogen Pulmonary embolism or deep venous thrombosis *[22.7% non-ICU and 27% in ICU patients* (15)]	Tang et al. (10) Han et al. (15) Klok et al. (16)
Acute myocarditis	*Indirect mechanism:* innate immunity activation ⇒inflammatory cascade and exaggerated cytokine release *Direct mechanism*: ACE2 receptor (used by SARS-CoV2 for binding, overexpressed in diseased hearts)	STEMI-like presentation with myocardial degenerative changes and necrosis	Zhou et al. (17) Yao et al. (18) Beri et al. (19) Tavazzi et al. (20) Hu et al. (21) Zeng et al. (22) Sala et al. (23)
Stress cardiomyopathy	Infective +/- emotional trigger ⇒catecholamine induced myocardial stunning or macro- and micro-vascular spasm	Tako-tsubo syndrome	Moderato et al. (24) Meyer et al. (25) Chadha et al. (26)

ACE2, angiotensin-converting enzyme-2; CAD, coronary artery disease; DIC, disseminated intravascular coagulation; ICU, intensive care unit; MOF, multi-organ failure; NSTEMI, non ST-elevation myocardial infarction; SARS-CoV-2, severe acute respiratory syndrome coronavirus 2; STEMI, ST-elevation myocardial infarction; TH1, T-helper lymphocytes 1; TH2, T-helper lymphocytes 2; VTE, venous thromboembolism.
+, plus; ++, above all; ↑, higher.

Differential Diagnosis in COVID-19 Patient

Differential diagnosis of COVID-AMI really became a challenge for clinicians. Commonly, a rise and/or fall of hs-cTn is not sufficient to ensure the diagnosis of myocardial infarction, but it should also be corroborated with clinical judgment, symptom and signs, ECG changes, and imaging studies (28). As recent documents of the European Association of Cardiovascular Imaging (EACVI) and the American College of Cardiology (ACC) highlighted, this is especially valid in case of COVID-19, considering that cardiac enzymes elevation could either be secondary to non-specific raise during COVID infection or to other acute pathologic complications (e.g., sepsis, acute kidney injury, stroke) (29, 30). Moreover, as troponin elevation in patients with COVID-19 infection seems to be lower than in most cases of ACS or acute myocarditis, EAPCI suggests considering marked elevation (e.g., >5 times the upper normal limit) in a patient who is not critically ill to suspect COVID-AMI (27).

As a matter of fact, the access to diagnostic resources is currently limited since, considering the high infective power of SARS-CoV2, performing unnecessary imaging tests should be avoided in order to limit healthcare personnel and devices exposure to the risk of contamination (31).

Sometimes, COVID-19 presentation could entail cardiovascular symptoms rather than fever, cough, dyspnoea, as shown in a small Italian report with 81% of patients presenting ST-elevation MI (STEMI) as COVID-19 first manifestation, of whom 78.6% referring to ED with acute chest pain. Interestingly, only 39.3% demonstrated absence of obstructive coronary artery disease (32). In fact, the EACVI recommendations on the use of cardiac imaging during COVID-19 pandemic suggest considering the optimization of computed tomography (CT), often used to confirm of COVID-pneumonia, with the addition of coronary CT methods to exclude ACS in case of raised troponin (30). Similarly, the use of CT completed with contrast enhanced sequences has been proposed by Hendren et al. to exclude acute myocarditis avoiding the additional use of cardiac magnetic resonance (CMR) and invasive endomyocardial biopsy, since patterns of delayed myocardial enhancement consistent with acute myocarditis revealed by cardiac CT have also been described (33).

As regards patients hospitalized for COVID-19 with suspected ACS, EACVI recommends to evaluate the pre-test probability (PTP) based on symptoms, ECG signs, age, sex, previous history, and cardiovascular risk factors, to use coronary CT angiography

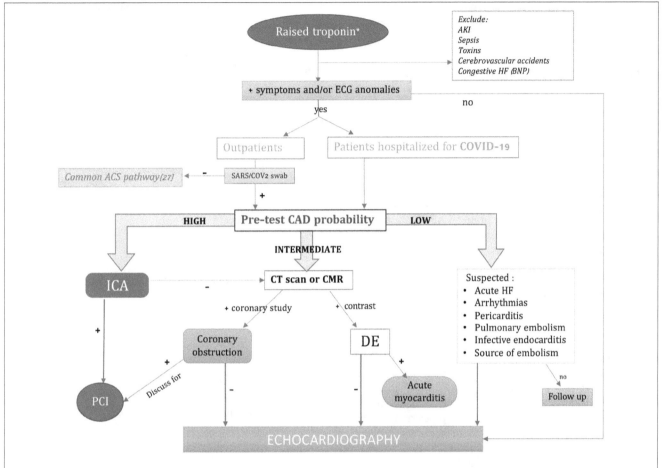

FIGURE 1 | Algorithm for the diagnosis of COVID-induced acute myocardial injury optimizing the available imaging techniques. *hs-cTn>99th percentile of its upper normal limit, or >5 times the upper normal limit in COVID patients. ACS, acute coronary syndromes; AKI, acute kidney injury; BNP, brain natriuretic peptide; CMR, cardiac magnetic resonance; CT, cardiac tomography; DE, delayed enhancement; HF, heart failure; ICA, invasive coronary angiography; PCI, percutaneous coronary intervention.

for intermediate PTP, and to reserve ICA only for cases with very high PTP or STEMI, high-risk non-STEMI (NSTEMI) or crescendo angina (34).

A schematic representation of the suggested pathway for differential diagnosis of COVID-AMI preventing from wasting unnecessary diagnostic resources is available in **Figure 1**. In that regard, two important messages deriving from the international societies' recommendations (27, 29, 30, 34), both for outpatients referring to ED and for hospitalized patients, should be highlighted:

- **ICA** should be performed only in patients with suspected type 1 MI (27) and who are expected to derive meaningful changes in outcome from invasive management; therefore, patients with high level of comorbidities, poor quality of life, and frailty should be early assigned to medical therapy, since additional investigations are futile;
- the use of **echocardiography**, which has always been regarded as a "gatekeeper" for differential diagnosis of cardiovascular disease, should be reconsidered in this emergency period. Transthoracic echocardiography should not be routinely

performed if patients are asymptomatic and stable, but it remains the first line approach in patients with high suspicion of COVID-AMI, in order to address diagnosis (35). Given its high aerosol-generating procedure, the use of transoesophageal echocardiography should be restricted to the selected cases of poorly feasible or informative transthoracic echocardiography, and when it would lead to change and optimization of the patient's management; when necessary, this procedure must be performed with FFP3 or N95 equipment.

Bearing all these recommendations and the possible poor availability of advanced imaging methods in some center, also due to the overwhelming requests of CT scan, for the purpose to determine the presence of an atypical COVID presentation with ACS, we would like to highlight the importance of performing accurate anamnesis, investigating symptoms occurrence and timing; a thorough ECG observation, seeking for ischemic abnormalities corresponding to coronary regions; rely on the dosage of troponin, after excluding troponin-affecting comorbidities which could act as confounders. In cases of extreme uncertainties, echocardiography should be applied with the use of appropriate PPE (**Figure 1**).

In-hospital ACS Management During COVID-19
Outpatients
The best therapeutic strategy for patients with ACS during the pandemic has been extensively discussed. Even though in early Chinese algorithms primary PCI was sacrificed in favor of the protection of healthcare personnel from contagion, opting for rapid testing for COVID-19 infection and immediate fibrinolysis, European societies recommend a halfway approach (34, 36). Accordingly, as stated in the EAPCI document on invasive management of ACS during COVID-19 (27), the COVID-19 infective danger should not change the first-line therapeutic approach to STEMI. Primary percutaneous coronary intervention (PCI) remains the standard of care for STEMI patients referred to Hub centers or transferred rapidly from non-PCI centers within 120 min from the first medical contact. For patients in whom a rapid reperfusion with primary PCI is not feasible, initial fibrinolysis is recommended, followed by consideration of transfer to a PCI center. More specifically, the consensus statement from the Society for Cardiovascular Angiography and Interventions (SCAI), ACC and the American College of Emergency Physicians (ACEP) suggests that for *STEMI patients with positive SARS-CoV2 swab* referred to a Spoke center, the transfer to a PCI center should be discussed, possibly preferring to perform fibrinolysis within 30 min of STEMI diagnosis, and eventually transfer to Hub Center for rescue PCI if needed (37), where this should be performed by experienced operators equipped with high-level PPE in dedicated rooms.

For NSTEMI management an approach based on individual risk is recommended (27):

- *very high risk NSTEMI* patients should follow a similar management of STEMI;
- *high risk NSTEMI* patients should follow medical treatment while waiting for SARS-CoV2 test results and planning an early invasive therapy, possibly < 24 h; in case of positive test, the patients should undergo ICA in a COVID-19 hospital;
- *low risk NSTEMI* could be firstly evaluated non-invasively, in order to exclude alternative etiology to type 1 MI, using coronary CT, if possible; if low risk is confirmed, they should follow conservative strategy.

Table 2 summarizes the criteria for risk stratification of NSTEMI patients based on the newest European Society of Cardiology (ESC) guidelines (38).

In case of necessary ICA approach, preventive strategies are of outmost importance to ensure protection to healthcare personnel and their relatives, hospital environment, and also other patients.

As regards high-risk patients whose COVID status is unknown, as soon as the patient arrives in the Cath-lab, vital signs should be assessed (with particular attention to body temperature and arterial oxygen saturation). Furthermore, blood gas analysis and biologic specimens (swab) collection for COVID-19 test

TABLE 2 | Risk stratification for non-ST-elevation myocardial infarction (NSTEMI) treatment (38).

Very high risk	High risk	Low risk
- Hemodynamic instability - Cardiogenic shock - Recurrent/refractory chest pain despite medical treatment - Life-threatening arrhythmias - Mechanical complications of myocardial infarction - Acute HF related to NSTEMI - ST-segment depression > 1 mm in 6 leads + ST-segment elevation in aVr and/or V1	- NSTEMI diagnosis already established - Symptomatic/asymptomatic - dynamic new (or presumably new) contiguous ST-T segment changes - Resuscitated cardiac arrest without ST-segment elevation or cardiogenic shock - GRACE risk score > 140	No recurrence of symptoms and none of the *very high* or *high-risk* criteria. Also includes patients with: - History of revascularization - Early post-infarction angina - LVEF<40% or congestive HF - GRACE risk score 109–140 - Diabetes mellitus Ruled out based on troponin levels

HF, heart failure, NSTEMI; LVEF, left ventricular ejection fraction; non-ST-elevation myocardial infarction.

should be performed using the necessary PPE according to the severity of respiratory symptoms (39):

- Low COVID-19 risk: surgical mask.
- High COVID-19 risk: PPE with FFP2 or FFP3 mask, depending on the gravity of respiratory impairment of the individual patient.

Operators should follow precise protocols of dressing/undressing (40) and, after the procedure, in patients with unknown or positive SARS-CoV2 Nucleic Acid test a sanitization of the Cath-lab is mandatory.

Inpatients
As for patients already hospitalized in a *COVID-Unit* with *suspected STEMI*, the risk and benefits of a possible coronary revascularization should be evaluated, weighting the individual patients' clinical conditions and comorbidities and the risks related to the transport in the Cath-lab. In case of risks overweight, fibrinolysis could be considered as an alternative to PCI (41, 42). However, the increased hemorrhagic and DIC risk in COVID-19 patients, especially those with severe conditions, should be considered.

Fibrinolytic Strategy
Even if bigger evidence is required in this field, the use of fibrinolysis as an alternative to PCI seemed to reach comparable results for in-hospital and 30-day clinical outcome (all-cause death, cardiac death, stroke, re-infarction/coronary re-occlusion, and revascularization) in patients during the COVID-19 pandemic with absence of major bleeding (43) and was proposed by several authors as a reasonable alternative to PCI, providing spare of medical resources (e.g., PPE and workflow) and of healthcare professionals exposure to the risk of contagion (41, 44, 45). However, we suggest that (1) the well-known superiority of PCI to definitely restore blood flow and in reducing

mortality, re-infarction, or stroke (46); (2) the risk of early re-thrombosis of the culprit lesion requiring rescue PCI if sufficient anticoagulation is not reached after the fibrinolytic treatment, resulting in longer hospitalization and possible complications; (3) the fatal/non-fatal bleeding risk of fibrinolysis itself (particularly if performed in patient with "STEMI-mimicker") should be taken into account both in COVID-19 and non-COVID-19 patients; therefore, in our view, fibrinolysis-lone strategy should be considered only in case of higher risks connected to patients' transfer to PCI-center or to the Cath lab outweighing incremental benefits of PCI, or in case of impossibility to provide timely PCI. Importantly, the bleeding risk of the single patient should be evaluated in the decision-making between primary PCI and fibrinolysis.

ACS METAMORPHOSIS IN COVID-19 ERA

Now that the control of COVID-19 contagion and management is improved, with resulting lower rates of morbidity, it is time for clinicians to look beyond COVID-19 and to care about the cardiovascular consequences of the pandemic. A serious concern regarding ACS is currently affecting global healthcare services: a downward trend in ACS incidence has been registered all over the world, awakening the interest of the scientific community. First, the Italian society of Cardiology multicenter register, which compared acute MI incidence in a week with the equivalent period in 2019, observed a drastic reduction of 48.4% ($p<0.001$), which was significant for both STEMI (26.5%, higher for women: 41.2% vs. 17.8%) and NSTEMI (65.1%) and was similar throughout Italy (52.1% Northern vs. 59.3% Central vs. 52.1% Southern). Importantly, they have also registered a substantial increase in STEMI fatality rate [risk ratio (RR) = 3.3, 1.7–6.6; $p< 0.001$] and complications (RR = 1.8; 1.1–2.8; p = 0.009) during the pandemic, compared to 2019 (46).

Then, Metzler et al. conducted an Austrian nationwide retrospective survey involving 17 primary PCI centers for 27 days during COVID-19 outbreak, founding a relative reduction from the beginning to the end of this period of 39.4% in admission for all subtypes of ACS (47). Huet et al. reported almost halved numbers of admission for acute MI or heart failure in 9 French ICU centers comparing 14 days periods before and after containment (4.8±1.6 vs. 2.6±1.5 patients per day, p = 0.0006) (48).

Furthermore, the impact of the pandemic on interventional cardiology procedures has been assessed by Garcia et al., who quantified STEMI activations in 9 high-volume (>100 PCI/year) United States cardiac Cath-labs from January 1, 2019, to March 31, 2020, and observed a 38% reduction in Cath-lab STEMI activations in the after-COVID period (49), similar to the 40% registered in Spain (50). Moreover, an analysis of the Italian Society of Interventional Cardiology (GISE) reported a decrease in interventional coronary and structural procedures of 48.5% for ICA, 45.7% for PCI, 84.7% for transcatheter aortic valve replacement, and 50% for Mitraclip in Piedmont (Italy), during the COVID-19 period (51).

In our experience, we have observed not only a reduction of hospitalization for AMI but also a dramatic increase of hospitalization for subacute myocardial infarction >72 h, with cases of malignant arrhythmias and severe heart failure resistant to conventional therapy and often requiring inotropic support; this unavoidably resulted in poor prognosis for patients and challenges for clinicians to select the best therapeutic strategy, due to the doubtful benefits of a late revascularization and the difficult selection of patients for the allocation of advanced therapeutic resources (such as mechanical assist devices).

Causative Factors

Altogether, these data depict a picture of almost half of patients with ACS not reaching the hospital and not receiving timely treatment. The embraceable opinion is that this worrisome phenomenon could be multifactorial:

❖ **Patient-related factors:** to start with, there was a reduced referral to ED of patients with chest discomfort or unclear ACS symptoms due to their fear of catching SARS-CoV-2 in the hospital, encouraged by in-hospital contagion described by the media and by the strict instructions to stay at home. These have led patients to underestimate their symptoms, such as in a case-report by Masroor et al. regarding a 48-year-old man who referred to the ED for chest pain started 2 days earlier, but not seeking attention until later, due to his reluctance to access the hospital for dreaded COVID-19 contagion. ECG clearly showed STEMI and he underwent ICA with successful PCI on the occluded right coronary artery; few hours later, he developed cardiogenic shock for postinfarction ventricular septal defect of 2 cm, initially treated with intra-aortic balloon pump to let the myocardium heal, and then with surgical repair using a pericardial patch (52). Other patient-related features explaining the reduction in hospital admissions for ACS during the COVID-19 era are a negative psychological response, emotional distress, distrust/avoidance behaviors, and reluctance to activate pre-hospital networks.

❖ **Healthcare-related factors:** during this period, the emergency services have focused on COVID-19, with most healthcare resources relocated to manage the pandemic and with possible fails in identification of MI, which could have led to an artificial decreasing of ACS diagnoses. First, the priority given to COVID-19 suspected or known patients could have finally distracted from cardiovascular emergencies. Then, it seems that, for patients presenting symptoms consistent with COVID-19, all the resources and clinical attention have been dedicated to excluding SARS-CoV-2 infection, with consequent overlooking of acute cardiovascular conditions, causing misdiagnosis and/or delayed treatment. A clear example was described by Yousefzai et al. in a case-report of a 56-year-old patient with cardiovascular risk factors presenting exertional dyspnea and left bundle branch block at ECG who at first hesitated to refer to the ED and was then misdiagnosed with COVID-19-induced acute myocarditis, though presenting STEMI. Meanwhile, he developed acute respiratory distress syndrome

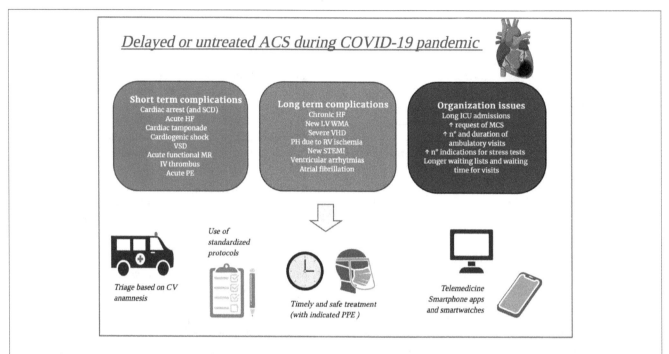

FIGURE 2 | Possible complications deriving from late or untreated acute coronary syndromes during COVID-19 pandemic and figurative hints for limiting them. ACS; acute coronary syndromes; HF, heart failure; ICU, intensive care unit; IV, intraventricular; LV, left ventricular; MCS, mechanical circulatory support; NSTEMI, non-ST elevation myocardial infarction; PE, pulmonary embolism; PH, pulmonary hypertension; PPE, personal protective equipment; RV, right ventricular; SCD, sudden cardiac death; STEMI, ST elevation myocardial infarction; VHD, valvular heart disease; VSD, ventricular septum defect; WMA, wall motion abnormalities.

requiring ventricular assistance and underwent late ICA with evidence of 99% left anterior descending coronary stenosis, 60% proximal circumflex artery stenosis, and moderate disease on right coronary artery; therefore, the clinicians opted not to perform revascularization. Then, after this completed anterior MI, he remained in ICU waiting for recovery or definitive ventricular assistance therapy (53).

Short- and Long-Term Consequences

The delay among symptoms presentation and revascularization could result in dramatic effects. Noteworthy, conjunction of the longer time from symptoms onset to first medical contact due to patients' reticence and waiting times for triaging, COVID-19 testing (since not all the healthcare facilities are equipped with ultra-rapid tests) and personnel precautions, would result in further delay for a needed PCI. This should represent an alarm for clinicians and public health, since the paramount importance of the timing of primary revascularization to save myocardial structure and function is well-known (53). In fact, in a recent study by Trabattoni et al., despite a regional optimization of the STEMI network through a re-structured Hub-Spoke model in Lombardy (Italy), a significant delay (> 24 h) in patients' referral to ED was present in 41% of STEMI patients in 2020, compared to 20% in 2019, resulting in in-hospital mortality rates of 38 vs. 10%, respectively (54). Similar results were shown by a Chinese group in an observational study on 149 patients

with MI before *(group 1, n = 85 patients)* and after *(group 2, n = 64 patients)* COVID-19 emergency measures; the second group not only had longer symptom-to-first medical contact time and higher presentation rates out of the PCI window (33 vs. 27.8%) but also showed a more elevated incidence of the composite outcome measure including in-hospital death, cardiogenic shock, sustained ventricular tachycardia/fibrillation, and use of mechanical circulatory support (29.7, vs. 14.1%, p = 0.02) (55).

These data, together with those previously mentioned (34), suggest that an increase in the incidence of late presenting MIs with chronic heart failure and sudden cardiac death is the most expectable eventuality in the near future, together with raised early and late morbidity and mortality. Short term-complications would require prolonged hospitalization in ICU, which could represent a serious concern in these times of poor resources. Over the long-term, suboptimal revascularization and large infarct size will result in maladaptive ventricular remodeling and dysfunction (56). Short and long-term complications and their impact on healthcare services are presented in **Figure 2**.

The earliest reports referred to cases with initially mild symptoms who experienced sudden cardiac death at home while in quarantine (57). Moreover, Baldi et al. described an increased incidence of out-of-hospital cardiac arrest during 40 days of COVID-19 pandemic in Italy compared to the same period in 2019, which such cumulative increased incidence being strongly associated with the diffusion of COVID-19 (58). Similarly, a

4.97-fold increase in out-of-hospital sudden cardiac arrest and a doubling of pronounced deaths on the scene was reported in New York City during the surge of pandemic, compared with the same period (March 20–April 22) of 2019 (59). These data could reflect the eventual consequences of medical care avoidance or distraction.

Possible Solutions

As the ESC guidance for the diagnosis and management of cardiovascular disease during the COVID-19 pandemic illustrates (60), it would be rational to triage patients with suspected or known COVID-19 according to the presence of underlying cardiovascular risk factors and co-morbidities, as well as to evidence of myocardial injury, in order to select those who deserve prioritized treatment and even more aggressive therapeutic strategies.

Organization of healthcare facilities should be improved with dedicated pathways and rapid SARS-CoV-2 testing, if available, allowing a timely supply of diagnostic and interventional procedures. ACS patients with highly suspected COVID-19 should be isolated and undergo necessary laboratory and imaging tests, with all healthcare workers wearing the appropriate PPE (34).

Besides, the most important issue is to educate the general population about the early recognition of high-risk ACS symptoms with promptly referral to ED (or at least to contact a physician) in such cases. This could be reached by social media, television, and journals. Interestingly, following this rationale, the Italian Society of Cardiology promoted a national campaign to raise public awareness about MI symptoms during the outbreak, showing encouraging results in terms of subsequent fall in the time from symptoms to ED admission (50).

Social education should emphasize the concept of an outweigh of untreated-MI consequences, rather than of COVID-19 in-hospital infection, since hospitals are now equipped with appropriate PPE and follow the preventive protocols to minimize the risk of contagion. The use of telemedicine and/or telemonitoring in doubtful cases would allow to obtain a close follow-up of patients' symptoms and clinical conditions and, sometimes, to perform some kinds of triaging in order to avoid unrecognized MI on one hand, and to optimize resources allocation on the other hand. More compliant patients could also be engaged in the use of smartwatches and smartphone apps, achieving rapid medical screening and/or self-monitoring.

CONCLUSIONS

During the COVID-19 pandemic, the topic of ACS has been widely discussed. Even if there is paucity of randomized data on the best methods for management, expert consensus and international society recommendation could help us in adopting a standardized approach. First of all, it is important to distinguish between primary ACS or COVID-AMI and, for the latter, discriminate the actual etiology and provide the optimal treatment. This should be done balancing timeliness of screening and conscious use of diagnostic resources and protective measures, in order to ensure safety conditions to all patients and healthcare professionals. COVID status should be assessed as soon as possible. Each primary PCI center should evaluate the feasibility of a timely primary PCI, based on staff, PPE and Cath-lab availability, and the need for additional testing. Otherwise, a first approach with fibrinolysis should be considered. The other important concern is the global registration of lower rates of admitted (and therefore treated) patients with ACS. This could lead to a substantial increase in early and late infarct-related morbidity and mortality. To face the possible collateral cardiac damage caused by COVID-19, every attempt should be done by the clinicians in means of avoiding delayed or missed diagnosis, re-organization of healthcare tools, and social education.

AUTHOR CONTRIBUTIONS

MC, MCP, GM, FD'A, PC, GP, GB, and MF performed the data search and drafted the manuscript. MC, FF, GP, SM, and SV critically revised the draft. All Authors contributed to the conception of this work and approved the final version of the manuscript.

REFERENCES

1. *COVID-19 Dashboard by the Center for Systems Science and Engineering (CSSE) at Johns Hopkins University (JHU).* Available online at: https://coronavirus.jhu.edu/map.html (accessed July 3, 2020).
2. Huang C, Wang Y, Li X, Ren L, Zhao J, Hu Y, et al. Clinical features of patients infected with 2019 novel coronavirus in Wuhan, China. *Lancet.* (2020) 395:497–506. doi: 10.1016/S0140-6736(20)30183-5
3. Richardson S, Hirsch JS, Narasimhan M, Crawford JM, McGinn T, Davidson KW, et al. Presenting characteristics, comorbidities, and outcomes among 5700 patients hospitalized with COVID-19 in the New York City Area. *JAMA.* (2020) 323:2052–9. doi: 10.1001/jama.2020.6775
4. De Filippo O, D'Ascenzo F, Angelini F, Bocchino PP, Conrotto F, Saglietto A, et al. Reduced rate of hospital admissions for acs during Covid-19 outbreak in Northern Italy. *N Engl J Med.* (2020) 383:88–9. doi: 10.1056/NEJMc2009166

5. Li B, Yang J, Zhao F, Zhi L, Wang X, Liu L, et al. Prevalence and impact of cardiovascular metabolic diseases on COVID-19 in China. *Clin Res Cardiol.* (2020) 109:531–8. doi: 10.1007/s00392-020-01626-9
6. Kang Y, Chen T, Mui D, Ferrari V, Jagasia D, Scherrer-Crosbie M, et al. Cardiovascular manifestations and treatment considerations in covid-19. *Heart.* (2020) 106:1132–41. doi: 10.1136/heartjnl-2020-317056
7. Zheng YY, Ma YT, Zhang JY, Xie X. COVID-19 and the cardiovascular system. *Nat Rev Cardiol.* (2020) 17:259–260. doi: 10.1038/s41569-020-0360-5
8. Tang N, Li D, Wang X, Sun Z. Abnormal coagulation parameters are associated with poor prognosis in patients with novel coronavirus pneumonia. *J Thromb Haemost.* (2020) 18:844–7. doi: 10.1111/jth.14768
9. Warren-Gash C, Hayward AC, Hemingway H, Denaxas S, Thomas SL, Timmis AD, et al. Influenza infection and risk of acute myocardial infarction in England and Wales: a CALIBER self-controlled case series study. *J Infect Dis.* (2012) 206:1652–9. doi: 10.1093/infdis/jis597

10. Sugiura M, Hiraoka K, Ohkawa S, Ueda K, Matsuda T. A clinicopathological study on cardiac lesions in 64 cases of disseminated intravascular coagulation. *Jpn Heart J.* (1977) 18:57–69. doi: 10.1536/ihj.18.57

11. Bangalore S, Sharma A, Slotwiner A, Yatskar L, Harari R, Shah B, et al. ST-segment elevation in patients with Covid-19—a case series. *N Engl J Med.* (2020) 382:2478–80. doi: 10.1056/NEJMc2009020

12. Xuan TM, Wang XX, Pu XY, Han WL, Guo XG. Primary percutaneous coronary intervention in a COVID-19 patient with ST-segment elevation myocardial infarction after lung transplantation: a case report. *J Zhejiang Univ Sci B.* (2020) 21:411–5. doi: 10.1631/jzus.B2000182

13. Shi S, Qin M, Shen B, Cai Y, Liu T, Yang F, et al. Association of cardiac injury with mortality in hospitalized patients with COVID-19 in Wuhan, China. *JAMA Cardiol.* (2020) 5:802–10. doi: 10.1001/jamacardio.2020.0950

14. Guo T, Fan Y, Chen M, Wu X, Zhang L, He T, et al. Cardiovascular Implications of Fatal Outcomes of Patients With Coronavirus Disease 2019 (COVID-19). *JAMA Cardiol.* (2020) 5:1–8. doi: 10.1001/jamacardio.2020.1017

15. Han H, Yang L, Liu R, Liu F, Wu KL, Li J, et al. Prominent changes in blood coagulation of patients with SARS-CoV-2 infection. *Clin Chem Lab Med.* (2020). 58:1116–20. doi: 10.1515/cclm-2020-0188

16. Klok FA, Kruip MJHA, van der Meer NJM, Arbous MS, Gommers DAMPJ, Kant KM, et al. Incidence of thrombotic complications in critically ill ICU patients with COVID-19. *Thromb Res.* (2020) 191:145–7. doi: 10.1016/j.thromres.2020.04.013

17. Zhou F, Yu T, Du R, Fan G, Liu Y, Liu Z, et al. Clinical course and risk factors for mortality of adult inpatients with COVID-19 in Wuhan, China: a retrospective cohort study. *Lancet.* (2020) 395:1054–62. doi: 10.1016/S0140-6736(20)30566-3

18. Yao XH, Li TY, He ZC, Ping YF, Liu HW, Yu SC, et al. [A pathological report of three COVID-19 cases by minimal invasive autopsies]. *Zhonghua Bing Li Xue Za Zhi.* (2020) 49:411–7. doi: 10.3760/cma.j.cn112151-20200312-00193

19. Beri A, Kotak K. Cardiac injury, Arrhythmia and Sudden death in a COVID-19 patient. *HeartRhythm Case Rep.* (2020) 6:367–9. doi: 10.1016/j.hrcr.2020.05.001

20. Tavazzi G, Pellegrini C, Maurelli M, Belliato M, Sciutti F, Bottazzi A, et al. Myocardial localization of coronavirus in COVID-19 cardiogenic shock. *Eur J Heart Fail.* (2020) 22:911–5. doi: 10.1002/ejhf.1828

21. Hu H, Ma F, Wei X, Fang Y. Coronavirus fulminant myocarditis saved with glucocorticoid and human immunoglobulin. *Eur Heart J.* (2020). doi: 10.1093/eurheartj/ehaa190. [Epub ahead of print].

22. Zeng JH, Liu YX, Yuan J, Wang FX, Wu WB, Li JX, et al. First case of COVID-19 complicated with fulminant myocarditis: a case report and insights. *Infection.* (2020) 48:1–5. doi: 10.1007/s15010-020-01424-5

23. Sala S, Peretto G, Gramegna M, Palmisano A, Villatore A, Vignale D, et al. Acute myocarditis presenting as a reverse Tako-Tsubo syndrome in a patient with SARS-CoV-2 respiratory infection. *Eur Heart J.* (2020) 41:1861–2. doi: 10.1093/eurheartj/ehaa286

24. Moderato L, Monello A, Lazzeroni D, Binno S, Giacalone R, Ferraro S, et al. [Takotsubo syndrome during SARS-CoV-2 pneumonia: a possible cardiovascular complication]. *G Ital Cardiol.* (2020) 21:417–20. doi: 10.1714/3359.33323

25. Meyer P, Degrauwe S, Van Delden C, Ghadri JR, Templin C. Typical takotsubo syndrome triggered by SARS-CoV-2 infection. *Eur Heart J.* (2020) 41:1860. doi: 10.1093/eurheartj/ehaa306

26. Chadha S. 'COVID-19 pandemic' anxiety-induced Takotsubo cardiomyopathy. *QJM.* (2020) 113:488–90. doi: 10.1093/qjmed/hcaa135

27. Chieffo A, Stefanini GG, Price S, Barbato E, Tarantini G, Karam N, et al. EAPCI position statement on invasive management of acute coronary syndromes during the COVID-19 pandemic. *Eur Heart J.* (2020) 41:1839–51. doi: 10.1093/eurheartj/ehaa381

28. Ibanez B, James S, Agewall S, Antunes MJ, Bucciarelli-Ducci C, Bueno H, et al. ESC Scientific Document Group. 2017 ESC Guidelines for the management of acute myocardial infarction in patients presenting with ST-segment elevation: The Task Force for the management of acute myocardial infarction in patients presenting with ST-segment elevation of the European Society of Cardiology (ESC). *Eur Heart J.* (2018) 39:119–77. doi: 10.1093/eurheartj/ehx393

29. American College of Cardiology. *Troponin and BNP Use in COVID-19.* Available online at: https://www.acc.org/latest-in-cardiology/articles/2020/03/18/15/25/troponin-and-bnp-use-in-covid19 (accessed July 3, 2020).

30. Skulstad H, Cosyns B, Popescu BA, Galderisi M, Salvo GD, Donal E, et al. COVID-19 pandemic and cardiac imaging: EACVI recommendations on precautions, indications, prioritization, and protection for patients and healthcare personnel. *Eur Heart J Cardiovasc Imaging.* (2020) 21:592–8. doi: 10.1093/ehjci/jeaa072

31. Cameli M, Pastore MC, Henein M, Aboumarie HS, Mandoli GE, D'Ascenzi F, et al. Safe performance of echocardiography during the COVID-19 pandemic: a practical guide. *Rev Cardiovasc Med.* (2020) 21:217–23. doi: 10.31083/j.rcm.2020.02.90

32. Stefanini GG, Montorfano M, Trabattoni D, Andreini D, Ferrante G, Ancona M, et al. ST-elevation myocardial infarction in patients with COVID-19: clinical and angiographic outcomes. *Circulation.* (2020) 141:2113–6. doi: 10.1161/CIRCULATIONAHA.120.047525

33. Hendren NS, Drazner MH, Bozkurt B, Cooper LT Jr. Description and proposed management of the acute COVID-19 cardiovascular syndrome. *Circulation.* (2020) 141:1903–14. doi: 10.1161/CIRCULATIONAHA.120.047349

34. Cosyns B, Lochy S, Luchian ML, Gimelli A, Pontone G, Allard SD, et al. The role of cardiovascular imaging for myocardial injury in hospitalized COVID-19 patients. *Eur Heart J Cardiovasc Imaging.* (2020) 21:709–14. doi: 10.1093/ehjci/jeaa136

35. Cameli M, Pastore MC, Soliman Aboumarie H, Mandoli GE, D'Ascenzi F, Cameli P, et al. Usefulness of echocardiography to detect cardiac involvement in COVID-19 patients. *Echocardiography.* (2020) 37:1278–86. doi: 10.1111/echo.14779

36. Jing ZC, Zhu HD, Yan XW, Chai WZ, Zhang S. Recommendations from the Peking Union Medical College Hospital for the management of acute myocardial infarction during the COVID-19 outbreak. *Eur Heart J.* (2020) 41:1791–4. doi: 10.1093/eurheartj/ehaa258

37. Mahmud E, Dauerman HL, Welt FG, Messenger JC, Rao SV, Grines C, et al. Management of acute myocardial infarction during the COVID-19 pandemic. *J Am Coll Cardiol.* (2020) 96:336–45. S0735-1097(20)35026-9. doi: 10.1016/j.jacc.2020.04.039

38. Collet J, Thiele H, Barbato E, Barthélémy O, Bauersachs J, Bhatt DL, et al. 2020 ESC Guidelines for the management of acute coronary syndromes in patients presenting without persistent ST-segment elevation. *Eur Heart J.* (2020) 1–79. doi: 10.1093/eurheartj/ehaa575. [Epub ahead of print].

39. Valente S, Anselmi F, Cameli M. Acute coronary syndromes during COVID-19. *Eur Heart J.* (2020) 41:2047–49. doi: 10.1093/eurheartj/ehaa457

40. Italian Society of Interventional Cardiology (GISE). *Management of cathetherization lab and interventional cardiology during COVID-19 emergency.* (2020). 41. Available online at: https://gise.it/Uploads/EasyCms/GM%20CF%20per%20PD%20gestione%20covid-19%20-_14892.pdf (accessed July 3, 2020).

41. Zeng J, Huang J, Pan L. How to balance acute myocardial infarction and COVID-19: the protocols from Sichuan Provincial People's Hospital. *Intensive Care Med.* (2020) 46:1111–3. doi: 10.1007/s00134-020-05993-9

42. Welt FGP, Shah PB, Aronow HD, Bortnick AE, Henry TD, Sherwood MW, et al. American College of Cardiology's Interventional Council and the Society for Cardiovascular Angiography and Interventions. Catheterization Laboratory Considerations During the Coronavirus (COVID-19) Pandemic: From the ACC's Interventional Council and SCAI. *J Am Coll Cardiol.* (2020) 75:2372–5. doi: 10.1016/j.jacc.2020.03021

43. Wang N, Zhang M, Su H, Huang Z, Lin Y, Zhang M. Fibrinolysis is a reasonable alternative for STEMI care during the COVID-19 pandemic. *J Int Med Res.* (2020) 48:300060520966151. doi: 10.1177/0300060520966151

44. Zhang L, Fan Y, Lu Z. Experiences and lesson strategies for cardiology from the COVID-19 outbreak in Wuhan, China, by 'on the scene' cardiologists. *Eur Heart J.* (2020) 41:1788–90. doi: 10.1093/eurheartj/ehaa266

45. Keeley EC, Boura JA, Grines CL. Primary angioplasty versus intravenous thrombolytic therapy for acute myocardial infarction: a quantitative review of 23 randomised trials. *Lancet.* (2003) 361:13–20. doi: 10.1016/S0140-6736(03)12113-7

46. De Rosa S, Spaccarotella C, Basso C, Calabrò MP, Curcio A, Filardi PP, et al. Società Italiana di Cardiologia and the CCU Academy investigators group. Reduction of hospitalizations for myocardial infarction in Italy in

the COVID-19 era. *Eur Heart J.* (2020) 41:2083–8. doi: 10.1093/eurheartj/ehaa610

47. Metzler B, Siostrzonek P, Binder RK, Bauer A, Reinstadler SJ. Decline of acute coronary syndrome admissions in Austria since the outbreak of COVID-19: the pandemic response causes cardiac collateral damage. *Eur Heart J.* (2020) 41:1852–3. doi: 10.1093/eurheartj/ehaa314

48. Huet F, Prieur C, Schurtz G, Gerbaud E, Manzo-Silberman S, Vanzetto G, et al. One train may hide another: acute cardiovascular diseases could be neglected because of the COVID-19 pandemic. *Arch Cardiovasc Dis.* (2020) 113:303–7. doi: 10.1016/j.acvd.2020.04.002

49. Garcia S, Albaghdadi MS, Meraj PM, Schmidt C, Garberich R, Jaffer FA, et al. Reduction in ST-segment elevation cardiac catheterization laboratory activations in the United States during COVID-19 pandemic. *J Am Coll Cardiol.* (2020) 75:2871–2. doi: 10.1016/j.jacc.2020.04.011

50. Rodriguez-Leor O, Cid-Alvarez B. ST-segment elevation myocardial infarction care during COVID-19: losing sight of the forest for the trees. *JACC Case Rep.* (2020) 2:1625–7. doi: 10.1016/j.jaccas.2020.04.011

51. Quadri G, Rognoni A, Cerrato E, Baralis G, Boccuzzi G, Brsic E, et al. Catheterization laboratory activity before and during COVID-19 spread: a comparative analysis in Piedmont, Italy, by the Italian Society of Interventional Cardiology (GISE). *Int J Cardiol.* (2020) 323:288–91. doi: 10.1016/j.ijcard.2020.08.072

52. Masroor S. Collateral damage of COVID-19 pandemic: delayed medical care. *J Card Surg.* (2020) 35:1345–7. doi: 10.1111/jocs.14638

53. Scott IA. "Time is muscle" in reperfusing occluded coronary arteries in acute myocardial infarction. *Med J Aust.* (2010) 193:493–5. doi: 10.5694/j.1326-5377.2010.tb04030.x

54. Trabattoni D, Montorsi P, Merlino L. Late STEMI and NSTEMI patients' emergency calling in COVID-19 outbreak. *Can J Cardiol.* (2020) 36:1161.e7–1161.e8. doi: 10.1016/j.cjca.2020.05.003

55. Tam CF, Cheung KS, Lam S, Wong A, Yung A, Sze M, et al. Impact of coronavirus disease 2019 (COVID-19) outbreak on outcome of myocardial infarction in Hong Kong, China. *Catheter Cardiovasc Interv.* (2020) 13:e006631. doi: 10.1002/ccd28943

56. Yousefzai R, Bhimaraj A. Misdiagnosis in the COVID-19 Era: when zebras are everywhere, don't forget the horses. *JACC Case Rep.* (2020) 2:1614–9. doi: 10.1016/j.jaccas.2020.04.018

57. Boukhris M, Hillani A, Moroni F, Annabi MS, Addad F, Ribeiro MH, et al. Cardiovascular implications of the COVID-19 pandemic: a global perspective. *Can J Cardiol.* (2020) 36:1068–80. doi: 10.1016/j.cjca.2020.05.018

58. Baldi E, Sechi GM, Mare C, Canevari F, Brancaglione A, Primi R, et al. Lombardia CARe researchers. Out-of-hospital cardiac arrest during the Covid-19 outbreak in Italy. *N Engl J Med.* (2020) 383:496–8. doi: 10.1056/NEJMc2010418

59. Mountantonakis SE, Saleh M, Coleman K, Kuvin J, Singh V, Jauhar R, et al. Out-of-hospital cardiac arrest and acute coronary syndrome hospitalizations during the COVID-19 surge. *J Am Coll Cardiol.* (2020) 76:1271–3. doi: 10.1016/j.jacc.2020.07.021

60. The European Society for Cardiology. *ESC Guidance for the Diagnosis and Management of CV Disease during the COVID-19 Pandemic.* Available online at: https://www.escardio.org/Education/COVID-19-and-Cardiology/ESC-COVID-19-Guidance (accessed June 10, 2020).

17

Mitigating the Risk of COVID-19 Deaths in Cardiovascular Disease Patients in Africa Resource Poor Communities

Ihunanya Chinyere Okpara[1]* and Efosa Kenneth Oghagbon[2]

[1] Cardiology Unit, Department of Internal Medicine, Benue State University Teaching Hospital, Makurdi, Nigeria, [2] Department of Chemical Pathology, Benue State University Teaching Hospital, Makurdi, Nigeria

*Correspondence:
Ihunanya Chinyere Okpara
iokparajubilee@gmail.com

The novel coronavirus disease 2019 (Covid-19) pandemic has affected millions of patients in almost all countries with over one million cases recorded in Africa where it is a major health challenge. Covid-19 is known to have significant implications for those with pre-existing cardiovascular disease (CVD) and their cardiologists. Patients with pre-existing CVD are at increased risk of morbidity and mortality from Covid-19 due to associated direct and indirect life threatening cardiovascular (CV) complications. Mitigating the risk of such Covid-19 deaths in resource poor communities requires the institution of preventive measures at the primary, secondary and tertiary levels of preventive phenomenon with emphasis at the first two levels. General preventive measures, screening and monitoring of CVD patients for complications and modification of drug treatment and other treatment methods will need to be implemented. Health policy makers and manager should provide required training and retraining of CV health care workers managing Covid-19 patients with CVD, provision of health education, personal protective equipment (PPE), and diagnostic kits.

Keywords: COVID-19 deaths, cardiovascular disease, levels of prevention, Africa, resource poor communities

INTRODUCTION

The novel corona virus disease referred to as Covid-19 was identified in December 2019 in Wuhan, China. It is caused by Severe Acute Respiratory Syndrome Coronavirus 2 (SARS-CoV-2) (1, 2) and the disease has since spread all over the world including resource poor communities in Africa (3).

Given the rapid spread of the virus in early 2020, the disease was declared a pandemic by the World Health Organization (WHO) on March 11, 2020 (2). Within a short time there was a litany of literature on the disease with physicians in all specialties expected to be aware of the impact of this disease in their respective clinical care areas and the medical community at large (4).

In Africa, the spread of Covid-19 was feared for so many reasons (5): Firstly, large and densely populated areas and townships with widespread poverty and high migration make such places vulnerable to airborne pandemics. Secondly, existing epidemics of human immunodeficiency virus (HIV), tuberculosis (TB), and malaria were thought to make Covid-19 more severe and thus lead to increased morbidity and mortality. Lastly, the high prevalence of non-communicable diseases in Africa such as hypertension, CVD and diabetes which are known risk factors for severe cases of Covid-19 portends a poor outcome (3), and this is of concern to the index authors.

The clinical presentation of this disease ranges from asymptomatic to mild, severe, and critical cases. Its symptoms which are similar to common viral and parasitic infections in sub-Saharan Africa include fever, cough, dyspnoea, myalgias, fatigue, and diarrhea. In severe and critical cases, it presents with pneumonia, acute respiratory distress syndrome (ARDS), cardiogenic, and septic shock. Over time, it was shown that elderly populations with pre-existing medical comorbidities are most vulnerable to severe disease (5–7).

In sub-Saharan Africa, the high prevalence of CVD and their relationship to the disease means cardiologists will be actively engaged in the management of Covid-19 patients. Aside Covid-19 infection being associated with CV complications, infected individuals with pre-existing CVD have elevated risk of severe disease and worse outcomes (8–10). Additionally, therapeutics for Covid-19 have potential adverse CV effects due to significant drug-drug interactions with regular CV medications. Finally, CVD drugs may interfere with the pathophysiology of Covid-19 especially with viral relationship to ACE2 receptors (11, 12).

The management of severe Covid-19 cases in patients with CVD and other high risk conditions is costly in resource poor countries of Africa, thus the need to activate primary and secondary levels of prevention. Presently, Covid-19 mortality in African countries are not as high as expected (5, 13). This is due to many factors including the implementation of primary and secondary preventive measures.

Hence, this review aim to discuss the need to mitigate Covid-19 deaths in CVD patients in resource poor countries of Africa, and the measures to be put in place toward realizing this goal.

VIROLOGY OF SARS-COV-2, EPIDEMIOLOGY AND PATHOPHYSIOLOGY OF COVID-19

The SARS-CoV-2 virus belongs to the family of Coronaviridae which are enveloped viruses with non-segmented, single stranded, positive-sense ribonucleic acid (RNA) genome (14). A number of the SARS—related coronaviruses have been found in bats, thus suggesting they may constitute the zoonotic host for SARS-CoV-2, especially given that the viral genome is 96.2% identical to a bat coronavirus (15). Typical of corona viruses such as SARS and the Middle East Respiratory syndrome virus (MERS-CoV), they commonly cause respiratory illnesses which are the predominant manifestation of Covid-19 disease. The infectivity of Covid-19 is greater than that of influenza with an estimated R_0 value of 2.28 (16). Similarly, death rate associated with Covid-19 is higher compared to <0.1% estimated recently for influenza by WHO, though it may be higher for the elderly, persons with comorbidities and persons in low resource settings (17). However, earlier coronaviruses infections such as SARS-CoV epidemic and MERS-CoV, had higher case fatality rates of 9.6 and 34.4%, respectively (18). Covid-19 disease however has spread more widely to affect larger populations and places than previous coronaviruses outbreaks (18, 19).

Since December 2019, Covid-19 disease has spread to all corners of the globe affecting over 37 million persons with more than 1 million deaths as of 11th October, 2020 (20) in over 100 countries across the world. Africa as of the same date has over 1 million cases with the highest number of 690,896 cases in South Africa and lowest of 414 in Eritrea. Nigeria with 60,103 cases of confirmed Covid-19 is the highest in West Africa sub-region (20). The crude case-fatality rate which was 3.8% in the USA in March 2020 (21, 22) fell to 2.8% in October, in same month it is 1.8% in Nigeria (20).

The clinical cases can either be asymptomatic or mild in a large proportion of patients and severe in a smaller portion (18). In China it was found that 81.4% of cases were mild requiring only symptomatic treatment and isolation, with severe disease in 13.9% of cases that needed supplemental oxygen therapy, and critical in 4.7% requiring intensive care unit (ICU) treatment including mechanical ventilation (22).

Studies show that SARS-CoV-2 as well as other coronaviruses use angiotensin-converting enzyme 2 (ACE2) protein; a homolog of ACE1 (9) for cell entry. ACE2 which is a type 1 integral membrane protein is highly expressed in lung alveolar cells and may expose humans to increased viral entry (15). After ligand binding, SARS-CoV-2 enters cells via receptor-mediated endocytosis in a manner akin to entry of HIV viruses in to body cells (23). The viral take-over of ACE2 receptors in Covid-19 infection deregulates lung protective pathway occasioned by uninfected receptors, thus contributing to viral pathogenicity (24). ACE2 is found primarily in the lower respiratory tract, rather than the upper airways (10). This distribution can explain the few upper respiratory tract symptoms typical of flu and why Covid-19 is not just a common cold (10, 17).

Clinicians are concerned about a possible link between SARS-CoV-2 and angiotensin 2 receptor blockers (ARBs) which could increase chances of adverse effects of the disease in CVD patients on this class of antihypertensives (17), Hence it is important that doctors understand clinical and preventive measures to reduce morbidity and mortality from Covid-19 among CVD patients.

REASONS TO MITIGATE THE RISK OF COVID-19 DEATHS IN CVD PATIENTS

Several reasons portend the need to mitigate the risk of Covid-19 deaths in CVD patients (**Table 1**) details of which are given below.

TABLE 1 | Reasons to mitigate the risk of Covid-19 deaths in CVD patients.

1.	Association between pre-existing CVD and severe Covid-19 disease.
2.	Life threatening CV complications are seen in Covid-19 patients with or without pre-existing CVD.
3.	Significant drug interactions exist between CVD medications and therapies under investigation for Covid-19.

Association Between Pre-existing CVD and Severe COVID-19 Disease

Different studies show the association between pre-existing CVD and severe Covid-19 disease. A meta-analysis of seriously ill Covid-19 patients found the prevalence of hypertension, cerebrovascular disease and diabetes to be 17.1, 16.4, and 9.7%, respectively, among them (8). The overall case fatality rate in Covid-19 patients is commonly <3% (18), but this increases to 10.5% in those with CVD, 7.3% in diabetes, and 6.3% in hypertensives (18). Similar findings showing more adverse events in CVD patients with Covid-19, have been reported in other investigations, whether in China, Europe, or sub-Saharan Africa (13, 25). In Ghana, the highest number of deaths occurred in Covid-19 patients with pre-existing hypertension and diabetes (13). This number will go up as more people become seriously ill with Covid-19 in the sub-region due to inadequate facilities and personnel.

Aside hypertension, other factors associated with increased deaths are age, diabetes, and hyperlipidemia. Age is a risk factor for hypertension, obesity, glucose intolerance, and reduced immunity (25–27); which are associated with increased risk of severe Covid-19 disease. Diabetes and hyperlipidemia causes dysregulation of the immune system in addition to deterioration of vascular integrity (27, 28). Thus, prevalent CVD may be a marker of accelerated immunologic aging/dysregulation and relate indirectly to Covid-19 prognosis. Other possible risk factors for severe disease in low income countries of sub-Saharan Africa include HIV, TB, Chronic Obstructive Pulmonary disease (COPD), Rheumatic Heart Disease (RHD), and cardiomyopathies (29).

Cardiovascular Complications of Covid-19 in Patients With or Without Pre-existing CVD

Several investigations suggest SARS-CoV-2 infection is associated with life threatening CV complications in those with or without pre-existing CVD (10, 18). The CV complications includes myocarditis, acute coronary syndromes, arrhythmias, heart failure, cardiogenic shock, and venous thromboembolism. The recognition of these complications must be possible in health facilities in Africa for improved survival of cardiac patients.

Myocarditis and Acute Coronary Syndromes

Myocardial injury is increased in patients with myocarditis and acute coronary syndrome as a results of ARDS and severe Covid-19 (10, 30, 31). Elevated serum troponin levels are seen in many Covid-19 patients, with significant differences noted in survivors and those who succumbed to the viral disease (32). Some authors found that mean cardiac troponin I levels was significantly higher in severe Covid-19-illness compared to non-severe disease (33).

Increased levels of troponin T (TnT) has been found to be associated with Covid-19 disease, especially in those with pre-existing CVD. Of note, the highest mortality rates were observed in those with elevated TnT levels whether due to Covid-19 or prior CVD.

Other markers of acute cardiac injury in Covid-19 patients are abnormal electrocardiographic and echocardiographic findings in patients.

Cardiac Arrhythmia and Cardiac Arrest

The arrhythmias observed in severe Covid-19 infections are cause for concern as it is a significant contributor to adverse outcomes (23). Arrhythmogenesis appears to be a feature of coronaviruses as these have been reported in SARS and MERS patients. The different forms of dysarrhythmias in coronaviruses infections include branch block, atrial fibrillation, premature beats, QT interval elongation, and even sudden cardiac death (34). In hospitalized Covid-19 patients, cardiac arrhythmias were noted in 16.7% of patients in a Chinese cohort especially in those in ICU (6). Up to 60% of fatal cases of Covid-19 have arrhythmias and in some patients the cardiac arrhythmias are independently associated with in-hospital mortality (35). This is more so as African Americans have been found to have genetic susceptibility for Covid-19 associated sudden cardiac death (36). It is advised that new onset of malignant tachyarrhythmias in the setting of troponin elevation should raise the suspicion of underlying myocarditis or acute coronary syndrome and potential arrhythmias (32, 37).

Arrhythmias should be considered a major complication of Covid-19 and be watched out for when medications are being considered in resource poor settings.

Cardiomyopathy and Heart Failure

Heart failure was reported in 23.0% of patients with Covid-19 presentations (10). Whether heart failure is most commonly due to exacerbations of pre-existing left ventricular (LV) dysfunction or new cardiomyopathy is unclear (38). Right heart failure and associated pulmonary hypertension should be considered, in particular in the context of severe parenchymal lung disease and ARDS, which are common findings in severe Covid-19 disease.

Cardiogenic and Mixed Shock

The appearance of ground glass opacities in severe Covid-19 patient similar to that in ARDS on chest imaging (39) should be distinguished from that of coexisting cardiogenic pulmonary oedema. A possibility of *in situ* cardiogenic or mixed cardiac plus primary pulmonary causes of respiratory manifestations in Covid-19 (mixed presentation), should be considered in clinical assessment of patients.

Venous Thromboembolic Disease

Patients with Covid-19 are at increased risk of venous thromboembolism and this is said to be as high as 31% in critically ill subjects (40). Studies suggest abnormal coagulation parameters like D-dimers are very useful in the diagnosis (41). In various places, elevated D-dimer levels (>1 g/l) are strongly associated with in-hospital death, even after multivariable adjustment (10, 41). The elevation of D-dimers and FDP (fibrin degradation products) are synonymous with poor survival in severely ill Covid-19 patients as this may indicate presence of disseminated intravascular coagulation (DIC) (41).

TABLE 2 | Drug therapy and Covid-19: interactions and cardiovascular complications.

1.	Therapies under investigation for Covid-19 may have significant drug-drug toxicity with CV medications.
2.	Therapies under investigation for Covid-19 have significant CV toxicities.
3.	Patient debilitation from severe Covid-19 may pose challenges in administering routine CV medications
4.	Drugs for patients with CVD could interfere with the pathophysiology of Covid-19

Drug Therapy and Covid-19: Interactions and Cardiovascular Complications

There are currently no specific effective therapies for Covid-19. However, it is worthy to note that significant drug interactions exist between CVD medications and therapies under investigation for Covid-19 (12, 42, 43) (**Table 2**).

MITIGATING THE RISK OF COVID-19 DEATHS IN CVD PATIENTS IN AFRICA RESOURCE POOR COMMUNITIES

Efforts to reduce Covid-19 deaths in CVD patients should involve three levels of prevention; primary, secondary, and tertiary levels. Primary prevention measures are those are put in place before the onset of illness. Secondary prevention refers to measures that ensure early diagnosis and prompt treatment, before development of CV complications. The tertiary prevention strategy is aimed at rehabilitation following significant illness.

In resource poor communities in sub-Saharan Africa, emphasis should be on primary and secondary preventive measures due to unsustainable financial requirements for tertiary measures of prevention.

Control measures will vary between:

1. Patients with CVD without Covid-19.
2. Patients with coexistence of CVD and Covid-19.
3. CV health workers.

Adequate consideration should be given to patients in resource poor communities where other immunosuppressive conditions such as HIV and TB could coexist with Covid-19 and CVD. Lifestyle measures, drug treatment and method of treatment modifications, as well as availability of necessary protective and medical equipment will all be required. Health care workers are also at risk of infection and should be protected.

Mitigating the Risk of Death in Patients With Pre-Existing CVD Without Covid-19

Measures to reduce the risk of death in resource poor settings should be emphasized at the primary and secondary levels of prevention for sustainability. Since disease transmission occurs most commonly via respiratory droplets and aerosols with the virus active on surfaces for several days (44), the recommendations are suggested for general prevention include:

a. All aged CVD patients should be taught to avoid close contact by practicing social distancing of at least 2 m away. They should be trained in community and personal hygiene and this should be more so with the uneducated subjects.
b. As much as possible, patients with known risk factors should avoid crowds, especially in door assembly. Possibly, very vulnerable subjects should practice voluntary isolation but be able to receive support from family members to prevent depressive events. This isolation is important for those in major congested cities in Africa (13).
c. Everyone must reduce or avoid touching their eyes, nose, and mouth, when up and about in their location where surfaces may be contaminated (44).
d. Subjects must wash their hands frequently under running water. The alternative is to use alcohol (65% w/v ethyl alcohol) based hand sanitizers for similar purpose.
e. The use of face masks should be mandatory for CVD subjects in resource poor settings.
f. Pseudo-telemedicine approaches such as use of internet based telephone consultations; these include WhatsApp and Facebook videos which are popular in Africa and can be used for patient consultations, during pandemics to reduce travels and social contacts at hospitals. This can help to promote viral containment (45).

Mitigating the Risk of Death in Covid-19 Patients With Pre-existing CVD in Sub-Saharan Africa

The majorly secondary and feasible tertiary levels of prevention features are as follows:

a. Screening for Covid-19 in all CVD patients for early diagnoses, especially when they are susceptible groups like health and other frontline workers, or those with immune compromise. This will enhance early diagnosis and closer monitoring for CV complications (10, 18) in resource poor communities.
b. Screening of Covid-19 patients for CVD and CV complications—The American College of Cardiology (ACC) has recommended the establishment of protocol for diagnosis, triage, and isolation of Covid-19 patients with CVD or CV complications (46).
c. Telemedicine and e-visits—as mentioned above, with the wide availability of cell phones in resource poor communities in sub-Saharan Africa consultations can be made by patients with specialty physicians without close contact.
d. Clear and prompt understanding of the effects of the virus and hypertension therapy in relation to ACE inhibitors and ARB therapy in Covid-19 patients, should be given early to reduce clinician and patient confusion (47). All CVD patients should be encouraged to continue their home blood pressure monitoring and medical regimen (48).
e. All drug—drug interactions with CV medications and direct CV toxicities should be avoided or reduced to the barest minimum, by retraining of clinicians and other healthcare workers.

f. As a tertiary measure, nationwide training of health workers on mechanical ventilatory support and Advanced Cardiac Life Support (ALCS) and all citizens on cardiac and vocational rehabilitation post Covid-19, should be commenced pending availability of resources for full implementation.

Recommendations for Healthcare Workers Managing CVD During Covid-19 Pandemic

a. Ensure the use of provided PPE and in the right manner as recommended by WHO, CDC and China's CDC, namely: facemask, goggles, disposable, or re-useable gowns and gloves (49–52).
b. Telemedicine and e-visits—this allows for triaging of patients and patient management while minimizing exposure of patients and health workers to potential infection.
c. Health care practitioners must be conversant with antiviral agents approved or under investigation for the treatment of Covid-19 and their CV toxicities (53).
d. Carefully managed rescheduling of elective procedures during the growth phase of the outbreak.
e. Ensure hospital equipment such as echocardiography, scanners et cetera are cleaned with antiseptic agents before and after each use.
f. When performing procedures that generates aerosol such as transesophageal echocardiography, endotracheal intubation, cardiopulmonary resuscitation, and bag mask ventilation, additional PPE may be required including controlled or powered air purifying respirators. Thorough infection control measures specific to the procedural cardiology specialty should be considered in light of Covid-19 outbreak.
g. In the event of cardiac arrest, use of external mechanical chest compression devices would help to minimize direct contact with infected patients.
h. The healthcare worker must self-report symptoms if present, and be excused from duty as health worker when symptomatic until tested and found negative.
i. Overall, as CV health workers are on the front lines treating Covid-19 patients, all possible measures should be implemented to reduce the risk of exposure (54).

Recommendations for Health Policy Officials and Manager

a. Provision of infrastructure for e-visits and telemedicine where possible.
b. Provision of sufficient PPEs for patient families and health care personnel.
c. Improving patient and public education concerning Covid-19 infection.
d. Provide adequate tests materials and personnel so that appropriate containment can be achieved.

CONCLUSION

The Covid-19 pandemic has affected thousands of patients globally, but its impact on resource poor communities in sub-Saharan Africa constitutes a major international health challenge. Where as many CVD patients have not died because of the virus, but a significant number had poor outcomes because of fear of going to the hospitals, or because hospitals have shut out routine care in most resource poor environment. Mitigating the risk of death from this disease will involve training and retraining of health care workers and ensuring provision of primary, secondary and tertiary levels preventions. Efficient resources channeled to combat this pandemic by health policy makers and managers will go a long way to mitigate risk of death, if actions are taken early and in right measures.

AUTHOR CONTRIBUTIONS

IO carried out data collection and manuscript writing. EO was involved in manuscript writing and editing of manuscript. All authors contributed to the article and approved the submitted version.

REFERENCES

1. Huang C, Wang Y, Li X, Ren L, Zhao J, Hu Y, et al. Clinical features of patients infected with 2019 novel coronavirus in Wuhan, China. *Lancet.* (2020) 395:497–506. doi: 10.1016/S0140-6736(20)30183-5
2. World Health Organization. *WHO Director-General's Opening Remarks at the Media Briefing on COVID-19- 11 March 2020.* (2020). Available online at: https://www.who.int/dg/speeches/detail/who-director-general-s-opening-remarks-at-the-media-briefing-on-covid-19-$-$11-march-2020 (accessed March 12, 2020).
3. Dong E, Du H, Gardner L. An interactive web-based dashboard to track COVID-19 in real time. *Lancet Infect Dis.* (2020) 20:533–4. doi: 10.1016/S1473-3099(20)30120-1
4. Biondi-Zoccai G, Landoni G, Carnevale R, Cavarretta E, Sciarretta S, Frati G, et al. SARS-CoV-2 and COVID-19: facing the pandemic together as citizens and cardiovascular practitioners. *Minerva Cardioangiol.* (2020) 68:61–4. doi: 10.23736/S0026-4725.20.05250-0

5. Nkengasong JN, Mankoula W. Looming threat of COVID-19 infection in Africa: act collectively and fast. *Lancet.* (2020) 395:841–2. doi: 10.1016/S0140-6736(20)30464-5
6. Wang D, Hu B, Hu C, Zhu F, Liu X, Zhang J, et al. Clinical characteristics of 138 hospitalized patients with 2019 novel coronavirus-infected pneumonia in Wuhan, China. *JAMA.* (2020) 323:1061–9. doi: 10.1001/jama.2020.1585
7. Murthy S, Gomersall CD, Fowler RA. Care for critically ill patients with COVID-19. *JAMA.* (2020) 323:1499–500. doi: 10.1001/jama.2020.3633
8. Li B, Yang J, Zhao F, Zhi L, Wang Y, Liu L, et al. Prevalence and impact of cardiovascular metabolic diseases on COVID-19 in China. *Clin Res Cardiol.* (2020) 109:531–8. doi: 10.1007/s00392-020-01626-9
9. Zheng YY, Ma YT, Zhang JY, Xie X. COVID-19 and the cardiovascular system. *Nat Rev Cardiol.* (2020) 17:1–2. doi: 10.1038/s41569-020-0360-5
10. Zhou F, Yu T, Du R, Fan G, Liu Y, Liu Z, et al. Clinical course and risk factors for mortality of adult in-patients with COVID-19 in Wuhan, China: a retrospective cohort study. *Lancet.* (2020) 395:1054–62. doi: 10.1016/S0140-6736(20)30566-3

11. Imai Y, Kuba K, Rao S, Huan Y, Gao F, Guan B, et al. Angiotensin-converting enzyme 2 protects from severe acute lung failure. *Nature*. (2005) 436:112–6. doi: 10.1038/nature03712

12. Ferrario CM, Jessup J, Chappell MC, Arerill DB, Brosnihan KB, Tallant EA, et al. Effect of angiotensin-converting enzyme inhibition and angiotensin II receptor blockers on cardiac angiotensin-converting enzyme 2. *Circulation*. (2005) 111:2605–10. doi: 10.1161/CIRCULATIONAHA.104.510461

13. Business Day. COVID-19: Sanofi to host 2-day virtual summit for healthcare practitioners. *Business Day* (2020, June 8).

14. Su S, Wong G, Shi W, Liu J, Lai ACK, Zhou J, et al. Epidemiology, genetic recombination, and pathogenesis of coronavirus. *Trends Microbiol*. (2016) 24:490–502. doi: 10.1016/j.tim.2016.03.003

15. Zhou P, Yang XL, Wang XG, Hu B, Zhang L, Zhang W, et al. A Pneumonia associated with a new coronavirus of probable bat origin. *Nature*. (2020) 579:270–3. doi: 10.1038/s41586-020-2012-7

16. Zhang S, Diao M, Yu W, Pei L, Lin Z, Chen D, et al. Estimation of the reproductive number of novel coronavirus (COVID-19) and the probable outbreak size on the Diamond Princess cruise ship: a data driven analysis. *Int J Infect Dis*. (2020) 93:201–4. doi: 10.1016/j.ijid.2020.02.033

17. Paules CI, Marston HD, Fauci AS. Coronavirus infections-more than just the common cold. *JAMA*. (2020) 323:707–8. doi: 10.1001/jama.2020.0757

18. Wu Z, McGoogan JM. Characteristics of and important lessons from the coronavirus disease 2019 (COVID-19) outbreak in China: summary of a report of 72,314 cases from the Chinese Centre for Disease Control and Prevention. *JAMA*. (2020) 323:1239–42. doi: 10.1001/jama.2020.2648

19. Mahase E. Coronavirus covid-19 has killed more people than SARS and MERS combined, despite lower case fatality rate. *BMJ*. (2020) 368:M641 doi: 10.1136/bmj.m641

20. Available online at: www.worldmeters.info

21. World Health Organization. *Coronavirus Disease 2019 (COVID-19) Situation Report – 46*. Available online at: https://20200306-sitrep-46-covid-19.pdf?sfvrsn=96b04adf_2 (accessed March 12, 2020).

22. CDC. *2019 Novel Coronavirus, Wuhan, China: 2019 Novel Coronavirus (2019 – nCoV) in the U.S Centres for Disease Control and Prevention (CDC)*. (2020). Available online at: https://www.cdc.gov/coronavirus/2019 -ncov/cases-in-us.html (accessed March 19, 2020).

23. Wang H, Yang P, Liu K, Guo F, Zhang Y, Zhang G, et al. SARS coronavirus entry into host cells through a novel clathrin- and caveolae-independent endocytic pathway. *Cell Res*. (2008) 18:290–301. doi: 10.1038/cr.2008.15

24. Zhang H, Penninger JM, Li Y, Zhong N, Slutsky AS. Angiotensin-converting enzyme 2 (ACE2) as a SARS-CoV-2 receptor: molecular mechanisms and potential therapeutic target. *Intensive Care Med*. (2020) 46:586–90. doi: 10.1007/s00134-020-05985-9

25. Porcheddu R, Serra C, Kelvin D, Kelvin N, Rubino S. Similarity in case fatality rates (CFR) of COVID-19/SARS-COV-2 in Italy and China. *J Infect Dev Ctries*. (2020) 14:125–8. doi: 10.3855/jidc.12600

26. Liu WM, van der Zeijst BA, Boog CJ, Soethout EC. Aging and impaired immunity to influenza viruses: implications for vaccine development. *Hum Vacc*. (2011) 7(Suppl):94–8. doi: 10.4161/hv.7.0.14568

27. Tall AR, Yvan-Charvet L. Cholesterol, inflammation and innate immunity. *Nat Rev Immunol*. (2015) 15:104–16. doi: 10.1038/nri3793

28. Saltiel AR, Olefsky JM. Inflammatory mechanisms linking obesity and metabolic disease. *J Clin Invest*. (2017) 127:1–4. doi: 10.1172/JCI92035

29. Thienemann F, Pinto F, Grobee DE, Boehm M, Bazargani N, Ge J, et al. World Heart Federation briefing on prevention: coronavirus disease 2019 (COVID-19) in low-income countries. *Global Heart*. (2020) 15:31. doi: 10.5334/gh.778

30. Sarkisian L, Saaby L, Poulsen TS, Gerke O, Jangaard N, Hosbond S, et al. Clinical characteristics and outcomes of patients with myocardial infarction, myocardial injury, and nonelevated troponins. *Am J Med*. (2016) 129:446. doi: 10.1016/j.amjmed.2015.11.006

31. Thygesen K, Alpert JS, Jaffe AS, Chaitman BR, Bax JJ, Morrow DA, et al. Fourth universal definition of myocardial infarction (2018). *J Am Coll Cardiol*. (2018) 72:2231–64. doi: 10.1016/j.jacc.2018.08.1038

32. Yang X, Yu Y, Xu J, Shu H, Xia J, Liu H, et al. Clinical course and outcomes of critically ill patients with SARS-CoV-2 pneumonia in Wuhan, China: a single-centred, retrospective, observational study. *Lancet Respir Med*. (2020) 8:475–81. doi: 10.1016/S2213-2600(20)30079-5

33. Lippi G, Lavie CJ, Sanchis-Gomar F. Cardiac troponin I in patients with coronavirus disease 2019 (COVID-19): evidence from a meta-analysis. *Prog Cardiovasc Dis*. (2020) 63:390–1. doi: 10.1016/j.pcad.2020.03.001

34. Wang Y, Wang Z, Tse G, Zhang L, Wan E, Guo Y et al. Cardiac arrhythmias in patients with COVID-19. *J Arrhythmia*. (2020) 36:1–10. doi: 10.1002/joa3.12405

35. Giudicessi JR, Roden DM, Wilde AMA, Ackerman MJ. Genetic susceptibility for COVID-19 associated sudden cardiac death in African Americans. *Heart Rhythm*. (2020) 17:1487–92. doi: 10.1016/j.hrthm.2020.04.045

36. Mehra MR, Desai SS, Kuy S, Henry TD. Cardiovascular Disease, drug therapy and mortality in Covid-19. *N Engl J Med*. (2020) 382:e102. doi: 10.1056/NEJMoa2007621

37. Chen C, Zhou Y, Wang DW. SARS-Cov-2: a potential novel etiology of fulminant myocarditis. *Herz*. (2020) 45:230–2. doi: 10.1007/s00059-020-04909-z

38. Buzon J, Roignot O, Lemoine S, Perez P, Kimmoun A, Levy B, et al. Takotsubo cardiomyopathy triggered by influenza A virus. *Intern Med*. (2015) 54:2017–9. doi: 10.2169/internalmedicine.54.3606

39. Zompatori M, Ciccarese F, Fasano L. Overview of current lung imaging in acute respiratory distress syndrome. *Eur Respir Rev*. (2014) 23:519–30. doi: 10.1183/09059180.00001314

40. Klok FA, Kruip MJ, van der Meer NJ, Arbous MS, Gommers DA, Kaptein FH, et al. Incidence of thrombotic complications in critically ill ICU patients with COVID-19. *Thrombosis Res*. (2020) 191:145–7. doi: 10.1016/j.thromres.2020.04.013

41. Tang N, Li D, Wang X, Sun Z. Abnormal coagulation parameters are associated with poor prognosis in patients with novel coronavirus pneumonia. *J Thromb Haemost*. (2020) 18:844–7. doi: 10.1111/jth.14768

42. Itkonen MK, Tornio A, Lapatto-Reiniluoto O, Neuvonen M, Neuvonen PJ, Niemi M, et al. Clopidogrel increases dasabuvir exposure with or without ritonavir, and ritonavir inhibits the bioactivation of clopidogrel. *Clin Pharmacol Ther*. (2019) 105:219–28. doi: 10.1002/cpt.1099

43. Tonnesmann E, Kandolf R, Lewalter T. Chloroquine cardiomyopathy – a review of the literature. *Immunopharmacol Immunotoxicol*. (2013) 35:434–42. doi: 10.3109/08923973.2013.780078

44. van Doremalen N, Bushmaker T, Morris D, Holbook M, Gamble A, Williamson B, et al. Aerosol and surface stability of SARS-CoV-2 as compared with SARS –COV-1. *N Engl J Med*. (2020) 382:1564–7. doi: 10.1056/NEJMc2004973

45. Hollander JE, Carr BG. Virtually imperfect? Telemedicine for Covid-19. *N Engl J Med*. (2020) 382:1679–81. doi: 10.1056/NEJMp2003539

46. American College of Cardiology. *COVID-19 Clinical Guidance for the Cardiovascular Care Team*. Available online at: https://www.acc.org/~/media/Non-Clinical/Files-PDFs-Excel-MS-Word-etc/2020/02/S20028-ACC-Clinical-Bulletin-Coronavirus.pdf (accessed March 10, 2020).

47. European Society of Cardiology. *Position Statement of the ESC Council on Hypertension on ACE-Inhibitors and Angiotensin Receptor Blockers*. (2020). Available online at: https://www.escardio.org/Councils/Council-on-Hypertension-(CHT)/News/position-statement-of-the-esc-council-on-hypertension-on-ace-inhibitors-and-ang (accessed March 27, 2020).

48. International Society of Hypertension. *A Statement From the International Society of Hypertension on COVID-19*. (2020). Available online at: https://ish-world.com/news/a/A-statement-from-the-International-Society-of-Hypertension-on-COVID-19/ (accessed March 27, 2020).

49. Welt FGP, Shah PB, Aronow HD, Bortnick AE, Henry TD, Sherwood MW, et al. Catheterization laboratory considerations during the coronavirus (COVID-19) pandemic: from tACC's Interventional Council and SCAI. *J Am Coll Cardiol*. (2020) 75:2372–5. doi: 10.1016/j.jacc.2020.03.021

50. *(CDC-1) Centres for Disease Control and Prevention. Coronavirus (COVID-19)*. Available online at: https://www.cdc.gov/coronavirus/2019-ncov/ (accessed May 1, 2020).

51. WHO/2019-nCoV/IPC_PPE_use/2020.4 Available online at: https://www.cdc.gov/coronavirus/2019-ncov/hcp

52. Livingstone E, Desai A, Berkwits M. Sourcing personal protective equipment during the COVID-19 pandemic. *JAMA.* (2020) 323:1912–4. doi: 10.1001/jama.2020.5317

53. Sanders JM, Monogue ML, Jodlowski TZ, Cutrell JB. Pharmacologic treatments for coronavirus disease 2019 (COVID-19): a review. *JAMA.* (2020) 323:1824–36. doi: 10.1001/jama.2020.6019

54. Adams JG, Wall RM. Supporting the health care workforce during the COVID-19 global epidemic. *JAMA.* (2020) 323:1439–40. doi: 10.1001/jama.2020.3972

18

Early vs. Late Onset Cardiac Injury and Mortality in Hospitalized COVID-19 Patients in Wuhan

Wei Sun [1,2,3†], Yanting Zhang [1,2,3†], Chun Wu [1,2,3†], Shuyuan Wang [1,2,3†], Yuji Xie [1,2,3],
Danqing Zhang [1,2,3], Hongliang Yuan [1,2,3], Yongxing Zhang [1,2,3], Li Cui [1,2,3], Meng Li [1,2,3],
Yiwei Zhang [1,2,3], Yuman Li [1,2,3], Jing Wang [1,2,3], Yali Yang [1,2,3], Qing Lv [1,2,3], Li Zhang [1,2,3*],
Philip Haines [4*], Wen-Chih Wu [5*] and Mingxing Xie [1,2,3*]

[1] Department of Ultrasound, Union Hospital, Tongji Medical College, Huazhong University of Science and Technology,
Wuhan, China, [2] Hubei Province Clinical Research Center for Medical Imaging, Wuhan, China, [3] Hubei Province Key
Laboratory of Molecular Imaging, Wuhan, China, [4] Rhode Island Hospital, Warren Alpert Medical School of Brown University,
Providence, RI, United States, [5] Department of Medicine, Providence VA Medical Center, Brown University Warren Alpert
Medical School, Providence, RI, United States

*Correspondence:
Mingxing Xie
xiemx@hust.edu.cn
Wen-Chih Wu
wen-chih_wu@brown.edu
Philip Haines
philip_haines@brown.edu
Li Zhang
zli429@hust.edu.cn

[†] These authors have contributed
equally to this work

Background: Increasing evidence points to cardiac injury (CI) as a common coronavirus disease 2019 (COVID-19) related complication. The characteristics of early CI (occurred within 72 h of admission) and late CI (occurred after 72 h of admission) and its association with mortality in COVID-19 patients is unknown.

Methods: This retrospective study analyzed patients confirmed with COVID-19 in Union Hospital (Wuhan, China) from Jan 29th to Mar 15th, 2020. Clinical outcomes (discharge, or death) were monitored to April 15, 2020, the latest date of follow-up. Demographic, clinical, laboratory, as well as treatment and prognosis were collected and analyzed in patients with early, late CI and without CI.

Results: A total of 196 COVID-19 patients were included for analysis. The median age was 65 years [interquartile range (IQR) 56–73 years], and 112 (57.1%) were male. Of the 196 COVID-19 patients, 49 (25.0%) patients had early and 20 (10.2%) patients had late CI, 56.6% developed Acute-Respiratory-Distress-Syndrome (ARDS) and 43 (21.9%) patients died. Patients with any CI were more likely to have developed ARDS (87.0 vs. 40.2%) and had a higher in-hospital mortality than those without (52.2 vs. 5.5%, $P < 0.001$). Among CI subtypes, a significantly higher risk of in-hospital death was found in patients with early CI with recurrence [19/49 patients, adjusted odds ratio (OR) = 7.184, 95% CI 1.472–35.071] and patients with late CI (adjusted OR = 5.019, 95% CI 1.125–22.388) compared to patients with early CI but no recurrence.

Conclusions: CI can occur early on or late after, the initial 72 h of admission and is associated with ARDS and an increased risk of in-hospital mortality. Both late CI and recurrent CI after the initial episode were associated with worse outcomes than patients with early CI alone. This study highlights the importance of early examination and periodical monitoring of cardiac biomarkers, especially for patients with early CI or at risk of clinical deterioration.

Keywords: COVID-19, cardiac injury, early, late, mortality

INTRODUCTION

Coronavirus disease 2019 (COVID-19) caused by the severe acute respiratory syndrome coronavirus 2 (SARS-CoV-2) has affected over 200 countries (1). With the increasing number of confirmed cases, the cardiovascular manifestations associated by this highly contagious viral infection have gained more and more attention. Several observational studies have found that between 7.2 and 37.5% of COVID-19 patients had cardiac injury (CI) which was associated with higher mortality in COVID-19 patients (2–11). However, a portion of CI does not occur on admission and the association of the timing of CI with prognosis is unknown. Furthermore, the clinical features and risk factors associated with early or late onset CI in COVID-19 patients have not been formally evaluated. The clinical sequence preceding and following CI at the time of admission may provide additional understanding of the pathogenesis associated with CI in COVID-19. Therefore, this study compared the clinical characteristics, risk factors and prognostic value of early vs. late onset of CI in COVID-19 patients.

METHODS

Study Design and Participants

We performed this retrospective study at Union Hospital (Affiliated Tongji Medical College, Huazhong University of Science and Technology) Wuhan, China. The West Branch of Union Hospital was one of the major designated hospitals for critically ill COVID-19 patients. We enrolled 429 consecutive patients with confirmed COVID-19, according to the WHO interim guidance criteria (12), who were either discharged alive or died during hospitalization from Jan 29th to April 15th, 2020. Only participants who had high-sensitivity troponin I (hs-TNI) measured before and after 72 h from admission during their hospitalization were included in the study (233 patients excluded). The study was approved by the ethics committee of the Union hospital, Tongji Medical College, Huazhong University of Science and Technology. Per institutional policy, written informed consent was waived for all participants with emerging infectious diseases.

Data Collection

Data were extracted from the electronic medical records including demographic information and clinical characteristics (i.e., vital signs, symptoms, laboratory findings, medical history, underlying comorbidities, treatments, complications, and outcomes) of the participants on admission and during hospitalization. The date of illness onset was defined as the day when symptoms of COVID-19 as defined by the World Health Organization (12) were appreciated. Laboratory measurements within and after 72 h of admission were collected. If multiple measurements were available, the patient's first abnormal measurements, both within and after 72 h, were recorded for the determination of the timing of the CI. The duration from the onset of admission to the onset of clinical complications and death in the hospital were also recorded. Clinical outcomes

(discharge and mortality) were monitored up to April 15, 2020, the last date of follow-up. Complete hospitalization data was available in all patients included in the study.

Timing of CI

The hs-TNI data for each patient were collected from admission to discharge or death. COVID-19 related CI was defined as the serum levels of cardiac high-sensitivity troponin I (hs-TNI) above the 99th percentile upper reference limit in a patient diagnosed with COVID-19 per Huang et al. and Shi et al. (2, 7–10). Early CI was defined as CI that occurred within 72 h of admission, whereas late CI was defined as occurring after 72 h of admission. We also defined a subgroup of recurrent CI within the early CI group as a second rise of hs-TNI value of >20% from its previous value after 72 h of admission.

Non-cardiac Complications

Acute respiratory distress syndrome (ARDS) was defined according to the World Health Organization interim guidance criteria (13). Acute kidney injury was identified according to the KDIGO clinical practice guidelines as an increase in serum creatinine by ≥ 0.3 mg/dl (≥ 26.5 μmol/l) within 48 h or by 1.5 times of the baseline values (14). Coagulation dysfunction was defined as a >3-s prolongation of prothrombin time (PT) or a 5-s prolongation of activated partial thromboplastin time (APTT). Thrombocytopenia was characterized by a platelet count <125 × 10^9/L (15).

Statistical Analysis

Categorical variables were expressed as number (%), and continuous variables were expressed as mean $\pm$ standard deviation (SD) or median [interquartile range (IQR)]. The normality of the distribution was tested with the Shapiro-Wilk normality test. Differences among the three groups (without CI, early CI or late CI) were assessed by ANOVA for normally distributed and Kruskal–Wallis H-test for non-normally distributed continuous variables. Categorical variables were compared by Chi-square or Fisher exact test where applicable. In-hospital survival curves of four groups of patients with early but no recurrent CI, early with recurrent CI, late CI, and no CI were estimated with the Kaplan-Meier method and the groups compared with the log-rank test. Univariate and multivariate logistic regression analyses were used to determine the independent risk associated with each of the four groups (early but no recurrent CI, early with recurrent CI, late CI, and no CI) of patients with in-hospital death, adjusted by known risk factors of COVID-19 mortality in the literature [age, sex, respiratory rate, heart rate, SpO_2, temperature, mean arterial pressure, coma, hypertension history, Lymphocyte count, C-reactive protein (CRP), and lactate dehydrogenase (LDH)] (16–18). All statistical analyses were performed with SPSS version 24.0 (Statistical Package for the Social Sciences, Chicago, Illinois), and STATA software version 10 (StataCorp, Texas, USA). A two-tailed P-value of <0.05 was considered statistically significant.

Early vs. Late Onset Cardiac Injury and Mortality in Hospitalized COVID-19 Patients in Wuhan

189

RESULTS

Clinical Characteristics, Laboratory Findings, and Treatments Within 72 h of Admission

Among the 429 patients, 100 patients were excluded due to missing hs-TNI data during the entire hospitalization, 133 patients were excluded due to missing hs-TNI data within 72 h of admission, the remaining 196 patients were included for analysis. The median age was 65.0 years (IQR: 56.0–73.0 years), and 112 (57.1%) were men. Of 196 COVID-19 patients, 69/196 (35.2%) had evidence of CI during hospitalization: 49/196 (25.0%) patients had early CI and 20/196 (10.2%) patients had late CI. In addition, 19/49 (38.8%) patients with early CI had recurrent CI after 72 h of admission. Compared with patients without CI, patients with early and late CI were more often older, and had lower SpO$_2$ on admission. They also had more comorbidities such as hypertension and underlying cardiac disease.

Compared with non-CI group, patients with early and late CI presented with more abnormal laboratory findings within 72 h of admission including lower lymphocyte and platelet counts, higher inflammation-related indices [CRP, procalcitonin (PCT)] and further elevations in liver and renal function indices.

Concerning the treatment of the 196 patients within 72 h of admission, there was no difference in the antiviral (P = 0.551) or antibiotic therapy (P = 0.235) among these three groups. However, compared with the non-CI group, more patients with early and late CI received glucocorticoid therapy (18.9 vs. 38.8% and 30.0%, P = 0.021), high-flow oxygen (18.1 vs. 69.4% and 80.0%, P <0.001), invasive mechanical ventilation (0.8 vs. 4.1% and 15.0%; P = 0.005), non-invasive mechanical ventilation (0.0 vs. 8.2% and 15.0%; P <0.001), and more subjects were transferred to the intensive care unit (ICU) (0.8 vs. 10.2% and 5.0%; P = 0.007) (Table 1).

Timing of CI and Non-cardiac Complications After 72 h of Admission

Major complications after 72 h included ARDS [111/196 (56.6%)], coagulation dysfunction [57/193 (29.5%)], late CI [20/196 (10.2%)] and acute kidney injury [33/193 (17.1%)]. Patients with early and late CI were more likely to have developed ARDS, ICU transfer and receive invasive mechanical ventilation (IMV) during their hospitalization compared to the non-CI group (Table 2). A majority, 87.0% (60/69) of patients with CI vs. 40.2% (51/127) without CI, developed ARDS. Overall, the median time from admission to ARDS was 4 days, to acute kidney injury was 7 days, to late CI was 11 days, and to coagulation dysfunction was 11 days for all patients.

For the early CI group (n = 49), the median time from admission to CI was 1 day (IQR 0–1 day), to the onset of ARDS (81.6%) was 2 days (IQR 1–8 days), and to the onset of recurrent CI [19/49 (38.8%)] was 7 days (IQR 5–16 days) for affected patients (Figure 1A). For the late CI group [20/196 (10.2%)], the median time from admission to the onset of ARDS (100%) was 7 days (IQR 2–8 days) and the onset of late CI was 11 days (IQR 5–22 days) (Figure 1B). Conversely, for the non-CI group [127/196 (64.8%)], the median time from admission to the onset of ARDS (40.2%) was 6 days (IQR 3–12 days) (Figure 1C).

Using the onset of ARDS as the temporal reference point, 15/20 (75%) patients with late CI had ARDS before their CI (Figure 2), with a median time between ARDS and CI of 4 days (IQR 3–17 days).

Cardiac Injury and Mortality

As of April 15, 2020, 153 patients (78.1%) were discharged and 43 patients (21.9%) died in the hospital. Patients with any CI had significantly higher in-hospital mortality than those without (52.2 vs. 5.5%, P < 0.001) (Figure 3). Among CI subtypes, multivariable regression modeling showed that compared to patients with early CI but no recurrence, a significantly higher risk of in-hospital death was found in patients with early CI with recurrence [odds ratio (OR) = 7.184, P = 0.015] and patients with late CI (OR = 5.019, P = 0.034) (Table 3).

DISCUSSION

In this cohort of 196 hospitalized COVID-19 patients from Wuhan, China, we found 35.2% had evidence of CI during hospitalization that included 25.0% of patients with early CI and 10.2% patients with late CI. In addition, there were 38.8% of patients with early CI who also had recurrent CI. Patients with any CI had significantly higher incidence of ARDS and in-hospital mortality than those without. Moreover, among CI subtypes, a significantly higher risk of in-hospital death was found in patients with early CI with recurrence and patients with late CI compared to patients with early CI and no recurrence.

Increasingly, researchers are reporting CI in COVID-19 patients, with the prevalence varying from 7.2 to 37.5% (4, 7, 8, 11). In our study, a remarkable 35.2% of patients had any CI. The pathogenesis of CI associated with COVID-19 is still unknown partly due to a dearth of autopsy or biopsy reported in these patients. The following potential mechanisms for CI have been proposed. The first possibility is direct myocardial damage by the virus, because angiotensin-converting enzyme 2 has been identified as a functional receptor for coronaviruses, which is also expressed abundantly in the myocardium (19, 20). Mixed literature from autopsy and biopsy case series were reported without conclusive evidence yet (21–25). The second mechanism is presumably the systemic inflammatory cytokine response, namely cytokine storm (26, 27). It can cause the proliferation of highly pro-inflammatory CCR4+CCR6+Th17 cells amongst the CD4+T cells, the expression of high concentrations of cytotoxic particles in CD8+T cells and over activation of T cells in general, all of which lead to a stronger inflammatory response in return (3, 21). Inflammation can in turn lead to thromboembolic complications (28). Our study showed that inflammation-related indices (CRP, PCT) were higher

TABLE 1 | Comparisons of demographics, clinical characteristics and laboratory examinations on admission within 72 h among the three groups.

	Total population (n = 196)	Without CI (n = 127)	Early CI (n = 49)	Late CI (n = 20)	P-value
Age (years)	65.0 (56.0, 73.0)	61.0 (49.0, 69.0)	71.0 (66.0, 77.0)*	69.0 (59.3, 72.8)	<0.001
Gender					0.458
Male, n (%)	112 (57.1)	70 (51.1)	28 (57.1)	14 (70.0)	
Female, n (%)	84 (42.9)	57 (44.9)	21 (42.9)	6 (30.0)	
Smoking, n (%)	22 (11.2)	16 (12.6)	5 (10.2)	1 (5.0)	0.537
Vital signs					
Temperature (°C)	38.0 (36.7, 38.7)	38.0 (36.7, 38.7)	37.9 (36.7, 38.5)	38.9 (38.1, 39.5)*#	0.004
Respiratory rate (breaths/min)	20.0 (20.0, 25.0)	20.0 (20.0, 24.0)	23.0 (20.0, 30.0)*	22.0 (20.0, 25.0)	0.008
Heart rate (bpm)	89.0 (80.0, 101.0)	87.0 (80.0, 98.0)	95.0 (81.0, 110.5)	92.0 (83.0, 106.5)	0.068
SBP (mmHg)	133.6 ± 19.9	132.7 ± 18.8	135.3 ± 22.6	135.5 ± 20.7	0.547
DBP (mmHg)	80.4 ± 13.1	81.3 ± 12.0	78.7 ± 15.5	79.0 ± 18.8	0.182
Mean arterial pressure (mmHg)	98.2 ± 13.9	98.4 ± 12.9	97.6 ± 16.2	98.6 ± 15.0	0.806
SpO_2 (%)	97.0 (94.0, 99.0)	98.0 (95.0, 99.0)	95.0 (89.5, 98.0)*	94.0 (87.5, 98.0)*	<0.001
Common initial symptoms					
Fever, n (%)	151 (77.0)	101 (79.5)	33 (67.3)	17 (85.0)	0.162
Cough, n (%)	113 (57.7)	78 (61.4)	23 (46.9)	12 (60.0)	0.214
Fatigue, n (%)	89 (45.4)	52 (40.9)	28 (57.1)	9 (45.0)	0.154
Dyspnea, n (%)	87 (44.4)	50 (39.4)	29 (59.2)	8 (40.0)	0.055
Chest tightness/chest pain, n (%)	75 (38.3)	50 (39.4)	17 (34.7)	8 (40.0)	0.837
Diarrhea, n (%)	21 (10.7)	17 (13.4)	4 (8.2)	0 (0.0)	0.056
Headache, n (%)	11 (5.6)	8 (6.3)	2 (4.1)	1 (5.0)	0.893
Coma, n (%)	9 (4.6)	2 (1.6)	6 (12.2)*	1 (5.0)	0.011
Comorbidities					
Hypertension, n (%)	87 (44.4)	48 (37.8)	30 (61.2)*	9 (45.0)	0.020
Diabetes mellitus, n (%)	29 (14.8)	14 (11.0)	10 (20.4)	5 (25.0)	0.130
Cardiac disease, n (%)	32 (16.3)	12 (9.4)	16 (32.7)*	4 (20.0)	0.001
Cerebral infarction, n (%)	15 (7.7)	7 (5.5)	6 (12.2)	2 (10.0)	0.234
Malignancy, n (%)	9 (4.6)	5 (3.9)	2 (4.1)	2 (10.0)	0.417
Chronic liver disease, n (%)	4 (2.0)	1 (0.8)	1 (2.0)	2 (10.0)*	0.037
Chronic kidney disease, n (%)	6 (3.1)	2 (1.6)	4 (8.2)	0 (0.0)	0.056
Chronic obstructive pulmonary disease, n (%)	8 (4.1)	3 (2.4)	4 (8.2)	1 (5.0)	0.173
Symptom onset to hospital admission (days)	14.0 (8.0, 20.0)	15.0 (10.0, 21.0)	10.0 (5.0, 14.5)*	10.0 (7.0, 15.0)*	<0.001
Laboratory findings on admission (within 72 h)					
White blood cells (×10^9/L)	7.0 (5.5, 9.2) 195/196	6.4 (5.2, 7.9) 126/127	8.9 (6.8, 10.9)* 49/49	7.0 (5.2, 9.6) 20/20	<0.001
Lymphocyte (%)	15.9 (7.4, 25.9) 195/196	22.1 (13.8, 29.3) 126/127	6.6 (4.6, 15.9)* 49/49	10.4 (6.0, 17.4)* 20/20	<0.001
Neutrophil (×10^9/L)	5.3 (3.7, 7.4) 195/196	4.3 (3.1, 6.0) 126/127	7.2 (5.9, 10.1)* 49/49	5.8 (4.5, 7.7) 20/20	<0.001
Platelets (×10^9/L)	205.0 (152.0, 262.0) 195/196	214.0 (174.5, 273.5) 126/127	179.0 (117.5, 262.5)* 49/49	167.5 (108.5, 245.0) 20/20	0.008
Hemoglobin (g/L)	124.0 (112.0, 135.0) 195/196	125.0 (110.8, 135.3) 126/127	121.0 (101.0, 135.0) 49/49	128.5 (116.3, 133.3) 20/20	0.452
CRP (mg/L)	32.0 (3.4, 75.9) 195/196	6.5 (1.9, 55.2) 126/127	62.4 (36.3, 109.9)* 49/49	71.0 (33.8, 114.6)* 20/20	<0.001
PCT (ng/ml)	0.11 (0.05, 0.24) 176/196	0.06 (0.04, 0.12) 114/127	0.40 (0.14, 0.60)* 42/49	0.15 (0.11, 0.28)* 20/20	<0.001
Coagulation function index					
D-dimer (µg/mL)	1.11 (0.35, 4.27) 186/196	0.75 (0.29, 2.39) 120/127	2.73 (1.28, 8.00)* 46/49	1.05 (0.46, 6.35) 20/20	<0.001

(Continued)

TABLE 1 | Continued

	Total population (n = 196)	Without CI (n = 127)	Early CI (n = 49)	Late CI (n = 20)	P-value
PT (s)	13.4 (12.6, 14.3) 186/196	13.1 (12.4, 14.0) 120/127	14.2 (13.2, 15.1)* 46/49	13.5 (13.0, 14.2) 20/20	<0.001
APTT (s)	37.4 (33.1, 42.2) 186/196	36.0 (32.5, 39.9) 120/127	38.7 (33.9, 44.9) 46/49	38.1 (32.4, 44.1) 20/20	0.274
Liver function index					
Total protein (g/L)	64.1 (58.9, 67.6) 196/196	64.4 (58.8, 67.7) 127/127	60.7 (56.2, 64.5)* 49/49	62.1 (60.0, 66.8) 20/20	0.002
Albumin (g/L)	31.7 (26.8, 37.4) 196/196	32.1 (27.3, 37.7) 127/127	28.2 (24.4, 32.1)* 49/49	27.4 (25.3, 31.8)* 20/20	<0.001
AST (U/L)	31.5 (23.0, 48.0) 196/196	28.0 (20.0, 43.0) 127/127	39.0 (29.0, 59.5)* 49/49	47.0 (33.8, 76.8)* 20/20	<0.001
ALT (U/L)	36.0 (23.0, 54.8) 196/196	32.5 (21.0, 50.0) 127/127	38.0 (23.0, 56.5) 49/49	38.5 (30.3, 78.8) 20/20	0.262
Total bilirubin (μmol/L)	11.2 (8.7, 16.9) 196/196	10.9 (8.3, 15.2) 127/127	14.2 (9.9, 21.3) 49/49	10.5 (7.8, 18.7) 20/20	0.110
Direct bilirubin (μmol/L)	3.8 (2.7, 5.6) 196/196	3.4 (2.5, 5.1) 127/127	4.8 (3.2, 7.6)* 49/49	4.3 (2.7, 5.9) 20/20	0.003
LDH (U/L)	250.5 (182.3, 403.0) 196/196	227.0 (174.3, 352.5) 127/127	388.0 (250.0, 597.0)* 49/49	492.0 (320.0, 665.3)* 20/20	<0.001
Kidney function index					
BUN (mmol/L)	5.2 (4.1, 7.3) 196/196	4.8 (3.7, 6.3) 127/127	7.0 (5.0, 11.2)* 49/49	5.7 (4.1, 7.5) 20/20	<0.001
Serum creatinine (μmol/L)	68.4 (56.4, 82.5) 196/196	64.3 (54.4, 75.2) 127/127	75.3 (61.4, 98.1)* 49/49	68.6 (62.5, 82.2) 20/20	0.008
K+ (mmol/L)	4.0 (3.5, 4.3) 195/196	3.9 (3.5, 4.2) 126/127	4.0 (3.5, 4.4) 49/49	4.0 (3.5, 4.6) 20/20	0.427
Na+ (mmol/L)	138.9 (136.9, 141.1) 195/196	139.0 (137.3, 141.2) 126/127	139.9 (136.1, 144.0) 49/49	138.8 (135.8, 140.5) 20/20	0.558
Cardiac injury index					
hs-TNI (ng/L)	8.3 (2.7, 27.0) 196/196	3.9 (2.0, 9.8) 127/127	86.4 (44.9, 378.8)* 49/49	10.8 (7.5, 16.2)*# 20/58	<0.001
CK-MB (U/L)	12.0 (10.0, 17.0) 170/196	11.0 (9.0, 15.0) 108/127	16.0 (10.0, 26.3)* 42/49	16.0 (10.3, 21.8)* 20/20	<0.001
BNP (pg/ml)	40.7 (15.0, 128.0) 152/196	30.1 (10.5, 84.1) 91/127	153.4 (46.0, 431.6)* 44/49	40.6 (22.9, 122.4)# 17/20	<0.001
Treatments on admission (within 72 h)					
Antiviral therapy, n (%)	147 (75.0)	94 (74.0)	36 (73.5)	17 (85.0)	0.551
Antibiotic therapy, n (%)	107 (54.6)	61 (48.0)	31 (63.3)	15 (75.0)	0.235
Glucocorticoid therapy, n (%)	49 (25.0)	24 (18.9)	19 (38.8)*	6 (30.0)	0.021
Immunoglobulin, n (%)	21 (10.7)	10 (7.9)	6 (12.2)	5 (25.0)	0.104
ACEI/ARB, n (%)	8 (4.1)	4 (3.1)	4 (8.2)	0 (0.0)	0.258
Oxygen therapy, n (%)	132 (67.3)	73 (57.5)	42 (85.7)*	17 (85.0)	<0.001
High-flow oxygen, n (%)	73 (37.2)	23 (18.1)	34 (69.4)*	16 (80.0)*	<0.001
IMV, n (%)	6 (3.1)	1 (0.8)	2 (4.1)	3 (15.0)*	0.005
NIMV, n (%)	7 (3.6)	0 (0.0)	4 (8.2)*	3 (15.0)*	<0.001
ICU transfer, n (%)	7 (3.6)	1 (0.8)	5 (10.2)*	1 (5.0)	0.007

*P < 0.05, vs. without CI; #P < 0.05, vs. early CI; ACE-I, angiotensin-converting enzyme inhibitors; ALT, alanine aminotransferase; APTT, activated partial thromboplastin time; ARB, angiotensin II receptor blockers; AST, aspartate aminotransferase; BNP, B-type natriuretic peptide; BUN, blood urea nitrogen; CI, cardiac injury; CK-MB, creatine kinase muscle-brain; CRP, C-reactive protein; DBP, diastolic blood pressure; hs-TNI, hypersensitive troponin I; ICU, intensive care unit; IMV, invasive mechanical ventilation; IQR, interquartile range; LDH, lactate dehydrogenase; NIMV, non-invasive mechanical ventilation; PCT, procalcitonin; PT, prothrombin time; SBP, systolic blood pressure; SD, standard deviation.

in the CI group compared to the non-CI group. Another mechanism is CI related to hypoxia. The balance between the oxygen demand and supply of the myocardium is disrupted during acute hypoxia. A cascade of cellular, biochemical and inflammatory reactions can occur during hypoxia, eventually causing myocardial apoptosis (29). Acute severe hypoxia can

TABLE 2 | Comparisons of additional treatment, complications, and prognosis after 72h of admission among the three groups.

Variables	Total population (n = 196)	Without CI (n = 127)	Early CI (n = 49)	Late CI (n = 20)	P-value
Additional treatment after admission					
Antiviral therapy, n (%)	36 (18.4)	24 (18.9)	9 (18.4)	3 (15.0)	1.000
Antibiotic therapy, n (%)	50 (25.5)	31 (24.4)	14 (28.6)	5 (25.0)	0.882
Glucocorticoid therapy, n (%)	48 (24.5)	26 (20.5)	11 (22.4)	11 (55.0)*#	0.007
Immunoglobulin, n (%)	49 (25.0)	22 (17.3)	14 (28.6)	13 (65.0)*#	<0.001
ACEI/ARB, n (%)	17 (8.7)	12 (9.4)	3 (6.1)	2 (10.0)	0.733
Oxygen therapy, n (%)	34 (17.3)	26 (20.5)	5 (10.2)	3 (15.0)	0.273
High-flow oxygen, n (%)	51 (26.0)	42 (33.1)	5 (10.2)*	4 (20.0)	0.006
IMV, n (%)	33 (16.8)	8 (6.3)	13 (26.5)*	12 (60.0)*#	<0.001
NIMV, n (%)	16 (8.2)	8 (6.3)	5 (10.2)	3 (15.0)	0.234
ICU transfer, n (%)	25 (12.8)	6 (4.7)	7 (14.3)	12 (60.0)*#	<0.001
Complications					
Cardiac injury (CI)					
Early CI, n (%)	49/196 (25.0)	/	49/49(100)	0/20 (0)	/
Recurrent CI, n (%)	19/49 (38.8)	/	19/49 (38.8)	/	/
Late CI, n (%)	20/196 (10.2)	/	/	20/20 (100)	/
ARDS, n (%)	111/196 (56.6)	51/127 (40.2)	40/49 (81.6)*	20/20 (100)*	<0.001
Coagulation dysfunction, n (%)	57/193 (29.5)	21/124 (16.9)	22/49 (44.9)*	14/20 (70.0)*	<0.001
Acute kidney injury, n (%)	33/193 (17.1)	8/125 (6.4)	17/48 (35.4)*	8/20 (40.0)*	<0.001
Time from admission to complications onset					
Cardiac injury (CI)					
Early CI (days)	1 (0, 1)	/	1 (0, 1)	/	/
Recurrent CI (days)	7 (5, 16)	/	7 (5, 16)	/	/
Late CI (days)	11 (5, 22)	/	/	11 (5, 22)	/
ARDS (days)	4 (2, 9)	6 (3, 12)	2 (1, 8)*	7 (2, 8)	0.014
Coagulation dysfunction (days)	11 (1, 20)	11 (1, 19)	8 (1, 15)	23 (8, 25)#	0.02
Acute kidney injury (days)	7 (3, 14)	10 (3, 17)	4 (2, 7)	12 (6, 21)	0.065
Prognosis					
Death, n (%)	43 (21.9)	7 (5.5)	23 (46.9)*	13 (65.0)*	<0.001

*Data are median (IQR) or n (%).*P < 0.05, vs. without CI; #P < 0.05, vs. early CI; ACE-I, angiotensin-converting enzyme inhibitors; ARB, angiotensin II receptor blockers; ARDS, acute respiratory distress syndrome; ICU, intensive care unit; IMV, invasive mechanical ventilation; IQR, interquartile range; NIMV, non-invasive mechanical ventilation.*

also trigger a systemic inflammatory response (30). In this study, patients with early or late CI had lower level of SpO_2 on admission and higher incidence of ARDS compared to the non-CI group. There was a large timing overlap between CI and ARDS in the early CI group and 75% of patients with late CI were preceded by ARDS which supports a strong relationship between CI and hypoxia. Lastly, antiviral drugs can cause cardiac insufficiency, arrhythmia or other cardiovascular disorders with variable individual susceptibility (4, 31). In the present study, almost all patients (93.4% of COVID-19 patients) were administrated with antiviral drugs either on admission or after admission for which the opportunity of individual susceptibility and/or interaction with the underlying comorbid conditions could contribute to onset of late CI or recurrence of the initial one. In addition, patients in the CI group were more likely to have received glucocorticoid therapy. The relationship between glucocorticoid therapy and cardiac injury remains controversial and is under investigation (32). On the other hand,

it is also likely that patients with any CI had higher disease severity for which more treatment was administered. This may suggest that the CI after admission was a sign of disease severity and/or progression.

Recent studies have demonstrated that CI was associated with increased mortality in COVID-19 patients (7, 8, 33). However, to the best of our knowledge, this is the first study to depict the clinical characteristics of both early CI and late CI and their association with in-hospital mortality. Our study showed that early CI was an independent predictor of death in COVID-19 patients even after accounting for variables that have proven prognostic value in the risk stratification of acutely ill patients, such as respiratory rate, heart rate, SpO_2, temperature, mean arterial pressure, and coma (16, 34). Cardiac injury remained significant after accounting for potential confounding laboratory variables with proven prognostic value in COVID hospitalizations such as lymphocyte count, LDH, CRP (17). This is important because clinicians should not consider patients

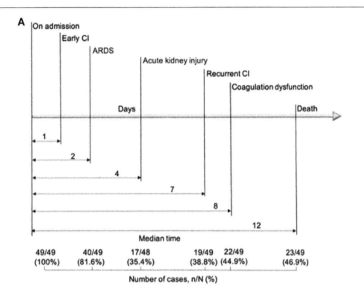

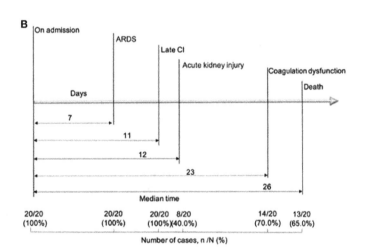

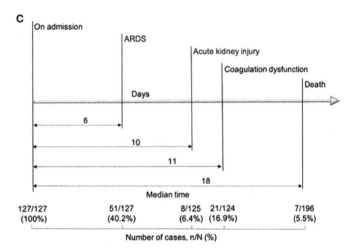

FIGURE 1 | Timeline of COVID-19 patients after admission. **(A)** Timeline of COVID-19 patients with early CI; **(B)** Timeline of COVID-19 patients with late CI; **(C)** Timeline of COVID-19 patients without CI. COVID-19, coronavirus disease 2019; CI, cardiac injury.

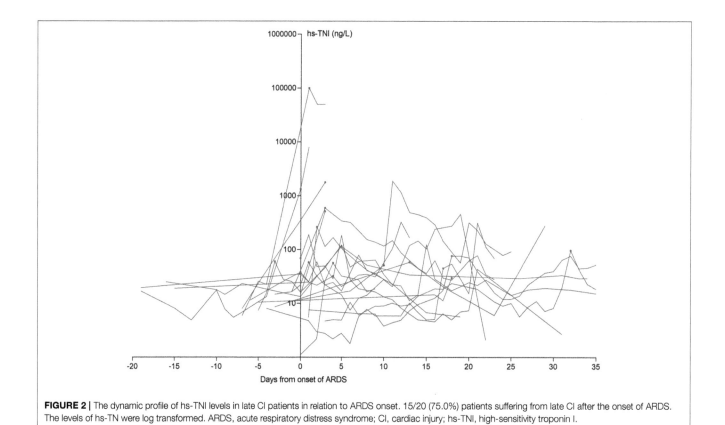

FIGURE 2 | The dynamic profile of hs-TNI levels in late CI patients in relation to ARDS onset. 15/20 (75.0%) patients suffering from late CI after the onset of ARDS. The levels of hs-TN were log transformed. ARDS, acute respiratory distress syndrome; CI, cardiac injury; hs-TNI, high-sensitivity troponin I.

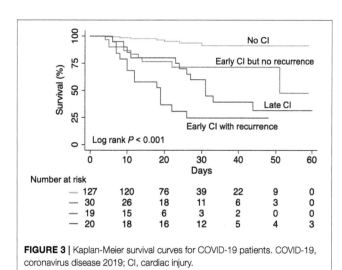

FIGURE 3 | Kaplan-Meier survival curves for COVID-19 patients. COVID-19, coronavirus disease 2019; CI, cardiac injury.

being out of danger despite absence of CI in the first 72 h since it can occur late. Similarly, a fall after the early rise in Trop I should not translate into a lower risk status since recurrence of CI can occur. Conversely, we also found that CI is closely related to the occurrence of ARDS as opposed to a primary cardiac event. Accordingly, our study suggested the need for a more systematic assessment of cardiac troponins for risk stratification of COVID-19 patients on admission, with repeat

measures for those who already have initial CI or who are at risk for clinical deterioration. With the advent of multiple therapies now to reduce the morbidity and mortality of COVID-19 (35–37), early identification of higher risk patients with cardiac biomarkers may be helpful to balance the cost vs. the effect of therapy.

LIMITATIONS

Our study has some limitations. First, this was a relatively small sample size and single-center retrospective observational study for which residual confounding cannot be excluded and we did not include all the potential factors associated with mortality in our study. Second, only 196 patients both had the data of hs-TNI within and after 72 h of admission, which may have underestimated the true incidence of CI in our study. Therefore, future studies should be multi-centered, with larger sample size and systematic data collection, in order to promote a more comprehensive understanding of the association between cardiac injury and mortality in hospitalized patients with COVID-19.

CONCLUSIONS

CI is a common condition that can occur early on or late after, the initial 72 h of admission and is associated with ARDS and an increased risk of in-hospital mortality. Both late CI

Early vs. Late Onset Cardiac Injury and Mortality in Hospitalized COVID-19 Patients in Wuhan

195

TABLE 3 | Univariate and multivariate logistic regression analysis of factors associated with in-hospital mortality of COVID-19 patients.

Factors	Univariate		Multivariate	
	Unadjusted OR (95% confidence interval)	P-value	Adjusted OR (95% confidence interval)	P-value
Age group (years)				
<45	1 (ref)			
45–54	0.680 (0.040, 11.632)	0.79		
55–64	4.675 (0.559, 39.116)	0.155		
65–74	7.650 (0.944, 61.980)	0.057		
>74	6.581 (0.787, 55.045)	0.082		
Sex				
Female	1 (ref)		1 (ref)	
Male	3.632 (1.632, 8.086)	0.002	8.828 (2.463, 31.643)	0.001
Respiratory rate (breaths/min)				
12–24	1 (ref)		1 (ref)	
>24	3.667 (1.804, 7.451)	<0.001	3.773 (1.188, 11.983)	0.024
Heart rate (bpm)				
70–109	1 (ref)			
40–69	2.321 (0.547, 9.845)	0.253		
110–139	3.095 (1.261, 7.600)	0.014		
140–179	4.643 (0.627, 34.377)	0.133		
SpO$_2$ (%)				
>89	1 (ref)		1 (ref)	
<75	24.833 (2.661, 231.712)	0.005	8.264 (0.694, 98.332)	0.095
75–85	31.042 (6.405, 150.435)	<0.001	11.129 (1.341, 92.388)	0.026
86–89	31.042 (3.474, 277.332)	0.002	74.421(3.121, 1774.444)	0.008
Temperature (°C)				
<37.2	1 (ref)			
37.2–38.9	1.991 (0.855, 4.633)	0.11		
>38.9	2.031 (0.741, 5.564)	0.168		
Mean arterial pressure (mmHg)				
70–109	1 (ref)			
50–69	8.065 (0.708, 91.829)	0.094		
110–129	1.578 (0.664, 3.748)	0.302		
130–159	1.008 (0.109, 9.340)	0.994		
Coma (yes vs. no) (9 vs. 320)	8.108 (1.937, 33.944)	0.004		
Hypertension (yes vs. no) (139 vs. 190)	2.974 (1.467, 6.029)	0.003		
Lymphocytes (%)				
≥20	1 (ref)			
<20	10.551 (3.594, 30.980)	<0.001		
CRP (mg/L)				
≤8	1 (ref)			
>8	17.500 (4.086, 74.956)	<0.001		
LDH (U/L)				
≤245	1 (ref)			
>245	8.129 (3.239, 20.398)	<0.001		
Type of CI				
Early CI but no recurrence	1 (ref)		1 (ref)	
Early CI with recurrence	6.533 (1.807, 23.627)	0.004	7.184 (1.472, 35.071)	0.015
Late CI	4.333 (1.298, 14.471)	0.017	5.019 (1.125, 22.388)	0.034
No CI	0.136 (0.046, 0.405)	<0.001	0.119 (0.030, 0.475)	0.003

OR, odds ratio; CI, cardiac injury; COVID-19, coronavirus disease 2019; CRP, C-reactive protein; LDH, lactate dehydrogenase.

and recurrent CI after the initial episode were associated with worse outcomes than patients with early CI alone. This study highlights the importance of early examination and periodical monitoring of cardiac biomarkers to identify predictors and markers of clinical deterioration in COVID-19 patients to guide intervention.

AUTHOR CONTRIBUTIONS

MX, W-CW, PH, and LZ: conception and design of study. WS, YaZ, CW, SW, DZ, HY, YoZ, LC, YL, JW, YY, and QL: acquisition of data. YaZ, WS, SW, ML, and YiZ: analysis and/or interpretation of data. LZ, WS, YaZ, and CW: drafting the manuscript. MX, W-CW, PH, and LZ: revising the manuscript critically for important intellectual content. All authors contributed to the article and approved the submitted version.

ACKNOWLEDGMENTS

The authors would like to express their appreciation for all of the emergency services, nurses, doctors, and other hospital staff for their efforts to combat the COVID-19 outbreak.

REFERENCES

1. World Health Organization. *Novel Coronavirus (2019-nCoV): Situation Report-88*. Available online at: https://www.who.int/docs/default-source/coronaviruse/situation-reports/20200417-sitrep-88-covid-191b6cccd94f8b4f219377bff55719a6ed.pdf (accessed December 22, 2020).
2. Huang C, Wang Y, Li X, Ren L, Zhao J, Hu Y, et al. Clinical features of patients infected with 2019 novel coronavirus in Wuhan, China. *Lancet*. (2020) 395:497–506. doi: 10.1016/S0140-6736(20)30183-5
3. Guan WJ, Ni ZY, Hu Y, Liang WH, Ou CQ, He JX, et al. Clinical characteristics of coronavirus disease 2019 in China. *N Engl J Med*. (2020) 382:1708–20. doi: 10.1056/NEJMoa2002032
4. Wang D, Hu B, Hu C, Zhu F, Liu X, Zhang J, et al. Clinical characteristics of 138 hospitalized patients with 2019 novel coronavirus-infected pneumonia in Wuhan, China. *JAMA*. (2020) 323:1061–9. doi: 10.1001/jama.2020.1585
5. Zhou F, Yu T, Du R, Fan G, Liu Y, Liu Z, et al. Clinical course and risk factors for mortality of adult inpatients with COVID-19 in Wuhan, China: a retrospective cohort study. *Lancet*. (2020) 395:1054–62. doi: 10.1016/S0140-6736(20)30566-3
6. Yang X, Yu Y, Xu J, Shu H, Xia J, Liu H, et al. Clinical course and outcomes of critically ill patients with SARS-CoV-2 pneumonia in Wuhan, China: a single-centered, retrospective, observational study. *Lancet Respir Med*. (2020) 8:475–81. doi: 10.1016/S2213-2600(20)30079-5
7. Shi S, Qin M, Shen B, Cai Y, Liu T, Yang F, et al. Association of cardiac injury with mortality in hospitalized patients with COVID-19 in Wuhan, China. *JAMA Cardiol*. (2020) 5:802–10. doi: 10.1001/jamacardio.2020.0950
8. Guo T, Fan Y, Chen M, Wu X, Zhang L, He T, et al. Cardiovascular implications of fatal outcomes of patients with coronavirus disease 2019 (COVID-19). *JAMA Cardiol*. (2020) 5:811–8. doi: 10.1001/jamacardio.2020.1017
9. Shi S, Qin M, Cai Y, Liu T, Shen B, Yang F, et al. Characteristics and clinical significance of myocardial injury in patients with severe coronavirus disease 2019. *Eur Heart J*. (2020) 41:2070–9. doi: 10.1093/eurheartj/ehaa408
10. Ferrante G, Fazzari F, Cozzi O, Maurina M, Bragato R, D'Orazio F, et al. Risk factors for myocardial injury and death in patients with COVID-19: insights from a cohort study with chest computed tomography. *Cardiovasc Res*. (2020) 116:2239–46. doi: 10.1093/cvr/cvaa193
11. Deng Q, Hu B, Zhang Y, Wang H, Zhou X, Hu W, et al. Suspected myocardial injury in patients with COVID-19: evidence from front-line clinical observation in Wuhan, China. *Int J Cardiol*. (2020) 311:116–21. doi: 10.1016/j.ijcard.2020.03.087
12. World Health Organization. *Clinical Management of Severe Acute Respiratory Infection When Novel Coronavirus (nCoV) Infection Is Suspected: Interim Guidance, 25 January 2020*. World Health Organization (2020). Available online at: https://apps.who.int/iris/handle/10665/330854 (accessed December 22, 2020).
13. World Health Organization. *COVID-19 Clinical Management: Living Guidance* (2020). Available online at: https://www.who.int/publications/i/item/WHO-2019-nCoV-clinical-2021-1 (accessed February 12, 2021).
14. Kidney Disease Improving Global Outcomes. Acute Kidney Injury Work Group: KDIGO clinical practice guideline for acute kidney injury. *Kidney Int*. (2012) 2:1–138. doi: 10.1038/kisup.2012.1
15. World Health Organization. *Nutritional Anaemias*. Report of a WHO Scientific Group. World Health Organization technical report series no. 405. Geneva: World Health Organization (1968). p. 5–37.
16. Hu H, Yao N, Qiu Y. Comparing rapid scoring systems in mortality prediction of critically ill patients with novel coronavirus disease. *Acad Emerg Med*. (2020) 27:461–8. doi: 10.1111/acem.13992
17. Yan L, Zhang H, Goncalves J, Xiao Y, Wang M, Guo Y, et al. An interpretable mortality prediction model for COVID-19 patients. *Nat Mach Intell*. (2020) 2:283–8. doi: 10.1038/s42256-020-0180-7
18. Shi Y, Yu X, Zhao H, Wang H, Zhao R, Sheng J. Host susceptibility to severe COVID-19 and establishment of a host risk score: findings of 487 cases outside Wuhan. *Crit Care*. (2020) 24:108. doi: 10.1186/s13054-020-2833-7
19. Turner AJ, Hiscox JA, Hooper NM. ACE2: from vasopeptidase to SARS virus receptor. *Trends Pharmacol Sci*. (2004) 25:291–4. doi: 10.1016/j.tips.2004.04.001
20. Gallagher PE, Ferrario CM, Tallant EA. Regulation of ACE2 in cardiac myocytes and fibroblasts. *Am J Physiol Heart Circ Physiol*. (2008) 295:H2373–9. doi: 10.1152/ajpheart.00426.2008
21. Xu Z, Shi L, Wang Y, Zhang J, Huang L, Zhang C, et al. Pathological findings of COVID-19 associated with acute respiratory distress syndrome. *Lancet Respir Med*. (2020) 8:420–2. doi: 10.1016/S2213-2600(20)30076-X
22. Tavazzi G, Pellegrini C, Maurelli M, Belliato M, Sciutti F, Bottazzi A, et al. Myocardial localization of coronavirus in COVID-19 cardiogenic shock. *Eur J Heart Fail*. (2020) 22:911–5. doi: 10.1002/ejhf.1828
23. Wichmann D, Sperhake JP, Lütgehetmann M, Steurer S, Edler C, Heinemann A, et al. Autopsy findings and venous thromboembolism in patients with COVID-19: a prospective cohort Study. *Ann Intern Med*. (2020) 173:268–77. doi: 10.7326/L20-1206
24. Lindner D, Fitzek A, Bräuninger H, Aleshcheva G, Edler C, Meissner K, et al. Association of cardiac infection with SARS-CoV-2 in confirmed COVID-19 autopsy cases. *JAMA Cardiol*. (2020) 5:1281–5. doi: 10.1001/jamacardio.2020.3551
25. Schaller T, Hirschbühl K, Burkhardt K, Braun G, Trepel M, Märkl B,

Early vs. Late Onset Cardiac Injury and Mortality in Hospitalized COVID-19 Patients in Wuhan

197

et al. Postmortem examination of patients with COVID-19. *JAMA.* (2020) 323:2518–20. doi: 10.1001/jama.2020.8907

26. Tang Y, Liu J, Zhang D, Xu Z, Ji J, Wen C. Cytokine storm in COVID-19: the current evidence and treatment strategies. *Front Immunol.* (2020) 11:1708. doi: 10.3389/fimmu.2020.01708

27. Mahmudpour M, Roozbeh J, Keshavarz M, Farrokhi S, Nabipour I. COVID-19 cytokine storm: the anger of inflammation. *Cytokine.* (2020) 133:155151. doi: 10.1016/j.cyto.2020.155151

28. Zhang L, Feng X, Zhang D, Jiang C, Mei H, Wang J, et al. Deep vein thrombosis in hospitalized patients with COVID-19 in Wuhan, China: prevalence, risk factors, and outcome. *Circulation.* (2020) 142:114–28. doi: 10.1161/CIR.0000000000000887

29. Han Q, Li G, Ip MS, Zhang Y, Zhen Z, Mak JC, et al. Haemin attenuates intermittent hypoxia-induced cardiac injury via inhibiting mitochondrial fission. *J Cell Mol Med.* (2018) 22:2717–26. doi: 10.1111/jcmm.13560

30. Eltzschig HK, Carmeliet P. Hypoxia and inflammation. *N Engl J Med.* (2011) 364:656–65. doi: 10.1056/NEJMra0910283

31. Ni C, Ma P, Wang R, Lou X, Liu X, Qin Y, et al. Doxorubicin-induced cardiotoxicity involves IFNγ-mediated metabolic reprogramming in cardiomyocytes. *J Pathol.* (2019) 247:320–32. doi: 10.1002/path.5192

32. Violi F, Calvieri C, Cangemi R. Effect of corticosteroids on myocardial injury among patients hospitalized for community-acquired pneumonia: rationale and study design. The colosseum trial. *Intern Emerg Med.* (2020) 15:79-86. doi: 10.1007/s11739-019-02117-0

33. Mumoli N, Cei M, Mazzone A, Conte G. Cardiac injury as prognostic value in COVID-19: more remains to be clarified. *Intern Emerg Med.* (2021) 16:267–8. doi: 10.1007/s11739-020-02540-8

34. Olsson T, Terent A, Lind L. Rapid emergency medicine score: a new prognostic tool for in-hospital mortality in nonsurgical emergency department patients. *J Intern Med.* (2004) 255:579–87. doi: 10.1111/j.1365-2796.2004.01321.x

35. Grein J, Ohmagari N, Shin D, Diaz G, Asperges E, Castagna A, et al. Compassionate use of remdesivir for patients with severe COVID-19. *N Engl J Med.* (2020) 382:2327–36. doi: 10.1056/NEJMc2015312

36. Wiersinga WJ, Rhodes A, Cheng AC, Peacock SJ, Prescott HC. Pathophysiology, transmission, diagnosis, and treatment of coronavirus disease 2019 (COVID-19): a review. *JAMA.* (2020) 324:782–93. doi: 10.1001/jama.2020.12839

37. Robbiani DF, Gaebler C, Muecksch F, Lorenzi JCC, Wang Z, Cho A, et al. Convergent antibody responses to SARS-CoV-2 in convalescent individuals. *Nature.* (2020) 584:437–42. doi: 10.1038/s41586-020-2456-9

19

Covid-19 Kills More Men than Women: An Overview of Possible Reasons

Annalisa Capuano[1]*, Francesco Rossi[1] and Giuseppe Paolisso[2]

[1] Department of Experimental Medicine, University of Campania Luigi Vanvitelli, Regional Centre of Pharmacovigilance, Campania Region, Naples, Italy, [2] Department of Advanced Medical and Surgical Sciences, University of Campania Luigi Vanvitelli, Naples, Italy

*Correspondence:
Annalisa Capuano
annalisa.capuano@unicampania.it

The high mortality observed in Covid-19 patients may be related to unrecognized pulmonary embolism, pulmonary thrombosis, or other underlying cardiovascular diseases. Recent data have highlighted that the mortality rate of Covid-19 seems to be higher in male patients compared to females. In this paper, we have analyzed possible factors that may underline this sex difference in terms of activity of the immune system and its modulation by sex hormones, coagulation pattern, and preexisting cardiovascular diseases as well as effects deriving from smoking and drinking habits. Future studies are needed to evaluate the effects of sex differences on the prevalence of infections, including Covid-19, its outcome, and the responses to antiviral treatments.

Keywords: Covid-19, mortality, gender difference, immune system, sex hormones, smoking habit, coagulation pattern, cardiovascular diseases

INTRODUCTION

All countries around the world are facing the COVID-19 emergency. As of June 22nd, more than 9,118,000 people have contracted the disease, and deaths have exceeded 471,000[1].

From a pathogenetic point of view, the progression of COVID-19 follows three main stages (1). The first stage, which approximately occurs in the initial 1–2 days, represents the phase in which the SARS-CoV-2 binds to epithelial cells and starts replicating. The human angiotensin-converting enzyme 2 (ACE2) receptor and TMPRSS2 are the main proteins involved in the cell entry of SARS-CoV-2 (2, 3). This phase is asymptomatic, and the innate immune response is limited. The second stage starts once the virus migrates down the respiratory tract. This phase is symptomatic with clear airway response and the innate immune response is triggered. An increase in the level of CXCL10 or other innate response cytokine is observed (4, 5). Indeed, this is the stage in which the so-called "cytokine storm" arises. Lastly, about 20% of patients with COVID-19 progress to a third stage, which is the most severe, and this stage is characterized by serious respiratory symptoms that include hypoxia, ground glass infiltrate, and progression to acute respiratory distress syndrome (ARDS). This stage can be further aggravated by organ failure and sepsis, potentially progressing to patient's death (6). At this stage, an aggressive immunomodulatory therapy is probably needed to prevent the onset of serious clinical consequences, such as the Disseminated intravascular coagulation (DIC) and the subsequent consumption coagulopathy (7). Indeed, as recently reported by a group of Italian researchers, the high mortality observed among Covid-19 patients may be somewhat due to unrecognized pulmonary embolism and pulmonary *in situ* thrombosis. Therefore, they suggested that a better understanding of Covid-19-related thromboembolic risk

---

[1]https://www.worldometers.info/coronavirus/ (accessed May 10, 2020).

would help to optimize diagnostic strategies but also the proper pharmacological management of patients with Covid-19 (8).

Data shared by Global Health 50/50, an internationally selected company that promotes gender equality in healthcare, revealed a higher proportion of deaths for Covid-19 in men than women in almost all countries. In Italy, according to data reported in the bulletin of integrated surveillance (update of April 23rd, 2020), deaths in men are approximately double compared to that of women (17.1 vs. 9.3%). Similar findings were reported in Greece, Holland, Denmark, Belgium, Spain, China, and the Philippines[2]. A study carried out by Liu et al. on 4,880 patients with respiratory symptoms or close contact with Covid-19 patients in a hospital in Wuhan showed that there was a significant higher rate in positivity to SARS-CoV-2 in males and the elderly population (>70 years), although only age was recognized as a risk factor (9). Similarly, a recent retrospective observational study showed that among critically ill patients with SARS-CoV-2, 67% were males and that the mortality rate was higher in males (10). In addition, a review of data related to 1,099 patients with Covid-19 showed that 58.1% were males. Furthermore, out of 173 severe cases, 57.8% concerned this population too (11). In addition, recent published data from a survival analysis (12) showed that men had a significantly higher mortality and exhibited worse symptoms than women. Lastly, Scully et al. recently reported that the case fatality rate for males is 1.7 times higher than for females ($P < 0.0001$) (13).

Considering that sex differences are frequently observed in many diseases, responses to drugs and the occurrence of adverse drugs reactions (14–17)—and that many reasons may underline these differences—in this paper, we aim to provide an overview of factors, including those influencing the immune system response, that possibly underline the sex and gender differences observed in Covid-19 patients. All those factors are summarized in **Table 1**.

SEX DIFFERENCES IN IMMUNE SYSTEM

Many studies, both preclinical and clinical, have analyzed the role of the sex in immune response patterns during viral infections. Few studies have proposed that the sex variability in the prevalence, pathogenesis, and response to viral infections can be related to the greater humoral and cell-mediated immune responses of females to viral antigens (18–20). This variability is probably the driver of a lower intensity and prevalence of viral infections in females than males. Indeed, female patients seem to be less susceptible to viral infections due to intense and prolonged innate, humoral, and cell-mediated immune responses. The higher activity of innate immune system in women, which is mediated by Toll-like receptors, retinoic acid-inducible gene I-like receptors, and nucleotide oligomerization domain-like receptors, may lead to a faster and higher recognition of viral components and consequently higher production of type 1 interferon (IFN) and inflammatory cytokines (IL-1, TNFs) (21).

[2]https://www.epicentro.iss.it/coronavirus/sars-cov-2-differenze-genere-importanza-dati-disaggregati

TABLE 1 | Overview of sex- and gender-differences that could be responsible of increased mortality rate in men with Covid-19.

Activity of the immune system	■ Female patients seem to have an intense and prolonged innate, humoral, and cell-mediated immune response, leading to a faster and higher recognition of viral components ■ Preclinical studies showed that females might recover to a greater extent and are better protected from death during infections
Role of sex hormones	■ Testosterone shows suppressive effect on the immune function, while estrogen may have both suppressive and not suppressive effects depending on their levels ■ In men androgens deficiency is associated with increased levels of inflammatory cytokines and increased CD4+/CD8+ T-cell ratio ■ Estrogens are able to induce an upregulation in the expression of ACE2 ■ Exogenous estrogen increases the clotting risk in women and in biological males undergoing gender-affirming hormonal therapy ■ Sex hormones could also affect the response to antiviral treatments or vaccines
Prevalence of cardiovascular diseases	■ Women seem to have a higher risk and incidence of symptomatic supraventricular tachycardia and long QT syndrome compared with men ■ Men show higher risk of atrial fibrillation and sudden cardiac death and they are more affected by atherosclerotic cardiovascular disease compared with women
Coagulation pattern	■ Men have a 3.6-fold higher risk of recurrent VTE than women ■ Women show higher risk of VTE during fertile years
Smoking and drinking habits	■ Smoking habit is higher in men than women ■ Drinking habit is higher in men than women

For instance, in the United States, the 1918 influenza pandemic was associated with a higher mortality rate in men than women (22). Male gender could also be associated with higher mortality rate in herpes simplex virus-1 (HSV-1) respiratory infection. Indeed, Brown et al. evaluated the effects of sex on susceptibility to HSV-1 respiratory infection after repeated exhaustive exercise (treadmill running at 36 m/min) in CD-1 mice (86 males and 89 females). The results showed that the exercise stress was associated with increased morbidity and mortality in male mice, while only an increase in morbidity was observed in females. Authors suggested that females might recover to a greater extent and are ultimately better protected from death (23). Similar findings were found by another preclinical study carried out by Han et al. (24), while no sex differences were found for ocular HSV-1 infection (25).

On the other hand, the higher immune responses observed in females may lead to increased development of symptoms of infection in this population (26). For instance, with regard to influenza A viruses, even though men seemed to be more exposed to this infection, women showed higher mortality rates

(27). During 2009 H1N1, a higher hospitalization rate was observed in young women (28). Furthermore, females had a 2-fold higher risk of death than males (29, 30). This could be the consequence of the higher immune response that leads to high levels of pro-inflammatory cytokines, including IL-1, IL-2, IL-6, G-CSF, IP-10, and TNFα, a condition that is defined as a "cytokine storm" and that seems to worsen symptoms of Covid-19 infections, such as ARDS, organ failure, and sepsis (31–33).

The Role of Sex Hormones

Apart from factors merely related to a higher/lower activity of innate, humoral, and cell-mediated immune responses and to the production of inflammatory cytokines, other factors, including sex hormones, may play a key role during response to viral infections (34). In women, the level of estrogen varies during the menstrual cycle and falls with menopause, while, in men, the level of testosterone remains stable up to 60 years of age. Sex hormones induce their effects through the binding with estrogen receptors (ERα and ERβ), the androgen receptor (AR), and progesterone receptors (PR-A and PR-B). Innate immune cells express those receptors to varying degrees (35). Some studies have demonstrated that testosterone exhibits a suppressive effect on the immune function, while estrogen may have both suppressive or not suppressive effects depending on their levels (36–38). Data from studies carried out in humans revealed that in men androgens deficiency is associated with increased levels of inflammatory cytokines and increased CD4+/CD8+ T-cell ratio compared to men with normal level of testosterone (39, 40). On the other hand, estrogens could affect several activities of the innate and adaptive immune responses, showing opposite effects on the immune system based on their level. Indeed, low doses of estrogens seem to induce monocyte differentiation into inflammatory DCs, leading to higher production of IL-4 and IFN-α and activate Th1-type and cell-mediated immune responses. On the contrary, high doses of estrogens show inhibitory activity on innate and pro-inflammatory immune responses and enhance Th2-type responses and humoral immune responses (36, 41). Given the multiple effects of female hormones on immune system functions, women may present different responses to viral infections during the course of their lives. For instance, during pregnancy, which represents a unique immunological state, women seem to undergo three different stages: an initial pro-inflammatory phase, a second one (corresponding to the second trimester of pregnancy), which is characterized by an anti-inflammatory state, and a third phase that is characterized by an increase of inflammatory processes, which are useful for uterine muscle contraction, for the delivery as well as for placenta rejection. The succession of these pro- and anti-inflammatory phases seems to be the results of T helper 1 (Th1)/T helper 2 (Th2) immune shifts that, in turn, could also reflect a change in sensitivity to infectious diseases among pregnant women (42). Indeed, the higher mortality rate of 2009 H1N1 in women was found for those in reproductive age (20–49 years), suggesting a role of gonadal hormones, especially during pregnancy (28).

Lastly, sex hormones could also affect the response to antiviral treatments or vaccines. As reported by Klein (26), the efficacy of the HSV-2 vaccine and of the recombinant glycoprotein D (gD)-based HSV-2 vaccine against the development of symptoms associated with genital herpes was found to be higher in women than in men.

SEX DIFFERENCE IN CARDIOVASCULAR DISEASES

Recent literature data showed a higher prevalence of hypertension and coronary artery disease in patients with severe forms of Covid-19 (43, 44), suggesting that preexisting cardiovascular diseases may lead to a worse prognosis. According to Wu et al. (45), an arrhythmogenic effect of Covid-19, with occurrence of long and short QT syndrome, Brugada syndrome, and catecholaminergic polymorphic ventricular tachycardia, could be expected (46). These life-threatening cardiac disorders can be the consequence of enhanced inflammation, which can increase the duration of ventricular repolarization, by affecting the QTc interval (47). On the other hand, heart injury can be induced by other mechanisms, including some deriving from the effects of ACE2 that is expressed in the lungs and in the cardiovascular system, while other deriving from the cytokine storm and hypoxaemia that results in myocardial cells damage[3]. Indeed, inflammatory cytokines, especially interleukin-6, increase the risk of QT interval prolongation and life-threatening arrhythmias (48). In addition, cytokines show a pro-atherogenic effect, including TNF-α, which activates NF-κB, p38 MAPK, and the transcription of proinflammatory genes for cytokines involved in the cytokine storm (49). Therefore, the role of cytokines in worsening the cardiovascular homeostasis of patients with Covid-19 cannot be excluded.

Some sex differences have been found in the incidence of cardiovascular diseases. Indeed, while women seem to have a higher risk and incidence of symptomatic supraventricular tachycardia and long QT syndrome, men show higher risk of atrial fibrillation and sudden cardiac death. Furthermore, epidemiological studies demonstrated that men are more affected by atherosclerotic cardiovascular disease compared with women. This difference can be imputable to the clinical risk profile, effects of sex hormones, and social attitude (50). Apart from sex differences in the production of inflammatory cytokines and in the incidence of cardiovascular diseases, recent evidence shows that a sex difference in virus-targeted mechanism could be hypothesized. As previously reported, the ACE2 receptor is essential for the cell entry of SARS-CoV-2, but it also represents an important enzyme of the renin-angiotensin system (RAS) that provides protective effects in many chronic conditions, like hypertension, cardiovascular diseases, and acute respiratory distress syndrome. All these clinical conditions represent risk factors for a worse prognosis in Covid-19 patients. Ruggieri and Gagliardi have recently reported that estrogens are able to

---

[3]https://www.nature.com/articles/s41569-020-0360-5#citeas

induce an upregulation in the expression of ACE2, which could explain better outcome and lower death rate in women compared to men[4]. Furthermore, as recently reported by Gagliardi et al., the gene that encodes for ACE2 is on the X chromosome, and XX cells over-express it (51). Furthermore, the results of a preclinical study that investigated the role of ACE2 in angiotensin (1–7)-induced hypertension and regulation of the RAS system in the kidney of wild type and Ace2 knockout mice revealed some sex differences in rising of mean arterial pressure, binding of glomerular AT1 receptor, and renal protein expression of the neutral endopeptidase neprilysin, suggesting that females may be protected from angiotensin (1–7)-induced hypertension (52).

Even though the ACE2 plays an essential role in the RAS system, it should be highlighted that a recent retrospective cohort study, carried out on 4,480 patients with Covid-19, showed that the prior use of ACE inhibitors or angiotensin receptor blockers (both acting on RAS) was not significantly associated with COVID-19 diagnosis neither with mortality or severe disease (53).

SEX DIFFERENCE IN COAGULATION PATTERN

The DIC is a life-threatening syndrome which leads to disseminated and uncontrolled activation of coagulation, thrombosis, and progressive consumption coagulopathy, leading to an increased bleeding risk. The DIC occurs frequently in almost 30–50% of patients with sepsis and 10% in patients with solid tumors, trauma, or obstetric calamities. Furthermore, the risk of DIC is higher in critically ill patients hospitalized in ICU, for whom the prevalence of DIC is about 8.5–34% (54). According to Tang et al., ~71.4% of the non-survivor patients with Covid-19 matched the grade of overt-DIC ($\geq$5 points) in later stages of SARS-Cov-2 pneumonia, and 76% of the non-survivors were males. On the contrary, only the 0.6% of survivors matched the DIC criteria during the hospital stay (55). Moreover, the DIC appears to be a driver of disease severity. As might be expected, it is a strong prognostic factor for poor outcome (55). Finally, *microthrombi* have been reported as autopsy findings in patients with Covid-19[5].

It is widely demonstrated that differential risks in men and women for cardiovascular disease exist, especially during premenopausal period due to female sex regulating hormones. Moreover, once reproductive risk factors are taken into account, men have a 3.6-fold higher risk of recurrent venous thromboembolism (VTE) than women (56). The pathophysiology behind this observation is unclear (57). Indeed, it is known that deficient coagulation problems, such as hemophilia, are under genetic control and sex-related, so one cannot exclude that hypercoagulability might be also affected by genetic factors (58). Furthermore, women show higher risk of VTE during fertile years, mainly as consequence of the effects mediated by pregnancy and oral contraceptive use. In this regard, literature data suggested that exogenous estrogen increases the clotting risk in women and in biological males undergoing gender-affirming hormonal therapy (59, 60).

GENDER DIFFERENCES IN SMOKING AND DRINKING HABITS

Compared to non-smokers, smokers generally show higher rates of respiratory diseases, including colds, influenza, bacterial pneumonia, and tuberculosis (61–64). Indeed, smoking habit leads to progressive lung damage, which exposes patients to higher risk of pulmonary bacterial and viral infections (65). This leads to higher risk of hospitalization due to influenza infection as well (66). Lastly, smoking represents the fourth leading cause of death in the world (67). In the context of Covid-19, smokers are more likely to contract the disease since the act of smoking implies that possibly contaminated fingers are in contact with lips, increasing the possibility of the SARS-CoV-2 virus being transmitted from hand to mouth (68, 69). Furthermore, smoking is also related to higher expression of ACE2, which is involved in the process of cell entry of the SARS-CoV-2 (70).

Generally, the percent of smoking habits is found to be higher in men than women, since the adolescent age, even though with differences among low- medium- and high-income countries (71, 72). In order to evaluate the association between smoking and Covid-19 outcomes, in terms of disease severity, need for mechanical ventilation or intensive care unit (ICU), hospitalization, and death, Vardavas et al. carried out a systematic review of studies on Covid-19 patients that included information on patients' smoking status. Authors highlighted that there were higher percentages of current and former smokers among patients who accessed to ICU, required mechanical ventilation, or who had died (73). Other studies are strongly needed to evaluate the prevalence of smokers among patients with severe Covid-19, but based on current knowledge it is possible to assume that smokers are likely to be at higher risk for severe SARS-CoV-2 infection. Therefore, smoking cessation awareness should be strongly encouraged in order to reduce the global impact of COVID-19 (74).

As for smoking habits, drinking is found to be higher in men than women. Indeed, women generally drink less and have a lower prevalence of drink problems than men (75). Alcohol-related liver disease represents one of the main causes of liver cirrhosis, associated with high mortality and morbidity. A recent study, which has analyzed the prevalence, severity and mortality of patients diagnosed with COVID-19 with underlying chronic liver diseases, showed that this disease is associated to higher severity and mortality also in Covid-19 patients[6].

---

[4]https://www.gendermedjournal.it/articoli.php?archivio=yes&vol_id=3351&id=33219

[5]https://www.preprints.org/manuscript/202002.0407/v2

[6]https://www.mdpi.com/2414-6366/5/2/80/htm

CONCLUSION

Covid-19 still represents a worldwide health emergency. In this paper, we have analyzed possible factors that may have contributed to a gender difference in Covid-19 clinical outcomes, especially in the rate of death. Among possible factors, those related to the activity of immune system and the role of sex hormones seem to be the most important. However, in our opinion, sex differences in cardiovascular diseases and coagulation patterns should be considered as well, especially considering the possible role of the cytokine storm in inducing vascular inflammation and atherosclerosis-related cardiovascular diseases but also gender differences in coagulation, which can be responsible of higher risk of thrombotic/thromboembolic phenomena in men compared to women. Further epidemiological studies will be needed to confirm this. Lastly, considering that women are often underrepresented in randomized clinical trials, future studies are needed to evaluate the effects of sex differences on the prevalence of infections, their outcome, and responses to antiviral treatments.

AUTHOR CONTRIBUTIONS

AC, FR, and GP drafted the work and revised it for important intellectual content, made substantial contributions to the acquisition, analysis, or interpretation of data for the work, approved the final version of the manuscript, developed the concept, and wrote the manuscript. All authors contributed to the article and approved the submitted version.

REFERENCES

1. Mason RJ. Pathogenesis of COVID-19 from a cell biology perspective. *Eur Respir J.* (2020) 55:2000607. doi: 10.1183/13993003.00607-2020
2. Fehr AR, Perlman S. Coronaviruses: an overview of their replication and pathogenesis. *Methods Mol Biol.* (2015) 1282:1–23. doi: 10.1007/978-1-4939-2438-7_1
3. Hoffmann M, Kleine-Weber H, Schroeder S, Krüger N, Herrler T, Erichsen S, et al. SARS-CoV-2 cell entry depends on ACE2 and TMPRSS2 and is blocked by a clinically proven protease inhibitor. *Cell.* (2020) 181: 271–280.e8. doi: 10.1016/j.cell.2020.02.052
4. Qian Z, Travanty EA, Oko L, Edeen K, Berglund A, Wang J, et al. Innate immune response of human alveolar type II cells infected with severe acute respiratory syndrome-coronavirus. *Am J Respir Cell Mol Biol.* (2013) 48:742–8. doi: 10.1165/rcmb.2012-0339OC
5. Wang J, Nikrad MP, Phang T, Gao B, Alford T, Ito Y, et al. Innate immune response to influenza A virus in differentiated human alveolar type II cells. *Am J Respir Cell Mol Biol.* (2011) 45:582–91. doi: 10.1165/rcmb.2010-0108OC
6. Guo YR, Cao QD, Hong ZS, Tan YY, Chen SD, Jin HJ, et al. The origin, transmission and clinical therapies on coronavirus disease 2019 (COVID-19) outbreak - an update on the status. *Mil Med Res.* (2020) 7:11. doi: 10.1186/s40779-020-00240-0
7. *COVID-19 and Haemostasis: A Position Paper From Italian Society on Thrombosis and Haemostasis (SISET).* Available online at: http://www.sah.org.ar/pdf/covid-19/083-20_pre-publishing.pdf
8. Lodigiani C, Iapichino G, Carenzo L, Cecconi M, Ferrazzi P, Sebastian T, et al. Venous and arterial thromboembolic complications in COVID-19 patients admitted to an academic hospital in Milan, Italy. *Thromb Res.* (2020) 191:9–14. doi: 10.1016/j.thromres.2020.04.024
9. Liu R, Han H, Liu F, Lv Z, Wu K, Liu Y, et al. Positive rate of RT-PCR detection of SARS-CoV-2 infection in 4880 cases from one hospital in Wuhan, China, from Jan to Feb 2020. *Clin Chim Acta.* (2020) 505:172–5. doi: 10.1016/j.cca.2020.03.009
10. Yang X, Yu Y, Xu J, Shu H, Xia J, Liu H, et al. Clinical course and outcomes of critically ill patients with SARS-CoV-2 pneumonia in Wuhan, China: a single-centered, retrospective, observational study. *Lancet Respir Med.* (2020) 8:475–481. doi: 10.1016/S2213-26002030079-5
11. Xie J, Tong Z, Guan X, Du B, Qiu H. Clinical characteristics of patients who died of coronavirus Disease 2019 in China. *JAMA New Open.* (2020) 3:e205619. doi: 10.1001/jamanetworkopen.2020.5619
12. Jin JM, Bai P, He W, Wu F, Liu XF, Han DM, et al. Gender differences in patients with COVID-19: focus on severity and mortality. *Front Public Health.* (2020) 8:152. doi: 10.3389/fpubh.2020.00152
13. Scully EP, Haverfield J, Ursin RL, Tannenbaum C, Klein SL. Considering how biological sex impacts immune responses and COVID-19 outcomes. *Nat Rev Immunol.* (2020) 20:442–7. doi: 10.1038/s41577-020-0348-8
14. Ferrajolo C, Sultana J, Ientile V, Scavone C, Scondotto G, Tari M, et al. Gender Differences in outpatient pediatric drug utilization: a cohort study from Southern Italy. *Front Pharmacol.* (2019) 10:11. doi: 10.3389/fphar.2019.00011
15. Sessa M, Mascolo A, Scavone C, Perone I, Di Giorgio A, Tari M, et al. Comparison of long-term clinical implications of beta-blockade in patients with obstructive airway diseases exposed to beta-blockers with different β1-adrenoreceptor selectivity: an Italian Population-Based Cohort Study. *Front Pharmacol.* (2018) 9:1212. doi: 10.3389/fphar.2018.01212
16. Scavone C, Di Mauro C, Ruggiero R, Bernardi FF, Trama U, Aiezza ML, et al. Severe cutaneous adverse drug reactions associated with allopurinol: an analysis of spontaneous reporting system in Southern Italy. *Drugs Real World Outcomes.* (2020) 7:41–51. doi: 10.1007/s40801-019-00174-7
17. Corrao S, Santalucia P, Argano C, Djade CD, Barone E, Tettamanti M, et al. Gender-differences in disease distribution and outcome in hospitalized elderly: data from the REPOSI study. *Eur J Intern Med.* (2014) 25:617–23. doi: 10.1016/j.ejim.2014.06.027
18. Klein SL, Jedlicka A, Pekosz A. The Xs and Y of immune responses to viral vaccines. *Lancet Infect Dis.* (2010) 10:338–49. doi: 10.1016/S1473-3099(10)70049-9
19. Khandaker G, Dierig A, Rashid H, King C, Heron L, Booy R. Systematic review of clinical and epidemiological features of the pandemic influenza A (H1N1) 2009. *Influenza Other Respir Viruses.* (2011) 5:148–56. doi: 10.1111/j.1750-2659.2011.00199.x
20. Puchhammer-Stöckl E, Aberle SW, Heinzl H. Association of age and gender with alphaherpesvirus infections of the central nervous system in the immunocompetent host. *J Clin Virol.* (2012) 53:356–9. doi: 10.1016/j.jcv.2011.12.015
21. Ruggieri A, Gagliardi MC, Anticoli S. Sex-dependent outcome of hepatitis B and C viruses infections: synergy of sex hormones and immune responses? *Front Immunol.* (2018) 9:2302. doi: 10.3389/fimmu.2018.02302
22. Noymer A. The 1918 influenza pandemic affected sex differentials in mortality: Comment on Sawchuk. *Am J Phys Anthropol.* (2010). 143:499–500. doi: 10.1002/ajpa.21405
23. Brown AS, Davis JM, Murphy EA, Carmichael MD, Ghaffar A, Mayer EP. Gender differences in viral infection after repeated exercise stress. *Med Sci Sports Exerc.* (2004) 36:1290–5. doi: 10.1249/01.MSS.0000135798.72735.B3
24. Han X, Lundberg P, Tanamachi B, Openshaw H, Longmate J, Cantin E. Gender influences herpes simplex virus type 1 infection in normal and gamma interferon-mutant mice. *J Virol.* (2001) 75:3048–52. doi: 10.1128/JVI.75.6.3048-3052.2001
25. Riccio RE, Park SJ, Longnecker R, Kopp SJ. Characterization of sex differences in ocular herpes simplex virus 1 infection and herpes stromal keratitis pathogenesis of wild-type and herpesvirus entry mediator knockout mice. *mSphere.* (2019) 4:e00073-19. doi: 10.1128/mSphere.00073-19

26. Klein SL. Sex influences immune responses to viruses, and efficacy of prophylaxis and treatments for viral diseases. *Bioessays.* (2012) 34:1050–9. doi: 10.1002/bies.201200099

27. Klein SL, Pekosz A, Passaretti C, Anker M, Olukoya P. *Sex, Gender and Influenza.* Geneva: World Health Organization (2010). p. 1–58.

28. Klein SL, Passaretti C, Anker M, Olukoya P, Pekosz A. The impact of sex, gender and pregnancy on 2009 H1N1 disease. *Biol Sex Differ.* (2010) 1:5. doi: 10.1186/2042-6410-1-5

29. Randolph AG, Vaughn F, Sullivan R, Rubinson L, Thompson BT, Yoon G, et al. Critically ill children during the 2009–2010 influenza pandemic in the United States. *Pediatrics.* (2011) 128:e1450–8. doi: 10.1542/peds.2011-0774d

30. Zarychanski R, Stuart TL, Kumar A, Doucette S, Elliott L, Kettner J, et al. Correlates of severe disease in patients with 2009 pandemic influenza (H1N1) virus infection. *CMAJ.* (2010) 182:257–64. doi: 10.1503/cmaj.091884

31. Capuano A, Scavone C, Racagni G, Scaglione F, Italian Society of Pharmacology. NSAIDs in patients with viral infections, including Covid-19: victims or perpetrators? *Pharmacol Res.* (2020) 157:104849. doi: 10.1016/j.phrs.2020.104849

32. Scavone C, Brusco S, Bertini M, et al. Current pharmacological treatments for COVID-19: what's next? *Br J Pharmacol.* (2020) 1–12. doi: 10.1111/bph.15072

33. di Mauro G, Scavone C, Rafaniello C, Rossi F, Capuano A. SARS-Cov-2 infection: response of human immune system and possible implications for the rapid test and treatment. *Int Immunopharmacol.* (2020) 84:106519. doi: 10.1016/j.intimp.2020.106519

34. Roved J, Westerdahl H, Hasselquist D. Sex differences in immune responses: hormonal effects, antagonistic selection, and evolutionary consequences. *Horm Behav.* (2017) 88:95–105. doi: 10.1016/j.yhbeh.2016.11.017

35. Kadel S, Kovats S. Sex Hormones regulate innate immune cells and promote sex differences in respiratory virus infection. *Front Immunol.* (2018) 9:1653. doi: 10.3389/fimmu.2018.01653

36. Khan D, Ansar Ahmed S. The immune system is a natural target for estrogen action: opposing effects of estrogen in two prototypical autoimmune diseases. *Front Immunol.* (2016) 6:635. 10.3389/fimmu.2015.00635

37. Foo YZ, Nakagawa S, Rhodes G, Simmons LW. The effects of sex hormones on immune function: a meta-analysis. *Biol Rev Camb Philos Soc.* (2017) 92:551–71. doi: 10.1111/brv.12243

38. Trigunaite A, Dimo J, Jørgensen TN. Suppressive effects of androgens on the immune system. *Cell Immunol.* (2015) 294:87–94. doi: 10.1016/j.cellimm.2015.02.004

39. Malkin CJ, Pugh PJ, Jones RD, Kapoor D, Channer KS, Jones TH. The effect of testosterone replacement on endogenous inflammatory cytokines and lipid profiles in hypogonadal men. *J Clin Endocrinol Metab.* (2004) 89:3313–8. doi: 10.1210/jc.2003-031069

40. Bobjer J, Katrinaki M, Tsatsanis C, Lundberg Giwercman Y, Giwercman A. Negative association between testosterone concentration and inflammatory markers in young men: a nested cross-sectional study. *PLoS ONE.* (2013) 8:e61466. doi: 10.1371/journal.pone.0061466

41. Seillet C, Laffont S, Trémollières F, Rouquié N, Ribot C, Arnal JF, et al. The TLR-mediated response of plasmacytoid dendritic cells is positively regulated by estradiol *in vivo* through cell-intrinsic estrogen receptor α signaling. *Blood.* (2012) 119:454–64. doi: 10.1182/blood-2011-08-371831

42. Mor G, Cardenas I. The immune system in pregnancy: a unique complexity. *Am J Reprod Immunol.* (2010) 63:425–33. doi: 10.1111/j.1600-0897.2010.00836.x

43. Guan WJ, Ni ZY, Hu Y, Liang W, Ou C, He J, et al. Clinical characteristics of coronavirus disease 2019 in China. *N Engl J Med.* (2020) 382:1708–20. doi: 10.1056/NEJMoa2002032

44. Wang D, Hu B, Hu C, Zhu F, Liu X, Zhang J, et al. Clinical characteristics of 138 hospitalized patients with 2019 novel coronavirus–infected pneumonia in Wuhan, China. *JAMA.* (2020) 323:1061–9. doi: 10.1001/jama.2020.1585

45. Wu CI, Postema PG, Arbelo E, Behr ER, Bezzina CR, Napolitano C, et al. SARS-CoV-2, COVID-19, and inherited arrhythmia syndromes. *Heart Rhythm.* (2020) S1547-5271(20)30285-X. doi: 10.1016/j.hrthm.2020.03.024

46. Baldi E, Sechi GM, Mare C, Canevari F, Brancaglione A, Primi R et al. Out-of-hospital cardiac arrest during the Covid-19 outbreak in italy. *N Engl J Med.* (2020) NEJMc2010418. doi: 10.1056/NEJMc2010418. [Epub ahead of print].

47. Lazzerini PE, Boutjdir M, Capecchi PL. COVID-19, arrhythmic risk and inflammation: mind the gap!. *Circulation.* (2020). doi: 10.1161/CIRCULATIONAHA.120.047293

48. Aromolaran AS, Srivastava U, Alí A, Chahine M, Lazaro D, El-Sherif N, et al. Interleukin-6 inhibition of hERG underlies risk for acquired long QT in cardiac and systemic inflammation. *PLoS ONE.* (2018) 13:e0208321. doi: 10.1371/journal.pone.0208321

49. Welsh P, Grassia G, Botha S, Sattar N, Maffia P. Targeting inflammation to reduce cardiovascular disease risk: a realistic clinical prospect? *Br J Pharmacol.* (2017) 174:3898–913. doi: 10.1111/bph.13818

50. Tian J, Wang X, Tian J, Yu B. Gender differences in plaque characteristics of nonculprit lesions in patients with coronary artery disease. *BMC Cardiovasc Disord.* (2019) 19:45. doi: 10.1186/s12872-019-1023-5

51. Gagliardi MC, Tieri P, Ortona E, Ruggieri A. ACE2 expression and sex disparity in COVID-19. *Cell Death Discov.* (2020) 6:37. doi: 10.1038/s41420-020-0276-1

52. Ji H, de Souza AMA, Bajaj B, Zheng W, Wu X, Speth RC, et al. Sex-specific modulation of blood pressure and the renin-angiotensin system by ACE (Angiotensin-Converting Enzyme) 2. *Hypertension.* (2020). doi: 10.1161/HYPERTENSIONAHA.120.15276

53. Fosbøl EL, Butt JH, Østergaard L, Andersson C, Selmer C, Kragholm K, et al. Association of angiotensin-converting enzyme inhibitor or angiotensin receptor blocker use with COVID-19 diagnosis and mortality. *JAMA.* (2020) e2011301. doi: 10.1001/jama.2020.11301

54. Papageorgiou C, Jourdi G, Adjambri E, Walborn A, Patel P, Fareed J, et al. Disseminated intravascular coagulation: an update on pathogenesis, diagnosis, and therapeutic strategies. *Clin Appl Thromb Hemost.* (2018) 24(9 Suppl.):1076029618806424. doi: 10.1177/1076029618806424

55. Tang N, Li D, Wang X, Sun Z. Abnormal coagulation parameters are associated with poor prognosis in patients with novel coronavirus pneumonia. *J Thromb Haemost.* (2020) 18:844–7. doi: 10.1111/jth.14768

56. Tagalakis V. Sex may matter when it comes to the presenting location of deep vein thrombosis. *Thromb Res.* (2019) 173:164–5. doi: 10.1016/j.thromres.2018.12.001

57. Roach RE, Cannegieter SC, Lijfering WM. Differential risks in men and women for first and recurrent venous thrombosis: the role of genes and environment. *J Thromb Haemost.* (2015) 12:1593–600. doi: 10.1111/jth.12678

58. Bushnell CD. Stroke and the female brain. *Nat Clin Pract Neurol.* (2008) 4:22–33. doi: 10.1038/ncpneuro0686

59. Bischof E, Wolfe J, Klein SL. Clinical trials for COVID-19 should include sex as a variable. *J Clin Invest.* (2020) 130:3350–3352. doi: 10.1172/JCI139306

60. Getahun D, Nash R, Flanders WD, Baird TC, Becerra-Culqui TA, Cromwell L, et al. Cross-sex hormones and acute cardiovascular events in transgender persons: a cohort study. *Ann Intern Med.* (2018) 169:205–213. doi: 10.7326/M17-2785

61. Atto B, Eapen MS, Sharma P, Frey U, Ammit AJ, Markos J, et al. New therapeutic targets for the prevention of infectious acute exacerbations of COPD: role of epithelial adhesion molecules and inflammatory pathways. *Clin Sci.* (2019) 133:1663–703. doi: 10.1042/CS20181009

62. Eapen MS, Sharma P, Moodley YP, Hansbro PM, Sohal SS. Dysfunctional immunity and microbial adhesion molecules in smoking-induced pneumonia. *Am J Respir Crit Care Med.* (2019) 199:250–1. doi: 10.1164/rccm.201808-1553LE

63. Eapen MS, Sharma P, Sohal SS. Mitochondrial dysfunction in macrophages: a key to defective bacterial phagocytosis in COPD. *Eur Respir J.* (2019) 54:1901641. doi: 10.1183/13993003.01641-2019

64. Eapen MS, Sohal SS. Understanding novel mechanisms of microbial pathogenesis in chronic lung disease: implications for new therapeutic targets. *Clin Sci.* (2018) 132:375–9. doi: 10.1042/CS20171261

65. Lawrence H, Hunter A, Murray R, Lim WS, McKeever T. Cigarette smoking and the occurrence of influenza—Systematic review. *J Infect.* (2019) 79:401–6. doi: 10.1016/j.jinf.2019.08.014

66. Han L, Ran J, Mak YW, Suen LK, Lee PH, Peiris JSM, et al. Smoking and influenza-associated morbidity and mortality: a systematic review and meta-analysis. *Epidemiology.* (2019) 30:405–17. doi: 10.1097/EDE.0000000000000984

67. *World Health Organisation Chronic Obstructive Pulmonary Disease (COPD).* (2020). Available online at: https://www.who.int/respiratory/copd/en/ (accessed March, 11 2020)

68. Istituto Superiore di Sanità. *Tobacco Smoking in the Age of COVID-19.* Available online at: https://www.epicentro.iss.it/en/coronavirus/sars-cov-2-addictions-smoking

69. Cai H. Sex difference and smoking predisposition in patients with COVID-19. *Lancet Respir Med.* (2020) 8:e20. doi: 10.1016/S2213-260020 30117-X

70. Li J, Zhang Y, Wang F, Liu B, Li H, Tang G, et al. Sex differences in clinical findings among patients with coronavirus disease 2019 (COVID-19) and severe condition. *medRxiv.* (2020) 02.27.20027524. doi: 10.1101/2020.02.27.200 27524

71. Zeman MV, Hiraki L, Sellers EM. Gender differences in tobacco smoking: higher relative exposure to smoke than nicotine in women. *J Womens Health Gend Based Med.* (2002) 11:147–53. doi: 10.1089/152460902753 645281

72. Han J, Chen X. A Meta-analysis of cigarette smoking prevalence among adolescents in China: 1981-2010. *Int J Environ Res Public Health.* (2015) 12:4617–30. doi: 10.3390/ijerph120504617

73. Vardavas CI, Nikitara K. COVID-19 and smoking: a systematic review of the evidence. *Tob Induc Dis.* (2020) 18:20. doi: 10.18332/tid/119324

74. Komiyama M, Hasegawa K. Smoking cessation as a public health measure to limit the coronavirus disease 2019 pandemic. *Eur Cardiol.* (2020) 15:e16. doi: 10.15420/ecr.2020.11

75. Ely M, Hardy R, Longford NT, Wadsworth ME. Gender differences in the relationship between alcohol consumption and drink problems are largely accounted for by body water. *Alcohol Alcohol.* (1999) 34:894–902. doi: 10.1093/alcalc/34.6.894

20

Prevalence of Venous Thromboembolism in Critically Ill COVID-19 Patients

Mouhand F. H. Mohamed[1]*, Shaikha D. Al-Shokri[1], Khaled M. Shunnar[1],
Sara F. Mohamed[1], Mostafa S. Najim[1], Shahd I. Ibrahim[1], Hazem Elewa[2],
Lina O. Abdalla[1], Ahmed El-Bardissy[3], Mohamed Nabil Elshafei[3], Ibrahim Y. Abubeker[4],
Mohammed Danjuma[1,5], Khalid M. Dousa[6] and Mohamed A. Yassin[7]

[1] Department of Medicine, Hamad Medical Corporation, Doha, Qatar, [2] College of Pharmacy, QU Health, Qatar University,
Doha, Qatar, [3] Clinical Pharmacy Department, Hamad General Hospital, Doha, Qatar, [4] Alpert Medical School, Brown
University, Providence, RI, United States, [5] College of Medicine, QU Health, Qatar University, Doha, Qatar, [6] Division of
Infectious Diseases and HIV Medicine, University Hospitals Cleveland Medical Center, Case Western Reserve University,
Cleveland, OH, United States, [7] Department of Hematology, Hamad Medical Corporation, Doha, Qatar

*Correspondence:
Mouhand F. H. Mohamed
dr.m.oraiby@hotmail.com

Background: Recent studies revealed a high prevalence of venous thromboembolism (VTE) events in coronavirus disease 2019 (COVID-19) patients, especially in those who are critically ill. Available studies report varying prevalence rates. Hence, the exact prevalence remains uncertain. Moreover, there is an ongoing debate regarding the appropriate dosage of thromboprophylaxis.

Methods: We performed a systematic review and proportion meta-analysis following the Preferred Reporting Items for Systematic Reviews and Meta-Analyses (PRISMA) guidelines. We searched PubMed and EMBASE for studies exploring the prevalence of VTE in critically ill COVID-19 patients till 25/07/2020. We pooled the proportion of VTE. Additionally, in a subgroup analysis, we pooled VTE events detected by systematic screening. Finally, in an exploratory analysis, we compared the odds of VTE in patients on prophylactic compared with therapeutic anticoagulation.

Results: The review comprised 24 studies and over 2,500 patients. The pooled proportion of VTE prevalence was 0.31 [95% confidence interval (CI) 0.24, 0.39; I^2 94%], of VTE utilizing systematic screening was 0.48 (95% CI 0.33, 0.63; I^2 91%), of deep venous thrombosis was 0.23 (95% CI 0.14, 0.32; I^2 96%), and of pulmonary embolism was 0.14 (95% CI 0.09, 0.20; I^2 90%). Exploratory analysis of few studies, utilizing systematic screening, VTE risk increased significantly with prophylactic, compared with therapeutic anticoagulation [odds ratio (OR) 5.45; 95% CI 1.90, 15.57; I^2 0%].

Discussion: Our review revealed a high prevalence of VTE in critically ill COVID-19 patients. Almost 50% of patients had VTE detected by systematic screening. Higher thromboprophylaxis dosages may reduce VTE burden in this patient's cohort compared with standard prophylactic anticoagulation; however, this is to be ascertained by ongoing randomized controlled trials.

Keywords: COVID-19, SARS-CoV-2, VTE, thrombosis, venous, ICU, DVT—deep vein thrombosis

INTRODUCTION

The pool of recent evidence suggests that coronavirus disease 2019 (COVID-19) is a thrombogenic condition. It leads to an increased incidence of both venous and arterial thromboembolic events (1). COVID-19 patients admitted to the intensive care units (ICU) seem to carry a higher risk (1). Venous thromboembolism (VTE) prevalence in the critically ill COVID-19 patients varied across individual studies. This is likely due to differences in screening methods (systematic vs. non-systematic screening), among other study-specific characteristics, leaving VTE's exact prevalence unknown. The prevalence of deep venous thrombosis (DVT) was considered low compared with pulmonary embolism (PE), which led researchers to consider microthrombosis as an additional mechanism of PE in COVID-19 patients (2).

VTE's heightened risk led to a wide chemoprophylaxis use for critically ill COVID-19 patients (3). Notwithstanding this, recent studies showed that even COVID-19 patients on chemoprophylaxis remain to carry a high risk of VTE compared with non-COVID-19 patients (4). As a result, guidance driven by expert opinions suggested utilizing higher doses of anticoagulation (1). However, this recommendation lacks robust, supporting systematic studies. Thus, we aimed to systematically review the literature and explore the pooled prevalence of VTE, PE, and DVT in critically ill COVID-19 patients. Additionally, we aimed to evaluate the yield of systematic VTE screening and its effect on the prevalence. Moreover, if data allow, we aimed to examine the odds of VTE in patients on prophylactic compared with therapeutic anticoagulation.

This review follows the Preferred Reporting Items for Systematic Reviews and Meta-Analyses (PRISMA) guidelines (5). It is pre-registered at the International Prospective Register of Systematic Reviews (PROSPERO) (registration number: CRD42020185916).

ELIGIBILITY CRITERIA

We limited our review to observational studies (cohort, cross-sectional, retrospective, or case series), estimating the proportion of VTE events in critically ill COVID-19 adult (>18 years) patients (admitted to the ICU). To facilitate a timely review, we limited our inclusion to articles written in the English language only. We excluded studies where the proportion of VTE could not be ascertained or if the population of interest is not ICU patients.

INFORMATION SOURCES AND LITERATURE SEARCH

For a timely review, we performed the search in PubMed, MEDLINE, and EMBASE. We used free text, emtree, and MeSH terms in our search. There were no language or date limitations implied in the search. The last date of the formal search was the 10th of July 2020; however, we performed a scoping search till the 25th of July 2020. Example of a utilized search strategy was [("venous thromboembolism" OR "deep vein thrombosis" OR "lung embolism" OR "vein thrombosis"/exp/mj) AND [embase]/lim] AND [("covid 19" OR (coronavirus AND disease AND 2019) OR (sars AND cov AND 2) OR "covid 19"/exp/mj) AND [embase]/lim]. We also performed relevant citations and reference searches.

SCREENING AND DATA EXTRACTION

Two reviewers (MM and SM) conducted the screening in two stages. The first stage was screening the retrieved articles' titles and abstracts independently. Secondly, the articles' full text was retrieved and assessed for inclusion. When disagreement occurred, a third reviewer (LA) settled the disagreement guided by the protocol. We used pre-made excel sheets to collect relevant articles data. This included the last author name, publication date, study country, sample size, events number (DVT, PE, and VTE), baseline characteristics (median age, gender frequency, average BMI, and other comorbidities), intubation frequency, thromboprophylaxis frequency, and follow-up duration.

STUDY QUALITY AND RISK OF BIAS ASSESSMENT

We used a validated tool for assessing the risk of bias of prevalence studies. The tool was devised by Hoy et al. and is composed of 10 items summarizing four domains (6). We additionally generated funnel plots to examine the risk of publication bias in our review.

DATA ANALYSIS

A scoping review revealed heterogeneity of the method of VTE screening, reporting, and detection. Additionally, there were varying follow-ups given the nature of ICU admitted patients. Hence, neither the true incidence (different follow-up times and some patients may already have the event of interest before the study) nor the true prevalence (varying follow-up times and absence of unifying screening for all individuals at risk) could be accurately pooled. We instead decided a priori to pool a proportion of VTE with a 95% confidence interval (CI). This proportion represents the number of patients with the event of interest divided by the study population at risk during the study regardless of their follow-up duration. We felt that this would be a proxy or an estimate of the prevalence. We used the validated method of double arcsine transformation to stabilize the variance and confine the CI between 0 and 1 (7). We generated forest plots to display the results of the analysis. We used the Cochrane Q test and I^2 to examine heterogeneity. I^2 >60% indicates significant heterogeneity. Regardless of the heterogeneity, we would use the random-effects model (REM) in our analysis. We used MetaXl software for statistical analysis (version 5.3©, EpiGear International Pty Ltd., ABN 51 134 897 411, Sunrise Beach, Queensland, Australia, 2011–2016).

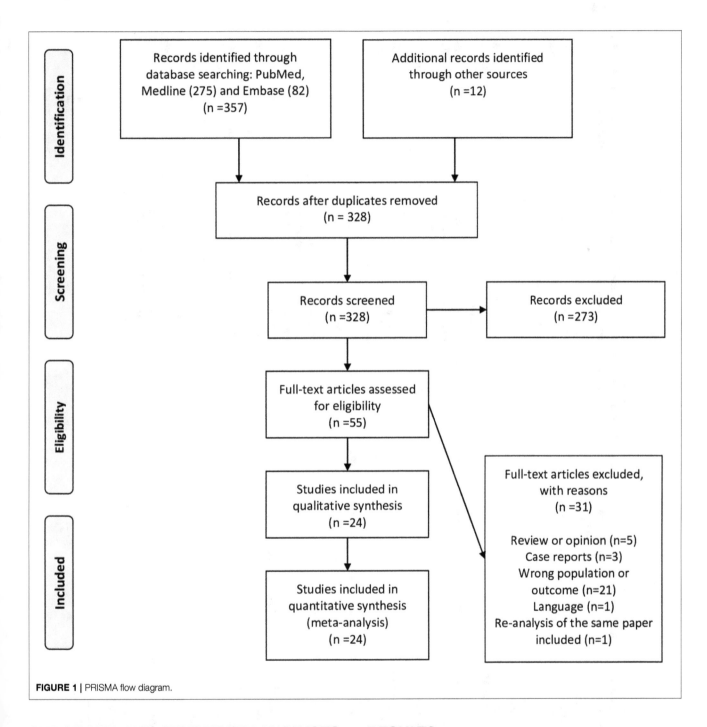

FIGURE 1 | PRISMA flow diagram.

SUBGROUP AND SENSITIVITY ANALYSES

We *a priori* decided to examine the proportion of DVT and PE. Additionally, we looked at the proportion of VTE in various populations (systematic screening vs. non-systematic screening, therapeutic vs. prophylactic anticoagulant dose). Moreover, we performed a sensitivity analysis to reflect the relative constituent studies' impact on the consistency of the pooled proportion of the primary endpoint.

RESULTS

Included Studies and Baseline Characteristics

Twenty-four studies describing a total of 2,570 patients were included in our final analysis (**Figure 1** shows the flow diagram) (4, 8–29). The studies were heterogeneous in terms of VTE events identification and screening (**Table 1**). In 10 studies, the screening for VTE was systematically done using lower and upper limb ultrasound (US) (systematic screening was only for

TABLE 1 | Summary of included studies.

Study (location)	Study design	Study duration in days	Total number	Age, mean, or median (males percentage %)	Intubated %	D-dimers (mean or median)	Pharmacologic prophylaxis %	Screening method	VTE proportion % (numbers)	Mortality %
Al-Samkari et al. (United States) (8)	Retrospective analysis	36 days (March–April 2020)	–	65 (males 64.7%)	–	–	98.6% (12.5% intermediate or full anticoagulation)	Clinical suspicion	10.4% (15/144)	18.8% (27/144)
Beun et al. (Netherlands) (19)	Retrospective analysis	24 days (March–April 2020)	75	–	–	–		Clinical suspicion	30.6% (23/75)	–
Bilaloglu et al. (United States)(23)	Retrospective analysis	48 days (March–April 2020)	829	–	–	–	Most patients (percentage not specified)	Clinical suspicion	13.6% (113/829)	54.4% (451/829)
Criel et al. (Belgium) (24)	Retrospective analysis	24 days (April 2020)	30	64.5 (males 67%)	70%	1,400 ng/ml	100% (intermediate prophylactic dose)	Systematic screening (Doppler US of upper and lower limbs)	13.3% (4/30)	13.3% (4/30)
Cui et al. (China) (25)	Retrospective analysis	53 days (Jan–March 2020)	81	59.9 (males 46%)	–	5,200 ng/ml	0%	Systematic screening (lower limb Doppler US)	24.6% (20/81)	10% (8/81)
Desborough et al. (United Kingdom) (26)	Retrospective analysis	31 days (March 2020)	66	59 (males 73%)	79%	1,200 ng/ml	100% (83% prophylactic, 17% therapeutic)	Clinical suspicion	16.6% (11/66)	30.3% (20/66)
Fraissé et al. (France) (27)	Retrospective analysis	–	92	61 (males 79%)	89%	2,400 ng/ml	100% (47% prophylactic, 53% therapeutic)	Clinical suspicion	33.6% (31/92)	–
Grandmaison et al. (Switzerland) (28)	Retrospective analysis	–	29	66 (males 64.7%)	–	8,760 ng/ml	93% (96% prophylactic, 4% therapeutic)	Systematic screening (Doppler US of upper and lower limbs)	58.6% (17/29)	–
Helms et al. (France) (29)	Retrospective analysis	29 days (March 2020)	150	63 (males 81%)	100%	2,270 ng/ml	100% (70% prophylactic, 30% therapeutic)	Clinical suspicion	18.6% (28/150)	8.70% (13/150)
Hippensteel et al. (United States) (9)	Retrospective analysis	28 days (March–April 2020)	91	55 (males 57%)	85%	1,071 ng/ml	54.3% therapeutic	Clinical suspicion	26.3% (24/91)	22% (22/91)
Klok et al. (Netherlands) (10)	Retrospective analysis	47 days (March–April 2020)	184	64 (males 76%)	–	–	100% (90.8% prophylactic, 9.2% therapeutic)	Clinical suspicion	36.9% (68/184)	22% (41/184)
Llitjos et al. (France) (4)	Retrospective analysis	24 days (March–April 2020)	26	68 (males 77%)	100%	1,750 ng/ml	100% (prophylactic 31%, therapeutic 69%)	Systematic screening (compression and Doppler US)	69.2% (18/26)	12% (3/26)
Lodigiani et al. (Italy) (11)	Retrospective analysis	58 days (February–April 2020)	48	61 (males 80.3%)	–	615 ng/ml	100% (40% weight adjusted or therapeutic)	Clinical suspicion	8.3% (4/48)	–

(Continued)

TABLE 1 | Continued

Study (location)	Study design	Study duration in days	Total number	Age, mean, or median (males percentage %)	Intubated %	D-dimers (mean or median)	Pharmacologic prophylaxis %	Screening method	VTE proportion % (numbers)	Mortality %
Iongchamp et al. (Switzerland) (12)	Retrospective analysis	26 days (March–April 2020)	25	68 (males 64%)	92%	2,071 ng/ml (953–3,606)	100% (prophylactic 23/25, therapeutic 2/25)	Systematic screening (proximal lower extremity DVT)	32% (8/25)	20% (5/25)
Maatman et al. (United States) (13)	Retrospective analysis	20 days (March 2020)	109	61 (males 57%)	94%	84,506 ng/ml	100% (prophylactic 102/109, therapeutic 7/109)	Clinical suspicion	28.4% (31/109)	25% (27/109)
Middeldorp et al. (Netherlands) (14)	Retrospective analysis	42 days (March–April 2020)	75	62 (males 58%)	100%	2,000 ng/ml	100%	Systematic screening (lower limb Doppler every 5 days)	46.6% (35/75)	
Moll et al. (United States) (15)	Retrospective analysis	38 days (March–April 2020)	102	64.61 (males 57.8%)	86.3%	3,964 ng/ml	97.1% (89.8% prophylactic, 10.1% therapeutic)	Clinical suspicion	8.8% (9/102)	27.5% (28/102)
Nahum et al. (France) (16)	Case series	Mid-March–April 2020	34	62.2 (males 78%)	100%	27,927 ng/ml	100% prophylactic anticoagulation	Systematic screening (lower limbs US for all patients)	79.4% (27/34)	Not mentioned
Pineton De Chambrun et al. (France) (17)	Retrospective analysis	26 days (March–April 2020)	25	47.7 (males 68%)	–	Highly elevated (NS)	100% therapeutic	Clinical suspicion	24% (6/25)	–
Poissy et al. (France) (18)	Retrospective analysis	34 days (February–March 2020)	107	57 (males 59%)	62.6%	–	100%	Clinical suspicion	22.4% (24/107)	14% (15/107)
Ren et al. (China) (22)	Cross-sectional	3 days (Feb–March)	48	70 (males 54.2%)	37.5%	3,480 ng/ml	97.9% prophylactic	Systematic screening (proximal and distal lower limbs compression US)	85.4% (41/48)	31.3% (15/48)
Stessel et al. (Belgium) (20)	Quasi-experimental	18 days (March 2020)	46	69.5 (males 73.9%)	–	970 ng/ml	100% Prophylactic standard dose	Systematic screening	41.3% (19/46)	39.13% (18/46)
Stessel et al. (Belgium) (20)	Quasi-experimental	21 days (March–April 2020)	26	62 (males 57.3%)	–	2,180 ng/ml	100% Intensive prophylactic dose	Systematic screening (Doppler US and compression US of the great veins in upper and lower limbs)	15.3% (4/26)	3.85% (1/26)
Thomas et al. (United Kingdom) (21)	Retrospective analysis	33 days (March–April 2020)	63	59 (males 69%)	83%	394 ng/ml	100% (prophylactic dose)	Clinical suspicion	9.5% (6/63)	8% (5/63)
Zhang et al. (China) (22)	Retrospective analysis	32 days (January February 2020)	65	–	–	–	–	Systematic screening (lower limbs US Doppler for DVT at proximal and distal levels)	66.1% (43/65)	–

(–) Refers to data unavailable for the ICU cohort.

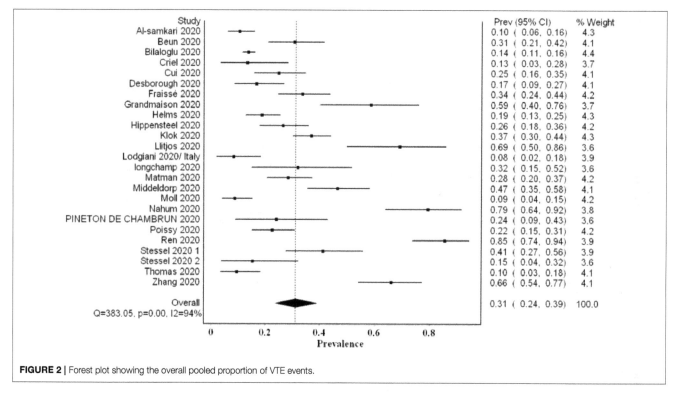

FIGURE 2 | Forest plot showing the overall pooled proportion of VTE events.

DVT and not PE). Fourteen studies evaluated for the presence of VTE based on clinical suspicion and further confirmation by imaging (non-systematic). Twenty-two studies reported the proportion of DVTs, and 17 studies reported the proportion of PE events. Out of the 10 studies where systematic screening was adopted, the screening was incomplete in one. In all studies but one (25), most patients were on thromboprophylaxis with varying doses.

THE PROPORTION OF VTE EVENTS

The overall pooled proportion of VTE from 24 studies examining a total of 2,570 was 0.31 (95% CI 0.24, 0.39; I^2 94%; Q 383) with significant heterogeneity (**Figure 2**). The funnel plot showed significant asymmetry suggestive of possible publication bias (**Supplementary 1**). The sensitivity analysis did not affect the final point estimate significantly (**Supplementary 2**).

THE PROPORTION OF VTE UTILIZING SYSTEMATIC SCREENING

Ten studies examining 478 patients using systematic screening revealed a higher VTE proportion of 0.48 (95% CI 0.33, 0.63; I^2 91%; Q 109) with significant heterogeneity (**Figure 3**). The funnel plot suggested a publication bias (**Supplementary 3**). The exclusion of Cui et al.'s study that did not utilize thromboprophylaxis resulted in a higher proportion of VTE events of 0.51. Additional sensitivity analyses revealed a lower VTE proportion with the exclusion of Ren et al.'s data (0.43); this proportion increased with the exclusion of Criel et al.'s study (0.52) (**Supplementary 4**). All the studies evaluated

systematically for the presence of DVT events only (PE was not a primary aim). Hence, this pooled proportion represents the proportion of DVT events and may underestimate the overall VTE proportion.

THE PROPORTION OF VTE UTILIZING NON-SYSTEMATIC SCREENING

In most studies utilizing non-systematic screening, the authors addressed the high threshold for screening and imaging due to infection control implications. They stated that this might have underestimated the true prevalence. The analysis of 14 studies examining 2,085 patients revealed a pooled proportion of VTE of 0.20 (95% CI 0.15, 0.26; I^2 87%; Q 98.4) (**Figure 4**). The funnel plot suggested a publication bias (**Supplementary 5**). On sensitivity analysis, the final point estimate did not significantly change with the ordered exclusion of the constituent studies (**Supplementary 6**).

THE PROPORTION OF DVT EVENTS

The overall pooled proportion of DVT from 22 studies examining a total of 2,401 was 0.23 (95% CI 0.14, 0.32; I^2 96%; Q 531) with significant heterogeneity (**Figure 5**). The funnel plot suggested a publication bias (**Supplementary 7**), whereas the sensitivity analysis suggested a consistency of the final point estimate with ordered-single-study exclusion (**Supplementary 8**). The pooled proportion of DVT from studies utilizing non-systematic screening was 0.08 (95% CI 0.04, 0.12; I^2 87%; Q 85) (**Supplementary 9**).

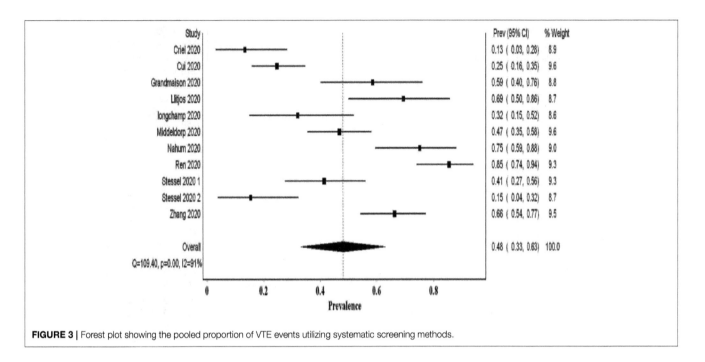

FIGURE 3 | Forest plot showing the pooled proportion of VTE events utilizing systematic screening methods.

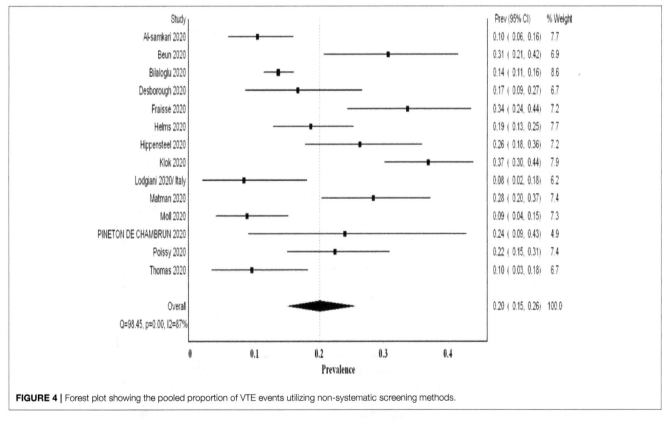

FIGURE 4 | Forest plot showing the pooled proportion of VTE events utilizing non-systematic screening methods.

THE PROPORTION OF PE EVENTS

PE was not screened systematically. The analysis of 2,096 patients (17 studies) revealed a pooled proportion of 0.14 (95% CI 0.09, 0.20; I^2 90%; Q 159) (**Figure 6**). The funnel plot revealed a major asymmetry suggestive of publication bias (**Supplementary 10**). Sensitivity analysis showed consistency of the results upon single-study-ordered exclusion.

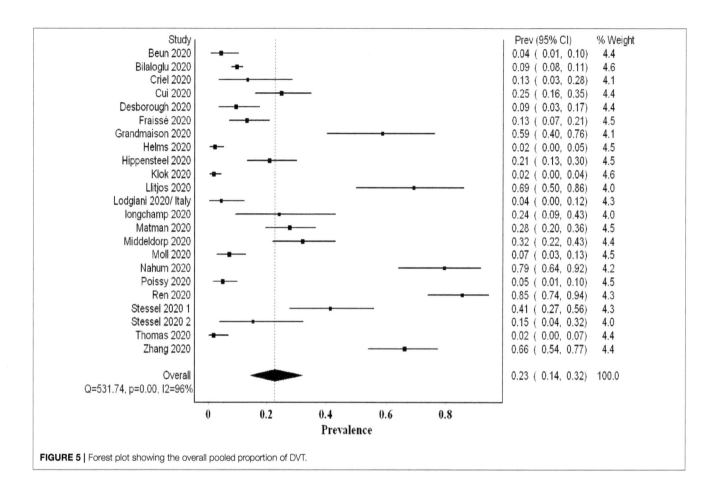

FIGURE 5 | Forest plot showing the overall pooled proportion of DVT.

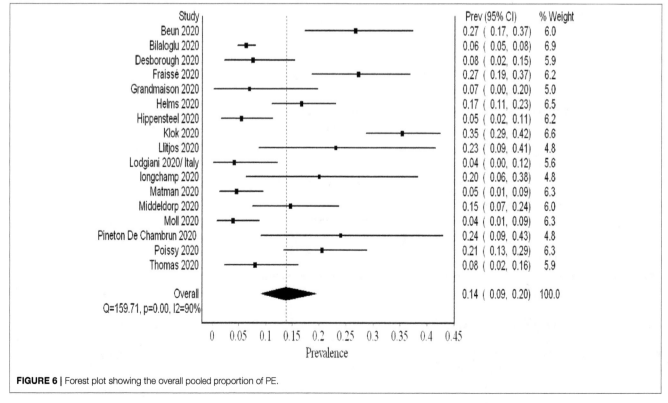

FIGURE 6 | Forest plot showing the overall pooled proportion of PE.

THROMBOPROPHYLAXIS STRATEGY

Six studies reported the number of VTE events in patients receiving prophylactic anticoagulation (479 patients) compared with therapeutic dosages (83 patients). The dosages and definitions varied across these studies. In one study (pre- and post-intervention), a higher prophylactic dosage of nadroparin with adjustment guided by factor X-a activity (labeled as semi-therapeutic) was compared with standard prophylactic dose (4, 14, 20). For synthesis, we considered this adjusted dosage therapeutic and analyzed it in the corresponding arm (due to the paucity of studies). The VTE odds ratio (OR) was increased in the prophylactic anticoagulation group with uncertainty in the final point estimate OR 2.34 (95% CI 0.77, 7.14; I^2 53%; Q 10). Three studies utilized systematic screening; hence, they provided a better estimate of the true VTE prevalence (20). In an exploratory analysis, we analyzed these studies separately, and the results showed significantly increased odds of VTE events with prophylactic dosing OR 5.45 (95% CI 1.90, 15.57; I^2 0%; Q 1.2), and there was no evidence of heterogeneity (**Figure 7**).

QUALITY ASSESSMENT AND RISK OF BIAS ASSESSMENT

Most of the constituent studies had a moderate or unclear risk of bias (**Table 2**). Although the number of included studies is adequate, the funnel plot suggested publication bias (its value is limited in assessing prevalence studies publication bias). There was also reporting bias, as the reporting of distal DVT, PE, and VTE, method of diagnosis, and dosing of chemoprophylaxis varied across studies.

DISCUSSION

Our meta-analysis comprised over 2,500 patients and revealed a high VTE prevalence of 0.31 (95% CI 0.24, 0.39) in critically ill COVID-19 patients. This prevalence increased to 0.48 (95% CI 0.33, 0.63) when systematic screening was utilized, meaning that almost one in two critical COVID-19 patients suffers from VTE. Furthermore, this heightened prevalence of VTE when systematic screening was used did not include PE since it was not part of systematic screening. Hence, screening for PE systematically could have possibly further increased VTE prevalence. Even when non-systematic screening was utilized, VTE prevalence remained high at 0.20 (95% CI 0.15, 0.26). Regarding PE and DVT prevalence, the overall prevalence of DVT (0.23) was higher than that of PE (0.14). This concurs with finding a high prevalence of undiagnosed DVT in an autopsy evaluation of COVID-19 patients (31). Additionally, it may argue against the earlier literature suggesting that PE prevalence was much higher than DVT, proposing that PE events can originate in the lung's vasculature in patients with severe acute respiratory syndrome coronavirus 2 (SARS-CoV-2) infection (32).

Our analysis revealed that approximately 40/100 additional DVTs are detected by systematic screening (0.48) compared with non-systematic screening (0.08). This is likely due to

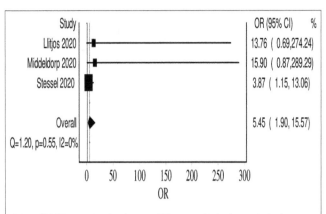

FIGURE 7 | Forest plot showing the VTE event odds in the prophylactic anticoagulation group, compared with therapeutic dosing.

the fact that asymptomatic DVT can be overlooked in non-systematic screening. On the opposite side, PE is more likely to be associated with easily detected signs (sudden deterioration, unexplained tachycardia or sudden changes in the ventilator settings) especially in the context of the ICU.

A recent study by Zhang et al. evaluated the utility of bedside ultrasonography in the diagnosis of DVT. It revealed a significantly higher DVT prevalence in deceased patients than in surviving COVID-19 critically ill patients [94% (33/35) vs. 47% (22/46), $P < 0.001$] (30). Moreover, Wichmann et al. analyzed autopsies of 12 COVID-19 patients. They found that 7 (58%) had undiagnosed VTE, whereas in 4 (33.3%), massive PE was the direct cause of death (31). Based on these data, we understand that the high mortality reported by many studies may actually be attributed to undiagnosed fatal VTE events. Consequently, studies with high mortality will likely underestimate the true VTE prevalence when deceased patients are excluded from screening. We additionally understand the impact of prevention and early identification on patient's morbidity and mortality.

Tang et al. showed that prophylactic dosing of heparin in high-risk COVID-19 patients is associated with significantly lower mortality (33). This led the International Society on Thrombosis and Hemostasis (ISTH) among other societies to recommend a prophylactic dosage of pharmacological anticoagulants (LMWH or fondaparinux) for all hospitalized COVID-19 patients (3, 34). However, it seemed that prophylactic anticoagulation is not sufficient for severe COVID-19 patients. This was concluded in a study by Llitjos et al. where they found a higher prevalence of VTE in patients on a prophylactic dose of anticoagulation (100%) compared with therapeutic anticoagulation (56%) (4). More recently, Stessel et al. attempted the first quasi-experimental trial (pre- and post-intervention) comparing the mortality and incidence of VTE between conventional prophylaxis (once-daily nadroparin calcium 2,850 IU) compared with an individualized semi-therapeutic, prophylactic dosage guided by factor Xa activity (semi-therapeutic dosing). Both mortality (3.8 vs. 39.1%, $P < 0.001$) and VTE (15.3 vs. 41.3%, $P = 0.03$) were significantly lower in the aggressive thromboprophylaxis group (20). Emerging evidence showed that even in COVID-19 patients receiving therapeutic anticoagulation, there is a high incidence

TABLE 2 | Table summarizing the risk of bias assessment.

Study	1	2	3	4	5	6	7	8	9
Al-Samkari et al. (8)	?	+	+	−	−	−	−	−	−
Beun et al. (19)	+	?	+	−	−	+	−	−	−
Bilaloglu et al. (23)	+	+	+	?	−	+	−	−	−
Criel et al. (24)	?	?	−	+	+	?	−	−	−
Cui et al. (25)	?	?	−	?	+	?	+	+	−
Desborough et al. (26)	+	+	+	+	−	+	−	−	−
Fraissé et al. (27)	+	?	−	+	−	+	−	−	−
Grandmaison et al. (28)	+	+	−	+	+	+	+	+	−
Helms et al. (29)	+	+	−	+	−	+	−	−	−
Hippensteel et al. (9)	+	+	−	+	−	+	−	−	−
Klok et al. (10)	+	+	+	+	−	+	−	−	−
Llitjos et al. (4)	+	+	−	+	+	+	+	+	−
Lodigiani et al. (11)	+	+	+	+	−	+	−	−	−
longchamp et al. (12)	?	−	−	−	−	?	+	−	−
Maatman et al. (13)	+	+	−	+	−	+	−	−	−
Middeldorp et al. (14)	+	+	+	+	−	+	−	−	−
Moll et al. (15)	+	+	−	+	+	+	+	+	−
Nahum et al. (16)	+	+	+	+	−	−	−	−	−
Pineton de Chambrun et al. (17)	+	+	+	+	−	−	−	−	−
Poissy et al. (18)	+	+	+	+	−	−	−	−	−
Ren et al. (22)	+	+	+	+	+	+	+	+	−
Stessel et al. (20)	+	+	+	+	?	+	+	+	−
Stessel et al. (20)	+	+	+	+	+	+	+	+	−
Thomas et al. (21)	+	+	−	−	−	+	−	−	−
Zhang et al. (30)	?	+	+	−	?	+	?	+	−

+ , low risk; − , high risk; ? , unclear risk assessment.

(1) Was the study's target population a close representation of the national population in relation to relevant variables, e.g., age, sex, occupation?; (2) was the sampling frame a true or close representation of the target population?; (3) was some form of random selection used to select the sample, OR, was a census undertaken?; (4) was the likelihood of non-response bias minimal?; (5) were data collected directly from the subjects (as opposed to a proxy)?; (6) was an acceptable case definition used in the study?; (7) was the study instrument that measured the parameter of interest (e.g., prevalence of low back pain) shown to have reliability and validity (if necessary)?; (8) was the same mode of data collection used for all subjects?; (9) were the numerator(s) and denominator r(s) for the parameter of interest appropriate?

of heparin resistance and sub-optimal peak in anti-Xa levels (19, 35). This may explain, in part, the high rate of VTE in patients on usual prophylactic doses and even in patients on therapeutic dosing (although relatively at a lower rate).

Our review also aimed to address the uncertainty of using higher vs. standard prophylactic doses. In an exploratory manner,

we limited our analysis to studies that only used systematic screening and thus reduce the chances of missing fatal VTE events; we found that prophylactic dosing was associated with increased odds of VTE compared with therapeutic dosing (one study was counted in the therapeutic side although it used subtherapeutic dosing, due to limited studies) (20). The results were homogenous. The reader should consider that the odds of VTE in the therapeutic arm were lower even in the likely event that those patients may have had VTE predisposing conditions, for which they were initiated on this therapeutic dosing (except Stessel et al.'s study, which was protocolized). This small exploratory unadjusted comparison suggests a value for a higher dosing or therapeutic chemoprophylaxis. Nonetheless, this will be ascertained by a number of ongoing trials aiming to address the efficacy and safety of various chemoprophylactic dosages (prophylactic, intermediates, weight-adjusted, or therapeutic); examples of such trials are IMPROVE (http://www.clinicaltrials.gov, NCT04367831), COVI-DOSE (http://www.clinicaltrials.gov, NCT04373707), and Hep-COVID (https:www.clinicaltrials.gov, NCT04401293). The safety of intensive thromboprophylaxis was not addressed in our review due to data paucity. Nonetheless, two recent observational studies suggested that this intensive thromboprophylaxis is safe in terms of inducing major bleeding events (36, 37). Thus, we believe that the intensive thromboprophylaxis protocol suggested by Stessel et al. seems promising as a chemoprophylaxis regimen until further data from ongoing randomized clinical trials (RCTs) become available (20).

Limitations of our review are the heterogeneity in the pooled prevalence in the constituent studies. This is likely due to varying detection methods (systematic vs. non-systematic, imaging modalities used, timing, etc.), screening threshold (many studies reported that the threshold was high due to infection control concerns), varying severity of illness, prophylaxis strategies, and dosage, missing VTE in deceased patients of fatal VTE events, and varying and insufficient follow-ups. Additionally, the inability to provide a mortality comparison between the VTE group and the non-VTE group due to data paucity (we contacted the primary authors; however, we could not get the data necessary for its computation) and limited conclusion provided by the comparison of VTE in the therapeutic vs. prophylactic anticoagulation groups (small number of studies, absence of adjustment, and varying doses between studies). Moreover, the retrospective nature of the included studies, inability to accurately compute the prevalence of PE (absence of systematic PE screening), and absence of autopsies to ascertain causes of death add to the limitations of our review.

Notwithstanding this, there are many strengths to our review that are worthy of mention. This is the most extensive review examining the prevalence of VTE exclusively in critically ill patients. Additionally, the review examines VTE prevalence based on the utilized screening method providing the readers with a better estimate of VTE prevalence. We also pooled

a proportion that reflects the prevalence; nonetheless, we acknowledged its limited accuracy. Finally, the results of the limited comparison between lower and higher dosing of chemoprophylaxis may help inform therapeutic decisions until further data from RCTs become available.

Future research direction should evaluate the utility of systematic screening and early therapeutic anticoagulation dosage on outcomes (VTE progression, ICU stay, and mortality). The utility of systematic screening with US at regular intervals to ascertain the exact prevalence of VTE is needed. In these studies, patients with distal DVT should be temporally followed up and compared with a non-DVT cohort to determine the incidence of proximal DVT, PE, and mortality events. This will ascertain the exact need for therapy in these patients.

In conclusion, our review of critically ill COVID-19 patients revealed a high prevalence of VTE events. This prevalence is higher when systematic screening is utilized. Our review suggested a potential for higher prophylactic or therapeutic dosages in reducing VTE burden. Data from ongoing RCTs are awaited to further confirm the findings of our review.

AUTHOR CONTRIBUTIONS

MM conceived the idea of the review and formed the team, performed the analysis, constructed the tables and figures, and wrote the initial draft. MM conducted the initial search and with SM conducted the screening. MM, KS, SA-S, SM, SI, MN, and LA extracted the data. The manuscript was then critically reviewed and revised by all the study authors. The final version was approved by all authors for publication.

ACKNOWLEDGMENTS

We acknowledge the editor and the reviewers for the timely review and constructive feedback.

REFERENCES

1. Klok FA, Kruip MJHA, van der Meer NJM, Arbous MS, Gommers DAMPJ, Kant KM, et al. Incidence of thrombotic complications in critically ill ICU patients with COVID-19. *Thromb Res.* (2020) 191:145–7. doi: 10.1016/j.thromres.2020.04.013

2. McFadyen JD, Stevens H, Peter K. The emerging threat of (micro)thrombosis in COVID-19 and its therapeutic implications. *Circ Res.* (2020) 127:571–87. doi: 10.1161/circresaha.120.317447

3. Thachil J, Tang N, Gando S, Falanga A, Cattaneo M, Levi M, et al. ISTH interim guidance on recognition and management of coagulopathy in COVID-19. *J Thromb Haemost.* (2020) 18:1023–6. doi: 10.1111/jth.14810

4. Llitjos JF, Chochois C, Monsallier JM, Ramakers M, Auvray M, Merouani K. High incidence of venous thromboembolic events in anticoagulated severe COVID-19 patients. *J Thromb Haemost.* (2020) 18:1743–6. doi: 10.1111/jth.14869

5. Moher D, Liberati A, Tetzlaff J, Altman DG. Preferred reporting items for systematic reviews and meta-analyses: the

PRISMA statement. *BMJ.* (2009) 339:332–6. doi: 10.1136/bmj. b2535

6. Hoy D, Brooks P, Woolf A, Blyth F, March L, Bain C, et al. Assessing risk of bias in prevalence studies: Modification of an existing tool and evidence of interrater agreement. *J Clin Epidemiol.* (2012) 65:934–9. doi: 10.1016/j.jclinepi.2011.11.014

7. Barendregt JJ, Doi SA, Lee YY, Norman RE, Vos T. Meta-analysis of prevalence. *J Epidemiol Community Health.* (2013) 67:974–8. doi: 10.1136/jech-2013-203104

8. Al-Samkari H, Dzik WH, Carlson JC, Fogerty AE, Waheed A, Goodarzi K, et al. COVID and coagulation: bleeding and thrombotic manifestations of SARS-CoV2 infection. *Blood.* (2020) 136:489–500. doi: 10.1182/blood.2020006520

9. Hippensteel JA, Burnham EL, Jolley SE. Prevalence of venous thromboembolism in critically ill patients with COVID-19. *Br J Haematol.* (2020) 190:e134–7. doi: 10.1111/bjh.16908

10. Kloka FA, Kruipb MJHA, van der Meercd NJM, Arbouse MS, Gommersf D, Kant KM, et al. Confirmation of the high cumulative incidence of thrombotic complications in critically ill ICU patients with COVID-19: An updated analysis. *Thromb Res.* (2020) 191:148–50. doi: 10.1016/j.thromres.2020.04.041

11. Lodigiani C, Iapichino G, Carenzo L, Cecconi M, Ferrazzi P, Sebastian T, et al. Venous and arterial thromboembolic complications in COVID-19 patients admitted to an academic hospital in Milan, Italy. *Thromb Res.* (2020) 191:9–14. doi: 10.1016/j.thromres.2020.04.024

12. Longchamp A, Longchamp J, Manzocchi-Besson S, Whiting L, Haller C, Jeanneret S, et al. Venous thromboembolism in critically ill patients with Covid-19: results of a screening study for deep vein thrombosis. *Res Pr Thromb Haemost.* (2020) 4:842–847. doi: 10.1002/rth2.12376

13. Maatman TK, Feizpour C, Douglas A II, McGuire SP, Kinnaman G, Hartwell JL, et al. Routine venous thromboembolism prophylaxis may be inadequate in the hypercoagulable state of severe coronavirus disease 2019. *Crit Care Med.* (2020) 48:e78–90. doi: 10.1097/CCM.0000000000004466

14. Middeldorp S, Coppens M, van Haaps TF, Foppen M, Vlaar AP, Müller MCA, et al. Incidence of venous thromboembolism in hospitalized patients with COVID-19. *J Thromb Haemost.* (2020) 18:1995–2002. doi: 10.1111/jth.14888

15. Moll M, Zon RL, Sylvester KW, Chen EC, Cheng V, Connell NT, et al. Venous thromboembolism in COVID-19 ICU Patients. *Chest.* (2020) 158:2130–5. doi: 10.1016/j.chest.2020.07.031

16. Nahum J, Morichau-Beauchant T, Daviaud F, Echegut P, Fichet J, Maillet JM, et al. Venous thrombosis among critically ill patients with coronavirus disease 2019 (COVID-19). *JAMA Netw Open.* (2020) 3:e2010478. doi: 10.1001/jamanetworkopen.2020.10478

17. Pineton de Chambrun M, Frere C, Miyara M, Amoura Z, Martin-Toutain I, Mathian A, et al. High frequency of antiphospholipid antibodies in critically-ill COVID-19 patients: a link with hypercoagulability? *J Intern Med.* (2020). doi: 10.1111/joim.13126. [Epub ahead of print].

18. Poissy J, Goutay J, Caplan M, Parmentier E, Duburcq T, Lassalle F, et al. Pulmonary embolism in COVID-19 patients: awareness of an increased prevalence. *Circulation.* (2020) 142:184–6. doi: 10.1161/CIRCULATIONAHA.120.047430

19. Beun R, Kusadasi N, Sikma M, Westerink J, Huisman A. Thromboembolic events and apparent heparin resistance in patients infected with SARS-CoV-2. *Int J Lab Hematol.* (2020) (42 Suppl. 1) (Suppl. 1):19–20. doi: 10.1111/ijlh.13230

20. Stessel B, Vanvuchelen C, Bruckers L, Geebelen L, Callebaut I, Vandenbrande J, et al. impact of implementation of an individualised thromboprophylaxis protocol in critically ill ICU patients with COVID-19: a longitudinal controlled before-after study. *Thromb Res.* (2020) 194:209–15. doi: 10.1016/j.thromres.2020.07.038

21. Thomas W, Varley J, Johnston A, Symington E, Robinson M, Sheares K, et al. Thrombotic complications of patients admitted to intensive care with COVID-19 at a teaching hospital in the United Kingdom. *Thromb Res.* (2020) 191:76–7. doi: 10.1016/j.thromres.2020.04.028

22. Ren B, Yan F, Deng Z, Zhang S, Xiao L, Wu M, et al. Extremely high incidence of lower extremity deep venous thrombosis in 48 patients with severe COVID-19 in Wuhan. *Circulation.* (2020) 142:181–3. doi: 10.1161/CIRCULATIONAHA.120.047407

23. Bilaloglu S, Aphinyanaphongs Y, Jones S, Iturrate E, Hochman J, Berger JS. Thrombosis in hospitalized patients with COVID-19 in a New York City Health System. *J Am Med Assoc.* (2020) 324:799–801. doi: 10.1001/jama.2020.13372

24. Criel M, Falter M, Jaeken J, Van Kerrebroeck M, Lefere I, Meylaerts L, et al. Venous thromboembolism in SARS-CoV-2 patients: only a problem in ventilated ICU patients, or is there more to it? *Eur Respir J.* (2020) 56. doi: 10.1183/13993003.01201-2020

25. Cui S, Chen S, Li X, Liu S, Wang F. Prevalence of venous thromboembolism in patients with severe novel coronavirus pneumonia. *J Thromb Haemost.* (2020) 18:1421–4. doi: 10.1111/jth.14830

26. Desborough MJR, Doyle AJ, Griffiths A, Retter A, Breen KA, Hunt BJ. Image-proven thromboembolism in patients with severe COVID-19 in a tertiary critical care unit in the United Kingdom. *Thromb Res.* (2020) 193:1–4. doi: 10.1016/j.thromres.2020.05.049

27. Fraissé M, Logre E, Pajot O, Mentec H, Plantefève G, Contou D. Thrombotic and hemorrhagic events in critically ill COVID-19 patients: a French monocenter retrospective study. *Crit Care.* (2020) 24:275. doi: 10.1186/s13054-020-03025-y

28. Grandmaison G, Andrey A, Périard D, Engelberger RP, Carrel G, Doll S, et al. Systematic screening for venous thromboembolic events in COVID-19 pneumonia. *TH Open.* (2020) 4:e113–5. doi: 10.1055/s-0040-1713167

29. Helms J, Tacquard C, Severac F, Leonard-Lorant I, Ohana M, Delabranche X, et al. High risk of thrombosis in patients with severe SARS-CoV-2 infection: a multicenter prospective cohort study. *Intensive Care Med.* (2020) 1089–98. doi: 10.1007/s00134-020-06062-x

30. Zhang P, Qu Y, Tu J, Cao W, Hai N, Li S, et al. Applicability of bedside ultrasonography for the diagnosis of deep venous thrombosis in patients with COVID-19 and treatment with low molecular weight heparin. *J Clin Ultrasound.* (2020) 48:522–6. doi: 10.1002/jcu.22898

31. Wichmann D, Sperhake J-P, Lütgehetmann M, Steurer S, Edler C, Heinemann A, et al. Autopsy findings and venous thromboembolism in patients with COVID-19. *Ann Intern Med.* (2020) 173:268–77. doi: 10.7326/m20-2003

32. Spyropoulos AC, Weitz JI. Hospitalized COVID-19 patients and venous thromboembolism: a perfect storm. *Circulation.* (2020) 142:129–32. doi: 10.1161/CIRCULATIONAHA.120.048020

33. Tang N, Bai H, Chen X, Gong J, Li D, Sun Z. Anticoagulant treatment is associated with decreased mortality in severe coronavirus disease 2019 patients with coagulopathy. *J Thromb Haemost.* (2020) 18: 1094–9. doi: 10.1111/jth.14817

34. Marietta M, Ageno W, Artoni A, De Candia E, Gresele P, Marchetti M, et al. COVID-19 and haemostasis: a position paper from Italian Society on Thrombosis and Haemostasis (SISET). *Blood Transfus.* (2020) 18:167–9. doi: 10.2450/2020.0083-20

35. White D, MacDonald S, Bull T, Hayman M, de Monteverde-Robb R, Sapsford D, et al. Heparin resistance in COVID-19 patients in the intensive care unit. *J Thromb Thrombolysis.* (2020) 50:287–91. doi: 10.1007/s11239-020-02145-0

36. Mattioli M, Benfaremo D, Mancini M, Mucci L, Mainquà P, Polenta A, et al. Safety of intermediate dose of low molecular weight heparin in COVID-19 patients. *J Thromb Thrombolysis.* (2020). doi: 10.1007/s11239-020-02243-z. [Epub ahead of print].

37. Kessler C, Stricker H, Demundo D, Elzi L, Monotti R, Bianchi G, et al. Bleeding prevalence in COVID-19 patients receiving intensive antithrombotic prophylaxis. *J Thromb Thrombolysis.* (2020) 50:833–6. doi: 10.1007/s11239-020-02244-y

21

Echocardiographic Characteristics and Outcome in Patients with COVID-19 Infection and Underlying Cardiovascular Disease

Yuman Li [1,2,3†], Lingyun Fang [1,2,3†], Shuangshuang Zhu [1,2,3†], Yuji Xie [1,2,3†], Bin Wang [1,2,3], Lin He [1,2,3], Danqing Zhang [1,2,3], Yongxing Zhang [1,2,3], Hongliang Yuan [1,2,3], Chun Wu [1,2,3], He Li [1,2,3], Wei Sun [1,2,3], Yanting Zhang [1,2,3], Meng Li [1,2,3], Li Cui [1,2,3], Yu Cai [1,2,3], Jing Wang [1,2,3], Yali Yang [1,2,3], Qing Lv [1,2,3], Li Zhang [1,2,3*], Amer M. Johri [4*] and Mingxing Xie [1,2,3*]

[1] Department of Ultrasound, Tongji Medical College, Union Hospital, Huazhong University of Science and Technology, Wuhan, China, [2] Clinical Research Center for Medical Imaging in Hubei Province, Wuhan, China, [3] Hubei Province Key Laboratory of Molecular Imaging, Wuhan, China, [4] Department of Medicine, Queen's University, Kingston, ON, Canada

*Correspondence:
Mingxing Xie
xiemx@hust.edu.cn
Amer M. Johri
amerschedule@gmail.com
Li Zhang
zli429@hust.edu.cn

† These authors have contributed equally to this work

Background: The cardiac manifestations of coronavirus disease 2019 (COVID-19) patients with cardiovascular disease (CVD) remain unclear. We aimed to investigate the prognostic value of echocardiographic parameters in patients with COVID-19 infection and underlying CVD.

Methods: One hundred fifty-seven consecutive hospitalized COVID-19 patients were enrolled. The left ventricular (LV) and right ventricular (RV) structure and function were assessed using bedside echocardiography.

Results: Eighty-nine of the 157 patients (56.7%) had underlying CVD. Compared with patients without CVD, those with CVD had a higher mortality (22.5 vs. 4.4%, $p = 0.002$) and experienced more clinical events including acute respiratory distress syndrome, acute heart injury, or deep vein thrombosis. CVD patients presented with poorer LV diastolic and RV systolic function compared to those without CVD. RV dysfunction (30.3%) was the most frequent, followed by LV diastolic dysfunction (9.0%) and LV systolic dysfunction (5.6%) in CVD patients. CVD patients with high-sensitivity troponin I (hs-TNI) elevation or requiring mechanical ventilation therapy demonstrated worsening RV function compared with those with normal hs-TNI or non-intubated patients, whereas LV systolic or diastolic function was similar. Impaired RV function was associated with elevated hs-TNI level. RV function and elevated hs-TNI level were independent predictors of higher mortality in COVID-19 patients with CVD.

Conclusions: Patients with COVID-19 infection and underlying CVD displayed impaired LV diastolic and RV function, whereas LV systolic function was normal in most patients. Importantly, RV function parameters are predictive of higher mortality.

Keywords: COVID-19, cardiovascular disease, echocardiography, cardiac injury, cardiac function

INTRODUCTION

Coronavirus disease 2019 (COVID-19) caused by the severe acute respiratory syndrome coronavirus 2 (SARS-CoV-2) has become a global pandemic causing an escalating number of cases and fatalities worldwide. A large proportion of COVID-19 patients have comorbidities, with cardiovascular disease (CVD) being the most frequent. It was present in approximately 30–48% of patients (1–3). Patients with CVD are more likely to be infected with SARS-CoV-2 and to develop severe cases. In SARS, the presence of comorbidity increased the risk of death 12-fold (4). Therefore, COVID-19 patients with underlying CVD may suffer from a higher risk of mortality after SARS-CoV-2 infection (3, 5). A recent study revealed that hospitalized COVID-19 patients with concomitant cardiac disease have an exceptionally poor prognosis compared with those without cardiac disease (6). Nevertheless, the detailed features of cardiac function were not yet established in the aforementioned study. In clinical practice, echocardiography is the first-line imaging modality in cardiac assessment and is an indispensable bedside tool, allowing non-invasive quantification of heart performance in COVID-19 patients in isolated wards (7). Currently, there are limited data regarding the cardiac manifestations of COVID-19 patients with CVD. Therefore, we aimed to investigate the echocardiographic characteristics and explore the prognostic value of echocardiographic parameters in COVID-19 patients with CVD.

METHODS

Study Population

This observational study was performed at the west branch of Union Hospital, Tongji Medical College, Huazhong University of Science and Technology of Wuhan, China, which was a designated hospital to treat patients with COVID-19. We enrolled a total of 157 consecutive adult patients who were confirmed to have COVID-19 infection according to the WHO interim guidance from February 12, 2020 to March 16, 2020 (8). Bedside echocardiography was performed in all patients from three wards managed by the investigators for evaluation of cardiac function. The study was approved by Union Hospital Tongji Medical College, Huazhong University of Science and Technology Ethics Committee (KY-2020-02.06). Written informed consent was waived for all participants with emerging infectious diseases as per the Ethics Committee.

Data Collection and Definitions

Epidemiological, medical history, comorbidities, laboratory, treatment, and outcomes data were collected from electronic medical records. The data were analyzed by a trained team of physicians. The timing of laboratory measurements was within 3 days of echocardiographic examination with a mean interval of 1 day [interquartile range (IQR), 1–2]. The median time from admission to echocardiographic examination was 7 days (IQR, 3–11). Clinical outcomes (death or discharge) were monitored through to April 7th, 2020.

Underlying CVD included a history of hypertension, coronary artery disease, heart failure, cardiomyopathy, and arrhythmia.

Acute cardiac injury was defined as serum levels of cardiac high-sensitivity troponin I (hs-TNI) above the 99th percentile upper reference limit.

Echocardiography

Bedside echocardiography examinations were performed with an EPIQ 7C machine (Philips Medical Systems, Andover, MA, USA) at the designated COVID-19 isolation wards or intensive care units (ICU). Two-dimensional and Doppler echocardiography were performed in standard views according to the American Society of Echocardiography (ASE) guidelines (9). All scans were conducted by trained individuals in full personal protective equipment (PPE) (B.W., L.H., D.Z., Y.Z., H.Y., C.W., and H.L.). Personal protection at the time of echocardiographic assessment included wearing protective clothing, double gloving, shoe covers, head covers, N95 respirator masks, goggles, face shields. All images were stored in the ultrasound machine. At the end of the day, images were copied to hard disk and saved in Digital Imaging for subsequent offline analysis to reduce exposure contamination. Echocardiographic image readers (S.Z., W.S., Y.C., and L.C.) were blinded to epidemiological, clinical, laboratory, treatment, and outcomes findings.

Left Heart Assessment

Left ventricular (LV) ejection fraction (LVEF) and volumes were calculated using Simpson's biplane method. LV mass was calculated according to Devereux's formula. LV diastolic function was estimated using the ratio of early transmitral flow velocity (E) to the late transmitral flow velocity (A) and the ratio of transmitral E to the early diastolic LV septal tissue velocity (e′). LV systolic dysfunction was defined as a LVEF <50%, and LV diastolic dysfunction was determined according to the published guideline of the American Society of Echocardiography (ASE) and the European Association of Cardiovascular Imaging (EACVI) (10).

Right Heart Evaluation

RV function was assessed by tricuspid annular plane systolic excursion (TAPSE), fractional area change (FAC), peak systolic velocity (S′) of the tricuspid lateral annulus, and myocardial performance index (MPI) (9). RV dysfunction was defined as the aforementioned parameters measured to be lower than the published reference values (9). Representative examples of RVFAC and TAPSE measurements from COVID-19 patients without and with CVD are shown in **Figure 1**. The degree of tricuspid regurgitation (TR) was defined as moderate, moderate to severe, or severe TR. Pulmonary artery systolic pressure (PASP) was estimated according to published guidelines (9).

Statistical Analysis

Continuous numeric variables are expressed as mean ± SD or medians (interquartile range), and categorical variables are expressed as frequency (percentage). Continuous variables were compared using a two-sample t-test or Mann–Whitney test. Categorical variables were compared using the χ^2-test or Fisher's exact test. Correlations between echocardiographic and biomarker parameters were examined using Spearman's correlation coefficient. Receiver operator characteristic (ROC)

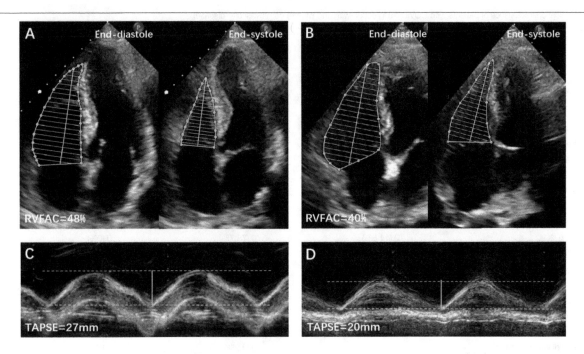

FIGURE 1 | Representative examples of RVFAC and TAPSE measurements from COVID-19 Patients without and with CVD. **(A)** RVFAC in COVID-19 patient without CVD. **(B)** RVFAC in COVID-19 patient with CVD. **(C)** TAPSE in COVID-19 patient without CVD. **(D)** TAPSE in COVID-19 patient with CVD. CVD, cardiovascular disease; RVFAC, right ventricular fractional area change; TAPSE, tricuspid annular plane systolic excursion.

curves were used to evaluate the optimal cutoff value (maximum Youden index) of LV and RV function parameters for detecting poor outcome. Survival curves were plotted using the Kaplan–Meier analysis and compared using the log-rank test. To investigate the risk factors associated with in-hospital death, univariate and multivariate Cox regression models were used. All potential explanatory variables entered into univariate analyses, including age, sex, laboratory findings, LV and RV echocardiographic parameters, and comorbidities. Variables with $p < 0.05$ in univariate Cox proportional hazard regression were included in the multivariate model. To assess the additional prognostic value of echocardiographic parameters over other clinical variables, likelihood ratio tests were performed, and Akaike information criterion (AIC) and Harrell's C statistic were calculated. All statistical analyses were performed using SPSS version 24.0 (SPSS Inc., Chicago, Illinois) and R version 3.6.3 (R Foundation for Statistical Computing, Vienna, Austria). Statistical charts were generated using Prism 7 (GraphPad) and Minitab (Version 18). A two-sided $p < 0.05$ was considered as statistically significant.

RESULTS

Clinical and Echocardiographic Characteristics in Patients With COVID-19 and CVD

Clinical characteristics of patients with COVID-19 with and without CVD are shown in **Table 1**. Among the 157 hospitalized patients with COVID-19, 134 (85.4%) patients were discharged and 23 (14.6%) patients died. The mean age was 62 ± 13 years, and 79 (50.3%) were men. Eighty-nine (56.7%) patients had underlying CVD. Among the CVD patients, hypertension, coronary artery disease, heart failure, and arrhythmia were present in 78.7, 29.2, 4.5, and 6.7% of the patients, respectively. Compared with patients without CVD, those with pre-existing CVD were older, and a higher proportion were men (42.7% female). Patients with underlying CVD were more likely to have a higher systolic arterial pressure, lower level of lymphocyte count and partial pressure of arterial oxygen to percentage of inspired oxygen ratio (PaO_2: FIO_2), higher levels of serum hs-TNI and B-type natriuretic peptide (BNP), more treatment with antibiotic, high-flow oxygen and mechanical ventilation, higher rate of ICU admissions, and higher incidence of acute respiratory distress syndrome (ARDS), acute heart injury, and deep vein thrombosis (DVT). Mortality was significantly higher in CVD compared with non-CVD patients (22.5 vs. 4.4%, $p = 0.002$).

Echocardiographic characteristics of COVID-19 patients with and without CVD are depicted in **Table 2**. Compared with patients without CVD, those with CVD had impaired LV diastolic and RV function and a higher PASP. No differences were identified in LV wall thickness and mass, LV volumes, LVEF, and mitral regurgitation (MR) or TR severity. The most frequent cardiac abnormality in CVD patients was RV dysfunction (27/89, 30.3%), followed by LV diastolic dysfunction (8/89, 9.0%) and LV systolic dysfunction (5/89, 5.6%).

At the time of echocardiographic examination, 27 (30%) COVID-19 patients with CVD were treated with

TABLE 1 | Clinical characteristics of patients with COVID-19 infection with and without cardiovascular disease.

Variables	All patients (*n* = 157)	With CVD (*n* = 89)	Without CVD (*n* = 68)	*P*-value
Clinical characteristic				
Age, years	62 ± 13	66 ± 11	58 ± 14	<0.001
Male, *n* (%)	79 (50.3%)	51 (57.3%)	28 (41.2%)	0.045
Body mass index, kg/m^2	24.1 ± 3.1	24.0 ± 3.0	24.3 ± 3.1	0.445
Heart rate, beats/min	90 ± 17	89 ± 16	92 ± 17	0.164
Respiratory rate, breaths/min	25 ± 6	25 ± 6	25 ± 6	0.780
Systolic arterial pressure, mm Hg	133 ± 81	138 ± 17	126 ± 17	<0.001
Diastolic arterial pressure, mm Hg	81 ± 12	82 ± 13	80 ± 10	0.096
Smoker, *n* (%)	17 (10.8%)	11 (12.4%)	6 (8.8%)	0.480
Comorbidities				
Hypertension, *n* (%)	70 (44.6%)	70 (78.7%)	0 (0%)	<0.001
Diabetes, *n* (%)	23 (14.6%)	17 (19.1%)	6 (8.8%)	0.071
Obesity, *n* (%)	24 (15.3%)	15 (16.9%)	9 (13.2%)	0.532
COPD, *n* (%)	9 (5.7%)	6 (6.7%)	3 (4.4%)	0.534
Coronary artery disease, *n* (%)	26 (16.6%)	26 (29.2%)	0 (0%)	<0.001
Heart failure, *n* (%)	4 (2.5%)	4 (4.5%)	0 (0%)	0.077
Arrhythmia, *n* (%)	6 (3.8%)	6 (6.7%)	0 (0%)	0.029
Chronic kidney disease, *n* (%)	3 (1.9%)	2 (2.2%)	1 (1.5%)	0.725
Chronic liver disease, *n* (%)	6 (3.8%)	2 (2.2%)	4 (5.8%)	0.234
Malignancy, *n* (%)	11 (7.0%)	3 (3.4%)	8 (11.8%)	0.041
Laboratory findings				
Lymphocyte count, ×10^9/L	1.0 (0.6, 1.4)	0.9 (0.5, 1.2)	1.0 (0.7, 1.5)	0.012
D-dimer, mg/L	1.1 (0.4, 2.7)	1.5 (0.4, 2.4)	1.0 (0.5, 4.2)	0.295
PT, s	13.5 (12.5, 15.0)	13.4 (12.6, 15.2)	13.7 (12.5, 14.5)	0.99
APTT, s	37.4 (33.3, 44.6)	38.0 (33.1, 45.6)	37.0 (33.7, 42.2)	0.555
CK-MB, U/L	11 (8, 18)	12 (8, 25)	10 (8, 13)	0.05
hs-TNI, ng/L	4.8 (2.2, 31.2)	10.6 (3.3, 53.7)	2.7 (1.7, 7)	0.043
BNP, pg/ml	79.1 (35.7, 163.9)	85.3 (34.6, 162.5)	57.9 (38.7, 153.2)	0.049
CRP, mg/L	26.5 (3.7, 67.6)	27.5 (7.1, 75.4)	25.3 (2.8, 63.2)	0.44
PCT, ng/ml	0.08 (0.05, 0.20)	0.10 (0.05, 0.20)	0.07 (0.05, 0.21)	0.244
IL-6, pg/ml	5.2 (2.4, 20.7)	8.9 (3.5, 21.6)	4.6 (2.5, 21.7)	0.269
PaO$_2$:FIO$_2$, mmHg	232.0 (151.0, 268.97)	212.1 (140.6, 241.5)	254.0 (212.1, 330.5)	0.016
Treatments				
Antiviral therapy, *n* (%)	150 (95.5%)	86 (96.6%)	64 (94.1%)	0.45
Antibiotic therapy, *n* (%)	119 (75.8%)	73 (82.0%)	46 (67.6%)	0.037
Glucocorticoid therapy, *n* (%)	65 (41.4%)	36 (40.4%)	29 (42.6%)	0.782
Intravenous immune globulin, *n* (%)	56 (35.9%)	37 (41.6%)	19 (27.9%)	0.089
Anticoagulant therapy, *n* (%)	81 (51.6%)	52 (58.4%)	29 (42.6%)	0.05
Diuretics, *n* (%)	39 (24.8%)	32 (36.0%)	7 (10.3%)	<0.001
Beta-blockers, *n* (%)	33 (21.0%)	28 (31.5%)	5 (7.4%)	<0.001
Calcium channel blockers, *n* (%)	48 (30.6%)	43 (48.3%)	5 (7.4%)	<0.001
ACE-I/ARB, *n* (%)	17 (10.8%)	15 (16.9%)	2 (2.9%)	0.005
Oxygen therapy, *n* (%)	139 (88.5%)	83 (93.3%)	56 (82.3%)	0.034
High-flow oxygen, *n* (%)	90 (57.3%)	61 (68.5%)	29 (42.6%)	0.001
Mechanical ventilation, *n* (%)	37 (23.6%)	27 (30.3%)	10 (14.7%)	0.022
IMV, *n* (%)	26 (16.6%)	19 (21.3%)	7 (10.3%)	0.065
NIMV, *n* (%)	11 (7.0%)	8 (9.0%)	3 (4.4%)	0.266
ICU admission, *n* (%)	27 (17.2%)	20 (22.5%)	7 (10.3%)	0.045
Complications				
Acute kidney injury, *n* (%)	20 (12.8%)	12 (13.5%)	8 (11.8%)	0.775

(Continued)

TABLE 1 | Continued

Variables	All patients (n = 157)	With CVD (n = 89)	Without CVD (n = 68)	P-value
ARDS, n (%)	64 (40.8%)	47 (52.8%)	17 (25.0%)	<0.001
Acute heart injury, n (%)	48 (20.6%)	35 (39.3%)	13 (19.1%)	0.006
Coagulation dysfunction, n (%)	29 (18.5%)	19 (21.3%)	10 (14.7%)	0.288
DVT, n (%)	63 (40.1%)	42 (47.2%)	21 (30.9%)	0.039
Shock, n (%)	1 (0.6%)	1 (1.1%)	0 (0%)	0.567
Prognosis				
Discharge, n (%)	134 (85.4%)	69 (77.5%)	65 (95.6%)	0.002
Death, n (%)	23 (14.6%)	20 (22.5%)	3 (4.4%)	0.002

Values are mean ± SD, n (%), median (interquartile range).
ACE-I, angiotensin-converting enzyme inhibitors; APTT, activated partial thromboplastin time; ARB, angiotensin II receptor blockers; ARDS, acute respiratory distress syndrome; BNP, B-type natriuretic peptide; CK-MB, creatine kinase muscle–brain; COVID-19, coronavirus disease 2019; COPD, chronic obstructive pulmonary disease; CRP, C-reactive protein; CVD, cardiovascular disease; DVT, deep vein thrombosis; FIO_2, fraction of inspiration oxygen; HF, heart failure; hs-TNI, high-sensitivity troponin I; ICU, intensive care unit; IL-6, interleukin-6; IMV, invasive mechanical ventilation; NIMV, non-invasive mechanical ventilation; PCT, procalcitonin; PT, prothrombin time; PaO_2, partial pressure of oxygen.

TABLE 2 | Echocardiographic characteristics of patients with COVID-19 with and without cardiovascular disease.

Variables	All patients (n = 157)	With CVD (n = 89)	Without CVD (n = 68)	P-value
Left heart				
LA dimension, mm	35.4 ± 5.5	36.7 ± 5.9	33.3 ± 4.3	< 0.001
LV dimension, mm	45.7 ± 5.1	45.7 ± 5.0	45.7 ± 5.2	0.967
IVS, mm	9.6 ± 1.2	9.7 ± 1.3	9.5 ± 1.0	0.125
PW, mm	9.1 ± 1.3	9.2 ± 1.4	8.9 ± 1.2	0.291
LVMI, g/m²	86.9 ± 21.0	88.4 ± 23.4	84.7 ± 16.9	0.331
Mitral DT, ms	203 ± 55	206 ± 53	200 ± 58	0.561
Mitral E/A	0.91 ± 0.36	0.88 ± 0.33	0.96 ± 0.39	0.473
Mitral E/e′	9.2 ± 3.2	9.7 ± 3.4	8.5 ± 2.8	0.043
LVEDVI, ml/m²	51.3 (43.8, 62.5)	53.5 (43.0, 64.7)	50.7 (44.0, 58.0)	0.173
LVESVI, ml/m²	19.3 (15.6, 25.7)	21.7 (15.6, 28.1)	18.6 (15.6, 23.8)	0.085
LVEF, %	63.4 ± 7.0	62.5 ± 8.3	64.7 ± 4.7	0.063
Moderate-severe MR, n (%)	6 (3.9%)	5 (5.6%)	1 (1.5%)	0.179
Right heart				
RA dimension, mm	35.8 ± 5.0	36.6 ± 5.3	34.9 ± 4.4	0.042
RV dimension, mm	34.6 ± 5.5	34.9 ± 5.6	34.2 ± 5.3	0.390
Tricuspid E/A	0.96 ± 0.29	0.92 ± 0.29	1.0 ± 0.29	0.134
Tricuspid E/e′	5.5 ± 1.8	5.7 ± 1.7	5.2 ± 2.0	0.577
TAPSE, mm	22.2 ± 3.8	21.5 ± 3.7	23.2 ± 3.9	0.007
RV FAC, %	47.5 ± 6.8	46.0 ± 5.3	49.3 ± 7.3	0.009
S′, cm/s	13.5 ± 3.2	13.4 ± 3.1	13.5 ± 3.4	0.946
RV MPI	0.46 ± 0.14	0.48 ± 0.16	0.43 ± 0.10	0.011
Moderate-severe TR, n (%)	6 (3.9%)	5 (5.6%)	1 (1.5%)	0.179
PASP, mmHg	32 (24, 47)	42 (27, 50)	28 (24, 39)	0.033

Values are mean ± SD, n (%), median (interquartile range). COVID-19, coronavirus disease 2019; CVD, cardiovascular disease; DT, deceleration time; IVS, interventricular septum; LA, left atrium; LV, left ventricular; LVEDVI, left ventricular end diastolic volume index; LVESVI, left ventricular end systolic volume index; LVEF, left ventricular ejection fraction; LVM, left ventricular mass; MR, mitral regurgitation; RA, right atrium; RV, right ventricular; TAPSE, tricuspid annular plane systolic excursion; RV FAC, RV fractional area change; RV MPI, RV myocardial performance index; TR, tricuspid regurgitation; PASP, pulmonary artery systolic pressure; PW, posterior wall of left ventricle.

mechanical ventilation. These mechanically ventilated patients had decreased TAPSE and RVFAC and higher PASP, suggesting impaired RV function (**Supplementary Table 1**).

In contrast, LV systolic or diastolic function was not different between patients with and without mechanical ventilation therapy.

Biomarker Levels and Echocardiography in COVID-19 Patients With CVD

Echocardiographic findings in COVID-19 patients with CVD stratified by hs-TNI level are shown in **Table 3**. Patients with high hs-TNI levels had worse RV function, as evidenced by lower TAPSE and RVFAC, and higher MPI, whereas LV diastolic or systolic function did not differ between patients with and without hs-TNI elevation. Correlations of hs-TNI level with LV and RV parameters are displayed in **Supplementary Table 2**. hs-TNI level negatively correlated with tricuspid E/A, TAPSE, and RVFAC and positively correlated with LA and right heart dimension, mitral E/e', and RVMPI.

Clinical and Echocardiographic Characteristics of Survivors and Non-survivors Among CVD Patients

Clinical characteristics of survivors and non-survivors among CVD patients are presented in **Supplementary Table 3**. Compared with CVD patients who were alive, those who died were more likely to have been male and have a lower lymphocyte count, higher levels of biomarkers, more likely to be treated with

TABLE 3 | Clinical and echocardiographic characteristics of COVID-19 patients with CVD stratified by hs-TNI level.

Variables	Normal hs-TNI (*N* = 58)	Elevated hs-TNI (*N* = 31)	*P*-value
Age, years	65 ± 11	68 ± 10	0.185
Male, *n* (%)	27 (46.6%)	24 (77.4%)	0.003
Body mass index, kg/m2	23.8 ± 2.9	24.2 ± 3.3	0.629
Heart rate, beats/min	88 ± 17	91 ± 15	0.426
Respiratory rate, times/min	25 ± 6	25 ± 7	0.637
Systolic arterial pressure, mm Hg	139 ± 18	134 ± 16	0.216
Diastolic arterial pressure, mm Hg	83 ± 13	80 ± 13	0.236
CK-MB, U/L	10 (7, 14)	22 (13, 33)	0.072
BNP, pg/ml	53.2 (26.6, 111.8)	138.6 (86.9, 279)	0.062
CRP, mg/L	16.2 (4.2, 16.2)	62.9 (22.7, 124.5)	0.002
PCT, ng/ml	0.07 (0.05, 0.11)	0.21 (0.08, 0.40)	0.003
IL-6, pg/ml	4.5 (3.0, 14.8)	14 (10.5, 71)	0.126
D-dimer, mg/L	0.9 (0.3, 2.1)	1.7 (0.9, 3.0)	0.262
Left heart			
LA dimension, mm	35.7 ± 5.2	38.6 ± 6.5	0.029
LV dimension, mm	45.7 ± 4.9	45.8 ± 5.3	0.913
IVS, mm	9.8 ± 1.2	9.7 ± 1.5	0.653
PW, mm	9.0 ± 1.4	9.4 ± 1.3	0.206
LVMI, g/m^2	87.4 ± 20.5	90.2 ± 28.3	0.628
Mitral E/A	0.82 ± 0.29	0.97 ± 0.38	0.050
Mitral E/e'	9.1 ± 3.0	10.5 ± 3.9	0.084
LVEDVI, ml/m^2	53.0 (42.1, 68.8)	53.5 (45.5, 62.5)	0.079
LVESVI, ml/m^2	21.6 (16.0, 31.1)	23.4 (15.0, 25.3)	0.061
LVEF, %	61.6 ± 8.9	64.2 ± 6.8	0.203
Right heart			
RA dimension, mm	35.6 ± 4.6	38.1 ± 6.1	0.038
RV dimension, mm	34.2 ± 5.3	36.1 ± 6.0	0.134
Tricuspid E/A	0.92 ± 0.30	0.92 ± 0.30	0.985
Tricuspid E/e'	4.8 ± 2.2	5.5 ± 2.4	0.147
TAPSE, mm	22.2 ± 3.7	20.1 ± 3.3	0.013
RVFAC, %	47.2 ± 6.1	43.6 ± 5.0	0.020
S', cm/s	13.5 ± 3.3	13.4 ± 2.8	0.855
RV MPI	0.45 ± 0.14	0.54 ± 0.17	0.018
PASP, mmHg	32 (26, 40)	47 (34, 56)	0.009

Data are mean ± SD, n (%), median (IQR). hs-TNI elevation was defined as higher than 26.5 ng/L.
SD, standard deviation; IQR, interquartile range. BNP, B-type natriuretic peptide; CK-MB, creatine kinase muscle-brain; CRP, C-reactive protein; hs-TNI, high-sensitivity troponin I; IL-6, interleukin-6; PCT, procalcitonin; COVID-19, coronavirus disease 2019; CVD, cardiovascular disease; IVS, interventricular septum; LA, left atrium; LV, left ventricular; LVEDVI, left ventricular end diastolic volume index; LVEF, left ventricular ejection fraction; LVESVI, left ventricular end systolic volume index; LVM, left ventricular mass; MPI, myocardial performance index; PW, posterior wall of left ventricle; RA, right atrium; RV, right ventricular; RVFAC, right ventricular fractional area change; RV MPI, RV myocardial performance index; TAPSE, tricuspid annular plane systolic excursion; PASP, pulmonary artery systolic pressure.

glucocorticoids, intravenous immune globulins, anticoagulants, diuretics, high-flow oxygen, and mechanical ventilation, and had a higher rate of admission to the ICU. Among the complications, acute kidney injury, acute heart injury, ARDS, coagulation dysfunction, and DVT were more common in non-survivors than survivor.

Echocardiographic characteristics of survivors and non-survivors among CVD patients are depicted in **Table 4**. Compared with survivors, non-survivors had enlarged left atrial size, lower RV function, and higher PASP, while LV systolic or diastolic function was similar between survivors and non-survivors. Of these non-survivors, 12/20 (60%) patients had RV dysfunction, while only 1/20 (5%) had LV diastolic dysfunction.

Predictors of Mortality in COVID-19 Patients With CVD

LV and RV function parameters were studied by a receiver operating characteristic (ROC) analysis to evaluate the probability of mortality. RV functional indices were associated with a higher risk of mortality in COVID-19 patients with CVD (**Figure 2**). Area under the curve was 0.74 for RVFAC and 0.81 for TAPSE.

Kaplan–Meier survival curves for mortality are displayed **Figures 3A,B**. When stratified by cutoff values, RVFAC <44.3% or TAPSE <18.6 mm was associated with higher mortality ($p < 0.001$). To determine the relationship between levels of hs-TNI, RV function parameters, and mortality, a contour plot was performed. Our findings revealed that decreased RV function was associated with increased mortality, which was pronounced in patients with higher levels of hs-TNI (**Figures 3C,D**).

In univariate and multivariate Cox analysis, higher level of hs-TNI, TAPSE, and RVFAC were independent predictors of higher risk of mortality (**Figures 4, 5**). To determine the incremental prognostic value of TAPSE over RVFAC and clinical variables in COVID-19 patients with CVD, a likelihood ratio test was performed. **Figure 6** compares the additional chi-square statistic value of TAPSE and RVFAC to increase predictive value for mortality. After the addition of RVFAC to the baseline model, an increase in the chi-square value was observed (chi-square difference = 4.9; $p = 0.027$). After the addition of TAPSE to the baseline model, an increased chi-square value was noted (chi-square difference = 10.4; $p = 0.001$). The incremental chi-square value of TAPSE was higher than that of RVFAC, demonstrating the additional prognostic value of TAPSE in COVID-19 patients

TABLE 4 | Echocardiographic characteristics of COVID-19 patients with CVD stratified by vital status.

	With CVD (*n* = 89)	Survivors (*n* = 69)	Non-survivors (*n* = 20)	*P*-value
Left heart				
LA dimension, mm	36.7 ± 5.9	36.2 ± 6.2	38.3 ± 4.3	0.035
LV dimension, mm	45.7 ± 5.0	46.0 ± 5.1	44.9 ± 4.6	0.460
IVS, mm	9.7 ± 1.3	9.9 ± 1.3	9.4 ± 1.3	0.230
PW, mm	9.2 ± 1.4	9.1 ± 1.4	9.3 ± 1.2	0.853
LVMI, g/m²	88.4 ± 23.4	90.8 ± 24.6	80.4 ± 17.4	0.141
Mitral DT	206 ± 53	210 ± 54	187 ± 45	0.142
Mitral E/A	0.88 ± 0.33	0.80 (0.67, 1.00)	0.72 (0.67, 0.80)	0.110
Mitral E/e'	9.7 ± 3.4	9.7 ± 3.5	9.7 ± 3.0	0.713
LVEDVI, ml/m²	53.5 (43.0, 64.7)	52.4 (40.3, 67.2)	53.6 (46.4, 59.4)	0.257
LVESVI, ml/m²	21.7 (15.6, 28.1)	20.9 (15.8, 28.1)	23.4 (14.6, 29.8)	0.505
LVEF, %	62.5 ± 8.3	61.7 ± 8.6	65.4 ± 6.6	0.083
Moderate-severe MR, *n* (%)	5 (5.6%)	2 (2.8%)	3 (15%)	0.073
Right heart				
RA dimension, mm	36.6 ± 5.3	36.0 ± 5.1	38.1 ± 5.8	0.136
RV dimension, mm	34.9 ± 5.6	33.4 ± 5.1	36.7 ± 6.7	0.198
Tricuspid E/A	0.92 ± 0.29	1.0 ± 0.33	1.06 ± 0.24	0.502
Tricuspid E/e'	5.7 ± 1.7	5.9 ± 2.0	5.4 ± 1.3	0.618
TAPSE, mm	21.5 ± 3.7	22.2 ± 3.5	19.1 ± 3.1	0.002
RV FAC, %	46.0 ± 5.3	47.2 ± 5.6	41.6 ± 5.5	0.001
S', cm/s	13.4 ± 3.1	13.6 ± 3.3	12.9 ± 2.7	0.340
RV MPI	0.48 ± 0.16	0.46 ± 0.15	0.54 ± 0.19	0.045
Moderate-severe TR, *n* (%)	5 (5.6%)	3 (4.3%)	2 (10%)	0.313
PASP, mmHg	42 (27, 50)	33 (27, 43)	48 (34, 59)	0.042

Values are mean ± SD, n (%), median (interquartile range).
COVID-19, coronavirus disease 2019; DT, deceleration time; IVS, interventricular septum; LA, left atrium; LV, left ventricular; LVEDVI, left ventricular end diastolic volume index; LVESVI, left ventricular end systolic volume index; LVEF, left ventricular ejection fraction; LVM, left ventricular mass; MR, mitral regurgitation; RA, right atrium; RV, right ventricular; TAPSE, tricuspid annular plane systolic excursion; RV FAC, RV fractional area change; RV MPI, RV myocardial performance index; TR, tricuspid regurgitation; PASP, pulmonary artery systolic pressure; PW, posterior wall of left ventricle.

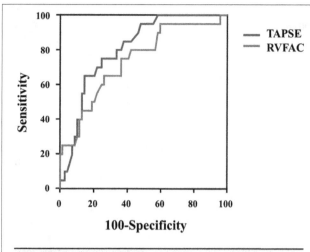

Variables	AUC	95%CI	Sensitivity	Specificity	P-value
RVFAC	0.74	0.64–0.83	65%	74%	<0.001
TAPSE	0.81	0.71–0.88	65%	86%	<0.001

FIGURE 2 | Receiver operating characteristic curves of RVFAC and TAPSE for adverse clinical outcome. RVFAC, right ventricular fractional area change; TAPSE, tricuspid annular plane systolic excursion.

with CVD. Moreover, the model with TAPSE (AIC = 129, C index = 0.86) was the best in predicting mortality compared with those with RVFAC (AIC = 137, C index = 0.84), and baseline model (AIC = 138, C index = 0.81).

DISCUSSION

To the best of our knowledge, this may be the first study describing the echocardiographic features and its prognostic value in patients with COVID-19 and CVD. COVID-19 patients with CVD displayed poorer LV diastolic and RV function than non-CVD patients. The most common cardiac abnormality in CVD patients was RV dysfunction, followed by LV diastolic dysfunction and LV systolic dysfunction. Furthermore, diminished RV function was associated with higher mortality in CVD patients, suggesting that RV measurements may be important for detecting COVID-19 patients with CVD who are at higher risk of mortality.

COVID-19 Patients With CVD and Cardiac Injury

Consistent with a previous study, we found that COVID-19 patients with CVD had a significantly higher mortality compared to those without (11). The mechanism of poor outcomes in patients of COVID-19 with CVD remains unknown. Previous reports suggest that coronavirus viral infections may trigger cardiovascular events and exacerbate heart failure (11–13). Direct viral damage, aggravation of a systemic inflammatory response, and hypoxemia may result in cardiac injury. Our study showed that COVID-19 patients with pre-existing CVD are more

susceptible to cardiac injury. Furthermore, CVD patients with hs-TNI elevation are more likely to develop severe illness. Prior studies demonstrated that cardiac injury was associated with poor clinical outcome, irrespective of a history of CVD (3, 14, 15). In the present study, CVD patients who died had a significantly higher incidence of cardiac injury compared to those who were alive. Moreover, our results further revealed that the level of hs-TNI could help identify patients at higher risk and requiring earlier or more aggressive treatment strategies.

Cardiac Characteristics of COVID-19 Patients With CVD

Our study showed that patients with COVID-19 infection and underlying CVD had impaired LV diastolic function. This is in keeping with the study of Li et al., which demonstrated that only subclinical LV diastolic impairment was identified in patients with severe acute respiratory syndrome (16). In line with the results of Inciardi et al. (6), no difference was observed in LVEF between patients with or without CVD. Furthermore, LVEF was preserved in the majority of hospitalized CVD patients, in agreement with the results of Churchill et al., demonstrating that LVEF was normal/hyperdynamic in most patients with COVID-19 (17). Several case reports also demonstrate that the majority of patients with uncomplicated myocarditis displays normal cardiac function (17–19). In addition, diminished RV performance was the most common in patients with CVD, consistent with recent reports in unselected COVID-19 patients (20–22).

Generally, the etiology of RV dysfunction in COVID-19 infection has not been well-established. In addition to myocardial injury, it is though that the RV dysfunction may be reflective of conditions that can increase RV afterload during this viral infection, including hypoxic pulmonary vasoconstriction, hypercarbia, excessive positive end-expiratory pressure (PEEP), pneumonia, elevated left atrial pressure, or combination of all these factors (21). In a recent study of 26 symptomatic patients with COVID-19 infection (and without a history of coronary artery disease or myocarditis), Huang et al. investigated cardiac involvement using magnetic resonance imaging and found that 58% of patients displayed impaired RV function (23). Furthermore, myocardial edema and fibrosis were observed in these patients. Indeed, 30% of COVID-19 patients with CVD required mechanical ventilation at the time of echocardiogram. RV dysfunction has been demonstrated to be a complication of hypoxemic injury including ARDS and may deteriorate following mechanical ventilation due to the presence of higher PEEP causing higher RV afterload (24, 25). Importantly, we noticed that LV diastolic and RV function was further diminished in patients with CVD compared with those without. Recent evidence suggests that patients with CVD are more likely to develop severe and critical illness that may partially explain why these patients present with worsening cardiac function (3). Another possible explanation may be that SARS-CoV-2 infection might aggravate a pre-existing cardiovascular condition (26). The poorer cardiac function in COVID-19 patients with CVD may alert physicians to pay greater attention to the management of these patients.

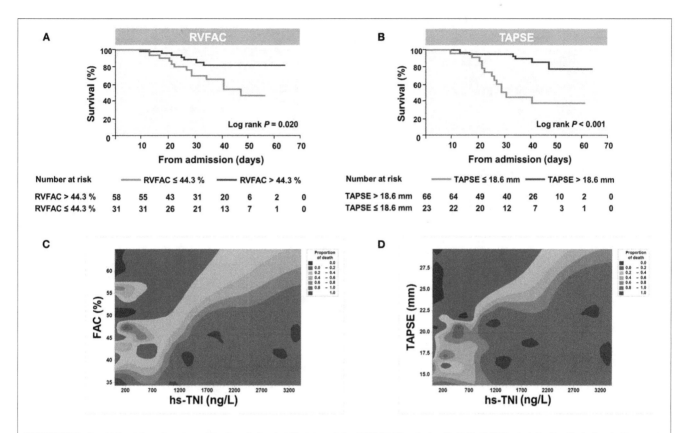

FIGURE 3 | Kaplan–Meier plots and contour plots of survival probability in hospitalized COVID-19 patients with CVD. **(A,B)** Survival significantly declined with diminished TAPSE and RVFAC. **(C,D)** Decreased TAPSE and RVFAC were associated with higher mortality, which were pronounced in patients with higher levels of hs-TNI. RVFAC, right ventricular fractional area change; TAPSE, tricuspid annular plane systolic excursion; hs-TNI, high-sensitivity troponin I.

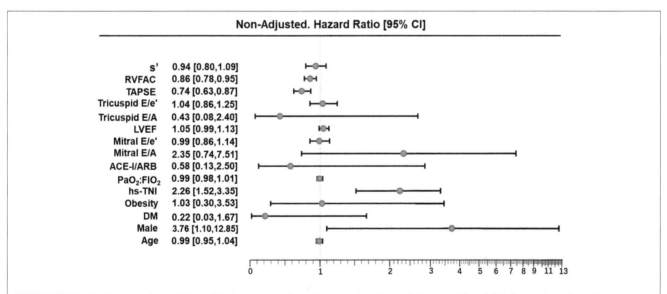

FIGURE 4 | Univariate Cox regression analysis of clinical and echocardiographic parameters. Forest plot for association of clinical and echocardiographic parameters with mortality. Impact of clinical and echocardiographic indicators on mortality in COVID-19 patients with CVD. ACE-I, angiotensin-converting enzyme inhibitors; ARB, angiotensin II receptor blockers; CI, confidence interval; COVID-19, coronavirus disease 2019; CVD, cardiovascular disease; DM, diabetes mellitus; FIO$_2$, fraction of inspiration oxygen; hs-TNI, hypersensitive troponin I; LVEF, left ventricular ejection fraction; RVFAC, right ventricular fractional area change; TAPSE, tricuspid annular plane systolic excursion; PaO$_2$, partial pressure of oxygen.

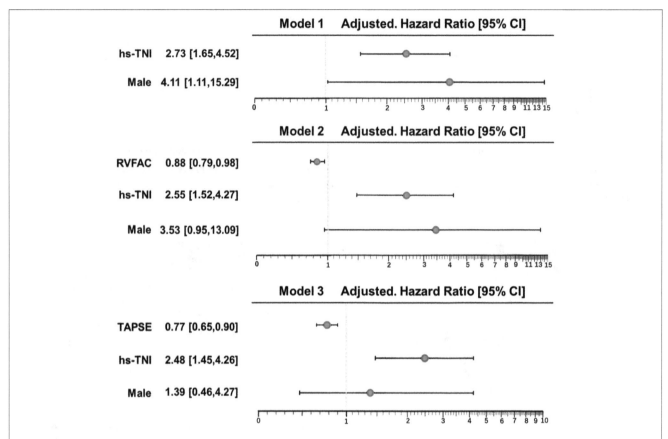

FIGURE 5 | Multivariate Cox regression analysis of clinical and echocardiographic parameters. Forest plot for association of clinical and echocardiographic parameters with mortality. Impact of clinical and echocardiographic indicators on mortality in COVID-19 patients with CVD. CI, confidence interval; COVID-19, coronavirus disease 2019; CVD, cardiovascular disease; hs-TNI, hypersensitive troponin I; RVFAC, right ventricular fractional area change; TAPSE, tricuspid annular plane systolic excursion.

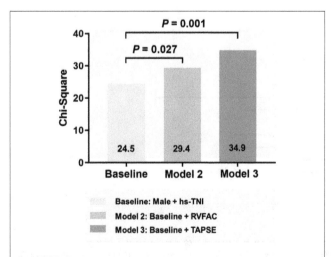

FIGURE 6 | Likelihood ratio test for the incremental prognostic value of TAPSE. The incremental value of TAPSE over clinical and RVFAC for the prediction of mortality. RVFAC, right ventricular fractional area change; TAPSE, tricuspid annular plane systolic excursion; hs-TNI, high-sensitivity troponin I.

Prognostic Value of Echocardiographic Parameters in COVID-19 Patients With CVD

Considering that patients with COVID-19 infection and underlying CVD are more likely to have a more severe course of their illness and a poorer clinical outcome, it is imperative to identify this high-risk group for consideration of earlier or more intensive therapy. Thus far, some prognostic indicators of poor outcome, in particular elevated level of hs-TNI, have been recognized (3, 27, 28). Our current study not only verified the role of these previously reported risk prognosticators but also reported the novel and additive prognostic value of RV measurements in patients with COVID-19 infection and underlying CVD.

In our study, patients found to have reduced RV function by echocardiography were at higher risk of deterioration and death. Our results demonstrate that RV function serves as a novel imaging biomarker that predicts higher mortality in patients with COVID-19 infection and underlying CVD. These findings were consistent with our previous work showing that RV dysfunction predicted poorer outcome in unselected patients with COVID-19 (with or without CVD) (25). Similarly, in a recent study of 110 patients with COVID-19, Argulian et al. demonstrated that RV dilation was an independent predictor of in-hospital mortality (29). Importantly, our study reveals that TAPSE appears to be the best predictor of higher mortality compared with RVFAC and other clinical variables. RVFAC depends on imaging quality, resulting in relatively poor inter- and intraobserver reproducibility in subjects with suboptimal endocardial definition. In contrast, TAPSE is less dependent upon image quality, is simple to perform, and is reproducible. TAPSE is widely used on a daily basis in most echocardiographic laboratories. Considering the reduced time of exposure during echocardiographic examination in patients with COVID-19, the present study revealed the key clinical implication of TAPSE, as it can be easily obtained during bedside echocardiography. Our results highlights that the additional prognostic value of TAPSE over the other clinical parameters and RVFAC is important for risk stratification in COVID-19 patients with CVD.

Limitations

Although our results demonstrated the presence of cardiac impairment in COVID-19 patients with underlying CVD, the time course for the development of these cardiac abnormalities remained unknown, as we did not have serial echocardiography available for these patients. Another limitation to consider is that although RV functional parameters were revealed to be important predictors of risk in this study, we only carried out the basic, commonly used measures of RV function such as TAPSE and RVFAC (30), as opposed to more advanced measures such as RV myocardial strain and RV three-dimensional imaging, which are now recommended for consideration by the ASE (31) and EACVI (32).

Finally, the main limitation of our study was that it was a single-center study, with a relatively limited sample size and a homogenous population. As a center designated to treat patients with COVID-19 in our region, our study subjects may not be representative of populations elsewhere, limiting extrapolation

of our results. Future studies, involving larger sample sizes, multiple centers, and international collaboration, are needed to determine the true prognostic value of echocardiographic parameters in patients with COVID-19 infection and allow for further refinement of stratification by determinants such as sex, age, and ethnicity.

CONCLUSIONS

Right ventricular dysfunction is more common than LV dysfunction among COVID-19 patients with underlying CVD. Importantly, RV function parameters are associated with higher mortality, suggesting that RV measurement may serve as a novel imaging biomarker for the risk stratification of patients with COVID-19 infection and underlying CVD. The study highlights the importance of bedside cardiovascular ultrasound in the assessment and prognostication of hospitalized patients with COVID-19 infection.

AUTHOR CONTRIBUTIONS

Conception and design of the study: YL, LF, SZ, YX, JW, YY, QL, AJ, MX, and LZ. Acquisition of data: BW, LH, DZ, YoZ, and HY. Analysis and interpretation of data: CW, HL, WS, YaZ, ML, YC, and LC. Drafting the article: YL, LF, SZ, and YX. Revising the article: YL, LF, SZ, YX, LZ, and MX. Final approval of the article: SZ, YX, LY, and LZ. All authors listed have made a substantial, direct and intellectual contribution to the work, and approved it for publication.

REFERENCES

1. Zhou F, Yu T, Du R, Fan G, Liu Y, Liu Z, et al. Clinical course and risk factors for mortality of adult inpatients with COVID-19 in Wuhan, China: a retrospective cohort study. *Lancet.* (2020) 395:1054–62. doi: 10.1016/S0140-6736(20)30566-3

2. Wang D, Hu B, Hu C, Zhu F, Liu X, Zhang J, et al. Clinical characteristics of 138 hospitalized patients with 2019 novel coronavirus–infected pneumonia in Wuhan, China. *JAMA.* (2020) 323:1061–9. doi: 10.1001/jama.2020.1585

3. Guo T, Fan Y, Chen M, Wu X, Zhang L, He T, et al. Cardiovascular implications of fatal outcomes of patients with coronavirus disease 2019 (COVID-19). *JAMA Cardiol.* (2020) 5:811–8. doi: 10.1001/jamacardio.2020.1017

4. Booth CM, Matukas LM, Tomlinson GA, Rachlis AR, Rose DB, Dwosh HA, et al. Clinical features and short-term outcomes of 144 patients with SARS in the greater Toronto area. *JAMA.* (2003) 289:2801–9. doi: 10.1001/jama.289.21.JOC30885

5. Liu PP, Blet A, Smyth D, Li H. The science underlying COVID-19: Implications for the cardiovascular system. *Circulation.* (2020) 142:68–78. doi: 10.1161/CIRCULATIONAHA.120.047549

6. Inciardi RM, Adamo M, Lupi L, Cani DS, Pasquale MD, Tomasoni D, et al. Characteristics and outcomes of patients hospitalized for COVID-19 and cardiac disease in Northern Italy. *Eur Heart J.* (2020) 41:1821–9. doi: 10.1093/eurheartj/ehaa388

7. Zhang L, Wang B, Zhou J, Kirkpatrick J, Xie MX, Johri AM. Bedside focused cardiac ultrasound in COVID-19 infection from the Wuhan epicenter: the role of cardiac point of care ultrasound (POCUS), limited transthoracic echocardiography and critical care echocardiography. *J Am Soc Echocardiogr.* (2020) 33:676–82. doi: 10.1016/j.echo.2020.04.004

8. Hendren NS, Drazner MH, Bozkurt B, Cooper LT. Description and proposed management of the acute COVID-19 cardiovascular syndrome. *Circulation.* (2020) 141:1903–14. doi: 10.1161/CIRCULATIONAHA.120.047349

9. Lang RM, Badano LP, Mor-Avi V, Afilalo J, Armstrong A, Ernande L, et al. Recommendations for cardiac chamber quantification by echocardiography in adults: an update from the American Society of Echocardiography and the European Association of Cardiovascular Imaging. *J Am Soc Echocardiogr.* (2015) 28:1–39. doi: 10.1016/j.echo.2014.10.003

10. Nagueh SF, Smiseth OA, Appleton CP, Byrd BF, Dokainish H, Edvardsen T, et al. Recommendations for the evaluation of left ventricular diastolic function by echocardiography: an update from the American Society of Echocardiography and the European Association of Cardiovascular Imaging. *J Am Soc Echocardiogr.* (2016) 29:277–314. doi: 10.1016/j.echo.2016.01.011

11. Madjid M, Safavi-Naeini P, Solomon SD, Vardeny O. Potential effects of coronaviruses on the cardiovascular system: a review. *JAMA Cardiol.* (2020) 5:831–40. doi: 10.1001/jamacardio.2020.1286

12. Udell JA, Rosamond W, Temte J, Udell JA, Rosamond W, Temte J, et al. Association of influenza-like illness activity with hospitalizations for heart failure: the atherosclerosis risk in communities study. *JAMA Cardiol.* (2019) 4:363–9. doi: 10.1001/jamacardio.2019.0549

13. Corrales-Medina VF, Madjid M, Musher DM. Role of acute infection in triggering acute coronary syndromes. *Lancet Infect Dis.* (2010) 10:83–92. doi: 10.1016/S1473-3099(09)70331-7

14. Shi S, Qin M, Shen B, Cai Y, Liu T, Yang F, et al. Association of cardiac injury with mortality in hospitalized patients with COVID-19 in Wuhan, China. *JAMA Cardiol.* (2020) 5:802–10. doi: 10.1001/jamacardio.2020.0950

15. Yang X, Yu Y, Xu J, Shu H, Xia J, Liu H, et al. Clinical course and outcomes of critically ill patients with SARSCoV-2 pneumonia in Wuhan, China: a single-centered, retrospective, observational study. *Lancet Respir Med.* (2020) 8:475–81. doi: 10.1016/S2213-2600(20)30079-5

16. Li SS, Cheng CW, Fu CL, Chan Y, Lee M, Chan J, et al. Left ventricular performance in patients with severe acute respiratory syndrome: a 30-day echocardiographic follow-up study. *Circulation.* (2003) 108: 1798–803. doi: 10.1161/01.CIR.0000094737.21775.32

17. Churchill TW, Bertrand PB, Bernard S, Namasivayam M, Churchill J, Crousillat D, et al. Echocardiographic features of COVID-19 illness and association with cardiac biomarkers. *J Am Soc Echocardiogr.* (2020) 33:1053–4. doi: 10.1016/j.echo.2020.05.028

18. Hu H, Ma F, Wei X, Fang Y. Coronavirus fulminant myocarditis saved with glucocorticoid and human immunoglobulin. *Eur Heart J.* (2021) 42:206. doi: 10.1093/eurheartj/ehaa190

19. Danzi GB, Loffi M, Galeazzi G, Gherbesi E. Acute pulmonary embolism and COVID-19 pneumonia: a random association. *Eur Heart J.* (2020) 41:1858. doi: 10.1093/eurheartj/ehaa254

20. Li Y, Li H, Zhu S, Wang B, He L, Zhang D, et al. Prognostic value of right ventricular longitudinal strain in patients with COVID-19. *JACC Cardiovasc Imaging.* (2020) 13:2287–99. doi: 10.1016/j.jcmg.2020.04.014

21. Szekely Y, Lichter Y, Taieb P, Banai A, Hochstadt A, Merdler I, et al. The spectrum of cardiac manifestations in coronavirus disease 2019 (COVID-19) - a systematic echocardiographic study. *Circulation.* (2020) 142:342–53. doi: 10.1161/CIRCULATIONAHA.120.047971

22. Mahmoud-Elsayed HM, Moody WE, Bradlow WM, Khan-Kheil AM, Senior J, Hudsmith LE, et al. Echocardiographic findings in Covid-19 pneumonia. *Can J Cardiol.* (2020) 36:1203–7. doi: 10.1016/j.cjca.2020.05.030

23. Huang L, Zhao P, Tang D, Zhu T, Han R, Zhan C, et al. Cardiac involvement in patients recovered COVID-19 patients identified by magnetic resonance imaging. *JACC Cardiovasc Imaging.* (2020) 13:2330–9. doi: 10.1016/j.jcmg.2020.05.004

24. Zochios V, Parhar K, Tunnicliffe W, Roscoe A, Gao F. The right ventricle in ARDS. *Chest.* (2017) 152:181–93. doi: 10.1016/j.chest.2017.02.019

25. Vieillard-Baron A, Millington SJ, Sanfilippo F, Chew M, Diaz-Gomez J, McLean A, et al. A decade of progress in critical care echocardiography: a narrative review. *Intensive Care Med.* (2019) 45:770–88. doi: 10.1007/s00134-019-05604-2

26. Zheng Y, Ma Y, Zhang J, Xie X. COVID-19 and the cardiovascular system. *Nat Rev Cardiol.* (2020) 17:259–60. doi: 10.1038/s41569-020-0360-5

27. Chen T, Wu D, Chen H, Yan W, Yang D, Chen G, et al. Clinical characteristics of 113 deceased patients with coronavirus disease 2019: retrospective study. *BMJ.* (2020) 368:m1091. doi: 10.1136/bmj.m1091

28. Capone V, Cuomo V, Esposito R, Canonico ME, Ilardi F, Prastaro M, et al. Epidemiology, prognosis, and clinical manifestation of cardiovascular disease in COVID-19. *Expert Rev Cardiovasc Ther.* (2020) 18:531–9. doi: 10.1080/14779072.2020.1797491

29. Argulian E, Sud K, Vogel B, Bohra C, Garg VP, Talebi S, et al. Right ventricular dilation in hospitalized patients with COVID-19 infection. *JACC Cardiovasc Imaging.* (2020) 13:2459–61. doi: 10.1016/j.jcmg.2020.05.010

30. Johri AM, Galen B, Kirkpatrick JN, Lanspa M, Mulvagh S, Thamman R, et al. ASE statement on point-of-care ultrasound during the 2019 novel coronavirus pandemic. *J Am Soc Echocardiogr.* (2020) 33:670–3. doi: 10.1016/j.echo.2020.04.017

31. Kirkpatrick JN, Grimm R, Johri AM, Kimura BJ, Kort S, Labovitz AJ, et al. Recommendations for echocardiography laboratories participating in cardiac point of care cardiac ultrasound (POCUS) and critical care echocardiography training: report from the American Society of Echocardiography. *J Am Soc Echocardiogr.* (2020) 33:409–22 e4. doi: 10.1016/j.echo.2020.01.008

32. Skulstad H, Cosyns B, Popescu BA, Galderisi M, Salvo GD, Donal E, et al. COVID-19 pandemic and cardiac imaging: EACVI recommendations on precautions, indications, prioritization, and protection for patients and healthcare personnel. *Eur Heart J Cardiovasc Imaging.* (2020) 21:592–8. doi: 10.1093/ehjci/jeaa072

22

Pulmonary Rehabilitation Accelerates the Recovery of Pulmonary Function in Patients with COVID-19

Pengfei Zhu[1†], Zhengchao Wang[2†], Xiaomi Guo[3†], Zhiyong Feng[4], Chaochao Chen[4], Ai Zheng[4], Haotian Gu[5‡] and Yu Cai[4*‡]*

[1] *Department of Cardiology, Wuhan Fourth Hospital, Puai Hospital, Tongji Medical College, Huazhong University of Science and Technology, Wuhan, China,* [2] *Tongji Hospital, Tongji Medical College, Huazhong University of Science and Technology, Wuhan, China,* [3] *Department of Ultrasound, Wuhan Asia General Hospital, Wuhan, China,* [4] *Department of Rehabilitation, Wuhan Fourth Hospital, Puai Hospital, Tongji Medical College, Huazhong University of Science and Technology, Wuhan, China,* [5] *British Heart Foundation Centre of Research Excellence, King's College London, London, United Kingdom*

*Correspondence:
Yu Cai
caiy_kf@163.com
Haotian Gu
haotian.gu@kcl.ac.uk

[†] *These authors share first authorship*

[‡] *These authors share senior authorship*

Objectives: To evaluate the effect of in-hospital pulmonary rehabilitation (PR) on short-term pulmonary functional recovery in patients with COVID-19.

Methods: Patients with COVID-19 ($n = 123$) were divided into two groups (PR group or Control group) according to recipient of pulmonary rehabilitation. Six-min walk distance (6MW), heart rate (HR), forced vital capacity (FVC), forced expiratory volume in 1 s (FEV$_1$), diffusing capacity of the lung for carbon monoxide (DL$_{CO}$), and CT scanning were measured at the time of discharge, 1, 4, 12, and 24 weeks.

Results: At week one, both PR group and Control group showed no significant changes in pulmonary function. At 4 and 12 weeks, 6MW, HR, FVC, FEV$_1$, and DL$_{CO}$ improved significantly in both groups. However, the improvement in the PR group was greater than the Control group. Pulmonary function in the PR group returned to normal at 4 weeks [FVC (% predicted, PR vs. Control): 86.27 ± 9.14 vs. 78.87 ± 7.55; FEV1 (% predicted, PR vs. Control) 88.76 ± 6.22 vs. 78.96 ± 6.91; DLCO (% predicted, PR vs. Control): 87.27 ± 6.20 vs. 77.78 ± 5.85] compared to 12 weeks in the control group [FVC (% predicted, PR vs. Control): 90.61 ± 6.05 vs. 89.96 ± 4.05; FEV1 (% predicted, PR vs. Control) 94.06 ± 0.43 vs. 93.85 ± 5.61; DLCO (% predicted, PR vs. Control): 91.99 ± 8.73 vs. 88.57 ± 5.37]. Residual lesions on CT disappeared at week 4 in 49 patients in PR group and in 28 patients in control group ($p = 0.0004$).

Conclusion: Pulmonary rehabilitation could accelerate the recovery of pulmonary function in patients with COVID-19.

Keywords: pulmonary training, corona virus disease 2019, pulmonary function, pulmonary rehabilitation, 2019-nCoV

INTRODUCTION

Corona Virus Disease (COVID-19) caused by a novel coronavirus named as Severe Acute Respiratory Syndrome (SARS)-CoV (Corona Virus)-2 has been rapidly occurring the world and is not completely controlled till now (1, 2). Transmissions through fecal-oral route and ocular are also considered to be possible while evidences are not sufficient till now (3, 4). All age groups are susceptible to SARS-CoV-2, while the elderlies and people with underlying diseases are more likely to develop severe conditions such as severe pneumonia and respiratory failure in a short period of time (2). The therapeutic principles of COVID-19 include general treatment (vital sign monitoring, mechanical ventilation, etc.), drug therapy (anti-infection drugs, traditional Chinese medicine, etc.), pulmonary rehabilitation (PR), nutrition management and mental support.

Pulmonary rehabilitation, as a comprehensive intervention including exercise training, education and behavioral changes that aims to improve the physical and psychological condition in patients with respiratory disease and to promote high long-term quality of life. It has also been confirmed to be an important part of the integrated care strategy for chronic obstructive pulmonary disease (COPD) (5, 6). Its positive effects in preoperative pulmonary rehabilitation were also discovered including reducing the sensation of dyspnea, reducing muscle strength loss associated with dyspnea, and improving psychologic states (7). As for infectious disease of respiratory system, Hsieh et al. (8) found that survivors of acute respiratory distress syndrome (ARDS) caused by influenza A (H1N1) who received pulmonary rehabilitation for 2 months had improved pulmonary function, exercise capacity, and quality of life.

Therefore, the aim of present study was to evaluate the effect of in-hospital pulmonary rehabilitation on short-term pulmonary functional recovery in patients with COVID-19.

METHODS

Patients and Data Collection

We conducted a perspective observational study in patients with COVID-19.

Participants were recruited from Puai Hospital, Wuhan Forth Hospital and Huazhong University of Science and Technology, and were divided into two groups according to whether patients received in-hospital pulmonary rehabilitation. Patients who underwent in-hospital pulmonary rehabilitation were based on the clinical judgements by attending physicians. No patients were directly involved in the design, planning and conception of this study. Inclusion criteria were: (1) patients with COVID-19; (2) able to receive pulmonary rehabilitation; (3) no co-infection of other pathogene; (4) sign the informed consent. Exclusion criteria include: (1) suffering from high blood pressure, diabetes, or other chronic or basic diseases; (2) COVID-19 recurrence during the follow-up period. (3) infection of other pathogene during the follow-up period. (4) pregnancy before or during the follow-up period. Data were collected at the time of discharge and 1, 4, 12, 24 weeks after discharge. The study was approved by Chinese Clinical Trial Registry (ChiCTR2000031751).

Pulmonary Rehabilitation

In the PR group, all patients underwent a standardized rehabilitation scheme (ref) when their clinical condition was stable and capable of PR. Detailed PR protocol as follow: (1) allow patients to maintain regular movement, such as chest expansion and ambulation, in the isolation ward for at least 1 h per day while monitoring heart rate and respiratory rate during movement to avoid overexertion in terms of heart and lung function; (2) provide respiratory control training: Help the patients sit in an upright position to avoid orthopnea. If the patients could not sit upright, lift the head of bed by 60 degrees. Let the patients relax their shoulder muscles by placing one hand on the chest and the other on the abdomen, instruct the patients to deeply breathe in through their nose and breathe out through their mouth to expand the lower chest. (3) pursed lip breathing: Keep the same patient position as with respiratory control. Let the patients breathe in through their nose, hold their breath for 2 s, then deeply breathe out using their abdomen for 3–5 s with their mouth pursed as if they are whistling; this increases the expiratory resistance and prolongs the expiratory time. For (2) and (3) above, the patients were trained repeatedly for 10–15 min each and 4 times per day. The patients could train along with light music if possible. If any discomfort occurred, the training should be stopped immediately.

Outcome Measures

Six-min walk distance (6MW), Heart rate (HR), forced vital capacity (FVC), forced expiratory volume in 1 s (FEV_1), and Diffusing capacity of the lung for carbon monoxide (DL_{CO}) were measured. CT scanning was conducted at discharge, 4, and 24 weeks. FVC and FEV_1 were measure using spirometry. Spirometry was performed using the Medical Graphics CPXD (Minneapolis, MN, US). Diffusing capacity of the lung for carbon monoxide (DL_{CO}) were assessed using the rebreathe technique and a mass spectrometer (Perkin Elmer, St. Louis, MO, USA) as previously described (9, 10). CT scan was conducted using a 64-slice spiral CT machine (NeuSoft, NeuViz64). The CT images was evaluated by two experienced imaging clinicians. If their opinions were different, a third clinician was invited to make the final decision.

Statistical Analysis

Statistical analysis was completed using SPSS 21.0. Baseline differences between groups were analyzed by Student's t-test for continuous data and by the χ^2 test for categorical data. Continuous data are expressed as the means $\pm$ SDs, and the normality of distribution was tested by a QQ plot. The data were analyzed using Student's t-test and repeated measures analysis of variance (ANOVA). As for repeated measures ANOVA, post-hoc test of p-value was adopted by Bonferroni correction and effect size was expressed as eta-square. A value of $p < 0.05$ was considered statistically significant. Because of a small sample size, p-valued between 0.05 and 0.1 was marked with specific value.

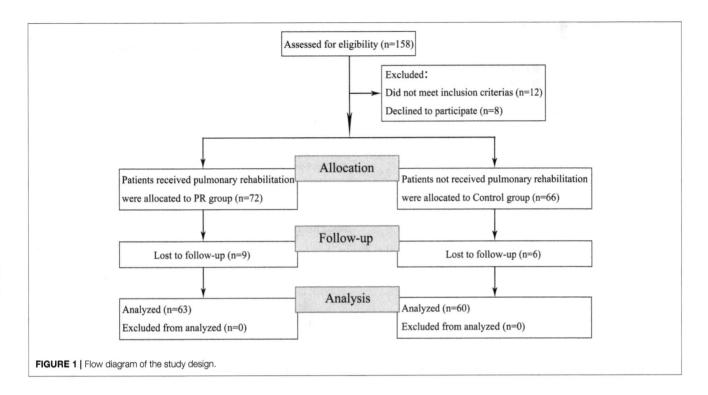

FIGURE 1 | Flow diagram of the study design.

RESULTS

A total of 158 participants were screened between February 1st 2020 to March 31st 2020, out of whom 20 patients were excluded because of not meeting the inclusion criteria or declined to participate in this study (**Figure 1**). Fifteen participants were lost to follow-up before 4 weeks follow-up. Baseline demographics were shown in **Tables 1–3**.

6MW and HR were shown in **Table 4**. At the time of discharge, 6MW distance in PR group was longer than the Control group and the HR was lower than the Control group, but did not reach significant. At the time of week 1 and 4, there were significant improvements of 6MW and HR in PR group compared to those at the time of discharge (week 1: 495.88 ± 34.67 vs. 470.83 ± 35.70 $p < 0.05$ and 83.24 ± 8.46 vs. 97.05 ± 14.24 $p < 0.001$; week 4: 557.94 ± 38.44 vs. 514.22 ± 43.47 $p < 0.01$ and 78.59 ± 6.73 vs. 88.61 ± 9.37 $p < 0.001$). However, in the Control group, only an improvement of 6MW was found at 4 weeks and was smaller than the PR group. At 12 and 24 weeks, 6MW and HR were similar in two groups.

The measurements of FVC and FEV_1 is shown in **Table 5**. At the time of discharge and week 1, FEV_1 in the PR group was significantly larger than that in the Control group. There was no significant difference in FVC between the two groups at week 1 (2.05 ± 0.26 vs. 1.91 ± 0.21, $p = 0.096$). Although FVC and FEV1 improved significantly in both groups, there was greater improvement in the PR groups than the Control group at week 4. FEV_1 and FVC in the PR group exceeded 80% of predicted values at 4 weeks [FVC (% predicted): 86.27 ± 9.14 vs. 78.87 ± 7.55, $p < 0.05$; FEV1 (% predicted) 88.76 ± 6.22 vs. 78.96 ± 6.91, $p < 0.001$]. At 12 and 24 weeks, there were no significant difference in

TABLE 1 | General characteristics in PR and control groups.

	No. (%)		p-value
	PR Group (n = 63)	Control Group (n = 60)	
Age (years)	36.59 ± 7.01	35.47 ± 7.58	0.40
Gender			0.53
Male	34	29	
Female	29	31	
Blood pressure (mmHg, at discharge)			
Systolic pressure	116.3 ± 4.4	115.8 ± 5.2	0.57
Diastolic pressure	78.7 ± 3.2	78.1 ± 3.5	0.32
Weight (kg, at discharge)	62.4 ± 11.3	64.0 ± 10.9	0.43
Height (cm, at discharge)	167.6 ± 13.2	167.8 ± 12.9	0.93
Personal habits			
Smoking	7 (11.1)	9 (15.0)	0.52
Drinking	4 (6.3)	3 (5.0)	0.75
Education			0.66
Junior high school or below	12	9	
High school or vocational school	19	24	
College degree	16	17	
Bachelor degree	12	8	
Postgraduate degree or above	4	2	

PR, pulmonary rehabilitation.

FEV_1 and FVC between two groups and FEV1 and FVC reached 90% of predicted values. There was no significant change in FEV_1 to FVC ratio during the entire follow-up period.

TABLE 2 | Clinical characteristics in PR and control groups.

Clinical Presentation	PR Group (n = 63)	Control Group (n = 60)	p-value
Fever	62 (98.8)	59 (98.3)	1.00
Dry cough	45 (71.4)	41 (68.3)	0.71
Headache	5 (7.9)	4(6.7)	1.00
Sore throat	7 (11.1)	5 (8.3)	0.40
Myalgia	21(33.3)	18 (30.0)	0.69
Fatigue	24 (38.1)	19 (31.7)	0.46
Dyspnoea	28 (44.4)	21 (35.0)	0.29
Rhinorrhoea	13 (20.6)	11 (18.3)	0.75
Nausea & vomiting	18 (28.6)	19 (31.7)	0.71
Diarrhea	12 (19.0)	10 (16.7)	0.73
Length of Hospital stay (days)	21.18 ± 4.98	21.94 ± 3.24	0.32

PR, pulmonary rehabilitation.

TABLE 3 | Results of laboratory examination at discharge.

	PR Group (n = 63)	Control Group (n = 60)	p-value
Blood Count			
WBC (×10^9/L)	7.14 ± 3.41	6.86 ± 2.99	0.63
Lymphocyte count (×10^9/L)	0.62 ± 0.08	0.66 ± 0.09	0.20
PLT at discharge (×10^9/L)	243 ± 99	216 ± 71	0.09
Hemoglobin (g/dL)	118 ± 23	125 ± 17	0.10
Coagulation Function			
PT (s)	14.1 ± 3.3	13.2 ± 1.4	0.08
APTT (s)	37.6 ± 9.0	37.2 ± 6.2	0.82
D-dimer (mg/L)	1.7 ± 2.4	1.3 ± 1.9	0.24
Blood Biochemistry			
TP (g/L)	64.5 ± 10.3	66.5 ± 7.2	0.21
Albumin (g/L)	34.6 ± 5.8	37.5 ± 6.4	0.10
ALT (U/L)	35 ± 19	40 ± 22	0.14
AST (U/L)	30 ± 15	34 ± 19	0.20
TB (μmol/L)	11.8 ± 5.5	12.5 ± 6.2	0.51
Sodium (mmol/L)	137.7 ± 5.3	138.5 ± 3.3	0.30
Potassium (mmol/L)	4.1 ± 0.5	3.9 ± 0.4	0.09
Creatinine (μmol/L)	71.2 ± 27.5	69.1 ± 20.4	0.62
BUN (mmol/L)	5.2 ± 2.1	5.4 ± 2.3	0.66
LDH (U/L)	239 ± 133	213 ± 127	0.27
CK-MB (U/L)	10.9 ± 8.5	11.8 ± 7.7	0.53
Infection-Related Biomarkers			
CRP (mg/L)	23 ± 34	18 ± 25	0.34
PCT (ng/ml)	0.18 ± 0.45	0.11 ± 0.18	0.21

PR, pulmonary rehabilitation; RBC, red blood cell, WBC, white blood cell; PT, prothrombin time; PLT, platelet; APTT, activated partial thromboplastin time; FBG, fasting blood glucose; TP, total protein; ALT, alanine transaminase; AST, aspertate aminotransfera; TB, total bilirubin; BUN, blood urea nitrogen; LDH, lactate dehydrogenase; CK-MB, creatine kinase–MB; CRP, hypersensitive C-reactive protein; PCT, procalcitonin.

DL_{CO} was shown in **Table 6**. At the first week after discharge, no improvements were discovered in DL_{CO}. Meanwhile, the DL_{CO} of PR group was higher than Control group (19.65 ± 2.12 vs. 17.03 ± 1.94, $p < 0.01$). Significant improvements were discovered at 4 weeks, while level of DL_{CO} in the PR group was higher than the Control group [DLCO (% predicted): 87.27 ± 6.20 vs. 77.78 ± 5.85, $p < 0.001$]. At 12 and 24 weeks, DL_{CO} reached normal level and had no significantly differences between two groups.

As shown in **Figure 2**, in the PR group, little parenchymal bands with group-glass opacity were observed at the time of discharge in all patients. The lesions of 49 patients (77.8%) in PR group basically disappeared at 4 weeks follow-up and no changes were discovered at 24 weeks. The CT images of 60 patients (95.2%) in PR group were basically normal at 24 weeks. In the control group, little parenchymal bands with more group-glass opacities were observed at the time of discharge in all patients. At 4 weeks follow-up, some group-glass opacities still existed in CT images of 32 patients (53.3%). The lesions of only 28 patients (46.7%, $p = 0.0004$ vs. PR group) in control group basically disappeared at 4 weeks follow-up and no changes were discovered at 24 weeks. The CT images of 56 patients (93.3%, $p = 0.65$ vs. PR group) in control group were basically normal at 24 weeks.

DISCUSSION

The main physiological change in patient recovery from COVID-19 is poorer cardio-pulmonary function, and lower FVC, FEV$_1$, and DL_{CO}. Meanwhile most of the values of FEV$_1$/FVC were still abnormal. The main imaging changes from CT scanning were little parenchymal bands with residual group-glass opacity. As a result, the pathologic changes in the lung of patients after discharge might be: (1) residual unabsorbed exudative lesion; (2) mild lung fibrosis. These changes result in the

functional disorders include: (1) decreasing in lung capacity; (2) decreasing in lung compliance; (3) decreasing in diffusion function. However, all impairments disappeared within 12 weeks, which means the pathological and functional changes are reversible.

The residual lesions of lung function are not rarely in viral pneumonia. Studies have discovered that survivors from SARS had significantly impaired pulmonary function, limited physical and psychology function, and reduced life quality (11, 12). Regarding influenza A virus H1N1, a study found that over half of these patients had signs of more severe abnormal pulmonary function, including diffusion disorders and small airway dysfunction, 1 year after discharge (13). From our results, we found that the residual lesions of lung function caused by SARS-CoV-2 is relatively short-term and reversible. It might attribute to the relatively lower virulence of the virus or the participants we included were not severe and critical.

Pulmonary rehabilitation is a comprehensive intervention that includes but is not limited to exercise training, education and behavioral changes with the aim to improve the physical and psychological conditions of people with respiratory disease

TABLE 4 | Six-min walk distance and heart rate.

	Discharge	1 week	4 weeks	12 weeks	24 weeks
6MW (m)					
PR group	462.12 ± 31.61	495.88 ± 34.67*	557.94 ± 38.44*†	584.41 ± 20.12*†	598.71 ± 22.35*†‡
Control group	448.56 ± 31.10	470.83 ± 35.70	514.22 ± 43.47*†	573.11 ± 29.20*†‡	590.33 ± 19.88*†‡
PR vs. control	$p > 0.05$	$p < 0.05$	$p < 0.01$	$p > 0.05$	$p > 0.05$
p and η^2 for ANOVA	$p_{time} < 0.001$, $\eta^2_{time} = 0.932$, $p_{group} < 0.05$, $\eta^2_{group} = 0.124$, $p_{time*group} < 0.001$, $\eta^2_{time*group} = 0.168$				
HR (beats/min)					
PR group	90.71 ± 9.30	83.24 ± 8.46*	78.59 ± 6.73*	76.06 ± 6.09†	76.06 ± 6.09*†
Control group	97.44 ± 10.39	97.05 ± 14.24	88.61 ± 9.37	78.61 ± 9.37*†‡	77.00 ± 6.16*†‡
PR vs. control	$p = 0.052$	$p < 0.001$	$p < 0.001$	$p > 0.05$	$p > 0.05$
p and η^2 for ANOVA	$p_{time} < 0.001$, $\eta^2_{time} = 0.778$, $p_{group} < 0.05$, $\eta^2_{group} = 0.143$, $p_{time*group} < 0.001$, $\eta^2_{time*group} = 0.332$				

PR, pulmonary rehabilitation; 6MW, 6-min walk distance; HR, heart rate.
P-value of PR. vs. Control was from Student's t-test between two groups.
P-value of the comparison between different times was from post-hoc test with Bonferroni correction for multiple comparisons [C5(2)]: *p <0.05/10 vs. discharge; †p < 0.05/10 vs. 1 week; ‡p < 0.05/10 vs. 4 weeks.

TABLE 5 | Forced vital capacity and forced expiratory volume in 1 s.

	Discharge	1 week	4 weeks	12 weeks	24 weeks
FVC (L)					
PR group	2.05 ± 0.26	2.11 ± 0.29	2.75 ± 0.30*†	2.89 ± 0.22*†	2.95 ± 0.15*†
Control group	1.91 ± 0.21	2.02 ± 0.19	2.51 ± 0.20*†	2.86 ± 0.12*†‡	2.91 ± 0.10*†‡
PR vs. control	$p = 0.096$	$p > 0.05$	$p < 0.05$	$p > 0.05$	$p > 0.05$
p and η^2 for ANOVA	$p_{time} < 0.001$, $\eta^2_{time} = 0.947$, $p_{group} = 0.053$, $\eta^2_{group} = 0.109$, $p_{time*group} < 0.05$, $\eta^2_{time*group} = 0.288$				
FVC (% predicted)					
PR group	64.25 ± 7.94	66.29 ± 9.14	86.27 ± 9.14*†	90.61 ± 6.05*†	92.64 ± 3.27*†
Control group	60.04 ± 6.28	63.46 ± 6.32	78.87 ± 7.55*†	89.96 ± 4.05*†‡	91.51 ± 2.62*†‡
PR vs. control	$p = 0.090$	$p > 0.05$	$p < 0.05$	$p > 0.05$	$p > 0.05$
p and η^2 for ANOVA	$p_{time} < 0.001$, $\eta^2_{time} = 0.946$, $p_{group} = 0.061$, $\eta^2_{group} = 0.102$, $p_{time*group} < 0.05$, $\eta^2_{time*group} = 0.295$				
FEV$_1$ (L)					
PR group	1.52 ± 0.12	1.54 ± 0.14	2.12 ± 0.11*†	2.25 ± 0.10*†‡	2.29 ± 0.14*†‡
Control group	1.43 ± 0.11	1.48 ± 0.09	1.88 ± 0.12*†	2.24 ± 0.10*†‡	2.31 ± 0.13*†‡
PR vs. control	$p < 0.05$	$p < 0.05$	$p < 0.001$	$p > 0.05$	$p > 0.05$
p and η^2 for ANOVA	$p_{time} < 0.001$, $\eta^2_{time} = 0.980$, $p_{group} < 0.01$, $\eta^2_{group} = 0.302$, $p_{time*group} < 0.001$, $\eta^2_{time*group} = 0.499$				
FEV$_1$ (% predicted)					
PR group	63.62 ± 5.82	64.54 ± 7.11	88.76 ± 6.22*†	94.06 ± 0.43*†	95.83 ± 5.29*†‡
Control group	59.81 ± 4.94	61.58 ± 5.29	78.96 ± 6.91*†	93.85 ± 5.61*†‡	97.01 ± 5.79*†‡
PR vs. control	$p < 0.05$	$p < 0.05$	$p < 0.001$	$p > 0.05$	$p > 0.05$
p and η^2 for ANOVA	$p_{time} < 0.001$, $\eta^2_{time} = 0.938$, $p_{group} < 0.05$, $\eta^2_{group} = 0.152$, $p_{time*group} < 0.001$, $\eta^2_{time*group} = 0.198$				
FEV$_1$/FVC (%)					
PR group	74.73 ± 5.89	73.67 ± 8.08	77.70 ± 6.70	78.15 ± 5.96	77.62 ± 4.25
Control group	74.99 ± 5.55	74.39 ± 6.63	75.32 ± 5.43	78.30 ± 4.37	78.55 ± 5.35
PR vs. control	$p > 0.05$	$p > 0.05$	$p > 0.05$	$p > 0.05$	$p > 0.05$
p and η^2 for ANOVA	$p_{time} < 0.001$, $\eta^2_{time} = 0.565$, $p_{group} > 0.05$, $\eta^2_{group} = 0.004$, $p_{time*group} > 0.05$, $\eta^2_{time*group} = 0.210$				

PR, pulmonary rehabilitation; FVC, forced vital capacity; FEV1, forced expiratory volume in 1s.
P-value of PR. vs. Control was from Student's t-test between two groups.
P-value of the comparison between different times was from post-hoc test with Bonferroni correction for multiple comparisons [C5(2)]: *p < 0.05/10 vs. discharge; †p < 0.05/10 vs. 1 week; ‡p < 0.05/10 vs. 4 weeks.

TABLE 6 | Diffusing capacity of the lung for carbon monoxide.

	Discharge	1 week	4 weeks	12 weeks	24 weeks
DL_{CO} [ml/(min·mmHg)]					
PR group	18.53 ± 2.03	19.65 ± 2.12	$21.76 \pm 2.19^*$	$22.88 \pm 2.12^{*\dagger}$	$22.94 \pm 2.33^{*\dagger}$
Control group	16.00 ± 1.46	$17.03 \pm 1.94^*$	$18.83 \pm 1.86^*$	$21.50 \pm 2.38^{*\dagger\ddagger}$	$22.72 \pm 2.16^{*\dagger\ddagger}$
PR vs. control	$p < 0.001$	$p < 0.01$	$p < 0.001$	$p = 0.079$	$p > 0.05$
p and η^2 for ANOVA	$p_{time} < 0.001$, $\eta^2_{time} = 0.753$, $p_{group} < 0.01$, $\eta^2_{group} = 0.271$, $p_{time^*group} < 0.01$, $\eta^2_{time^*group} = 0.145$				
DL_{CO} (% predicted)					
PR group	74.36 ± 6.59	78.81 ± 6.57	$87.27 \pm 6.20^{*\dagger}$	$91.99 \pm 8.73^{*\dagger}$	$92.12 \pm 8.32^{*\dagger}$
Control group	66.24 ± 6.20	70.32 ± 7.46	$77.78 \pm 5.85^{*\dagger}$	$88.57 \pm 5.037^{*\dagger\ddagger}$	$93.94 \pm 8.29^{*\dagger\ddagger}$
PR vs. control	$p < 0.01$	$p < 0.01$	$p < 0.001$	$p > 0.05$	$p > 0.05$
p and η^2 for ANOVA	$p_{time} < 0.001$, $\eta^2_{time} = 0.740$, $p_{group} < 0.01$, $\eta^2_{group} = 0.283$, $p_{time^*group} < 0.01$, $\eta^2_{time^*group} = 0.143$				

PR, pulmonary rehabilitation; FVC, forced vital capacity; DL_{CO}, diffusing capacity of the lung for carbon monoxide.
P-value of PR. vs. Control was from Student's t-test between two groups.
P-value of the comparison between different times was from post-hoc test with Bonferroni correction for multiple comparisons [C5(2)]: $^*p < 0.05/10$ vs. discharge; $^\dagger p < 0.05/10$ vs. 1 week; $^\ddagger p < 0.05/10$ vs. 4 weeks.

and promote long-term quality of life (6). Previous studies have confirmed the positive effects of pulmonary rehabilitation on pulmonary diseases such as COPD and H1N1 pneumonia (8, 12, 14). Besides, pulmonary rehabilitation has been proved to benefit the lung function and life quality in interstitial lung diseases such as idiopathic pulmonary fibrosis and interstitial pneumonias (15–17). Based on clinical practice, the program of pulmonary mainly contained three aspects: (1) physical training, (2) respiratory training, and (3) psychological regulation. Therefore, there are three main benefits of PR: (1) improve the patients' exercise capacity, (2) improve the patients' pulmonary function, and (3) improve the patients' psychological state. During the whole follow-up from the time of discharge to 24 weeks later, we can find that the pulmonary function of PR group was basically normal at 4 weeks, while Control group was basically normal at 12 weeks. As a result, the pulmonary rehabilitation could accelerate the recovery of pulmonary lesions and cardio-pulmonary function. According to the changes in CT imaging, we suspected that the effects of pulmonary rehabilitation may attribute to the promotion in absorption of exudation and fibrosis lesions, result in improvement of lung capacity, compliance, and diffusion function.

Because of the flexibility, feasibility and low cost, pulmonary rehabilitation could be a relatively practical way to improve patient condition. Most of patients suffered from COVID-19 are mild and common type, which makes it easy to carry out pulmonary rehabilitation. As for critical patient, whether, when, and how to carry out pulmonary rehabilitation should be further considered. Moreover, the intensity of training relies on the patients' condition; hence, the therapists should pay more attention each patient's vital signs and subjective feelings to not only maximize the effectiveness of the training but also avoid adverse events.

The main limitation of our study is that we only reported the results of 24 weeks follow-up, whether COVID-19 have sequela in respiratory system or other systems should be further studied.

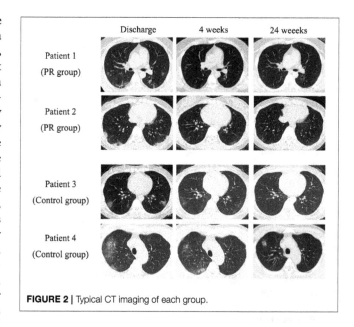

FIGURE 2 | Typical CT imaging of each group.

On the other hand, the characteristics of socio-economic of patients might affect patients' choice for accepting pulmonary rehabilitation, which might also lead to a better recovery. However, the socio-economic data were not available, which could be another limitation for this research.

In conclusion, pulmonary rehabilitation could accelerate the recovery of pulmonary function for COVID-19 patients.

AUTHOR CONTRIBUTIONS

PZ, HG, and YC conceived and designed the study. YC and PZ contributed to the literature search. CC, ZF, and AZ contributed to data collection. AZ, ZF, and XG contributed to data analysis. PZ and XG contributed to data interpretation. ZW contributed to the figures. ZW, HG, and PZ drafted the article. All authors contributed to the article and approved the submitted version.

ACKNOWLEDGMENTS

We are grateful for all our colleagues for their support of the present study. We are also grateful to the many front-line medical staffs for their dedication in the face of this outbreak, despite the potential threat to their own lives and the lives of their families.

REFERENCES

1. Chan JF, Yuan S, Kok KH, To KK, Chu H, Yang J, et al. A familial cluster of pneumonia associated with the 2019 novel coronavirus indicating person-to-person transmission: a study of a family cluster. *Lancet.* (2020) 395:514–23. doi: 10.1016/S0140-6736(20)30154-9

2. Chen ZM, Fu JF, Shu Q, Chen YH, Hua CZ, Li FB, et al. Diagnosis and treatment recommendations for pediatric respiratory infection caused by the 2019 novel coronavirus. *World J Pediatrics.* (2020) 16:240–6. doi: 10.1007/s12519-020-00345-5

3. Zhang H, Kang Z, Gong H, Xu D, Wang J, Li Z, et al. The digestive system is a potential route of 2019-nCov infection: a bioinformatics analysis based on single-cell transcriptomes. *bioRxiv.* 2020.2001.2030.927806 (2020). doi: 10.1101/2020.01.30.927806

4. Lu CW, Liu XF, Jia ZF. 2019-nCoV transmission through the ocular surface must not be ignored. *Lancet.* (2020) 395:e39. doi: 10.1016/S0140-6736(20)30313-5

5. Spruit MA, Pulmonary rehabilitation. *Eur Respir Rev.* (2014) 23:55–63. doi: 10.1183/09059180.00008013

6. Spruit MA, Singh SJ, Garvey C, ZuWallack R, Nici L, Rochester C, et al. An official American thoracic society/european respiratory society statement: key concepts and advances in pulmonary rehabilitation. *Am J Respir Crit Care Med.* (2013) 188:e13–64. doi: 10.1164/rccm.201309-1634ST

7. Pehlivan E, Balci A, Kilic L, Kadakal F. Preoperative pulmonary rehabilitation for lung transplant: effects on pulmonary function, exercise capacity, and quality of life; first results in Turkey. *Exp Clin Transp.* (2018) 16:455–60. doi: 10.6002/ect.2017.0042

8. Hsieh MJ, Lee WC, Cho HY, Wu MF, Hu HC, Kao KC, et al. Recovery of pulmonary functions, exercise capacity, and quality of life after pulmonary rehabilitation in survivors of ARDS due to severe influenza A (H1N1) pneumonitis. *Influenza Respir Viruses.* (2018) 12:643–8. doi: 10.1111/irv.12566

9. Snyder EM, Johnson BD, Beck KC. An open-circuit method for determining lung diffusing capacity during exercise: comparison to rebreathe. *J Appl Physiol.* (2005) 99:1985–91. doi: 10.1152/japplphysiol.00348.2005

10. Wheatley CM, Baker SE, Daines CM, Phan H, Martinez MG, Morgan WJ, et al. Influence of the Vibralung Acoustical Percussor on pulmonary function and sputum expectoration in individuals with cystic fibrosis. *Ther Adv Respir Dis.* (2018) 12:1753466618770997. doi: 10.1177/1753466618770997

11. Ngai JC, Ko FW, Ng SS, To KW, Tong M, Hui DS. The long-term impact of severe acute respiratory syndrome on pulmonary function, exercise capacity and health status. *Respirology.* (2010) 15:543–50. doi: 10.1111/j.1440-1843.2010.01720.x

12. Herridge MS, Tansey CM, Matte A, Tomlinson G, Diaz-Granados N, Cooper A, et al. Functional disability 5 years after acute respiratory distress syndrome. *N Engl J Med.* (2011) 364:1293–304. doi: 10.1056/NEJMoa1011802

13. Liu W, Peng L, Liu H, Hua S. Pulmonary function and clinical manifestations of patients infected with mild Influenza A virus subtype H1N1: a one-year follow-up. *PloS ONE.* (2015) 10:e0133698. doi: 10.1371/journal.pone.0133698

14. Carreiro A, Santos J, Rodrigues F. Impact of comorbidities in pulmonary rehabilitation outcomes in patients with chronic obstructive pulmonary disease. *Rev Port Pneumol.* (2013) 19:106–113. doi: 10.1016/j.rppnen.2012.12.001

15. Dowman L, Hill CJ, Holland AE. Pulmonary rehabilitation for interstitial lung disease. *Cochrane Database Syst Rev.* (2014) Cd006322. doi: 10.1002/14651858.CD006322.pub3

16. Vainshelboim B, Oliveira J, Yehoshua L, Weiss I, Fox BD, Fruchter O, et al. Exercise training-based pulmonary rehabilitation program is clinically beneficial for idiopathic pulmonary fibrosis. *Respir.* (2014) 88:378–88. doi: 10.1159/000367899

17. Yu X, Li X, Wang L, Liu R, Xie Y, Li S, et al. Pulmonary rehabilitation for exercise tolerance and quality of life in IPF patients: a systematic review and meta-analysis. *BioMed Res Int.* (2019) 2019:8498603. doi: 10.1155/2019/8498603

Heart Failure Probability and Early Outcomes of Critically Ill Patients with COVID-19

Weibo Gao [1†], Jiasai Fan [2†], Di Sun [2†], Mengxi Yang [2], Wei Guo [3], Liyuan Tao [4],
Jingang Zheng [2], Jihong Zhu [1], Tianbing Wang [3*] and Jingyi Ren [2*]

[1] Department of Emergency, Peking University People's Hospital, Beijing, China, [2] Department of Cardiology, Heart Failure
Center, China-Japan Friendship Hospital, Beijing, China, [3] Trauma Center, Peking University People's Hospital, Beijing, China,
[4] Research Center of Clinical Epidemiology, Peking University Third Hospital, Beijing, China

*Correspondence:
Jingyi Ren
renjingyi1213@hotmail.com
Tianbing Wang
wangtianbing@pkuph.edu.cn

†These authors have contributed
equally to this work

Background: The relationship between cardiac functions and the fatal outcome of coronavirus disease 2019 (COVID-19) is still largely underestimated. We aim to explore the role of heart failure (HF) and NT-proBNP in the prognosis of critically ill patients with COVID-19 and construct an easy-to-use predictive model using machine learning.

Methods: In this multicenter and prospective study, a total of 1,050 patients with clinical suspicion of COVID-19 were consecutively screened. Finally, 402 laboratory-confirmed critically ill patients with COVID-19 were enrolled. A "triple cut-point" strategy of NT-proBNP was applied to assess the probability of HF. The primary outcome was 30-day all-cause in-hospital death. Prognostic risk factors were analyzed using the least absolute shrinkage and selection operator (LASSO) and multivariate logistic regression, further formulating a nomogram to predict mortality.

Results: Within a 30-day follow-up, 27.4% of the 402 patients died. The mortality rate of patients with HF likely was significantly higher than that of the patient with gray zone and HF unlikely (40.8% vs. 25 and 16.5%, respectively, $P < 0.001$). HF likely [Odds ratio (OR) 1.97, 95% CI 1.13–3.42], age (OR 1.04, 95% CI 1.02–1.06), lymphocyte (OR 0.36, 95% CI 0.19–0.68), albumin (OR 0.92, 95% CI 0.87–0.96), and total bilirubin (OR 1.02, 95% CI 1–1.04) were independently associated with the prognosis of critically ill patients with COVID-19. Moreover, a nomogram was developed by bootstrap validation, and C-index was 0.8 (95% CI 0.74–0.86).

Conclusions: This study established a novel nomogram to predict the 30-day all-cause mortality of critically ill patients with COVID-19, highlighting the predominant role of the "triple cut-point" strategy of NT-proBNP, which could assist in risk stratification and improve clinical sequelae.

Keywords: COVID-19, heart failure, NT-ProBNP, nomogram, prognosis

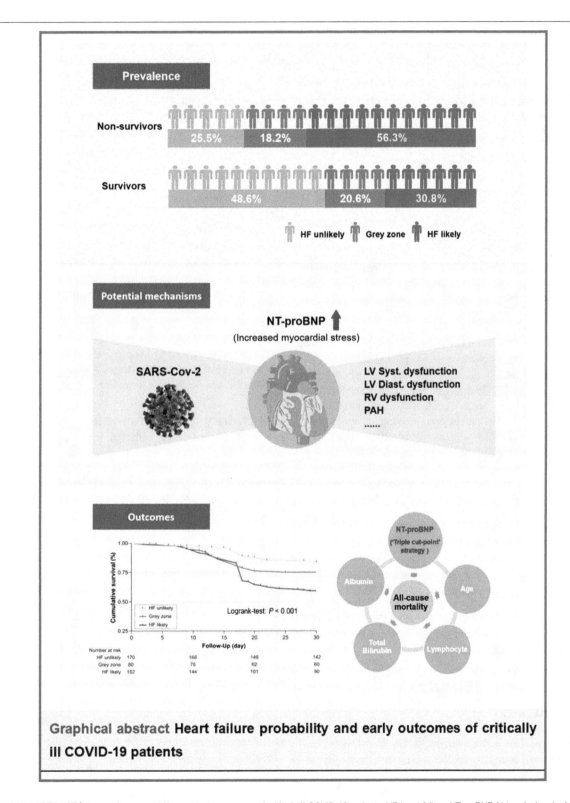

Graphical abstract **Heart failure probability and early outcomes of critically ill COVID-19 patients**

GRAPHICAL ABSTRACT | Heart failure probability and early outcomes of critically ill COVID-19 patients. HF, heart failure; NT-proBNP, N-terminal probrain natriuretic peptide; LV, left ventricular; RV, right ventricular; PAH, pulmonary arterial hypertension.

INTRODUCTION

An outbreak of novel infectious pneumonia, now known as coronavirus disease 2019 (COVID-19) caused by severe acute respiratory syndrome coronavirus 2, has been quickly spreading around the world since December 2019. To date, more than 168 million confirmed cases of COVID-19 have been identified worldwide, with over 3.49 million deaths. Despite the advancement of learning the etiology and clinical characteristics of COVID-19, there have been no effective strategies to wipe out the global COVID-19 epidemic, and it is still a public health threat.

The average mortality rate was estimated globally at 3.4% by the WHO, while it is 26–52% significantly higher for patients admitted to intensive care units (ICUs) (1, 2). Moreover, no medications have been proven definitely effective for curing COVID-19 (3). Thus, early evaluation and identification of individuals with high-risk mortality are of paramount importance to further guide optimal intervention strategies. Of note, critically ill patients with COVID-19 usually have multiple organ dysfunctions (4), among which cardiac involvement is prevalent, especially acute heart failure (AHF) (5). However, the role of AHF in the prognosis of COVID-19 has not been fully elucidated in prior studies, partially because comprehensive evaluations of cardiac dysfunction that utilize imaging examinations were usually unavailable in real-world practice. Hence, we proposed a "triple cut-point" strategy of N-terminal pro-brain natriuretic peptide (NT-proBNP) as a reliable and easy-to-use diagnostic tool for AHF in this study (6). Moreover, although previous studies have explored the risk factors of prognosis among critically ill patients with COVID-19 (7–9), a user-friendly and clinically relevant short-time outcome prediction model for patients with COVID-19 in ICU is still lacking.

Therefore, to address the gaps mentioned above, this multicenter study aims to (1) explore the potential prognostic value of the "triple cut-point" strategy of NT-proBNP and AHF in critically ill patients with COVID-19; and (2) construct and validate a simplified and effective nomogram to predict all-cause in-hospital death risk individually.

MATERIALS AND METHODS

Study Population

This multicenter, prospective, and observational study consecutively enrolled 1,050 patients with clinical suspicion of COVID-19 from four ICUs in Wuhan taken over by China-Japan Friendship Hospital, Peking University People's Hospital, Peking University First Hospital, and Peking University Third Hospital from January to May 2020. Patients who met one of the following criteria would be considered to be transferred to the ICU: (1) respiratory rate >30 breath/min; (2) blood oxygen (SpO$_2$) <93%; (3) PaO$_2$/FiO$_2$ <300 mmHg; (4) presented with respiratory failure; (5) presented with shock; or (6) other conditions that need to be monitored

in the ICU. Patients were diagnosed as COVID-19 with a positive result of real-time reverse transcriptase-polymerase chain reaction assay from nasal swab specimens according to WHO guidance (10). Exclusion criteria included patients who were not diagnosed with COVID-19, younger than 18 years of age, and had incomplete data, or died within 24 h of admission to the ICU. As a result, 402 patients were included in the final analysis. The study was conducted in accordance with the Declaration of Helsinki, and the protocol was approved by the Ethics Committee of Peking University People's Hospital.

Data Collection

The clinical data from each patient were recorded by experienced physicians following ICU admission and included demographic features, preexisting comorbidities, symptoms, vital signs, and length of ICU stay. The comorbidities included hypertension, coronary heart disease (CHD), diabetes mellitus (DM), chronic kidney disease (CKD), asthma, chronic obstructive pulmonary disease, chronic bronchitis, transient ischemic attack, ischemic stroke, and hemorrhagic stroke.

All the patients, during hospitalization, were followed up for 30-days or until discharge or death. The primary outcome was 30-day all-cause death after admission.

Laboratory Measurements

Laboratory values were collected including complete blood count, high-sensitivity cardiac troponin I (hs-cTNI), NT-proBNP, biochemical tests, d-dimer, and procalcitonin (PCT). Complete blood count was measured with a Sysmex XN-9000 (Sysmex, Kobe, Japan) automatic hematology analyzer. Coagulation parameters, such as d-dimer, were measured with a Stago STA-R automatic blood coagulation analyzer (Stago, Paris, France). Biochemical tests, namely, alanine aminotransferase (ALT), aspartate aminotransferase (AST), total bilirubin, albumin, blood urea nitrogen (BUN), and creatinine were performed using Roche Cobas 8000 automatic biochemical analyzer (Roche, Rotkreuz, Switzerland). Hs-cTNI was measured with an Abbott ARCHITECT i2000SR chemiluminescence immunoanalyzer (Abbott Laboratories, Illinois, United States). Elevated hs-cTNI was defined as plasma levels of hs-cTNI above the 99th-percentile upper reference limit. NT-proBNP was analyzed with a

TABLE 1 | Classification of patients using the "triple cut-point" strategy of NT-proBNP.

Setting	Cut-off levels of NT-proBNP (pg/mL)		
	Age < 50	Age 50–75	Age > 75
HF unlikely	<300		
Gray zone	300–450	300–900	300–1,800
HF likely	>450	>900	>1,800

NT-proBNP, N-terminal pro-B type natriuretic peptide; HF, heart failure.

Roche Cobas e602 electrochemical luminescence analyzer (Roche, Germany).

"Triple Cut-Point" Strategy of NT-proBNP

According to the recent guideline for HF, novel NT-proBNP cut-off values have been proposed to assist with AHF diagnosis. Hence, we classified the cases into three groups using this "triple cut-point" strategy of NT-proBNP to define the probability of AHF, as shown in **Table 1**. In detail, HF likely was defined as plasma NT-proBNP level > 450 pg/ml in patients below 50 years, >900 pg/ml in patients between 50 and 75 years, and >1,800 pg/ml in patients over 75 years (6). HF unlikely was defined as plasma NT-proBNP level <300 pg/ml regardless of age, while the

stratified approach of 300 pg/ml to 450/900/1,800 pg/ml for ages <50/50–75/>75 years were considered as "gray zone."

Statistical Analysis

Continuous variables were presented as mean $\pm$ SD if normally distributed, and median and interquartile range otherwise. The differences between the two groups were compared by the Student t-test and Mann–Whitney U test appropriately. Categorical variables were shown as n (%) and compared by χ^2 test or Fisher exact test when necessary.

Kaplan–Meier survival estimates were calculated, and the log-rank test was performed to compare the groups in terms of survival. The least absolute shrinkage and selection operator (LASSO) method (glmnet package), which is appropriate for

TABLE 2 | Baseline characteristics of the cohort.

Demographics	Total n = 402 (100.0)	Survivors n = 292 (72.6)	Non-survivors n = 110 (27.4)	P-value
Age, years	67.5 ± 13.7	65.6 ± 13.6	72.4 ± 12.8	<0.001
Sex				0.070
Female, n (%)	183 (45.5)	141 (48.3)	42 (38.2)	
Male, n (%)	219 (54.5)	151 (51.7)	68 (61.8)	
Vital signs				
Temperature, °C	38.7 ± 3.7	38.6 ± 4.3	39.0 ± 1.0	0.332
Respiratory rate, breath/min	25.1 ± 6.1	25.0 ± 5.6	25.4 ± 7.2	0.603
SpO2, %	91.2 ± 6.7	92.2 ± 5.7	88.6 ± 8.3	<0.001
Heart rate, beat/min	94.7 ± 17.0	93.7 ± 15.6	97.3 ± 20.0	0.002
SBP, mm/Hg	133.0 ± 23.0	132.6 ± 22.4	134.0 ± 24.5	0.570
DBP, mm/Hg	79.0 ± 14.4	78.9 ± 14.0	79.2 ± 15.3	0.883
Comorbidities				
Hypertension, n (%)	209 (52.0)	152 (52.1)	57 (51.8)	0.966
Coronary heart disease, n (%)	72 (17.9)	48 (16.4)	24 (21.8)	0.210
Diabetes mellitus, n (%)	96 (23.9)	69 (23.6)	27 (24.5)	0.848
Respiratory system diseases, n (%)	51 (12.7)	37 (12.7)	14 (12.7)	0.988
Chronic kidney disease, n (%)	37 (9.2)	25 (8.6)	12 (10.9)	0.468
Cerebrovascular diseases, n (%)	19 (4.7)	11 (3.8)	8 (7.3)	0.140
Cardiac comorbidities or risk factors, n (%)	258 (64.2)	187 (64.0)	71 (64.5)	0.925
No. of comorbidities ≥2, n (%)	139 (34.6)	95 (32.5)	44 (40.0)	0.161
Laboratory values				
Lymphocyte, ×10⁹ /L	0.8 (0.5, 1.1)	0.8 (0.7, 1.2)	0.6 (0.4, 0.8)	<0.001
Platelet, ×10⁹ /L	217.0 (141.8, 289.0)	235.0 (157.0, 307.2)	160 (106.0, 225.2)	<0.001
ALT, U/L	30.0 (16.4, 47.0)	28.5 (16.0, 46.0)	33.1 (18.0, 48.3)	0.291
AST, U/L	34.0 (21.0, 52.8)	29.2 (20.0, 50.8)	43.5 (26.4, 57.0)	<0.001
Albumin, g/L	32.2 ± 5.9	33.0 ± 5.2	29.9 ± 6.9	<0.001
Total bilirubin, μmol/L	12.2 (8.6, 16.9)	11.4 (8.3, 15.3)	14.5 (9.7, 20.4)	<0.001
eGFR, ml/ min/l.73 m²	73.2 ± 31.7	76.0 ± 31.8	65.7 ± 30.2	0.003
Glucose, mmol/L	8.6 ± 4.1	8.3 ± 4.0	9.5 ± 5.8	0.021
D-dimer, μg/mL	2.5 (0.7, 20.1)	1.7 (0.5, 15.7)	7.3 (2.4, 20.1)	<0.001
PCT, ug/L	0.3 (0.1, 1.8)	0.2 (0.1, 1.2)	1.5 (0.3, 1.8)	<0.001
hs-cTNI, pg/mL	12.0 (2.4, 503.7)	10.2 (2.3, 80.1)	274.4 (6.0, 659.6)	<0.001
NT-proBNP, pg/mL	393.2 (121.5, 2774.8)	321.0 (105.0, 2774.8)	1563.5 (240.7, 2775.8)	<0.001

Data are expressed as mean ± SD, median (25th–75th percentile), or n (%). SpO2, oxygen saturation; SBP, systolic blood pressure; DBP, diastolic blood pressure; ALT, alanine aminotransferase; AST, aspartate aminotransferase; eGFR, estimated glomerular filtration rate; PCT, procalcitonin; hs-cTNI, higher sensitivity cardiac troponin I; NT-proBNP, N-terminal pro-brain natriuretic peptide.

regression of high-dimensional data, was used to select the most useful predictive variables from the data set. Then, the multivariate logistic regression analysis was performed to identify independent risk factors. Odds ratios (ORs) were shown with a 95% CI.

The nomogram was established based on the multivariate logistic regression analysis (rms package). A likelihood ratio test approach for model selection was performed. Nomogram performance was quantified with respect to discrimination and calibration. Discrimination (the ability of a nomogram to separate patients with all-cause in-hospital death) was quantified with the concordance index (C-index) and 95% CI. Calibration was assessed graphically by plotting the relationship between actual (observed) probabilities and predicted probabilities (calibration plot) by Hosmer goodness-of-fit test. The internal validation of performance was estimated

with the bootstrapping method (500 replications). Integrated discrimination improvement (IDI) and net reclassification improvement (NRI) (survival package) were used to assess the improved ability of the "triple cut-point" strategy of NT-proBNP for the predictive value of the model.

All the tests were two-tailed, and a $P < 0.05$ was considered significant. The statistical analyses were performed with the SPSS version 25.0 software (SPSS Inc., Chicago, IL, United States), R programming language, and environment version 3.6.0 (http:// cran.r-project.org).

RESULTS

Baseline Characteristics

This study finally included 402 critically ill patients with laboratory-confirmed COVID-19 and their baseline

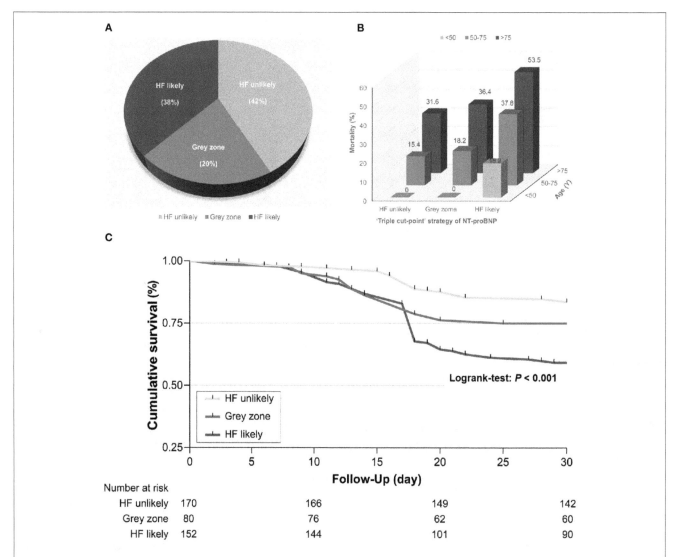

FIGURE 1 | Relationship between the "triple cut-point" strategy of N-terminal pro-brain natriuretic peptide (NT-proBNP) and death. **(A)** Distribution of the "triple cut-point" strategy of NT-proBNP (*n* = 402). **(B)** The mortality rate increased with aging and heart failure. **(C)** Kaplan–Meier survival curves stratified by the "triple cut-point" strategy of NT-proBNP. HF, heart failure.

characteristics are shown in **Table 2**. Overall, the mean age of the whole cohort was 67 years, and 54.5% ($n = 219$) were men. At the 30-day follow-up, 110 patients had died with a 27.4% mortality risk. Compared to the survivors, the non-survivors were more likely to be older, having decreased SpO$_2$ and elevated heart rate (HR) (all $P < 0.05$). Of note, there was no significance between the two groups regarding gender and comorbidities, irrespective of hypertension, CHD, DM, and respiratory system disease. Furthermore, we compared the laboratory data between the two groups and found that the non-survivors had significantly increased AST, total bilirubin, blood glucose, d-dimer, and PCT as well as decreased lymphocytes, platelets, and estimated glomerular filtration rate (eGFR) (all $P < 0.05$).

"Triple Cut-Point" Strategy of NT-proBNP and 30-Day Mortality

According to the "triple cut-point" strategy of NT-proBNP, the patients were divided into three groups, and the overall distribution of HF unlikely, gray zone, and HF likely was 170 (42.3%), 80 (19.9%), and 152 (37.8%), respectively (**Figure 1A**). As shown in **Table 3**, the non-survivor group has a significantly higher percentage of patients with HF likely (56.3 vs. 30.8%), and the distribution of the three groups (HF unlikely, gray zone, and HF likely) between the non-survivor and survivor groups was significantly different ($P < 0.001$). Otherwise, within the 30-day follow-up, we observed a mortality rate of 16.5 (28/170), 25 (20/80), and 40.8% (62/152) in group HF unlikely, gray zone, and HF likely, respectively ($P < 0.001$). Importantly, the mortality rate increased sharply, accompanied by the increased likelihood of AHF (**Figure 1B**). The Kaplan-Meier curves of short-time survival were shown in the central illustration, illustrating a significantly shorter mean survival time for patients with HF likely (**Figure 1C**). The overall cumulative risk of death at 30-days was significantly higher for the HF likely group than for HF unlikely and gray zone ($P < 0.001$).

TABLE 3 | Distribution of "triple cut-point" strategy of NT-proBNP in critically ill patients with coronavirus disease 2019 (COVID-19).

Setting	Total n = 402 (100.0)	Survivors n = 292 (72.6)	Non-survivors n = 110 (27.4)	P-value
HF unlikely, n (%)	170 (42.3)	142 (48.6)	28 (25.5)	<0.001
Gray zone, n (%)	80 (19.9)	60 (20.6)	20 (18.2)	
HF likely, n (%)	152 (37.8)	90 (30.8)	62 (56.3)*	

Data are expressed as n (%). NT-proBNP, N-terminal pro-brain natriuretic peptide; HF, heart failure.

*The distribution of HF likely between survivors and non-survivors was confirmed to be significantly different by post-hoc test (p < 0.001).

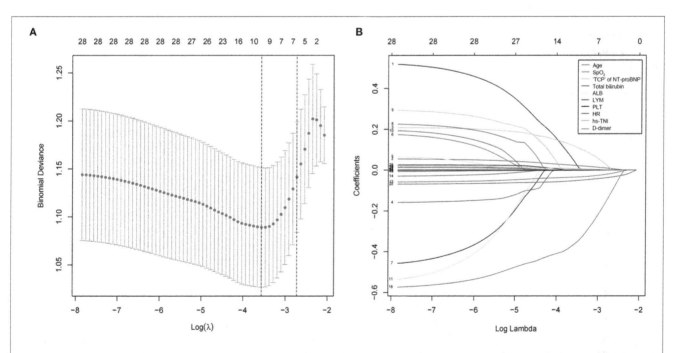

FIGURE 2 | Clinical feature selection using a least absolute shrinkage and selection operator (LASSO) binary logistic regression model. **(A)** Selection of optimal parameters (lambda) from the LASSO model using 10-fold cross-validation and minimum criteria. The partial likelihood deviance (binomial deviance) curve was plotted vs. log (lambda). Dotted vertical lines were drawn at the optimal values using the minimum criteria and the 1 standard error of the minimum criteria (1-SE criteria). **(B)** LASSO coefficient profiles of the 28 texture features. A vertical line was drawn at the value selected using 10-fold cross-validation, where optimal I resulted in nine non-zero coefficients. LASSO, least absolute shrinkage and selection operator; hs-cTNI, higher sensitivity cardiac troponin I; "TCP" of NT-proBNP, "triple cut-point" strategy of NT-proBNP; SpO$_2$, blood oxygen; HR, heart rate.

TABLE 4 | Multivariate logistic regression analyses of risk factors for 30-day mortality.

Variable	Univariate analysis*		Multivariate analysis	
	OR (CI 95%)	*P*-value	OR (CI 95%)	*P*-value
Age, years	1.042 (1.022, 1.061)	<0.001	1.040 (1.018, 1.061)	<0.001
SpO_2, %	0.926 (0.894, 0.959)	<0.001	—	
HR, beat/min	1.012 (1.000, 1.025)	0.060	—	
PLT, $\times 10^9$ /L	0.994 (0.992, 0.996)	<0.001	—	
LYM, $\times 10^9$ /L	0.224 (0.120, 0.418)	<0.001	0.361 (0.191, 0.681)	0.002
Albumin, g/L	0.878 (0.837, 0.921)	<0.001	0.915 (0.870, 0.963)	0.001
Total bilirubin, μmol/L	1.032 (1.010, 1.054)	0.005	1.022 (1.002, 1.042)	0.032
hs-cTNI, pg/mL	1.010 (1.001, 1.023)	0.048	—	
"TCP" of NT-proBNP		<0.001		0.013
HF unlikely	Reference	—	Reference	—
Gray zone	1.367 (0.718, 2.584)	0.343	1.011 (0.425, 1.725)	0.665
HF likely	2.773 (1.678, 4.583)	<0.001	1.970 (1.133, 3.424)	0.016
D-dimer, μg/mL	1.053 (1.027, 1.080)	<0.001	—	

*The variables of the univariate analysis were from the least absolute shrinkage and selection operator (LASSO) binary logistic regression model.
SpO_2, blood oxygen; HR, heart rate; hs-cTNI, higher sensitivity cardiac troponin I; "TCP" of NT-proBNP, "triple cut-point" strategy of NT-proBNP.

Predictors of 30-Day in-hospital Death of Critically Ill Patients With COVID-19

The least absolute shrinkage and selection operator was used to select the potential prognostic factors from numerous parameters. Finally, 28 indexes were reduced to 10 potential predictors, namely, age, lymphocyte, platelet, total bilirubin, "triple cut-point" strategy of NT-proBNP, SpO_2, HR, albumin, hs-cTNI, and d-dimer, based on the 402 patients, and were indexes with non-zero coefficients in the LASSO regression model (**Figures 2A,B**). Furthermore, as shown in **Table 4**, the multivariate logistic regression analysis displays five independent predictors for the short-time fatal outcome, namely, HF likely (OR 1.97, 95% CI 1.133–3.424), older age (OR 1.04, 95% CI 1.018–1.061), lymphocyte (OR 0.361, 95% CI 0.191–0.681), total bilirubin (OR 1.022, 95% CI 1.002–1.042), and albumin (OR 0.915, 95% CI 0.87–0.963) (all *P* <0.05).

Development and Validation of a Novel Nomogram for Predicting Prognosis

An optimal nomogram comprising all the above independent predictors was established to individualize the risk of 30-day in-hospital death (**Figure 3A**). The ratios of calculated β were used to decide the proportional prognostic effect of these variables. Projections from total points on the scales below indicated the estimated probability of death.

Performance accuracy was evaluated by the area under the curve (AUC) of the receiver operating characteristic (ROC) analysis. The AUC for in-hospital death was 0.781 (95% CI 0.733–0.827) (**Figure 3B**). The calibration curve of the nomogram for the probability of death demonstrated good agreement between prediction and observation in the primary cohort (**Figure 3C**). Hosmer-Lemeshow goodness-of-fit was satisfied (*P* = 0.354). The C-index for the prediction nomogram was 0.798 (95% CI 0.742–0.857). The decision curve analysis (DCA) for the clinical

laboratory index nomogram is presented in **Figure 3D**. It showed that this nomogram had more benefits than the treat-all-patients scheme or the treat-none scheme in predicting the risk of 30-day in-hospital death of critically ill patients with COVID-19. Moreover, the bootstrap validation method was used to verify the predictive accuracy of the nomogram. The C-index for the nomogram of 30-day in-hospital death was 0.779 (95% CI 0.721–0.834), suggesting the accuracy of this predictive nomogram.

Incremental Predictive Value of "Triple Cut-Point" Strategy of NT-proBNP

To investigate the role of the "triple cut-point" strategy of NT-proBNP in the predictive value of the current model, NRI and IDI were calculated. Compared with the model without the "triple cut-point" strategy of NT-proBNP, the addition of the "triple cut-point" strategy of NT-proBNP resulted in a significantly improved discrimination [IDI 7.3% (95% CI 1.1–14.5%) and NRI 4.9% (95% CI 2.6–7.2%), both with *P* < 0.05].

DISCUSSION

In this prospective multicenter study, we recruited 402 critically ill patients with COVID-19 from four ICUs in China and established a novel nomogram to predict the 30-day all-cause mortality risk in these patients. To the best of our knowledge, there have been few risks score models for predicting the prognosis of critically ill patients with COVID-19. This study has developed a user-friendly and relatively personalized model incorporating five variables, age, "triple cut-point" strategy of NT-proBNP, albumin, lymphocyte count, and total bilirubin, to predict short-time mortality risk in critically ill Chinese patients with COVID-19, which could assist risk stratification and provide insights for timely interventions upon admission. Furthermore, it is highlighted that the "triple cut-point" strategy of NT-proBNP

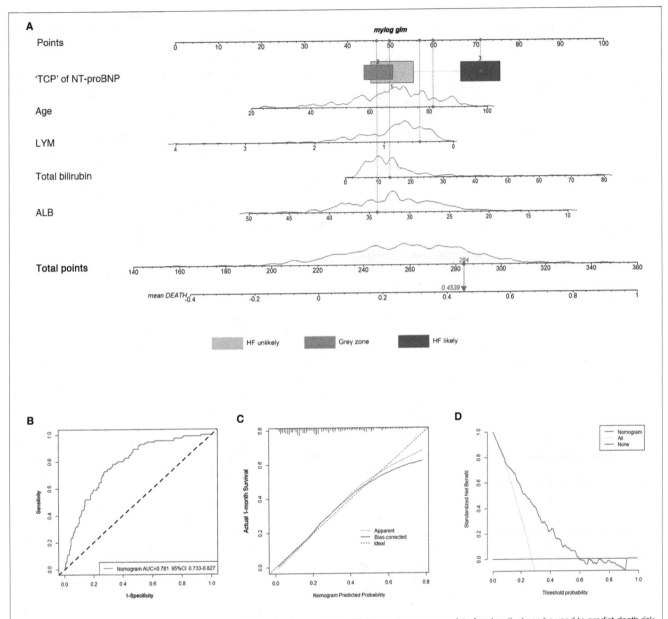

FIGURE 3 | Construction and validation of the nomogram for 30-day all-cause death. **(A)** The total nomogram point of each patient can be used to predict death risk on an individual basis. To predict patient death risk at 30-days, take the following as an example: an 81-year-old patient (60 points) who belonged to HF likely (71 points) had albumin of 34 g/L (46.5 points); his lymphocyte was .5 × 10⁹ /L (56.5 points), and total bilirubin was 14 μmol/L (50 points) at admission. He has a total point score of 284, corresponding to a 45.39% risk of death at 30-days. **(B)** ROC curves of the nomogram. **(C)** Calibration plot of observed proportion vs. predicted probability of 30-day death of the nomogram. **(D)** DCA for the nomogram and the model with subtracting of HF. The y-axis measures the net benefit. The dotted pink line represents the nomogram. The thin gray line represents the assumption that all patients will die. The bold black line represents the assumption that no patient will die. "TCP" of NT-proBNP, "triple cut-point" strategy of NT-proBNP; HF, heart failure; AUC, the area under the curve; ROC, receiver operating characteristic; DCA, decision curve analysis.

demonstrated the predominant role of AHF in the clinical course and prognosis in COVID-19.

The mortality risk of COVID-19 has been proven high, with 28-day mortality ranging from 26–53.8% in critically ill adult patients worldwide (1, 11), indicating the imperative of proposing an easy-to-use prediction model to assist risk-stratify and therapeutic optimization in clinical practice for ICU patients. Emerging evidence has tried to explore the

risk factors and construct diagnostic and prognostic models in COVID-19 populations (12, 13). However, previous reports regarding prognosis prediction have mainly focused on disease progression or mortality risk of the whole group without further distinguishing critically ill patients in ICU (14). The sample selection bias of the prior models could lead to poor adaptions. In line with existing data, this study reported a 27.6% mortality risk, and further constructed and validated a novel nomogram for the prediction of 30-day all-cause death. Variables referring to older age, higher level of total bilirubin, lower level of lymphocyte count and albumin, and "triple cut-point" strategy of NT-proBNP were likely to recognize individuals who are at high risk with high sensitivity and specificity. More importantly, the quantitative appraisal made it possible to estimate the likelihood of death more accurately and individually with easy and rapid access in clinical practice.

It has been widely confirmed that cardiac involvement, such as cardiac injury, arrhythmias, myocarditis, and cardiac dysfunction, was prevalent and prognostic in hospitalized patients with COVID-19 (15–17), among which HF is responsible for substantial morbidity and mortality (10). New-onset HF was observed in nearly 23% of hospitalized patients with COVID-19 and as much as one-third of those admitted to the ICU (2, 9). Recent reports revealed that HF was the most frequent cause of death just after acute respiratory distress syndrome (ARDS) and sepsis, accounting for 27.4% of the proximate causes of death in patients with COVID-19 (18). However, the role of HF in the prognosis of critically ill patients with COVID-19 has not been fully elucidated, partially because of high diagnostic uncertainty. A complete diagnosis of HF usually includes symptoms, signs, biomarkers (BNP/NT-proBNP), and imaging examinations, while it is impractical and unavailable to evaluate cardiac function by echocardiography for each critically ill patient with COVID-19 in the clinical practice. Although BNP/NT-proBNP levels are easily interfered with and obscured by considerable factors, the utility of these biomarkers performed well in the emergency setting as an adjunct tool for the diagnosis and triage of dyspneic patients. As such, the guidance has recommended BNP/NT-proBNP as a diagnostic aid for HF with comparable diagnostic accuracy.

As the widely admitted biomarker in HF, NT-proBNP quantitatively reflects hemodynamic myocardial stress (19), indicating not only left ventricular (LV) systolic dysfunction but also cardiac abnormalities, such as LV diastolic dysfunction, right ventricular (RV) dysfunction, valvular dysfunction, increased pulmonary pressures, and atrial arrhythmias. Prior studies have observed ambiguous results that higher levels of BNP or NT-proBNP were found in patients with severe COVID-19 and that they were independently associated with high mortality, maybe because of single-center design, patient population selection bias, and small sample size (20–23). This multicenter study demonstrated that the non-survivors had a significantly higher level of NT-proBNP than the survivors (1,564 vs. 321 ng/ml), with reasonable sample size. Consistently, a recent study described the characterization of NT-proBNP in patients with COVID-19, and 48.5% of their cohort presented NT-proBNP levels above the recommended cut-off for the identification of HF (24).

Furthermore, considering the fact that the plasma level of NT-proBNP is largely affected by age and renal functions, it seems to be not rigorous enough to use NT-proBNP as a simple continuous variable alone to predict the prognosis of patients with COVID-19. Thus, we reclassified the subjects into three groups (HF likely, gray zone, and HF unlikely) according to the recent HF guidance as to the "triple cut-point" strategy of

NT-proBNP, and observed that patients with HF likely occupied 37.8% of the total cohort, of which 56.3% were non-survivors (6). Moreover, we found that patients in the HF likely group had a significantly higher risk (OR 1.97, 95% CI 1.133–3.424) for 30-day all-cause death. Concerning the clinical presentations and biomarkers of HF on time would help make optimal individual treatment plans to prevent further deterioration efficiently.

It is worth noting that our prediction model did not incorporate troponin, as it was not independently associated with the outcome unexpectedly, while prior studies have suggested that troponin was a significant prognostic indicator in COVID-19 (15, 25). Similarly, Dong et al. conducted a retrospective study and built a nomogram assessing the 14-day and 21-day in-hospital survival of all the general patients with COVID-19. The final model was constructed based on hypertension, neutrophil-to-lymphocyte ratio, and NT-proBNP (26). Elevated troponin may be a possible confounder for NT-proBNP as they were postulated to share the same pathophysiological processes and found to be both elevated in pneumonia, sepsis, ARDS, and several other non-cardiac illnesses. Hence, we speculated that an accurate classification using the "triple cut-point" strategy of NT-proBNP may decrease the confounding effect of troponin. Notably, liver injuries, such as elevated total bilirubin and decreased albumin, have also been demonstrated to be common and associated with disease severity and poor outcomes for critically ill patients in this study, in accordance with previous studies (27). Furthermore, elevated total bilirubin may also be associated with cardiac dysfunctions as a significant and independent predictor of poor cardiovascular prognosis in patients with HF (28).

Critically ill conditions with COVID-19 were usually complicated by multiple organ dysfunctions with complex pathophysiological processes involving numerous parameters, including but not limited to hypoxemia, inflammation, thromboembolism, renal failure, and cardiac damage (29). Therefore, it is of vital importance to bring all reasonable possible variables into analysis and construct a scientific prediction model relying on appropriate statistical analysis awfully. In the current study, LASSO, a machine learning algorithm, was applied to shrink the regression coefficients from amounting clinical and laboratory indicators to 10 potential predictors. Thus, this algorithm could conquer common confusing collinearity issues and yield more robust results than traditional variable screening methods.

Some cautions should be considered when interpreting our results. First, although our study is observational and the sample size is relatively small, it has a multicenter and prospective design emphasizing critically ill patients. Further investigations with a larger sample size are warranted. Second, this study did not apply other diagnostic tools to make a complete HF diagnosis. However, it is impractical and unavailable to evaluate cardiac functions by echocardiography for each critically ill patient with COVID-19. Conversely, rapid measurements of NT-proBNP have substantial medical aids to fulfill the clinical need underlying this extraordinary stressful setting, although it should never be a stand-alone test for HF diagnosis. Third, our nomogram model lacks validation in an external population. Nevertheless, internal verification indicated the predictive strength in our study.

CONCLUSIONS

In this study, we explored the independent predictors for short-time prognosis in critically ill patients with COVID-19 in China and established a novel nomogram to predict the 30-day all-cause mortality risk for the first time, highlighting the predominant role of the "triple cut-point" strategy of NT-proBNP. This easy-to-use prognostication nomogram can provide survival estimations and help identify patients with COVID-19 with a high-risk trajectory, further advancing clinical management and ultimately improving outcomes.

AUTHOR CONTRIBUTIONS

JR and TW conceived and designed the study and coordinated to complete the study. JR critically revised the manuscript.

WG contributed to data collection and completed the project. JF and DS analyzed and interpreted the data and wrote the manuscript. LT assisted in performing statistical analysis. MY, WG, JZhe, and JZhu helped revise the manuscript for important intellectual content and language polishing. All the authors have read and approved the final version of the manuscript.

ACKNOWLEDGMENTS

We sincerely acknowledge the healthcare workers from Zhongfaxincheng campus and Guanggu campus of Tongji Hospital Affiliated with Huazhong University of Science and Technology in Wuhan. They contributed tremendously to blocking the spread and prevalence of COVID-19 in Wuhan, Hubei Province, China, and the whole country.

REFERENCES

1. Grasselli G, Zangrillo A, Zanella A, Antonelli M, Cabrini L, Castelli A, et al. Baseline characteristics and outcomes of 1591 patients infected with SARS-CoV-2 admitted to ICUs of the Lombardy Region, Italy. *JAMA.* (2020) 323:1574–81. doi: 10.1001/jama.2020.5394
2. Arentz M, Yim E, Klaff L, Lokhandwala S, Riedo FX, Chong M, et al. Characteristics and outcomes of 21 critically ill patients with COVID-19 in Washington state. *JAMA.* (2020) 323:1612–4. doi: 10.1001/jama.2020.4326
3. Casadevall A, Joyner MJ, Pirofski L-A. A Randomized trial of convalescent plasma for COVID-19—potentially hopeful signals. *JAMA.* (2020) 324:455–7. doi: 10.1001/jama.2020.10218
4. Wang T, Du Z, Zhu F, Cao Z, An Y, Gao Y, et al. Comorbidities and multi-organ injuries in the treatment of COVID-19. *Lancet.* (2020) 395:e52. doi: 10.1016/S0140-6736(20)30558-4
5. Aboughdir M, Kirwin T, Abdul Khader A, Wang B. Prognostic value of cardiovascular biomarkers in COVID-19: a review. *Viruses.* (2020) 12:527. doi: 10.3390/v12050527
6. Mueller C, McDonald K, de Boer RA, Maisel A, Cleland JGF, Kozhuharov N, et al. Heart Failure Association of the European Society of Cardiology practical guidance on the use of natriuretic peptide concentrations. *Eur J Heart Fail.* (2019) 21:715–31. doi: 10.1002/ejhf.1494
7. Yang X, Yu Y, Xu J, Shu H, Xia J, Liu H, et al. Clinical course and outcomes of critically ill patients with SARS-CoV-2 pneumonia in Wuhan, China: a single-centered, retrospective, observational study. *Lancet Respir Med.* (2020) 8:475–81. doi: 10.1016/S2213-2600(20)30079-5
8. Yu Y, Xu D, Fu SZ, Zhang J, Yang XB, Xu L, et al. Patients with COVID-19 in 19 ICUs in Wuhan, China: a cross-sectional study. *Crit Care.* (2020) 24:219–28. doi: 10.1186/s13054-020-02939-x
9. Haase N, Plovsing R, Christensen S, Poulsen LM, Brøchner AC, Rasmussen BS, et al. Characteristics, interventions, and longer term outcomes of COVID-19 ICU patients in Denmark—a nationwide, observational study. *Acta Anaesthesiol Scand.* (2021) 65:68–75. doi: 10.1111/aas.13701
10. WHO. *Clinical Management of Severe Acute Respiratory Infection When Novel Coronavirus (nCoV) Infection Is Suspected: Interim Guidance, 25 January 2020* (2020).
11. Xie J, Wu W, Li S, Hu Y, Hu M, Li J, et al. Clinical characteristics and outcomes of critically ill patients with novel coronavirus infectious disease (COVID-19) in China: a retrospective multicenter study. *Intensive CareMed.* (2020) 46:1863–72. doi: 10.1007/s00134-020-06211-2
12. Feng Z, Yu Q, Yao S, Luo L, Zhou W, Mao X, et al. Early prediction of disease progression in COVID-19 pneumonia patients with chest CT and clinical characteristics. *Nat Commun.* (2020) 11:4968–76. doi: 10.1038/s41467-020-18786-x
13. Wynants L, Van Calster B, Collins GS, Riley RD, Heinze G, Schuit E, et al. Prediction models for diagnosis and prognosis of covid-19: systematic review and critical appraisal. *BMJ.* (2020) 369:m1328. doi: 10.1136/bmj.m1328
14. Vultaggio A, Vivarelli E, Virgili G, Lucenteforte E, Bartoloni A, Nozzoli C, et al. Prompt predicting of early clinical deterioration of moderate-to-severe COVID-19 patients: usefulness of a combined score using IL-6 in a preliminary study. *J Allergy Clin Immunol Pract.* (2020) 8:2575–81.e2. doi: 10.1016/j.jaip.2020.06.013
15. Inciardi RM, Adamo M, Lupi L, Cani DS, Di Pasquale M, Tomasoni D, et al. Characteristics and outcomes of patients hospitalized for COVID-19 and cardiac disease in Northern Italy. *Eur Heart J.* (2020) 41:1821–9. doi: 10.1093/eurheartj/ehaa388
16. Wang D, Hu B, Hu C, Zhu F, Liu X, Zhang J, et al. Clinical characteristics of 138 hospitalized patients with 2019 novel coronavirus–infected pneumonia in Wuhan, China. *JAMA.* (2020) 323:1061–9. doi: 10.1001/jama.2020.1585
17. Liu PP, Blet A, Smyth D, Li H. The science underlying COVID-19: implications for the cardiovascular system. *Circulation.* (2020) 142:68–78. doi: 10.1161/CIRCULATIONAHA.120.047549
18. Zhang S, Guo M, Duan L, Wu F, Hu G, Wang Z, et al. Development and validation of a risk factor-based system to predict short-term survival in adult hospitalized patients with COVID-19: a multicenter, retrospective, cohort study. *Crit Care.* (2020) 24:438–50. doi: 10.1186/s13054-020-03123-x
19. Ibrahim NE, Burnett JC, Butler J, Camacho A, Felker GM, Fiuzat M, et al.

Natriuretic peptides as inclusion criteria in clinical trials. *JACC Heart Fail.* (2020) 8:347–58. doi: 10.1016/j.jchf.2019.12.010

20. Gao L, Jiang D, Wen X, Cheng X, Sun M, He B, et al. Prognostic value of NT-proBNP in patients with severe COVID-19. *Respir Res.* (2020) 21:83–9. doi: 10.1186/s12931-020-01352-w

21. Pranata R, Huang I, Lukito AA, Raharjo SB. Elevated N-terminal pro-brain natriuretic peptide is associated with increased mortality in patients with COVID-19: systematic review and meta-analysis. *Postgrad Med J.* (2020) 96:387–91. doi: 10.1136/postgradmedj-2020-137884

22. Sorrentino S, Cacia M, Leo I, Polimeni A, Sabatino J, Spaccarotella CAM, et al. B-type natriuretic peptide as biomarker of COVID-19 disease severity—a meta-analysis. *J Clin Med.* (2020) 9:2957–63. doi: 10.3390/jcm9092957

23. Shi S, Qin M, Shen B, Cai Y, Liu T, Yang F, et al. Association of cardiac injury with mortality in hospitalized patients with COVID-19 in Wuhan, China. *JAMA Cardiol.* (2020) 5:802–10. doi: 10.1001/jamacardio.2020.0950

24. Caro-Codón J, Rey JR, Buño A, Iniesta AM, Rosillo SO, Castrejon-Castrejon S, et al. Characterization of NT-proBNP in a large cohort of COVID-19 patients. *Eur J Heart Fail* (2021) 23:456–64. doi: 10.1002/ejhf.2095

25. Guo T, Fan Y, Chen M, Wu X, Zhang L, He T, et al. Cardiovascular implications of fatal outcomes of patients with Coronavirus Disease 2019 (COVID-19). *JAMA Cardiol.* (2020) 5:811–18. doi: 10.1001/jamacardio.2020.1017

26. Dong YM, Sun J, Li YX, Chen Q, Liu QQ, Sun Z, et al. Development and validation of a nomogram for assessing survival in patients with COVID-19 pneumonia. *Clin Infect Dis.* (2020) 72:652–60. doi: 10.1093/cid/ciaa963

27. Bloom PP, Meyerowitz EA, Reinus Z, Daidone M, Gustafson J, Kim AY, et al. Liver biochemistries in hospitalized patients with COVID-19. *Hepatology.* (2021) 73:890–900. doi: 10.1002/hep.31326

28. Suzuki K, Claggett B, Minamisawa M, Packer M, Zile MR, Rouleau J, et al. Liver function and prognosis, and influence of sacubitril/valsartan in patients with heart failure with reduced ejection fraction. *Eur J Heart Fail.* (2020) 22:1662–71. doi: 10.1002/ejhf.1853

29. Gupta S, Hayek SS, Wang W, Chan L, Mathews KS, Melamed ML, et al. Factors associated with death in critically ill patients with coronavirus disease 2019 in the US. *JAMA Intern Med.* (2020) 180:1–12. doi: 10.1001/jamainternmed.2020.3596

Permissions

List of Contributors

Angelo Zinellu and Salvatore Sotgia
Department of Biomedical Sciences, University of Sassari, Sassari, Italy

Ciriaco Carru
Department of Biomedical Sciences, University of Sassari, Sassari, Italy
Quality Control Unit, University Hospital of Sassari, Sassari, Italy

Arduino A. Mangoni
Discipline of Clinical Pharmacology, College of Medicine and Public Health, Flinders University, Adelaide, SA, Australia
Department of Clinical Pharmacology, Flinders Medical Centre, Southern Adelaide Local Health Network, Adelaide, SA, Australia

Ana Ferrer-Gómez, Irene Carretero-Barrio and Antonia Navarro-Cantero
Pathology Department, University Hospital Ramón y Cajal, Madrid, Spain
Faculty of Medicine, Alcalá University, Alcalá de Henares, Spain

Héctor Pian-Arias
Pathology Department, University Hospital Ramón y Cajal, Madrid, Spain

David Pestaña
Faculty of Medicine, Alcalá University, Alcalá de Henares, Spain
Anaesthesiology and Surgical Critical Care Department, Hospital Universitario Ramón y Cajal, Madrid, Spain

Raúl de Pablo
Faculty of Medicine, Alcalá University, Alcalá de Henares, Spain
Instituto Ramón y Cajal for Health Research (IRYCIS), Madrid, Spain
Medical Intensive Care Unit, Hospital Universitario Ramón y Cajal, Madrid, Spain

José Luis Zamorano
Faculty of Medicine, Alcalá University, Alcalá de Henares, Spain
Instituto Ramón y Cajal for Health Research (IRYCIS), Madrid, Spain
Cardiology Department, Hospital Universitario Ramón y Cajal, Madrid, Spain
Centro de Investigación Biomédica en Red de Enfermedades Cardiovasculares (CIBERCV), Instituto de Salud Carlos III, Madrid, Spain

Juan Carlos Galán
Instituto Ramón y Cajal for Health Research (IRYCIS), Madrid, Spain
Microbiology Department, Hospital Universitario Ramón y Cajal, Madrid, Spain
Centro de Investigación Biomédica en Red en Epidemiología y Salud Pública (CIBERESP), Madrid, Spain

Belén Pérez-Mies and José Palacios
Pathology Department, University Hospital Ramón y Cajal, Madrid, Spain
Faculty of Medicine, Alcalá University, Alcalá de Henares, Spain
Instituto Ramón y Cajal for Health Research (IRYCIS), Madrid, Spain
Centro de Investigación Biomédica en Red de Cáncer (CIBERONC), Instituto de Salud Carlos III, Madrid, Spain

Ignacio Ruz-Caracuel
Pathology Department, University Hospital Ramón y Cajal, Madrid, Spain
Instituto Ramón y Cajal for Health Research (IRYCIS), Madrid, Spain

Frédéric Chagué
Service de Cardiologie, Centre Hospitalier Universitaire, Dijon, France
Réseau Français d'Excellence de Recherche sur le tabac, la nicotine et les produits connexes, Paris, France

Mathieu Boulin and Amélie Cransac
Département de Pharmacie, Centre Hospitalier Universitaire, Dijon, France

Jean-Christophe Eicher, Florence Bichat, Maïlis Saint-Jalmes, Gabriel Laurent and Yves Cottin
Service de Cardiologie, Centre Hospitalier Universitaire, Dijon, France

Agnès Soudry
Département de Recherche Clinique, Centre Hospitalier Universitaire, Dijon, France

Nicolas Danchin
Service de Cardiologie, Hôpital Européen Georges Pompidou, Paris, France

Marianne Zeller
Réseau Français d'Excellence de Recherche sur le tabac, la nicotine et les produits connexes, Paris, France
PEC2, EA 7460, Université Bourgogne Franche-Comté, Dijon, France

Alvaro Petersen-Uribe, Alban Avdiu, Katja Witzel, Philippa Jaeger, Monika Zdanyte, David Heinzmann, Elli Tavlaki, Verena Warm, Tobias Geisler, Karin Müller, Meinrad Gawaz and Dominik Rath
Department of Cardiology and Angiology, University Hospital Tübingen, Eberhard Karls Universität Tübingen, Tübingen, Germany

Peter Martus
Institute for Clinical Epidemiology and Applied Biostatistics, University Hospital Tübingen, Eberhard Karls Universität Tübingen, Tübingen, Germany

Georgina M. Ellison-Hughes
Faculty of Life Sciences & Medicine, Centre for Human and Applied Physiological Sciences, School of Basic and Medical Biosciences, King's College London Guy's Campus, London, United Kingdom

Liam Colley
School of Sport, Health, and Exercise Sciences, Bangor University, Bangor, United Kingdom

Katie A. O'Brien
Department of Physiology, Development, and Neuroscience, University of Cambridge, Cambridge, United Kingdom

Kirsty A. Roberts
Research Institute for Sport and Exercise Sciences, Liverpool John Moores University, Liverpool, United Kingdom

Thomas A. Agbaedeng
Faculty of Health & Medical Sciences, Centre for Heart Rhythm Disorders, School of Medicine, The University of Adelaide, Adelaide, SA, Australia

Mark D. Ross
School of Applied Sciences, Edinburgh Napier University, Edinburgh, United Kingdom

Hossein Mohammad-Rahimi
Dental Research Center, Research Institute of Dental Sciences, Shahid Beheshti University of Medical Sciences, Tehran, Iran

Mohadeseh Nadimi and Azadeh Ghalyanchi-Langeroudi
Department of Medical Physics and Biomedical Engineering, Tehran University of Medical Sciences (TUMS), Tehran, Iran

Research Center for Biomedical Technologies and Robotics (RCBTR), Tehran, Iran

Mohammad Taheri
Urology and Nephrology Research Center, Shahid Beheshti University of Medical Sciences, Tehran, Iran

Soudeh Ghafouri-Fard
Department of Medical Genetics, Shahid Beheshti University of Medical Sciences, Tehran, Iran

Zuwei Li
Cardiology Department, The Affiliated Hospital of Jiangxi University of Chinese Medicine, Nanchang, China

Wen Shao, Shanshan Huang and Peng Yu
Endocrine Department, The Second Affiliated Hospital of Nanchang University, Nanchang, China

Jing Zhang
Anesthesiology Department, The Second Affiliated Hospital of Nanchang University, Nanchang, China

Jianyong Ma
Department of Pharmacology and Systems Physiology, University of Cincinnati College of Medicine, Cincinnati, OH, United States

Wengen Zhu
Department of Cardiology, The First Affiliated Hospital of Sun Yat-sen University, Guangzhou, China

Xiao Liu
Cardiology Department, The Sun Yat-sen Memorial Hospital of Sun Yat-sen University, Guangzhou, China
Guangdong Province Key Laboratory of Arrhythmia and Electrophysiology, Guangzhou, China

Wael Al Mahmeed
Cleveland Clinic, Heart and Vascular Institute, Abu Dhabi, United Arab Emirates

Khalid Al-Rasadi
Medical Research Center, Sultan Qaboos University, Muscat, Oman

Yajnavalka Banerjee
Department of Biochemistry, Mohamed Bin Rashid University, Dubai, United Arab Emirates

Antonio Ceriello
IRCCS MultiMedica, Milan, Italy

Francesco Cosentino
Unit of Cardiology, Karolinska Institute and Karolinska University Hospital, University of Stockholm, Stockholm, Sweden

Massimo Galia
Department of Biomedicine, Neurosciences and Advanced Diagnostics (Bind), University of Palermo, Palermo, Italy

Su-Yen Goh
Department of Endocrinology, Singapore General Hospital, Singapore, Singapore

Peter Kempler
Department of Medicine and Oncology, Semmelweis University, Budapest, Hungary

Nader Lessan
Imperial College London Diabetes Centre, The Research Institute, Abu Dhabi, United Arab Emirates

Nikolaos Papanas
Second Department of Internal Medicine, Diabetes Center, University Hospital of Alexandroupolis, Democritus University of Thrace, Alexandroupolis, Greece

Ali A. Rizvi
Department of Medicine, University of Central Florida College of Medicine, Orlando, FL, United States
Division of Endocrinology, Diabetes and Metabolism, University of South Carolina School of Medicine, Columbia, IN, United States

Raul D. Santos
Heart Institute (InCor) University of São Paulo Medical School Hospital, São Paulo, Brazil
Hospital Israelita Albert Einstein, São Paulo, Brazil

Anca P. Stoian
Faculty of Medicine, Diabetes, Nutrition and Metabolic Diseases, Carol Davila University, Bucharest, Romania,

Peter P. Toth
Cicarrone Center for the Prevention of Cardiovascular Disease, Johns Hopkins University School of Medicine, Baltimore, MD, United States

Manfredi Rizzo
Division of Endocrinology, Diabetes and Metabolism, University of South Carolina School of Medicine, Columbia, IN, United States
Faculty of Medicine, Diabetes, Nutrition and Metabolic Diseases, Carol Davila University, Bucharest, Romania
Department of Health Promotion, Mother and Child Care, Internal Medicine and Medical Specialties (Promise), University of Palermo, Palermo, Italy

Jia Teng Sun, Peng Nie, Heng Ge, Long Shen, Fan Yang, Xiao Long Qu, Xiao Ying Ying, Yong Zhou, Wei Wang and Min Zhang
Division of Cardiology, Renji Hospital, Shanghai Jiao Tong University School of Medicine, Shanghai, China
Division of Pulmonary and Critical Care Medicine, Leishenshan Hospital, Wuhan, China

Zhongli Chen
Institute of Cardiovascular Disease, Ruijin Hospital, Shanghai Jiao Tong University School of Medicine, Shanghai, China

Jun Pu
Division of Cardiology, Renji Hospital, Shanghai Jiao Tong University School of Medicine, Shanghai, China

Dario Winterton
Department of Anesthesia and Intensive Care Medicine, ASST Monza, Monza, Italy

Giacomo Maria Cioffi
Division of Cardiology, Fondazione Cardiocentro Ticino, Lugano, Switzerland
Department of Cardiology, Kantonsspital Luzern, Lucerne, Switzerland

Simone Ghidini
Dyspnea Lab, Department of Clinical Sciences and Community Health, University of Milan, Milan, Italy

Luigi Biasco
Division of Cardiology, Azienda Sanitaria Locale Torino 4, Ospedale di Ciriè, Ciriè, Italy
Department of Biomedical Sciences, University of Italian Switzerland, Lugano, Switzerland

Jeroen Dauw
Department of Cardiology, Ziekenhuis Oost-Limburg, Genk, Belgium
Doctoral School for Medicine and Life Sciences, Hasselt University, Diepenbeek, Belgium

Marco Vicenzi
Dyspnea Lab, Department of Clinical Sciences and Community Health, University of Milan, Milan, Italy
Cardiovascular Disease Unit, Fondazione IRCCS Ca' Granda Ospedale Maggiore Policlinico, Milan, Italy

Gregorio Tersalvi
Division of Cardiology, Fondazione Cardiocentro Ticino, Lugano, Switzerland
Department of Internal Medicine, Hirslanden Klinik St. Anna, Lucerne, Switzerland

Marco Roberto
Division of Cardiology, Fondazione Cardiocentro Ticino, Lugano, Switzerland

Giovanni Pedrazzini
Division of Cardiology, Fondazione Cardiocentro Ticino, Lugano, Switzerland
Department of Biomedical Sciences, University of Italian Switzerland, Lugano, Switzerland

Pietro Ameri
Cardiovascular Diseases Unit, IRCCS Ospedale Policlinico San Martino, Genoa, Italy
Department of Internal Medicine, University of Genoa, Genoa, Italy

Manuel Rattka, Lina Stuhler, Claudia Winsauer, Kevin Thiessen, Michael Baumhardt, Sinisa Markovic, Wolfgang Rottbauer and Armin Imhof
Clinic for Internal Medicine II, University Hospital Ulm - Medical Center, Ulm, Germany

Jens Dreyhaupt
Institute of Epidemiology and Medical Biometry, Ulm University, Ulm, Germany

Anum S. Minhas, Nisha A. Gilotra, Erin Goerlich, Thomas Metkus, Garima Sharma, Nicole Bavaro, Susan Phillip, Erin D. Michos and Allison G. Hays
Division of Cardiology, Department of Medicine, Johns Hopkins University School of Medicine, Baltimore, MD, United States

Brian T. Garibaldi
Division of Pulmonary and Critical Care Medicine, Department of Medicine, Johns Hopkins University School of Medicine, Baltimore, MD, United States

Qi Mao, Jianhua Zhao, Youmei Li, Li Xie, Han Xiao, Ke Wang, Youzhu Qiu, Jun Jin, Lan Huang and Xiaohui Zhao
Department of Cardiology, Institute of Cardiovascular Research, Xinqiao Hospital, Army Medical University, Chongqing, China

Jianfei Chen
Department of Cardiology, People's Hospital of Banan District, Chongqing, China

Qiang Xu
Department of Cardiology, The Fifth People's Hospital, Chongqing, China

Zhonglin Xu
Department of Cardiology, The Ninth People's Hospital, Chongqing, China

Yang Yu
Department of Cardiology, People's Hospital of Dianjiang District, Chongqing, China

Ying Zhang
Department of Cardiology, Emergency Medical Center, Chongqing, China

Qiang Li
Department of Cardiovascular Medicine, People's Hospital of Nanchuan District, Chongqing, China

Xiaohua Pang
Department of Cardiovascular Medicine, The Three Gorges Central Hospital, Chongqing, China

Zhenggong Li
Department of Cardiac Intervention Therapy, Zhongshan Hospital District, Chongqing General Hospital, University of Chinese Academy of Sciences, Chongqing, China

Boli Ran
Department of Cardiology, The Third Hospital District, Chongqing General Hospital, University of Chinese Academy of Sciences, Chongqing, China

Zhihui Zhang
Department of Cardiology, Southwest Hospital, Army Medical University, Chongqing, China

Zhifeng Li
Department of Cardiology, Yongchuan Hospital, Chongqing Medical University, Chongqing, China

Chunyu Zeng
Department of Cardiology, Daping Hospital, Army Medical University, Chongqing, China

Shifei Tong
Department of Cardiology, The Third Affiliated Hospital of Chongqing Medical University, Chongqing, China

Nobuko Kojima, Hayato Tada, Hirofumi Okada, Shohei Yoshida, Kenji Sakata, Soichiro Usui, Masa-aki Kawashiri and Masayuki Takamura
Department of Cardiovascular Medicine, Kanazawa University Graduate School of Medical Sciences, Kanazawa, Japan

Hiroko Ikeda
Diagnostic Pathology, Kanazawa University Hospital, Kanazawa, Japan

Masaki Okajima
Department of Emergency Medicine, Kanazawa University Hospital, Kanazawa, Japan

Sherry-Ann Brown
Cardio-Oncology Program, Division of Cardiovascular Medicine, Medical College of Wisconsin, Milwaukee, WI, United States

June-Wha Rhee
Stanford Cardiovascular Institute, Stanford University, Stanford, CA, United States

Avirup Guha
Harrington Heart and Vascular Institute, Case Western Reserve University, Cleveland, OH, United States

Vijay U. Rao
Franciscan Health, Indianapolis, Indiana Heart Physicians, Indianapolis, IN, United States

Matteo Cameli, Giulia Elena Mandoli, Flavio D'Ascenzi, Marta Focardi, Giulia Biagioni, Sergio Mondillo and Serafina Valente
Department of Medical Biotechnologies, Division of Cardiology, University of Siena, Siena, Italy,

Maria Concetta Pastore
Department of Medical Biotechnologies, Division of Cardiology, University of Siena, Siena, Italy
University of Eastern Piedmont, Maggiore della Carità Hospital, Novara, Italy

Paolo Cameli
Department of Clinical Medical and Neurosciences, Respiratory Disease and Lung Transplantation Section, Le Scotte Hospital, University of Siena, Siena, Italy

Giuseppe Patti
University of Eastern Piedmont, Maggiore della Carità Hospital, Novara, Italy

Federico Franchi
Department of Medical Biotechnologies, Anesthesia and Intensive Care, University of Siena, Siena, Italy

Ihunanya Chinyere Okpara
Cardiology Unit, Department of Internal Medicine, Benue State University Teaching Hospital, Makurdi, Nigeria

Efosa Kenneth Oghagbon
Department of Chemical Pathology, Benue State University Teaching Hospital, Makurdi, Nigeria

Philip Haines
Rhode Island Hospital, Warren Alpert Medical School of Brown University, Providence, RI, United States

Wei Sun, Shuyuan Wang, Yuji Xie, Danqing Zhang, Yiwei Zhang and Yuman Li
Department of Ultrasound, Union Hospital, Tongji Medical College, Huazhong University of Science and Technology, Wuhan, China
Hubei Province Clinical Research Center for Medical Imaging, Wuhan, China
Hubei Province Key Laboratory of Molecular Imaging, Wuhan, China

Wen-Chih Wu
Department of Medicine, Providence VA Medical Center, Brown University Warren Alpert Medical School, Providence, RI, United States

Annalisa Capuano and Francesco Rossi
Department of Experimental Medicine, University of Campania Luigi Vanvitelli, Regional Centre of Pharmacovigilance, Campania Region, Naples, Italy

Giuseppe Paolisso
Department of Advanced Medical and Surgical Sciences, University of Campania Luigi Vanvitelli, Naples, Italy

Mouhand F. H. Mohamed, Shaikha D. Al-Shokri, Khaled M. Shunnar, Sara F. Mohamed, Mostafa S. Najim, Shahd I. Ibrahim and Lina O. Abdalla
Department of Medicine, Hamad Medical Corporation, Doha, Qatar

Hazem Elewa
College of Pharmacy, QU Health, Qatar University, Doha, Qatar

Ahmed El-Bardissy and Mohamed Nabil Elshafei
Clinical Pharmacy Department, Hamad General Hospital, Doha, Qatar

Ibrahim Y. Abubeker
Alpert Medical School, Brown University, Providence, RI, United States

Mohammed Danjuma
Department of Medicine, Hamad Medical Corporation, Doha, Qatar
College of Medicine, QU Health, Qatar University, Doha, Qatar

Khalid M. Dousa
Division of Infectious Diseases and HIV Medicine, University Hospitals Cleveland Medical Center, Case Western Reserve University, Cleveland, OH, United States

Mohamed A. Yassin
Department of Hematology, Hamad Medical Corporation, Doha, Qatar

Yuman Li, Lingyun Fang, Shuangshuang Zhu, Bin Wang, Lin He, Yongxing Zhang, Hongliang Yuan, Chun Wu, He Li, Wei Sun, Yanting Zhang, Meng Li, Li Cui, Jing Wang, Yali Yang, Qing Lv, Li Zhang and Mingxing Xie
Department of Ultrasound, Tongji Medical College, Union Hospital, Huazhong University of Science and Technology, Wuhan, China
Clinical Research Center for Medical Imaging in Hubei Province, Wuhan, China
Hubei Province Key Laboratory of Molecular Imaging, Wuhan, China

Amer M. Johri
Department of Medicine, Queen's University, Kingston, ON, Canada

Pengfei Zhu
Department of Cardiology, Wuhan Fourth Hospital, Puai Hospital, Tongji Medical College, Huazhong University of Science and Technology, Wuhan, China

Zhengchao Wang
Tongji Hospital, Tongji Medical College, Huazhong University of Science and Technology, Wuhan, China

Xiaomi Guo
Department of Ultrasound, Wuhan Asia General Hospital, Wuhan, China

Zhiyong Feng, Chaochao Chen, Ai Zheng and Yu Cai
Department of Rehabilitation, Wuhan Fourth Hospital, Puai Hospital, Tongji Medical College, Huazhong University of Science and Technology, Wuhan, China

Haotian Gu
British Heart Foundation Centre of Research Excellence, King's College London, London, United Kingdom

Weibo Gao and Jihong Zhu
Department of Emergency, Peking University People's Hospital, Beijing, China

Jiasai Fan, Di Sun, Mengxi Yang, Jingyi Ren and Jingang Zheng
Department of Cardiology, Heart Failure Center, China-Japan Friendship Hospital, Beijing, China

Wei Guo and Tianbing Wang
Trauma Center, Peking University People's Hospital, Beijing, China

Liyuan Tao
Research Center of Clinical Epidemiology, Peking University Third Hospital, Beijing, China

Index

Printed in the USA
CPSIA information can be obtained
at www.ICGtesting.com
JSHW051414091023
49903JS00006B/414